ORAL MICROBIOLOGY AND IMMUNOLOGY

ORAL MICROBIOLOGY AND IMMUNOLOGY

Second Edition

Russell J. Nisengard, DDS, PhD
Associate Dean for Research and Advanced Education
Distinguished Teaching Professor
School of Dental Medicine
Professor
School of Medicine
State University of New York at Buffalo
Attending, Buffalo General Hospital and Buffalo VA Hospital
Buffalo, New York

Michael G. Newman, DDS, FACD
Adjunct Professor
School of Dentistry
University of California, Los Angeles
Diplomate American Board of Periodontology
Past President, American Academy of Periodontology
Los Angeles, California

W.B. SAUNDERS COMPANY
A Division of Harcourt Brace & Company
Philadelphia London Toronto Montreal Sydney Tokyo

W.B. SAUNDERS COMPANY

A Division of Harcourt Brace & Company

The Curtis Center
Independence Square West
Philadelphia, PA 19106

Library of Congress Cataloging-in-Publication Data

Oral microbiology and immunology / [edited by] Russell J. Nisengard,
  Michael G. Newman. — 2nd ed.
      p.   cm.
    Includes bibliographical references and index.
    ISBN 0-7216-6753-8
    1. Mouth—Microbiology. 2. Mouth—Immunology. I. Nisengard,
  Russell J. II. Newman, Michael G.
    [DNLM: 1. Mouth Diseases—microbiology. 2. Mouth Diseases—
  immunology. 3. Mouth—microbiology. 4. Mouth—immunology.   QW 65
  0618 1994]
  QR47.068   1994
  617.5′22—dc20
  DNLM/DLC   93-33973

ORAL MICROBIOLOGY AND IMMUNOLOGY   ISBN   0–7216–6753–8

2nd Edition

Last digit is the print number: 9   8   7   6   5   4   3   2   1

This book is dedicated to our wives, children, and families who have accepted our commitment to dentistry and have provided love, support, and encouragement and to our teachers and colleagues who have stimulated our interests in microbiology and immunology.

Contributors

Michael A. Apicella, MD
Professor and Chairman, Department of
Microbiology, University of Iowa,
Iowa City, Iowa

Neisseria

Cynthia G. Bloomquist, BA
Scientist, School of Dentistry, University of
Minnesota, Minneapolis, Minnesota

Normal Microbial Flora of the Human Body

Anthony A. Campagnari, PhD
Research Associate Professor of Medicine/
Microbiology, State University of New York at
Buffalo, Buffalo, New York

Neisseria

Sebastian G. Ciancio, DDS
Professor and Chairman, Department of
Periodontology, Clinical Professor of
Pharmacology, State University of New York at
Buffalo; Consultant, Veterans Administration
Medical Center and Erie County Medical Center,
Buffalo, New York

Control and Prevention of Periodontal Disease
Antimicrobials and Antibiotics

Richard P. Ellen, DDS
Professor and Head, Department of Periodontics,
Faculty of Dentistry, University of Toronto,
Toronto, Canada

Genus Actinomyces *and Other Filamentous*
Bacteria

Richard T. Evans, MS, PhD
Associate Professor of Oral Biology and
Microbiology, School of Dental Medicine, State
University of New York at Buffalo,
Buffalo, New York

Oral Infection and Immunity

Sydney M. Finegold, MD
Professor of Medicine and Microbiology and
Immunology, School of Medicine, University of
California, Los Angeles; Staff Physician,
Medical Service, VA Medical Center,
West Los Angeles, California

Bacillus *and* Clostridium

Colin K. Franker, PhD
Professor of Microbiology, School of Dentistry,
University of California, Los Angeles,
Los Angeles, California

Oral Mycology

M. Jane Gillespie, MS, PhD
Senior Research Scientist, Department of Oral
Biology, State University of New York at
Buffalo, Buffalo, New York

Haemophilus *and* Pasturella

Anthony D. Goodman, DDS, MScD
(Deceased)

Periapical Infections

Eugene A. Gorzynski, PhD
Professor of Microbiology and of Pathology,
School of Medicine and Biomedical Sciences,
State University of New York at Buffalo; Chief
Microbiologist, Pathology and Laboratory
Medicine, VA Medical Center,
Buffalo, New York

Enterobacteriaceae and Vibrionaceae

Violet Haraszthy, DDS
Instructor, Department of Periodontics, School of
Dental Medicine, State University of New York
at Buffalo, Buffalo, New York

Bacterial Classification
Mycoplasmas, Chlamydiae, and Rickettsiae

Stanley C. Holt, PhD
Professor of Microbiology and Periodontics,
The University of Texas Health Science Center
at San Antonio, San Antonio, Texas

General Microbiology, Metabolism, and Genetics

William F. Liljemark, DDS, PhD
Professor, School of Dentistry, University of
Minnesota, Minneapolis, Minnesota

Normal Microbial Flora of the Human Body

Walter J. Loesche, DMD, PhD
Professor of Dentistry, School of Dentistry, and
Professor of Microbiology, School of Medicine,
University of Michigan, Ann Arbor, Michigan

The Spirochetes
Ecology of the Oral Flora

Philip T. LoVerde, PhD
Professor of Microbiology and of Pathology,
School of Medicine and Biomedical Sciences,
State University of New York at Buffalo,
Buffalo, New York

Parasitology

Michael G. Newman, DDS, FACD
Adjunct Professor, School of Dentistry,
University of California, Los Angeles; Diplomate
American Board of Periodontology; Past
President, American Academy of Periodontology,
Los Angeles, California

Dental Plaque and Calculus
Periodontal Disease
Medical Infections of Interest
Diagnostic Microbiology and Immunology

Russell J. Nisengard, DDS, PhD
Associate Dean for Research and Advanced
Education, Distinguished Teaching Professor,
School of Dental Medicine, and Professor,
School of Medicine, University of New York at
Buffalo; Attending, Buffalo General Hospital and
Buffalo VA Hospital, Buffalo, New York

Pseudomonadaceae
Black-Pigmenting Bacteria
Periodontal Disease
Control and Prevention of Periodontal Disease
Periapical Infections
Medical Infections of Interest
Diagnostic Microbiology and Immunology

Joan Otomo-Corgel, DDS, MPH
Adjunct Assistant Professor, Department of
Periodontics, School of Dentistry, University of
California, Los Angeles; Faculty, School of
Dental Hygiene, West Los Angeles City College;
Staff, VA Medical Center, West Los Angeles;
Staff, Rancho los Amigos Hospital, GPR
Program, Los Angeles, California

Legionella

No-Hee Park, DMD, PhD
Professor, Section of Oral Biology, School of
Dentistry, University of California, Los Angeles,
Los Angeles, California

Virology

Ann Progulske, PhD
Associate Professor, University of Florida
College of Dentistry, Gainesville, Florida

General Microbiology, Metabolism, and Genetics

W. Eugene Rathbun, DDS, PhD
Professor, Department of Periodontics,
School of Dentistry, Loma Linda University,
Loma Linda, California

Sterilization and Asepsis

Burton Rosan, DDS, MSc
Professor of Microbiology, School of Dental
Medicine, University of Pennsylvania,
Philadelphia, Pennsylvania

The Streptococci
The Staphylococci

Mariano Sanz, MD, DDS
Professor and Vice Dean, Faculty of Odontology,
University of Complutense, Madrid, Spain

Dental Plaque and Calculus

Benjamin Schein, DDS, MScD
Formerly Assistant Professor, University of
California, San Francisco,
San Francisco, California

Periapical Infections

Jørgen Slots, DMD, DDS, PhD, MS, MBA, FACD
Professor and Chairperson of the Department of
Periodontology, Associate Dean for Research,
School of Dentistry, University of Southern
California, Los Angeles, California

Actinobacillus actinomycetemcomitans

Paulette J. Tempro, DDS
Assistant Professor of Periodontology, University
of Connecticut School of Dental Medicine,
Farmington, Connecticut

Corynebacterium and Mycobacterium
Brucella, Yersinia, and Francisella
Veillonella, Wolinella, and Campylobacter

Mark E. Wilson, PhD
Associate Professor, Department of Oral Biology,
State University of New York at Buffalo,
Buffalo, New York

The Immune System and Host Defense

Lawrence E. Wolinsky, PhD, DMD
Associate Professor of Oral Biology, School of
Dentistry, University of California,
Los Angeles, California

Caries and Cariology

Joseph J. Zambon, DDS, PhD
Professor of Periodontics and Oral Biology,
School of Dental Medicine, State University of
New York at Buffalo, Buffalo, New York

Bacterial Classification
Corynebacterium and Mycobacterium
Pseudomonadaceae
Brucella, Yersinia, and Francisella
Black-Pigmenting Bacteria
Veillonella, Wolinella, and Campylobacter
Mycoplasmas, Chlamydiae, and Rickettsiae
Periodontal Disease
Medical Infections of Interest

Preface

The fields of microbiology and immunology continue to expand with added significance and influence on the clinical practice of dentistry. Since the previous edition, there has been an increased understanding of the cause, diagnosis, and treatment of microbial and immunologic diseases. In addition, nomenclature changes have occurred for several important oral microorganisms. This second edition includes pertinent new information, particularly about oral diseases and infection control. The book provides a basis for adapting evolving knowledge as it becomes available to clinical dentistry in the future.

Recently, the dental profession has applied more stringent methods of infection control because of the acquired immunodeficiency syndrome (AIDS) epidemic, hepatitis, and drug-resistant tuberculosis. Advances in our knowledge of these and other systemic microbial diseases and host responses must be understood for effective protection.

This book is intended for students and practitioners of dentistry and other health-related fields. It provides an up-to-date survey with emphasis on microbial and immunologic diseases of dental origin or diseases with secondary oral manifestations. Whenever possible, the chapters include specific dental applications. This book is not an all-inclusive "bible." Its focus is on basic principles. With this in mind, the bibliographies include review articles and selected key references.

For ease in use of this book, it has been divided into five sections:

Section I: General Principles. This section includes basic up-to-date information about microbiology and immunology. Oral infection and immunity, host resistance and immune function, general microbiology, metabolism and genetics, and bacterial classification provide a framework for the specific areas of microbiology and immunology considered in the rest of the book.

Section II: General Bacteriology. The most significant bacteria in dentistry and medicine are discussed, including examples related to dental practice.

Section III: Virology and Parasitology. One of the fastest and most significant areas of relevance for all health care workers is presented. The information in these chapters prepares the reader for assimilation of new data and their clinical implementation in this rapidly evolving area.

Section IV: Oral Health and Disease. This section includes the ecology of the oral flora, dental plaque and calculus, caries and cariology, periodontal disease, control and prevention of periodontal disease, periapical infections, and medical infections of concern to the dental professional.

Section V: Applied Microbiology and Immunology. Sterilization and asepsis with currently accepted methods, antimicrobials and antibiotics, and diagnostic microbiology and immunology are discussed in this section.

Russell J. Nisengard, DDS, PhD
Michael G. Newman, DDS, FACD

Acknowledgment

The conceptual development of this textbook was a result of input from many individuals. The editors wish to thank all contributors for their efforts on this second edition, particularly Dr. Joseph Zambon, our friend and contributor, who had significant input in this text.

Contents

1 *Oral Infection and Immunity*

Richard T. Evans

CHAPTER OUTLINE

Origin, development, and history of infections

Studies in immunity

Developments in understanding the role of infectious agents in the oral cavity closely parallel those in medical microbiology. Indeed, several key initial observations of medical importance were made while describing an oral condition. Equally important were the technical advances made during these studies, which provided an understanding of basic principles of infection and immunity and suggested methods of control. Examples are the early descriptions of bacterial forms found in the mouth by van Leeuwenhoek, studies of oral bacteria by W. D. Miller and G. V. Black, caries studies using gnotobiotic animals, and the occurrence of secretory antibody in oral secretions.

ORIGIN, DEVELOPMENT, AND HISTORY OF INFECTIONS

Among ancient civilizations, epidemic diseases occurred where the nature or source of infection was unknown but the need for quarantine and hygiene was accepted. Only disease transmission by contact was understood. Generally, disease was ascribed to a natural occurrence such as the appearance of a comet or to a mystical event that would displease a deity. The Old Testament contains references to laws to avoid disease. The Book of Leviticus contains detailed descriptions of leprosy:

[I]f the hairs in it have turned white and the sore appears to be deeper than the surrounding skin it is the dreaded skin disease [leprosy] . . . but if the sore is white and does not appear deeper than the skin around it and the hairs have not turned white, the priest shall isolate him for seven days [the concept of quarantine].

In Hebrew, the word for "dreaded skin disease [leprosy]" and "mildew" are the same, suggesting the ancients associated mildew and leprosy:

[I]f the mildew has spread, the object [in this case cloth] is unclean. The priest shall burn it, because it is a spreading mildew which must be destroyed by fire.

Preventive measures to be instituted, personal hygiene, and cleaning or removal of mildew from the home environment were also dealt with.

Hippocrates, a Greek physician, codified concepts of disease that influenced thinking well into the Middle Ages. He believed disease required (1) intrinsic factors that equated with the host and the host's condition and (2) extrinsic factors, or "miasms." While the extrinsic factor did not equate with an infectious agent, it embodied the concept that an influence outside the body could induce a disease. An Italian, Girolamo Fracastoro, in 1546, defined contagion as occurring (1) by contact, (2) through fomites or objects, and (3) from a distance (airborne). Fracastoro (or Fracastorius in the Latinized form of his name) also used the term "seminaria," or seeds, to denote an infectious agent. It is not clear whether he considered "seminaria" as living or not.

During the 17th century, the first direct observations of living bacteria were made by Antony van Leeuwenhoek. The microscope had been used in its rudimentary form from around 1600 to describe fibers and small worms. Van Leeuwenhoek perfected a lens to observe objects the size of bacteria. Since he studied living organisms whose refractive index is close to that of water, and the objects were generally smaller than the resolving power of his lens, it is believed that he used a form of darkfield illumination to achieve the contrast and magnification required. To determine the size of the "little animalcules," he made comparative estimates based on larger objects such as strands of hair or grains of sand. Using these reference points he was able to give remarkably accurate estimates of size.

Van Leeuwenhoek's letters to the Royal Society in London in 1683 and again in 1695 give a clear description of bacteria found in the mouth. These letters were illustrated with accurate drawings of the three morphologic shapes—rods, cocci, and spiral forms—used to describe bacteria today (Fig. 1–1). He also described motility of the rod-shaped "animalcules" as "a very strong and swift motion and shot through the spittle like a pike through the water." He estimated that "there are more animals in the scum on the teeth in a man's mouth than there are men in the whole kingdom." He tried to kill them by rinsing his mouth with a strong wine vinegar but afterward found as many of them as before.

The observations of van Leeuwenhoek and of later microscopists raised questions as to the role of these unseen animals in disease. Without experimental evidence, Benjamin Marten, a London physician, wrote in 1720 that

> Certain species of animalcules may . . . [be] capable of existing in our juices and vessels . . . may by their spontaneous motion and injurious parts . . . cause . . . obstruction, inflammation, exulceration and all other phenomena and deplorable symptoms of disease.

Marten's writings, however, did not reflect the popular thinking of the day.

Since the processes of putrefaction and decay were readily seen, there was great interest as to how they occurred. Early speculation centered around the development of insects in putrefying meat. Francesco Redi in the late 17th century demonstrated that flies were attracted to decaying food, where they deposited their eggs and also found nourishment. In other experiments, he covered vessels containing meat with lids that allowed exchange of air but excluded flies. Naturally, no maggots or adult flies developed. These experiments helped exclude spontaneous generation for macroscopic organisms but did not eliminate this concept for microscopic animals. In 1776, approximately 100 years after Redi, Lazzaro Spallanzani furthered the demise of spontaneous generation by observing that heating meat infusions prevented "animalcules." He concluded that the organisms were airborne and the exclusion of air kept the infusions free of organisms for long periods of time. Still the debate continued because the experimental methods could be attacked since so many of the underlying principles and variables were poorly understood. Even so, practical applications were made. In the early 1800s Nicolas Appert proposed an early form of canning that preserved food by heating.

Finally, in 1860 Louis Pasteur performed his classic experiments, which totally disproved spontaneous generation. Following the lead of an earlier investigator, Theodor Schwann (1837), he prepared a series of flasks containing growth media that were sterilized by boiling. The necks of the flasks had curved elbows, which allowed air to enter but excluded particles. Other flasks were sealed after similar treatment. If left undisturbed the flasks remained growth free. If, however, the flasks were opened the media soon became overgrown. Other experiments confirmed these results. While Pasteur's results were definitive, those of John Tyndall (1881) also contributed to our knowledge. Tyndall removed particles from the air in a closed chamber by burning them in a flame. Media placed in the chamber remained uncontaminated as long as the particles were excluded from the chamber.

Fermentation of bread, wine, and beer was originally thought to be a chemical process rather than a biologic one. Charles Cagniard-Latour (1836) and Schwann (1837) independently discovered the yeast cell in wine and beer, respectively. Despite their descriptions of these cells and their presumed role in fermentation, chemical theories continued to dominate. Pasteur, a chemist, entered his studies from 1857 onward into this debate on fermentation. Although his ideas were not original, his experiments were definitive, giving him the credit for placing fermentation on a sound biologic basis. In his view, fermentation was essentially life without the presence of oxygen. How this occurred remained for others to describe.

Pasteur also studied the role of microorganisms in diseases of humans and animals. In 1880 he

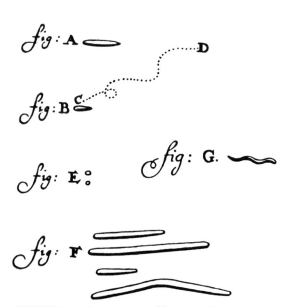

FIGURE 1–1 ✦ Drawings of bacterial forms seen by Antony van Leeuwenhoek (1695).

discovered that attenuated bacteria conferred protection in chicken cholera, and in 1884 he reported that attenuated virus was protective against rabies. These and studies of others introduced animal experimentation to microbiology, which led to many fundamental observations. Among the earliest studies regarding infectivity and disease induction by microorganisms are those of Devaine (1863) and Koch (1877). Devaine, using blood from animals infected with anthrax, transmitted infections to healthy mice, sheep, and cattle. Normal blood was unable to induce disease. Filtration of the infected blood on clay filters removed the organisms from the filtrate so it would not induce disease while the deposit on the filter would. Devaine and coworkers also showed that organisms found in pustules could transmit the disease. These experiments showed the association of organisms with the disease. The classic experiment of Robert Koch (1877) described the formation of resistant spores in anthrax, cultivation of the organism in vitro, and the reintroduction of the disease by injection of the pure culture.

Staining procedures and isolation culture techniques allowed the study of individual organisms. While others attempted to stain bacteria with varied results, Koch in 1877 was the first to use crystal violet with consistent success on the anthrax bacilli. Paul Ehrlich used methylene blue and F. Ziehl and F. Neelsen developed the use of acid staining, which allowed Koch to visualize the tubercle bacilli. One of the most widely used stains in medicine is the gram-modification of Ehrlich's aniline stain. Developed by Christian Gram in 1884, it remains one of the most powerful diagnostic procedures employed in microbiology today. Culturing of bacteria had its beginnings with liquid media. Usually this consisted of either meat infusions or yeast byproducts with added sugar. The results on such media were highly variable and depended on the skill of the investigator for reproducibility. One of the first studies into the composition of media was made by Carl von Nageli, who in 1882 described the effects of sugars, complex carbohydrates, and peptones on the growth of bacteria. This work was soon followed by the use of meat extracts as a nitrogen source. Solid media was used as early as 1872 by Joseph Schroeter, who employed potato slices, bread, coagulated egg albumin, meat, and starch pastes to isolate his organisms. As a result, Schroeter was the first investigator to work with pure bacterial cultures.

While ingenious, these methods were limited to pigmented organisms and were laborious to perform, producing erratic results. The fundamental importance of pure cultures, however, was clearly established. Oscar Brefeld, a mycologist of the time, extended this concept indicating that inoculation of media should be from one spore and that the culture should be protected from contamination. Working with pure cultures of waterborne bacteria, Koch developed the pour plate, in which the water samples were incorporated into gelatin as the plates were poured. The use of agar-containing medium was also introduced in Koch's laboratory. This major step allowed the use of solid medium at temperatures at which gelatin would melt. Koch also pioneered the use of coagulated serum media for culturing tuberculosis bacteria.

Robert Koch's accomplishments in the field of microbiology are numerous and varied. He identified the tubercule bacillus, described the differences between the human and bovine forms of the disease, and was the first to isolate the causative bacteria of anthrax and Asiatic cholera. Koch provided criteria for identifying an organism as the causative agent of a disease. While working with Jacob Henle early in his career, he became exposed to Henle's views that an organism must be isolated from the disease and studied in pure culture. To this, Koch added that the organism grown in pure culture must produce the disease in an experimental animal, and in turn must be reisolated from the infected experimental animal in pure culture. These rigorous criteria were applied by Koch in all of his studies of human and animal diseases. Although they have been restated and modified many times, they stand today as the definitive criteria and are known as the Koch-Henle postulates.

History of Oral Infection

One of Koch's students was an American, Willoughby D. Miller, who obtained his D.D.S. from the University of Pennsylvania and continued his studies at the University of Berlin. His major work, published in 1890, was entitled "The Microorganisms of the Human Mouth." He proposed that carbohydrates from food were broken down by oral bacteria and the resulting acids caused dissolution of the enamel. He further stated that bacteria from plaque could enter the initial lesion and continue to damage the underlying tooth structures. Because of the staining and pure culture methods available to him in Koch's laboratory, Miller was able to isolate and describe many of the oral forms. Contemporary with Miller, another American dentist working with less formal training was also describing the oral flora and speculating on its effects in the mouth. Greene V. Black from Jacksonville, Illinois, taught himself both dentistry and microbiology. Fully aware of Miller's work, he speculated in 1883 in his book, *The Formation of Poisons by Microorganisms,* that "all life including microorganisms produce injurious waste and they were responsible for disease including dental caries." In a description of his work published in 1886, "Microorganisms of the Oral Cavity," Black wrote in

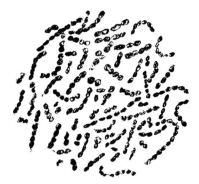

STREPTOCOCCUS MEDIA (Fungus of Dental Caries).

FIGURE 1–2 ✦ Drawing by G. V. Black (1886) of streptococci grown in broth from a carious lesion.

the following manner regarding the oral streptococci, which he refers to as the caries fungus (Fig. 1–2):

> We have found the product of the caries fungus to be lactic acid . . . you saw the gelatine formed by the microorganisms . . . in a crevice or anywhere a lodgement can be obtained this fungus begins its growth . . . growing against the side of the tooth it will form this gelatine and protect itself until it works its way through. . . .

This description of the bacterial attack on the tooth by the organisms found in the mouth is still accurate today.

Miller isolated organisms from saliva and decayed teeth, which produced acid when grown with carbohydrates. Generally, it was felt that the oral acid-producing bacteria alone could cause caries. Many dentists had observed a salivary drop in pH following meals with a gradual return to normal some hours later. It was also observed that some individuals were more prone to decay than others. A search was begun to identify specific organisms associated with caries. Lactobacilli, which predominate in saliva, were considered, as were several other acid formers.

In 1924 J. K. Clark identified a coccus from a caries lesion, which he named *Streptococcus mutans*. This organism was present in higher numbers in the caries lesion, adhered to the tooth, and was acidogenic. At that time, other investigators were not able to reproduce his findings. However, it was believed that a variety of streptococci in plaque and lactobacilli in saliva produced sufficient acid to cause enamel caries. Animal experiments of the time did not help clarify the situation. Organisms similar to those found orally in humans could be isolated orally from rodents. When placed on "cariogenic" diets some animals developed caries, but not in all instances, even among the same strains of animals.

During the 1930s and 1940s, lactobacilli were thought to be the principal acid-producing oral bacteria, even though the streptococci were numerically superior. A conceptual change regarding bacteria found in plaque began with the work of Robert Stephan. He measured the plaque pH with special antimony electrodes and found that within minutes following a glucose rinse the pH fell in the plaque of all subjects, but more markedly in plaque from caries-active subjects than from caries-free or caries-inactive subjects (Fig. 1–3). Moreover, the pH in the plaque of caries-active individuals fell to levels necessary for enamel dissolution. Stephan

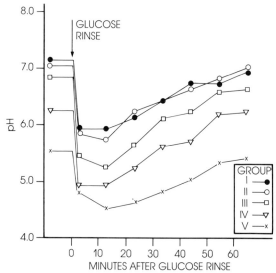

FIGURE 1–3 ✦ pH Curves showing increase in acid production following a glucose rinse. Group I = caries free; groups II through IV = increasing levels of caries activity; group V = extreme caries activity. (From Stephan, R. M.: Intraoral hydrogen-ion concentrations associated with dental caries activity. J. Dent. Res. 23:257, 1944, with permission.)

believed there must be qualitative differences in the plaque bacteria from the subject groups. Stephan and his coworkers further confirmed the specific nature of the caries-inducing bacteria by treating rats with antibiotics. Those rats receiving penicillin, an antibiotic most effective against gram-positive bacteria, had a greater than 90 percent reduction in caries.

In 1960 investigators working with caries-prone animals demonstrated that caries infections were transmissible. Paul Keyes treated hamsters with either penicillin or erythromycin to prevent caries. Offspring of antibiotic-treated animals did not develop caries, while offspring of the untreated animals did. When offspring of the antibiotic-treated animals were caged with the caries-active animals, they also developed caries. Feces from caries-prone animals added to the drinking water of offspring from antibiotic-treated animals also induced caries, demonstrating the transmission of the infectious agent. Thus began the search for the specific bacteria responsible for these observations, culminating in the rediscovery of *S. mutans* (described further in Chapter 6).

The early descriptions of periodontal disease frequently mentioned deposits surrounding the teeth involved in disease. Pierre Fauchard in 1745 described tartar and soft viscous deposits (plaque) in what appeared to be acute periodontal disease. The description, however, leads one to believe he considered the deposits diseases rather than the initiator of the disease. In his "Natural History of the Teeth," John Hunter (1773), the famous British physician, described gingivitis and pyorrhea and accurately stated that these diseases could serve as sources of infection elsewhere in the body. As mentioned earlier, W. D. Miller, in 1890, described the bacteria associated with soft tissue disease. He could not ascribe a specific bacterium as the cause of periodontal disease and thus he felt that these conditions were multifactorial. He stated:

> [A]s far as we know there is no bacterium which, inoculated under the gums, is able to provoke the disease in healthy persons . . . and . . . according to this conception, pyorrhea alveolaris is not caused by any specific bacterium.

Nevertheless, continued study of diseases of soft tissue revealed associations of certain bacteria with given conditions. Plaut in 1894 and Vincent in 1896 published accurate, detailed descriptions of fusiform bacteria and spirochetes and related them to an acute disease of oral soft tissues. Although anaerobic bacteria were known prior to this time, the work of H. A. Gins (1934) was first to reveal the anaerobic nature of many of the bacteria found in the mouth and recovered from oral infections. Gins' study discusses the increase in numbers and types of anaerobic bacteria found in the mouth with increasing age and disease. He isolated *Leptothrix, Streptobacillus, Actinomyces,* and *Spirillum* species, as well as anaerobic cocci. He also noted the frequent finding of *Bacterium (Bacteroides) melaninogenicum* associated with his isolates. As will be discussed in Chapter 16, black-pigmented bacterial species are often associated with forms of human periodontal disease.

Lack of information regarding a specific bacterium associated with periodontal disease led to several groups of organisms being implicated. During the 1920s and 1930s ameba and spirochetes were thought to be involved, since they were commonly found in material taken from periodontal pockets. Their numbers and motility undoubtedly influenced investigators. Because of their numbers and ease of isolation, streptococci were also considered to be involved. Most investigators at that time used only aerobic culturing techniques and were thus unable to study the majority of microorganisms. Failure to culture specific organisms associated with disease led to the "nonspecific plaque" hypothesis, which considered most bacteria found in plaque to be possible instigators. Interest waned in isolating plaque bacteria and identifying their role in periodontal disease.

Renewed interest occurred, however, when MacDonald and colleagues (1956) described mixed infections, which included black-pigmented bacterial species. These studies, while not identifying a specific organism, were notable for several reasons. First, anaerobic methods were routinely employed. Second, the products of organisms were recognized as playing a role in disease pathogenesis. Last, spirochetes, fusiforms, and anaerobic streptococci were no longer considered as pathogens. Knowledge obtained with the advent of improved cultural methods, and with sophisticated biochemical and serologic identification methods, has led to the conclusion that specific bacteria are responsible for adult and juvenile periodontitis (see Chapter 28).

STUDIES IN IMMUNITY

The field of immunology developed from the early studies in bacteriology, although some immunologic practices predated an understanding of the infectious process. The Chinese, Brahmins of India, and Persians during the Middle Ages practiced a form of immunization, called variolation, against smallpox. The technique consisted of deliberately exposing susceptible (unscarred) individuals to dried crusts taken from lesions of patients recovering from the disease. This form of immunization was not widely accepted, however, because of its danger. In 1776, Edward Jenner, a

British physician, recognized that milkmaids recovering from cowpox were protected against smallpox. With this observation, Jenner introduced the practice of active immunization, using an antigen to evoke protection against a subsequent infection. In this case, he deliberately exposed patients to a milder disease to protect them against the more virulent smallpox.

Approximately 100 years later, the concept of active immunization was extended by Pasteur, who observed that chicken cholera could be prevented by injecting bacteria that had been aged in culture to weaken their virulence. Pasteur developed this method of protecting against disease with attenuated cultures and prepared protective vaccines against anthrax, swine erysipelas, and rabies. In 1886, Theobald Smith and others showed that killed bacteria could protect against living infectious agents. Finally, von Behring and Kitasato (1890) showed that toxins of tetanus and diphtheria, free of bacteria, also induced protection. Shortly thereafter, antitoxins were used for passive immunization. The field of immunology was early divided into that which studied practical therapeutic and preventive uses for immunizations and that which studied theoretical and basic principles.

While interest in serum effects on microorganisms continued, the host's cellular reaction to infection was also studied. The classic example of cell-mediated immunity was the original observation by Koch that intradermal injections of tuberculin, an antigen derived from the tuberculosis organism, elicited delayed inflammatory responses in humans and animals previously exposed to the organism. This reaction could not be transferred by serum, but could be transferred by cells. Elie Metchnikoff (1884) observed that leukocytes took up bacteria (phagocytosis) and destroyed them by intracellular digestion. Metchnikoff proposed that cellular immunity acted as the principal host-protective defense against disease mechanism. His ideas, however, were not widely accepted. It was not until the studies of contact allergy by Landsteiner and Chase in the 1940s that cell-mediated immunity was fully recognized as a major immune mechanism.

Early attempts were made to control periodontal disease by immunologic means. Joseph Head in 1914 reported at the first annual meeting of the American Association of Immunologists on the use of either autogenous or stock bacterial vaccines, usually consisting of staphylococci and streptococci, as treatment combined with oral hygiene. Although many dental investigators felt encouraged, it soon was apparent that results obtained from such therapy were mixed, and the practice was soon discarded.

Of particular interest in oral microbiology and immunology is the description of the secretory immune system. Experiments of Kiyoshi Shiga (1908) examined the feeding of killed bacteria to rabbits, which were later challenged with an intravenous injection of toxin taken from the same bacteria. The animals were protected from the intestinal effects of the toxin even though no agglutinating activity was found in the serum. Similar experiments were performed throughout the ensuing two decades. In 1927, A. Besredka at the Pasteur Institute published a monograph entitled "Local Immunization," in which he asked the question ". . . will animals resist a fatal dose of virus (i.e., bacteria) after previous preparation by the buccal route?" Repeating and extending the previous work of Shiga, he concluded that "ingestion of heated cultures confers an immunity against a fatal dose of dysentery virus when inoculated intravenously." He further stated ". . . . the plan in artificial vaccination therefore is to follow the route which the virus takes in its penetration into the body." Burrows, in 1948, working with Asiatic cholera in guinea pigs, demonstrated the protective role of coproantibody. The concept of local protective immunity became clear when Fazekas de St. Groth in the 1950s demonstrated the presence of experimentally induced local antibody to influenza on the respiratory membranes of mice following stimulation by aerosols of the antigen. The stage was thus set for Heremans' descriptions in the 1960s of the IgA class of antibody in serum and for Tomasi's work on the predominance of this class of antibody in a variety of secretions such as saliva and colostrum. Today the secretory immune system is recognized as playing a major protective role against diseases which are acquired via the respiratory and oral routes. As will be seen in Chapter 27, the role of secretory immunity against caries and other oral diseases is currently an active field of investigation.

BIBLIOGRAPHY

Black, G. V.: Microorganisms of the Oral Cavity. Journal Illinois Dental Soc., pp. 180–208, 1886.

Bulloch, W.: The History of Bacteriology. Oxford Press, London, 1938.

Conant, J. B.: Pasteur's and Tyndall's Study of Spontaneous Generation. Harvard University Press, Cambridge, 1953.

Dayton, D. H., Small, P. A., Jr., Chanock, R. M., Kaufmann, H. E., and Tomasi, T. B. (eds.): The Secretory Immune System. U. S. Government Printing Office, Washington, D.C., 1970.

Dobell, C.: Antony van Leeuwenhoek and His "Little Animals." Staples Press, London, 1932.

Fouchard, P.: The Surgeon Dentist, or Treatise on the Teeth. Trans. Lindsay, L. from ed. 2, 1746. Milford House, New York, 1969.

Gins, H. A.: Die nichtversporenden Anaerobier der Mundhöhle und der Zähne. Zentralbl. f. Bakt. Parasit. u. Infekt. 132:129–145, 1934.

Head, J.: Society reports: American Association of Immunologists. Medical Record 86:942–946, 1914.

Keyes, P. H.: The infectious nature and transmissible nature of experimental dental caries. Arch. Oral Biol. 1:304–320, 1960.

Kobler, J.: The Reluctant Surgeon, A Biography of John Hunter. Doubleday, New York, 1960.

MacDonald, J. B., Sutton, R. M., Knoll, M. C., Madliner, E. M., and Grainger, R. M.: The pathogenic components of an experimental fusospirochetal infection. J. Infect. Dis. 98:15–20, 1956.

Miller, W. D.: The Microorganisms of the Human Mouth. S. S. White Dental Mfg. Co., Philadelphia, 1890.

Pappas, C. N.: The Life and Times of G. V. Black. Quintessence Publishing, Chicago, 1983.

Ring, M. E.: Dentistry–An Illustrated History. C. V. Mosby, St. Louis, 1985.

Stephan, R. M.: Intraoral hydrogen-ion concentrations associated with dental caries activity. J. Dent. Res. 23:257–266, 1944.

Vallery-Radot, R.: The Life of Pasteur. Doran and Co., New York, 1928.

Wilson, G., Miles, A., and Parker, M. T.: Principles of Bacteriology, Virology, and Immunity, ed. 7. Williams and Wilkins, Baltimore, 1983.

2 The Immune System and Host Defense

Mark E. Wilson

CHAPTER OUTLINE

Cellular elements of the immune system
Effector mechanisms of host immunity
Adverse immunologic responses: hypersensitivity reactions
Autoimmunity

The immune system has the formidable task of protecting the host against infection by potentially pathogenic microorganisms and in preventing the development and dissemination of malignant tumors. Ideally these objectives are met under conditions in which minimal injury to normal host tissues occurs. Moreover, the immune system must differentiate between "self" and "nonself" and only respond to the latter. Fortunately, immune responses to the majority of microbial infections are able to eradicate the foreign body with minimal damage to the host. However, prolonged or exuberant immune responses are often associated with significant tissue pathology.

Immune responses may be subdivided into two broad divisions, termed *innate* (or natural) *immunity* and *adaptive* (or acquired) *immunity*. These two types of immunity differ in certain key properties including specificity and immunologic memory. Innate immunity represents an important first line of defense against infectious agents. This type of immunity (1) is present from birth, (2) is not enhanced by prior exposure to an infectious agent, (3) lacks immunologic memory, and (4) does not display antigenic specificity. Innate immune responses entail a number of elements, both cellular and noncellular. Physical barriers such as skin and mucous membranes represent a component of innate immunity that infectious agents must breach to gain access to the host. When this initial obstacle has been overcome, the organism then may encounter phagocytic cells present in blood and tissues. These include polymorphonuclear leukocytes, monocyte/macrophages, and a class of lymphocytes termed *natural killer (NK) cells.* A number of soluble factors also contribute to innate immunity. For example, lysozyme, an enzyme found in mucous secretions, can damage the cell walls of many bacteria. Acute phase proteins found in serum, including C-reactive protein, also contribute to clearance of many bacteria and fungi. The proteins of the complement system (especially the alternative pathway, as discussed later in this chapter) contribute to innate immunity by generating products that recruit phagocytes into infected tissues, enhance phagocytosis and killing of bacteria, and lyse some organisms directly. The α and β interferons play an important role in eradication of virus-infected host cells. These proteins render host cells resistant to infection by viruses, and also enhance NK cytotoxicity toward cells already infected by viruses. Interferon-activated NK cells also exhibit increased cytotoxicity toward tumor cells.

Persistence of an infection in spite of an innate immune response typically leads to induction of an adaptive immune response. Adaptive immune responses, unlike innate responses, are characterized by (1) exquisite *specificity* for the offending antigen(s), (2) *memory* (a rapid and heightened response following subsequent encounter with the same or a closely related antigen), (3) *diversity* (the capacity to respond to millions of different antigens present in the environment), and (4) *self versus nonself recognition*. The characteristics of specificity and memory associated with adaptive immunity often are exploited in the development of vaccines designed to provide long-lived protection against pathogenic microorganisms.

CELLULAR ELEMENTS OF THE IMMUNE SYSTEM

The introduction of a foreign molecule or organism into an immunocompetent host typically results in the activation of lymphocytes. This adaptive immune response is manifested by an increase in the production of antibodies (humoral immunity), effector lymphocytes (cellular immunity), or both. In general, humoral immunity plays an important role in host defense against infections due to extracellular pathogens, while cellular immunity contributes to eradication of intracellular pathogens (e.g., virus-infected cells). However, humoral and cellular immune responses often function in concert to eliminate infectious agents. Thus, cell-mediated reactions help eliminate virus-infected cells, whereas antibodies can block the spread of viruses and prevent re-infection of the host. The key cell types involved in the acquired immune response include (1) B (bone marrow-derived) lymphocytes, (2) T (thymus-derived) lymphocytes, and (3) antigen presenting cells (APC).

B Lymphocytes

B lymphocytes are the principal cell types involved in antibody-mediated, or humoral, immunity. These cells comprise approximately 15 to 30 percent of the total lymphocyte population in peripheral blood, and are readily identified by virtue of their expression of surface immunoglobulins which serve as a receptor for specific antigen. Following their interaction with antigen, these cells are induced to differentiate into antibody-secreting plasma cells. These antibody molecules exhibit a diverse array of biologic activities that contribute to host immune defense against many species of extracellular bacteria, certain viruses and tumors. Antibodies also are able to neutralize a number of microbial products, particularly toxins, which may be injurious to host tissues.

B lymphocytes are thought to arise from pluripotential stem cells which subsequently form stem cells committed to differentiation into lymphoid (both T and B cells) or myeloid (granulocytes, erythrocytes, mononuclear phagocytes, and megakaryocytes) cells. The liver is the primary site of B lymphocyte production during the first trimester of life. Beyond this period, however, the bone marrow is the principal site for production of B lymphocytes.

The development of committed stem cells into mature B lymphocytes and, subsequently, into antibody-secreting plasma cells, involves antigen-independent and antigen-dependent phases (Fig. 2–1). During antigen-independent maturation, B lymphocyte precursors undergo a series of changes involving DNA rearrangement of genes encoding for the heavy (H) and light (L) chains that comprise all immunoglobulin molecules. Rearrangements of H and L chain genes occur independently, with H chain genes rearranging first. Because expression of surface immunoglobulin re-

quires synthesis and assembly of both the H and L chains, pre-B cells, which have rearranged and synthesized H chains but not L chains, are negative for surface immunoglobulin. However, pre-B cells contain cytoplasmic H chains of the IgM class (designated μ chain). Once L chain gene rearrangements are completed, the immature B cells are able to express surface IgM monomers. More mature B lymphocytes subsequently express both surface IgM and IgD. All of these events occur in the absence of antigen. Virgin B lymphocytes expressing surface immunoglobulin are now poised to bind antigen, which initiates a series of antigen-dependent changes leading to the differentiation of these cells into immunoglobulin-secreting plasma cells. Plasma cells are capable of secreting several thousand immunoglobulin molecules per second for a period of several days. Mature plasma cells are seldom found in the peripheral circulation, being primarily located in lymphoid tissues. These cells express few surface immunoglobulin molecules (consistent with the fact that plasma cells are geared toward immunoglobulin synthesis rather than antigen binding activity).

The differentiation of mature B lymphocytes into plasma cells requires multiple signals, the first of which is provided by antigen interaction with surface immunoglobulin (Fig. 2–1). Activated B lymphocytes are able to internalize and process the antigen and subsequently re-express the antigen on the cell surface in conjunction with glycoproteins encoded in the major histocompatibility complex (see Antigen Processing and Presentation below). In this manner, the activated B lymphocyte is able to "present" the antigen to T-helper lymphocytes with specificity for the antigen. The T-helper cells in turn secrete growth and differentiation factors (particularly IL-4 and IL-5) for antigen-stimulated B lymphocytes, which express membrane receptors for these molecules. An additional B cell differentiation factor, IL-6, is required for terminal differentiation into plasma cells. This factor is produced by a variety of lymphoid and nonlymphoid cells. Thus, although B lymphocytes are the only cells capable of producing antibodies, T lymphocytes play an important role in the process of B cell activation and differentiation into plasma cells.

GENERATION OF ANTIBODY DIVERSITY

For antibodies to be an effective component of host defense, these molecules must be capable of recognizing a diverse array of antigens. Fortunately, normal individuals produce antibodies capable of combining with more than 10^7 different antigens. This is possible due to variability and even hypervariability in the primary amino acid sequences of the antigen-combining sites of im-

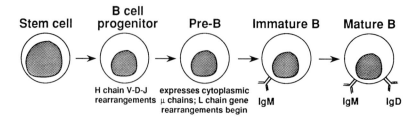

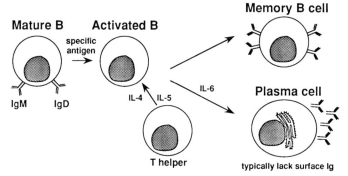

FIGURE 2–1 ✦ Antigen-independent and antigen-dependent phases of B lymphocyte development.

munoglobulin molecules. On the other hand, certain regions of the antibody molecule are structurally conserved. These regions are involved in many of the effector functions of antibodies. The information necessary to produce immunoglobulins of greater than 10^7 different antigenic specificities is encoded in DNA. However, individual genes encoding the heavy and light chains which form each unique antibody do not exist. Rather, B lymphocytes use an elaborate scheme involving somatic DNA rearrangements. Through this genetic mechanism, fewer than 10^4 gene segments can be combined in various ways sufficient to generate more than 10^7 antibodies of unique antigenic specificity.

The gene loci encoding sequences for the heavy chain and the two types of light chain (κ and λ) are found on different chromosomes (Fig. 2–2). The heavy and light chain loci are divided into multiple gene segments encoding the variable and constant regions of each chain. In the case of the κ and λ light chains, two segments encode the variable region and one segment encodes the constant region. Heavy chain synthesis involves three gene segments encoding the variable region and one segment encoding the constant region. The amino-terminal portions of the variable region of heavy and light chains are encoded in one of several variable (V) region gene segments. Each V region gene is preceded by a leader sequence involved in

the generation of a relatively hydrophobic signal peptide necessary for intracellular transport and secretion of immunoglobulins. Downstream (or in the 3′ direction) of the V region gene segments are located the constant (C) region genes. Whereas the κ L chain locus has a single C region gene, the λ L chain locus has three to six such segments. Between the V and C region genes are a variable number of joining (J) region genes and, in the case of heavy chains, a series of diversity (D) segments. Located in the 3′ end of the heavy chain locus is a cluster of constant gene segments encoding the different classes and subclasses of immunoglobulins. As shown in Figure 2–2, there are some differences in manner in which J segments are distributed in the κ and λ light chain loci.

The immunoglobulin gene segments are arranged in a similar germline configuration in all cells. It is only in B lymphocytes, however, that these genes are sequentially rearranged. Light chain rearrangements begin with the combination of one of several hundred κ V region genes or one of approximately one hundred λ V region genes with a J segment. The intervening segments between the combined V and J segments are deleted. These combined V-J segments form the variable region of a light chain gene. A primary, or nuclear, transcript is generated in which the C region genes remain separated from the rearranged V-J segments. Through a process termed *RNA splicing,* the intervening sequences separating the V-J and C genes are eliminated, resulting in formation of a "mature" messenger RNA. This mRNA can then be translated to yield a single polypeptide containing variable and constant region amino acid sequences. In the case of heavy chains, the process is similar but involves additional gene segments not found in the light chain loci. The process begins when one of approximately 5 to 15 D segments recombines with a J segment, during which time any intervening sequences are deleted. This D-J complex then combines with one of nearly 100 V region gene segments. Again, intervening sequences between the V and D segments are deleted. After a primary RNA transcript is formed, the VDJ complex is combined with one of several C region genes through RNA splicing. This mature mRNA is then translated into a complete heavy chain.

Rearrangement of V, D, J, and C genes is sufficient to generate substantial antibody diversity. However, other factors also contribute to this process. For example, *junctional site diversity* can extend the antibody repertoire by virtue of the fact that slight differences in the point of joining between V-J and V-D-J segments can lead to generation of new codons and, thus, altered amino acid sequences in the variable regions of the heavy and light chains. Secondly, inasmuch as the heavy and light chains are synthesized independently, the way in which heavy and light chains combine to form

a complete immunoglobulin molecule can lead to *combinatorial diversity*. Finally, *somatic mutation* of rearranged genes can extend antibody diversity. The latter mechanism is considered to be an important factor in the phenomenon of affinity maturation, as discussed below.

HEAVY CHAIN ISOTYPE SWITCHING

The constant region of the heavy chain defines the class, or isotype, of immunoglobulin. Five such classes have been defined including IgG, IgA, IgM, IgD, and IgE. A number of studies demonstrated that a single variation region can be associated with different constant regions. Recognition of this fact led to the concept of isotope switching. Recall that mature, resting B lymphocytes display IgM and IgD on their surface. As shown in Figure 2–2, the constant region genes for the IgM (μ) and IgD (δ) heavy chains are in closer proximity to the V, D, and J segments than are the remaining constant region genes. In fact, V-D-J complexes are first transcribed together with the μ constant region gene.

Following initial (primary) exposure to antigen, there is a lag period in which little or no antibody is present in serum. This is followed by an exponential increase in antibody production, particularly of the IgM isotype. Antibody production reaches a plateau and subsequently declines gradually. Upon subsequent encounters with the same antigen, the nature of the antibody response is

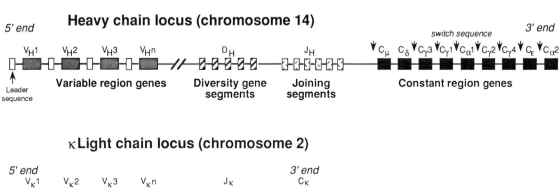

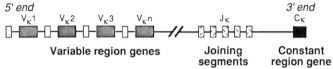

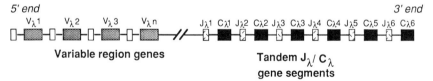

FIGURE 2–2 ✦ Germline organization of the heavy and light chain immunoglobulin genes.

markedly altered. First, the lag period is considerably shortened. Secondly, the magnitude of antibody production is substantially greater. Both of these effects are thought to be attributable to the presence of memory B and T lymphocytes. Further, there is a significant increase (100-fold or greater) in the average affinity of serum antibodies reactive toward the relevant antigen. This has been termed *affinity maturation,* and has been attributed to selection and clonal expansion of B lymphocytes whose surface immunoglobulins exhibit the greatest affinity for the antigen, as well as to somatic mutation of immunoglobulin variable region genes.

Apart from the aforementioned quantitative changes, which occur during the secondary or *anamnestic* response, there is often a qualitative change in which antibody isotypes other than IgM are produced in significant amounts. This latter effect is attributable to isotype switching, a process in which one or more constant heavy chain genes is irreversibly deleted. The process appears to be mediated by switch sequences (see Fig. 2–2) located on the 5' side of each constant heavy region gene (except for the δ chain), under the control of cytokines produced by T lymphocytes. Activation of a particular switch sequence results in deletion of all constant region genes located 5' to the expressed heavy chain gene. The fact that the μ and δ heavy chain genes are not separated by a switch sequence is consistent with the ability of B lymphocytes to co-express IgM and IgD.

Isotype switching is dependent on the presence of cytokines elaborated by T lymphocytes. Accordingly, the ability of a given antigen to induce isotype switching is dependent on the ability of that antigen to activate T lymphocytes. Many carbohydrate antigens, including bacterial lipopolysaccharides and pneumococcal polysaccharides, exhibit little or no ability to interact with T lymphocytes via their antigen receptors. Such antigens are termed *T-independent antigens.* Immunization with T-independent antigens typically results in the production of IgM antibody, with little or no evidence of isotype switching. On the other hand, many protein antigens can be processed and presented to T lymphocytes, resulting in T lymphocyte activation and elaboration of cytokines involved in B lymphocyte growth and isotype switching. These types of antigens are termed *T-dependent antigens.*

T Lymphocytes

A second population of lymphocytes, T lymphocytes, also arises from a pluripotential stem cell in bone marrow. Unlike B lymphocytes, which undergo continued maturation in bone marrow, T lymphocytes differentiate in the thymus. Whereas B lymphocytes recognize antigens via surface immunoglobulins, T lymphocytes are surface-negative for immunoglobulin and do not exhibit DNA rearrangements in immunoglobulin genes. Rather, T lymphocytes express a distinct membrane receptor for antigen that recognizes antigen in conjunction with membrane glycoproteins encoded in the major histocompatibility complex (see below). T lymphocytes play a major role in the initiation and regulation of immune responses, and are key elements of cell-mediated immune responses against viruses, intracellular bacteria, and tumors.

T lymphocytes express different surface membrane antigens at various stages of development and/or cell activation. These surface markers have been useful in the identification of phenotypic and functional diversity among T lymphocytes. These markers previously were identified by means of monoclonal antibodies, which recognize specific antigenic determinants (termed *epitopes*) within a given surface membrane protein. Hence, T lymphocyte markers were formerly referred to according to their reactivity toward different monoclonal antibodies (e.g., OKT4, Leu-15). Due to the structural complexity of membrane proteins, it is possible to generate a number of different monoclonal antibodies that recognize different epitopes within the same molecule. This led to a brief period in which scientific papers were published that described T lymphocyte on the basis of their reactivity toward a specific monoclonal antibody, rather than on lymphocyte expression of the entire surface membrane protein. This situation was resolved after a series of International Human Leukocyte Differentiation Antigen Workshops, commencing in 1982. As a consequence of these workshops, a leukocyte surface marker, which is reactive toward a group (or cluster) of monoclonal antibodies, is now identified according to a cluster of differentiation (CD) number (e.g., CD2, CD8).

Certain CD markers are expressed by virtually all peripheral blood T lymphocytes. This is the case with respect to CD2, a 50-kilodalton glycoprotein through which T lymphocytes form rosettes with sheep red blood cells. Other CD markers are useful in segregating T lymphocytes into a number of distinct subpopulations. Thus, approximately 60 percent of peripheral blood T lymphocytes express CD4, a glycoprotein expressed on T cells whose activation is dependent on recognition of antigen in conjunction with class II major histocompatibility complex (MHC) molecules (see below). Approximately 30 percent of peripheral blood T lymphocytes express CD8, a membrane protein expressed by T cells whose activation is dependent on recognition of antigen in conjunction with class I MHC molecules. The majority of circulating T lymphocytes express either CD4 or CD8, but not both. These two surface markers define subsets of

T lymphocytes with significantly different effector functions. Notably, CD4$^+$ T lymphocytes typically function as *helper* (designated T$_H$) cells, providing "help" to other T lymphocytes as well as to immunoglobulin-producing B lymphocytes. On the other hand, CD8$^+$ T cells exhibit *cytotoxic/suppressor* (T$_C$ or T$_S$) activity. These cells elaborate factors that inhibit T$_H$ activity, thereby suppressing immune responses. CD8$^+$ T lymphocytes also display cytotoxic activity toward numerous virally-infected or tumor cells. It is not clear whether the suppressor and cytotoxic activities are mediated by the same or distinct subpopulations of CD8$^+$ T cells.

T-LYMPHOCYTE ONTOGENY

T lymphocytes undergo differentiation in the thymus, irrespective of whether they express the CD4 or CD8 phenotype. The process of T lymphocyte maturation begins with the migration of T-cell precursors from the bone marrow to the cortical regions of the thymus. It is thought that these cells are attracted to the thymus by chemical signals provided by thymic epithelial cells. The earliest recognizable thymocyte committed to the T cell lineage is the pro-T cell (Fig. 2–3). These cells bear CD2 (the sheep erythrocyte receptor) but do not express the T cell antigen receptor. Pro-T cells are also surface-negative for CD4 and CD8. During the next phase of development, maturing cortical

thymocytes proceed along one of two alternative pathways. In one instance, the thymocytes begin to rearrange DNA segments encoding for the variable and constant regions of an alternative form of the T-cell antigen receptor (designated λ/δ TCR), and express this receptor in conjunction with a tightly associated complex of five membrane glycoproteins that form the CD3 complex. Most cells expressing the λ/δ TCR fail to express either CD4 or CD8 during further development and release into the peripheral circulation as "double-negative" T lymphocytes. The precise function of these λ/δ TCR–expressing cells has not been defined. The majority of pro-T cells follow a different pathway of differentiation. These pre-T cells co-express both CD4 and CD8, but do not yet express an antigen receptor. Subsequently, these cells undergo DNA rearrangements of genes encoding the constant and variable regions of the α/β TCR, which is expressed by the majority of mature T lymphocytes in the periphery. At this stage, the thymocytes are CD4$^+$, CD8$^+$, and express the α/β TCR in conjunction with the CD3 complex. During the first stages of development, which occur in the thymic medulla, two important events take place. First, the cells progressively lose either CD4 or CD8. Secondly, these cells are "educated" by thymic epithelial cells to learn to differentiate between "self" and "nonself"-MHC gene products. Those cells, which are autoreactive toward self-MHC mole-

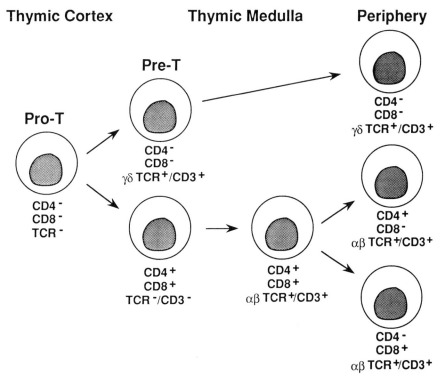

FIGURE 2–3 ✦ Intrathymic development of T lymphocyte subpopulations.

cules, are eliminated by a process of clonal deletion, an important mechanism of self-tolerance. As a consequence of this selection process, only about 10 percent of the immature T cells which enter the thymus ever reach the peripheral circulation. Mature T cells which survive this selection process leave the thymic medulla through the walls of post-capillary venules. After circulating for a time, these T lymphocytes distribute among various peripheral lymphoid tissues including thymus-dependent regions of the inner cortex of lymph nodes, the spleen, and mucosa-associated lymphoid tissue (e.g., Peyer's patches in the colon).

It is presently unknown what signal(s) drives proliferation and differentiation of immature thymocytes. These cells do express receptors for certain cytokines, which exhibit growth factor activity, including interleukin-2 (IL-2) and interleukin-7 produced by thymocytes and stromal cells, respectively. Alternatively, thymic epithelial cells may induce thymocyte activation via the CD2 molecule, which recognizes a cell adhesion molecule (LFA-3) expressed on the epithelial cells.

THE T-CELL ANTIGEN RECEPTOR COMPLEX

Unlike B lymphocytes, which recognize soluble antigens through membrane-associated immunoglobulin receptors, T lymphocytes only recognize antigens when displayed on the surface of antigen-presenting cells. The T cell antigen receptor is a heterodimer consisting of a 50-kilodalton acidic α chain and a 42-kilodalton basic β chain, which are linked through an interchain disulfide bond. Genes encoding the α chain are located on chromosome 14, while those encoding the β chain reside on chromosome 7. Each chain is comprised of a variable region, which interacts with the associated complex of immunogenic peptide plus a histocompatibility molecule, and a constant region. Antigenic diversity among T-lymphocyte antigen receptors is generated through a process of DNA rearrangements similar to those described for the immunoglobulin genes. There are more than 50 V region genes and roughly 100 J region genes that may encode the α chain. A single constant region gene for the α chain is located "downstream" of the J region segments. The β chain locus consists of some 75–100 V region genes, followed by two structurally similar C region genes. Upstream of each C_β gene is a cluster of 6–7 J region gene segments preceded by a diversity (D) region segment not found in the α chain locus. Through a series of DNA rearrangements, alternative V, D, J, and C region segments are brought into juxtaposition. A primary RNA transcript is formed, which is subsequently processed through RNA splicing to remove intervening gene sequences.

The mature messenger RNA thus formed is translated to generate a continuous α or β chain containing variable and constant region sequences. Such DNA rearrangements, as well as variable combinations of translated α and β chains, can give rise to a diversity of T cell antigen receptors capable of recognizing up to 1.7 million different antigenic specificities.

The variable regions of the α/β T cell antigen receptor define antigenic specificity. However, as noted previously, T lymphocytes do not recognize antigen alone, but rather "see" processed antigen presented in conjunction with membrane glycoproteins encoded in the major histocompatibility complex. In the case of $CD4^+$ T lymphocytes, antigen is recognized in conjunction with a class II MHC molecule, whereas $CD8^+$ T lymphocytes recognize antigen presented by class I MHC–bearing cells. As shown in Figure 2–4, certain regions of the T-cell antigen receptor recognize processed antigen, while others recognize variable regions of the class I or class II MHC molecule. In close proximity to the TCR complex is either a CD4 or CD8 molecule. These molecules do not exhibit structural polymorphism, and do not recognize antigen. These cell adhesion molecules recognize conserved regions in either a class I (CD8) or class II (CD4) molecule. The interaction between CD4 or CD8 and the corresponding MHC molecule appears to stabilize TCR interactions with the antigen-MHC complex.

The T-cell antigen receptor contains a short cytoplasmic tail (Fig. 2–4). It is thought that this cytoplasmic domain is insufficient to participate in signal transduction through the TCR molecule. However, tightly associated with the TCR molecule is a group of five molecules which comprise the CD3 complex. Three of the CD3 proteins (γ, δ, and ε) are members of the immunoglobulin superfamily, each containing a single immunoglobulin-like domain. Two additional proteins, typically consisting of a disulfide-linked homodimer of two ζ chains, comprise the remainder of the CD3 complex. In contrast to the TCR, the proteins of the CD3 complex contain substantial cytoplasmic tails, which are thought to play a major role in signal transduction initiated through the T cell antigen receptor.

FUNCTIONAL PROPERTIES OF T LYMPHOCYTES

T lymphocytes are broadly divided into two subpopulations, T_H and $T_C T_S$, which exhibit distinct functional characteristics. T_H lymphocytes (which typically display CD4) are essential elements in the development of cell-mediated immunity. Moreover, these cells provide important signals to B lymphocytes producing antibodies. The critical role

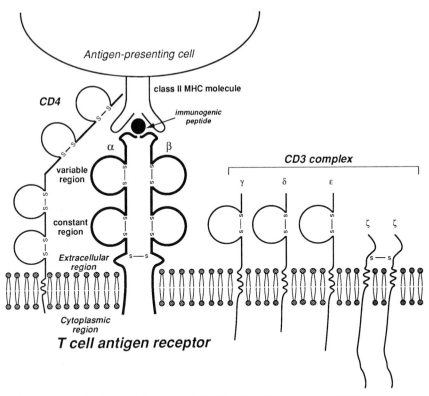

FIGURE 2–4 ✦ General features of the T cell antigen receptor/CD3 complex.

played by the T_H cell in orchestrating various aspects of the adaptive immune response is demonstrated in patients afflicted with the human immunodeficiency virus (HIV), a member of the lentevirus family of animal retroviruses. The envelope of HIV contains a 120-kilodalton surface glycoprotein (abbreviated gp120) which exhibits high affinity binding to CD4-bearing cells, including macrophages and T_H lymphocytes. Binding of gp120 to CD4 facilitates insertion of a second viral envelope protein, gp41, into the target cell membrane, thereby initiating viral fusion. This process ultimately leads to the destruction of a substantial number of CD4-bearing lymphocytes, a hallmark of HIV-infected subjects. Depletion of $CD4^+$ lymphocytes leads to development of the acquired immune deficiency syndrome (AIDS), in which the patient is markedly susceptible to opportunistic infections (especially pneumonia due to *Pneumocystis carinii*) and neoplastic disease (e.g., Kaposi's sarcoma). These clinical manifestations result from defects in cytotoxic T-cell, NK-cell, and B-lymphocyte functions attributed to the loss of T_H activity.

Activation of T_H lymphocytes requires two distinct signals. The first signal is provided by antigen-presenting cells displaying processed antigen in conjunction with a class II MHC molecule. This signal initiates a series of biochemical changes that lead to formation of a number of second messengers (including inositol trisphosphate and diacylglycerol), which cause an increase in cytosolic calcium level and protein kinase c activity. These events are necessary but not sufficient to induce T_H activation in the absence of a second signal. This second activation signal is referred to as a *co-stimulator molecule* and is provided by the antigen-presenting cell. A number of cytokines, including interleukin-1, tumor necrosis factor, and interleukin-6, have been found to exhibit costimulator activity, but it remains unclear which of these provides the critical second signal. In any case, T_H lymphocytes respond to these two signals by activating genes encoding for growth factors and growth factor receptors, particularly IL-2 and the IL-2 receptor. IL-2 produced by the activated T_H cell exerts autocrine activity on the same cell that produced it. Expression of IL-2 receptors on the activated T_H cell permits this cell to respond to IL-2 (formerly termed *T-cell growth factor*), resulting in increased cell proliferation. In this way, antigen stimulation of T_H cells leads to an expansion of the T cell population capable of responding to the antigen. This clonal expansion is a key factor in the development of heightened immune responses following secondary and subsequent exposure to the same antigen.

Activation of CD4$^+$ T$_H$ lymphocytes also results in the secretion of other cytokines that act upon other elements of the immune system. Thus, interferon-γ (also called immune interferon) is a potent activator of macrophage microbicidal and tumoricidal activity. CD4$^+$ lymphocytes also secrete IL-4 and IL-5, which are key growth factors for B lymphocytes. IL-2 also provides the second activation signal for CD8$^+$ T lymphocytes, which have been triggered through their T cell antigen receptors. Under the influence of IL-2 provided by the T$_H$ cell, CD8$^+$ T lymphocytes differentiate into cytotoxic T lymphocytes capable of lysing virus-infected and tumor cells.

Recent evidence suggests that CD4$^+$ T$_H$ lymphocytes may be subdivided into two subsets, based primarily on differences in the patterns of cytokines secreted by human and mouse CD4$^+$ cell lines. CD4$^+$ cells of the T$_H$1 phenotype secrete IL-2, lymphotoxin, and interferon-γ, but not the B-lymphocyte growth factors IL-4 and IL-5. In contrast, CD4$^+$ cells of the T$_H$2 phenotype secrete IL-4 and IL-5, but not IL-2, lymphotoxin, or interferon-γ. Cells of the T$_H$1 phenotype secrete cytokines, which appear to be important in delayed-type hypersensitivity and cytotoxic T cell reactions, whereas cytokines secreted by cells of the T$_H$2 phenotype appear to mediate immediate hypersensitivity (allergic) reactions in which B lymphocytes are induced to elaborate IgE. Distinct patterns of cytokines produced in allergic subjects and patients with certain forms of parasitic infections lend further support to the concept that functional subsets of T$_H$ cells exist. However, presently there are no definitive surface markers available that distinguish CD4$^+$ lymphocytes secreting different patterns of cytokines. Thus, it remains unclear whether the T$_H$1 and T$_H$2 phenotypes represent distinct subsets of CD4$^+$ T lymphocytes or merely reflect different stages of activation of a single cell type.

MEMORY B AND T LYMPHOCYTES

The development of a secondary, or anamnestic, humoral immune response is dependent on the generation of a population of B and T lymphocytes termed *memory cells*. It is unclear whether these cells arise during the normal process of antigen-induced clonal expansion and activation or are a distinct subset of lymphocytes predestined to become memory cells. Both memory B and T cells appear to be long-lived, in some instances surviving for as long as three decades. Memory B cells may be distinguished from resting B cells by the isotypes of immunoglobulin displayed on their surface. Notably, whereas resting B cells express surface IgM and IgD, memory B cells express other isotypes including IgG, IgA, and IgE. Differential binding of monoclonal antibodies to two distinct T

cell surface markers, designated CD44 and CD45, has been used to distinguish virgin T lymphocytes from memory T lymphocytes. Memory B and T cells are quite responsive to secondary exposure to antigen. In the case of memory B cells, this may be attributable to expression of surface immunoglobulin of higher affinity than occurs on resting B cells. Memory T cells, on the other hand, express high affinity receptors for IL-2.

Antigen Processing and Presenting Cells

Studies evaluating the specificity of antigen recognition by B and T lymphocytes revealed that there are some fundamental differences in the way these two leukocyte populations recognize various antigens. First, B lymphocytes (via their membrane-bound immunoglobulins) are capable of recognizing carbohydrates, proteins, and nucleic acids, as well as low molecular weight chemical (haptens) coupled to carrier proteins. In contrast, T lymphocytes preferentially recognize protein antigens. Secondly, B lymphocytes often recognize conformational determinants in protein antigens, whereas T lymphocytes preferentially recognize linear (sequential) determinants. Finally, B lymphocytes (and secreted antibodies) recognize soluble protein antigens, while T lymphocytes only respond to protein antigens displayed on the surface of other cells.

It is now clear that the T cell antigen receptor recognizes peptide fragments of protein antigens, rather than native proteins. Moreover, the T cell antigen receptor "sees" the peptide fragment in conjunction with membrane glycoproteins encoded in the major histocompatibility complex, or MHC. The latter conclusion was based on evidence that antigen-specific T lymphocytes only interact with cells expressing the appropriate antigen if the two cells share the same MHC, a phenomenon termed *MHC restriction*. Thus, for a T lymphocyte to recognize a protein antigen, the antigen must first be denatured, partially catabolized into small peptide fragments, become physically associated with a self–MHC-encoded molecule, and be displayed (or presented) on the surface of a cell as a peptide-MHC complex. This series of events is referred to as *antigen processing*.

The MHC molecules that play such a critical role in T cell antigen recognition are encoded in a multiallelic gene cluster located in the short arm of chromosome 6. The MHC complex in humans is known as the human leukocyte antigen (HLA) complex. The organization of genes associated with the HLA complex is depicted in Figure 2–5. This complex contains loci that encode for two major classes of membrane glycoproteins, termed

The Human Leukocyte Antigen (HLA) Complex

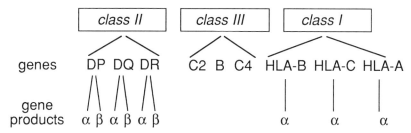

FIGURE 2–5 ✦ Organization of major histocompatibility complex (MHC)-encoded molecules in the human leukocyte antigen (HLA) complex.

class I and *class II MHC molecules*. The class I and class II gene regions are separated by a region containing genes which encode for certain complement components (C2, C4 and factor B), as well as for certain cytokines (tumor necrosis factor and lymphotoxin). Class I molecules are expressed on the surface of virtually all nucleated cells, and include the classical transplantation antigens, which are important in allograft rejection. In contrast, class II molecules are expressed in a restricted set of leukocytes termed *antigen-presenting cells,* or APCs. The region of HLA complex encoding class II molecules (HLA-D) was found to control immunologic responsiveness to certain antigens, and was termed the *immune response (or I) region.* Hence, the products of these genes often were referred to as *I region-associated, or Ia, antigens.*

The general structural features of the MHC class I and II molecules encoded in the HLA complex are depicted in Figure 2–6. Class I MHC mole-

cules have a two-chain structure consisting of a 43-kilodalton α chain encoded in the HLA-A, -B, and -C regions and a noncovalently associated 12-kilodalton chain, called β_2-microglobulin, which is encoded outside the HLA complex. The α chain is organized into a series of three extracellular domains (α_1, α_2, and α_3), a single transmembrane domain, and a short cytoplasmic tail. The greatest structural polymorphism among class I molecules is found in the α_1 and α_2 domains. It is this region that forms the "groove" that serves as the antigen-binding site for processed peptide fragments. β_2-microglobulin, on the other hand, does not exhibit structural polymorphism and does not participate in antigen binding. The association between β_2-microglobulin and the α chain appears to be important in maintaining class I molecules in their proper conformation.

Class II MHC molecules also possess a two-chain structure that is organized in a manner anal-

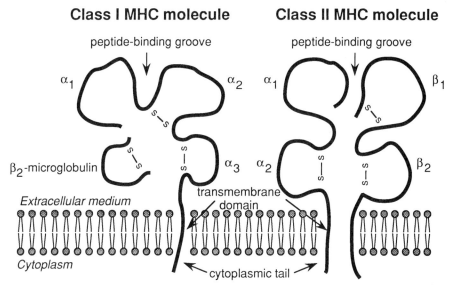

FIGURE 2–6 ✦ General structural features of major histocompatibility complex (MHC) class I and class II molecules involved in antigen presentation to T lymphocytes.

ogous to that of class I molecules. These molecules contain a 31–35 kilodalton α chain and a 27–30 kilodalton β chain, each of which contributes two extracellular domains, a transmembrane domain, and a cytoplasmic tail. Both chains are encoded in the HLA-D region. As is the case with class I molecules, the two most extracellular domains (α_1 and β_1) of class II molecules exhibit the most structural polymorphism and form a groove that appears to participate in peptide binding.

The physical dimensions of the groove present in the extracellular region of MHC class I and II molecules are consistent with the ability of these molecules to bind small peptides (8–10 amino acids) but not large molecules such as globular proteins or complex polysaccharides. Structural polymorphism in the most external regions of MHC class I and II molecules appears to enable these molecules to bind antigenically distinct peptide fragments. The antigenic specificities of MHC class I and II are, however, lower than for T cell antigen receptors or immunoglobulins.

Despite the fact that MHC class I and class II molecules share certain structural features, these molecules differ in one very significant way. This regards the nature of the T lymphocytes capable of recognizing class I-peptide and class II-peptide complexes. Specifically, MHC class I molecules present antigen to CD8-bearing T lymphocytes, whereas MHC class II molecules present antigen to CD4-bearing T lymphocytes. There also are differences in the intracellular routes followed by MHC molecules and antigens before their interaction with T lymphocytes, as discussed below.

PATHWAYS OF ANTIGEN PROCESSING

The immune system exhibits the capacity to respond to antigens of intracellular as well as extracellular origin. However, the nature of the immune response in each instance can differ significantly. It is not surprising to find that divergent mechanisms have evolved for the processing and presentation of intracellular and extracellular antigens. In the following discussion, it will become clear that intracellular antigens are presented to CD8[+] T lymphocytes by MHC class I molecules, while extracellular antigens are presented to CD4[+] T lymphocytes by MHC class II molecules.

The processing of intracellular protein antigens (either of host cell origin or encoded by viral nucleic acids) begins in the cytosol (Fig. 2–7). These protein antigens are "shuttled" to the lumen of the endoplasmic reticulum (ER) by transporter proteins. Cleavage of intracellular proteins into smaller peptide fragments is thought to occur during transport through the cytosol, within the lumen of the ER, or both. Peptide fragments of suitable size and composition associate with the peptide-

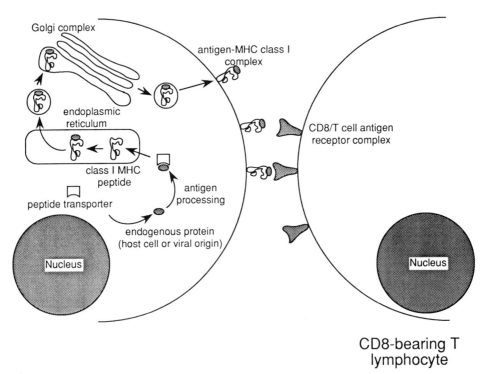

FIGURE 2–7 ✦ Schematic representation of events involved in processing and presentation of intracellular antigens to CD8[+] T lymphocytes.

binding groove in MHC class I molecules located in the lumen of the ER. The class I-peptide complexes are moved to the Golgi apparatus via transport vesicles and subsequently exported to the cell surface. The MHC molecules are anchored to the cell surface by their transmembrane domain. Since virtually all nucleated cells express MHC class I molecules, any cell is capable of processing and presenting intracellular protein antigens in this manner. Intracellular antigens handled via this route are presented to CD8+ T lymphocytes (typically of the cytotoxic/suppressor phenotype) whose antigen receptors have specificity for the antigenic peptide fragment displayed by the MHC molecule. Inasmuch as CD8+ cytotoxic T lymphocytes are key effectors against viruses and tumor cells, it makes sense teleologically that intracellular antigens would be presented to CD8+ T cells in this manner.

An alternative pathway is utilized in the processing of extracellular antigens (Fig. 2–8). As presently envisioned, extracellular antigens are first internalized by antigen-presenting cells by means of coated pits, and are subsequently shuttled to the endosomal compartment. Within the ER, newly synthesized MHC class II molecules associate with a 30-kilodalton invariant chain, which occupies the peptide-binding groove. This interaction prevents class II molecules from binding endogenous peptides. The MHC class II-invariant chain complex is transported to the endosomal compartment, whereupon lysosomal enzymes proteolytically degrade the invariant chain and enable the class II molecule to associate with processed antigen in this same compartment. The peptide-class II complex is transported to the cell surface, where it is available for interaction with CD4+ T lymphocytes bearing T cell antigen receptors of appropriate specificity.

Whereas intracellular antigens are presented to CD8+ T lymphocytes by MHC class I molecules, which are found on all nucleated cells, extracellular antigens are presented to CD4+ T lymphocytes by class II molecules found only on a specialized group of antigen-presenting cells (Table 2–1). These cells express class II molecules constitutively. Other cell types, including glial, mesenchymal, and vascular endothelial cells, normally do not express class II molecules unless induced by cytokines such as interferon-γ. Once induced in this manner, these cells can also function as antigen-presenting cells for CD4+ T lymphocytes.

MHC-restricted antigen presentation is biologically significant for a number of reasons. First, MHC-encoded molecules, by virtue of the structure of their antigen-binding grooves, determine which

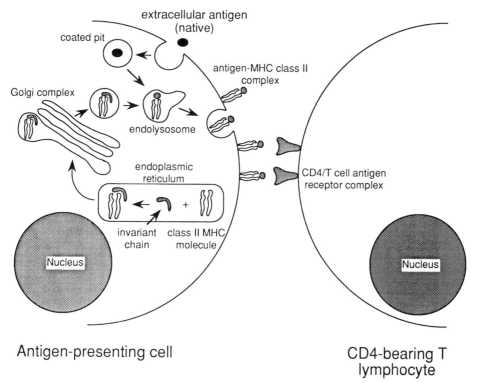

Antigen-presenting cell   CD4-bearing T lymphocyte

FIGURE 2–8 ✦ Schematic representation of events involved in processing and presentation of extracellular antigens to CD4+ T lymphocytes.

TABLE 2–1 ✦ Types of Antigen-Presenting Cells (APC) Expressing Class II MHC Molecules

CELL TYPE	COMMENTS
Mononuclear phagocytes	Fixed and wandering mononuclear phagocytes found in most tissues; constitutively express class II major histocompatibility complex (MHC) molecules, but levels can be markedly increased by mediators such as interferon-γ; antigen uptake facilitated by opsonization
Langerhans-dendritic cells (LDC)	Found in high numbers in thymus-dependent regions of peripheral lymphoid organs, as well as skin and epithelia; constitutively express high levels of class II MHC molecules; LDC in skin can process antigen and migrate to lymphoid tissues for subsequent antigen presentation; may be important in processing antigens introduced via skin or epithelia
B lymphocytes	Constitutively express class II MHC molecules; increased class II expression induced by IL-4 but not by interferon-γ; antigen uptake may be nonspecific or via membrane immunoglobulin; "resting" B lymphocytes are poor APCs in comparison with B lymphocytes activated by lymphokines or polyclonal B cell activators

antigens will be available for presentation to T lymphocytes. Second, the class of MHC molecule with which the immunogenic peptide fragment is associated determines the phenotype (CD4$^+$ or CD8$^+$) of T cell that is ultimately stimulated. Finally, MHC restriction necessitates that intimate contact exist between the antigen-presenting cell and the T lymphocyte. This assures that signals provided by the antigen-presenting cell are directed to appropriate antigen-specific T cell clones, which preferentially expand. For example, macrophages present antigen to CD4$^+$ T cells in conjunction with class II molecules. However, this is insufficient to cause activation of the T cell. A second signal is provided in the form of interleukin-1 (IL-1), a protein secreted by activated macrophages. These two signals induce activation of the CD4$^+$ T cell, which then secretes a number of cytokines, which promote growth and differentiation of other lymphocytes. Moreover, these cytokines exert an autocrine effect on the T cell that secreted them, thereby inducing clonal expansion of antigen-specific T cells. In this way, MHC restriction requires that cellular interactions necessary for optimal immune responsiveness take place.

Antigen presenting cells also play a key role in the development of immature T cells within the thymus. Thymic epithelial cells express both MHC class I and class II molecules on their surface, and present these molecules to thymocytes through direct cell-to-cell contact. This interaction appears to be important in "educating" maturing thymocytes with respect to differentiation of self- versus non-self-MHC gene products. Those thymocytes capable of recognizing self-MHC molecules are clonally deleted and fail to leave the thymus.

EFFECTOR MECHANISMS OF HOST IMMUNITY
Immunoglobulins
GENERAL FEATURES

It has been recognized for many years that a major component of acquired immunity is the production of antibody activity in the fluid phase (plasma) of blood. Antibody activity resides in a heterogeneous group of serum proteins that migrate principally as γ-globulins (and, to a lesser degree, as β-globulins) upon electrophoresis in agarose gels. It was for this reason that the term *gamma-globulins* was formerly used to describe the antibody-containing fraction of serum. This terminology has been abandoned in favor of the term *immunoglobulin*, which is more descriptive of the biologic properties of these molecules.

Immunoglobulins are glycoproteins containing 82 to 96 percent polypeptide and 4 to 18 percent carbohydrate, and are heterogeneously distributed in various biological fluids and on the surface of some populations of lymphocytes. These molecules are produced as a consequence of foreign substances with antigen-specific B lymphocytes, and are the mediators of humoral immunity. Immunoglobulins are bifunctional molecules capable of (1) recognizing specific antigenic determinants and (2) eliciting a diverse array of effector functions that promote neutralization and/or elimination of the antigen. Almost all of the biologic activity of immunoglobulins appears to be attributable to the polypeptide component. The role of the carbohydrate moiety in immunoglobulin function is not completely understood. It may, however, be involved in immunoglobulin secretion by plasma cells, as well as in modulation of some of the effector functions of immunoglobulins.

The basic structure of immunoglobulins was elucidated through a number of approaches, including the use of proteolytic enzymes (especially pepsin and papain) and chain dissociation techniques (unfolding proteins in 6 M urea and reducing disulfide bonds with mercaptoethanol). The results of these studies indicated that all immunoglobulins contain a basic monomer structure consisting of two heavy chains and two light chains (Fig. 2–9). The heavy chains contain approximately twice as many amino acid residues as the light chains. Each chain is organized into a series of domains, each consisting of approximately 110 amino acids, generated by intrachain disulfide linkages. The "loop" structure formed through such disulfide bonding is a common characteristic of a broad array of proteins belonging to the immunoglobulin superfamily. Immunoglobulins also contain interchain disulfide linkages (heavy-light and heavy-heavy), which can vary in position and number. Comparison of the amino acid sequences of numerous immunoglobulin molecules indicates that the amino termini of each H and L chain contain a V region sequence, whereas the carboxy termini contain more conserved constant (C) region sequences. Hence, the light chain contains a V_L and C_L region. The heavy chain also contains a single variable region (V_H), but contains multiple constant (C_H) domains. The

latter are numerically ordered from the amino terminus of the H chain (e.g., C_H1, C_H2, etc.). The region of the H chain between the first (C_H1) and second (C_H2) domains exhibits increased flexibility and susceptibility to proteolytic attack, and is termed the *hinge region*.

Within the variable region of each H and L chain there exists certain stretches of amino acids which exhibit marked sequence variation. Such regions are termed *hypervariable regions*. Other segments of the variable region show much less variation and are termed *framework regions*. It is now recognized that the hypervariable regions of the H and L chains form the antigen-binding site of the immunoglobulin molecule. Inasmuch as the hypervariable regions possess a structure complementary to that of the antigen they recognize, these regions also are referred to as *complementarity-determining regions,* or CDRs. There are three CDRs in each V_L and V_H segment.

Studies involving limited enzymatic cleavage provided additional insight into the general structure and function of the immunoglobulin molecule. Two enzymes, papain and pepsin, were particularly useful in this regard. Both enzymes cleave the immunoglobulin molecule in the area between the C_H1 and C_H2 domains, but differ with respect to the precise site of attack relative to the inter-heavy chain disulfide linkages (Fig. 2–9). Papain cleaves immunoglobulins on the amino-terminal side (i.e.,

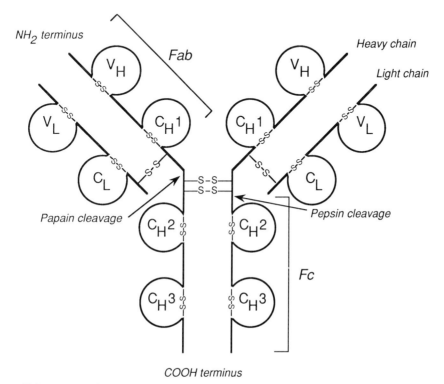

FIGURE 2–9 ✦ General features of a prototypical immunoglobulin monomer.

closer to the variable region domain) of the disulfide bonds that link the two H chains together. Digestion of the immunoglobulin molecule in this manner yields three fragments. Two of the fragments are of equal molecular mass, each containing all of the L chain and the V_H and C_H1 domains. These fragments were found to contain structures capable of binding specific antigen and were thus termed *fragment antigen-binding (Fab)*. The remaining fragment, which lacks antigen-binding activity, has a somewhat larger mass than the Fab fragment and tends to crystallize. This fragment has been termed *fragment-crystallizable (Fc)*. Pepsin cleaves immunoglobulins on the carboxy-terminal side of the inter-heavy chain disulfide bonds, producing a single large fragment containing both Fab fragments linked by disulfide bonds that is termed $F(ab)'_2$. The Fc fragment is extensively degraded by pepsin. The results of these studies indicated that the basic structure of the immunoglobulin monomer is comprised of two antigen-binding (Fab) fragments and a single Fc fragment, the latter of which is associated with many of the effector functions of immunoglobulins.

Immunoglobulin H Chain Classes (Isotypes)

As noted above, the constant region of the immunoglobulin heavy chain exhibits considerably less sequence variation than does the variable region. There are, however, subtle structural variations in the C_H regions of different immunoglobulin molecules. On the basis of serologic and chemical properties, human immunoglobulins can be differentiated into five distinct classes (or isotypes), each containing a different H chain. Thus, immunoglobulins are classified as belonging to the IgG, IgA, IgM, IgD, or IgE isotype. The H chain associated with each isotype is designated by a Greek letter. Hence, IgG contains a γ heavy chain, IgA an α chain, IgM a μ chain, IgD a δ chain, and IgE an ε chain. It is important to remember that the immunoglobulin isotype is determined by the structure of the C_H domain. The γ, δ, and α H chains each contain a hinge region between the C_H1 and C_H2 domains. The μ and ε H chains do not have a hinge region, but rather contain an extended C_H2 domain with hingelike flexibility. Moreover, μ and ε H chains contain five domains (one variable and four constant), whereas α and γ H chains contain four domains (one variable and three constant).

Immunoglobulin L Chain Types

Structural and antigenic differences in the constant region of L chains also are sufficient to differentiate these molecules into two types (analogous to H chain classes), designated κ and λ. A single immunoglobulin molecule always has two identical κ or λ L chains, rather than a mixture of the two types. Both L chain types are represented in all five immunoglobulin classes, although not equally. Approximately 65 percent of IgG, IgA, and IgM molecules contain κ L chains, while the remaining 35 percent contain λ L chains (the proportions of these two L chain types in IgD and IgE are less clear). In general, the κ:λ ratio among human immunoglobulins is considered to be 2:1.

Heavy Chain Subclasses

Based on minor physicochemical and serologic differences in the C_H regions of IgG and IgA, the H chains of these immunoglobulin isotypes may be further subdivided into a number of subclasses. IgG consists of four subclasses (IgG1, IgG2, etc.), while IgA consists of two subclasses (IgA1, IgA2). The IgG and IgA subclasses differ in their proportional representation in serum. The percentage of each IgG and IgA subclass in serum of normal adults is as follows: IgG1, 60 to 70 percent, IgG2, 19 to 31 percent, IgG3, 5 to 8 percent, and IgG4, 1 to 4 percent; IgA1, 93 percent, IgA2, 7 percent. Immunoglobulin A and G subclasses also differ in number and arrangement of interchain disulfide linkages (Fig. 2–10). Note, for example, that the L chains of IgA2 are covalently linked to each other rather than to the H chains. Although all four IgG subclasses contain covalently linked H and L chains, the location of the interchain disulfide link-

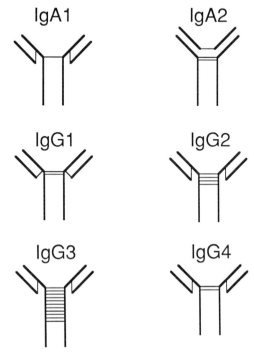

FIGURE 2–10 ✦ Distribution of interchain disulfide linkages in human IgA and IgG subclasses.

age varies somewhat. The L chain of IgG1 is linked to the γ H chain between the C_H1 and C_H2 domains (i.e., closer to the hinge region), whereas the L chains of the remaining three IgG subclasses are attached to the H chain between the V_H and C_H1 domains. Also note that the number of inter-heavy chain disulfide linkages among the IgG subclasses can vary from two (IgG1, IgG4) to eleven (IgG3). Structural variations can significantly influence the biological properties of the immunoglobulin subclasses, as will be discussed shortly.

Light Chain Subtypes

Minor differences in amino acid sequence of the constant region of the L chain also have been identified in humans, permitting classification into subtypes (analogous to H chain subclasses). Four subtypes of λ L chains have been identified. Kappa L chains, on the other hand, do not exhibit such C_L variation.

Allotypic and Idiotypic Determinants

All normal individuals inherit the set of genes that encode the antigenic determinants in the constant regions of the immunoglobulin molecule that define H chain isotype and subclass and L chain type and subtype. There are other antigenic determinants expressed in immunoglobulins of some members of the species but not others. Antigenic variations in the constant regions of some H and L chains that differentiate members of the same species are termed *allotypic determinants*. Allotypic variations arise because multiple alleles exist for some constant region genes, and these alleles are inherited in a Mendelian fashion. Allotypes have been identified on all four human IgG subclasses, for IgA2 subclass antibodies, and for the κ L chain. Allotypic markers on the γ and α H chains and the κ L chain are designated as Gm, Am, and Km determinants. Some 20 Gm, 3 Km, and 2 Am allotypes have been identified. Certain allotypic markers are restricted to the constant region of a single IgG subclass, whereas others are shared by two or more subclasses (these are termed isoallotypes). IgA2 molecules bearing the m(1) marker do not contain H-L interchain disulfide linkages (see Fig. 2–10), while those bearing the m(2) marker do.

Allotypic determinants are found on the immunoglobulin molecules of some, but not all, members of a given species. There are yet other antigenic determinants that distinguish one immunoglobulin molecule from another, even within a single individual. These antigenic markers are termed *idiotypic determinants,* and are found in the variable region of the immunoglobulin molecule. Many of these idiotypic determinants arise as a consequence of the unique amino acid sequences found in the hypervariable regions of the H and L chains and are involved in generating the antigen-binding site.

Monomeric Versus Polymeric Immunoglobulins

All five classes of immunoglobulin consist of the basic four chain (two heavy and two light chains) structure. Nevertheless, the molecular mass of different immunoglobulins can vary considerably, from approximately 150,000 to more than 900,000 daltons. This is due to the fact that certain immunoglobulin classes (IgM, IgA) exist as polymers. IgM is a macroglobulin (molecular mass ~900,000 daltons) containing five monomer subunits each containing two L chains and two μ chains. IgA can be found in serum in both monomeric (160,000 daltons) and dimeric (415,000 daltons) form, approximately 20 percent of the total serum IgA being in the latter form. All polymeric immunoglobulins are associated with an additional polypeptide approximately 15,000 daltons in size, which is termed the *joining (J) chain*. The J chain is synthesized by B lymphocytes producing polymeric immunoglobulins. Although it is not entirely clear how the J chain facilitates assembly of immunoglobulin monomers, it appears that this protein forms a disulfide linkage with cysteine residues located in the C-terminal region of the α or μ chain of two adjacent monomer units. Additional monomer subunits (in the case of IgM) then are added and polymerize through Fc-Fc interactions. All polymeric immunoglobulins, regardless of the number of monomer subunits involved, contain a single J chain molecule.

Secretory Component

IgA comprises only about 20 percent of the total serum immunoglobulins, but is the principal class of immunoglobulin found in external secretions (saliva, tracheobronchial secretions, genitourinary secretions, sweat, tears, breast milk, and colostrum). IgA present in such secretions possesses a dimeric structure, in which the two IgA monomers are connected via a J chain. However, secretory IgA contains an additional component not found in other immunoglobulins, regardless of whether they are monomeric or polymeric (Fig. 2–11). This protein, termed *secretory component,* is a 70,000-dalton polypeptide produced by epithelial cells (not by B lymphocytes, as is true for the J chain). The secretory component is covalently added to dimeric IgA during its transport across mucosal epithelial cells, and appears to protect secretory IgA from proteolytic cleavage by enzymes present in external secretions.

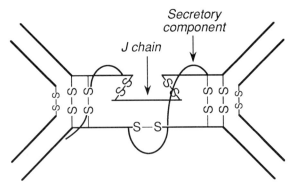

FIGURE 2–11 ✦ General structure of human secretory IgA.

BIOLOGIC PROPERTIES OF IMMUNOGLOBULINS

The bifunctional nature of immunoglobulins permits these molecules to bind antigens specifically and to initiate a number of biologic effector functions. Some of these effector functions are mediated through the antigen-binding region (Fab), while others are initiated through the Fc moiety. Moreover, distinct immunoglobulin classes and subclasses are often associated with different biologic activities. A number of the key effector functions performed by immunoglobulins are summarized in Table 2–2.

Fab-mediated binding of immunoglobulin to microbial toxins and certain viruses often results in their effective neutralization. For example, if an immunoglobulin molecule binds to a viral surface

TABLE 2–2 ✦ **Biologic Effector Functions of Immunoglobulins**

BIOLOGIC PROPERTY	ANTIBODY ISOTYPE(S)
Toxin neutralization	IgG, IgA, IgM
Virus neutralization	IgG, IgA, IgM
Bacterial agglutination	IgA, IgM
Bacterial opsonization	IgG, IgM
Complement fixation	IgG1, IgG2, IgG3, IgM
Increased vascular permeability	IgE
Antibody-dependent cell-mediated cytotoxicity (ADCC)	
Natural killer (NK) activity toward virus-infected and tumor cells	IgG
Eosinophil-mediated killing of parasites	IgA, IgE
B lymphocyte antigen receptor	IgD, IgM (monomeric)

antigen that is involved in the attachment of the virion to a host cell, the ability of the virus to infect the host is impaired. Similarly, immunoglobulin binding to toxins can inhibit the ability of the toxin to interact with membrane receptors on the host target cell. In both instances, Fab or F(ab)$'_2$ fragments suffice in mediating these effects.

Other immunoglobulin effector functions are dependent on an intact immunoglobulin molecule and are mediated through the Fc moiety. Formation of antigen-antibody complexes involving IgG (but not IgG4) or IgM can lead to activation of the complement system, resulting in a number of hematologic and hemodynamic changes associated with the inflammatory response. Complement activation via the classical pathway (see below) results from the interaction between complement component C1 with the C_H2 domain of IgG or the C_H3 domain of IgM. The interaction between immunoglobulins and isotype-specific Fc receptors on various host cells initiates other biologic effects. For example, deposition of IgG on bacterial surfaces can promote recognition and ingestion of these organisms by host phagocytic cells, which bear membrane Fc receptors for IgG. The process through which immunoglobulin binding enhances phagocytic cell function is termed opsonization. Antibody-dependent cell-mediated cytotoxicity (ADCC) plays an important role in the elimination of virus-infected host cells and tumor cells, as well as some types of parasites. In the first instance, IgG binding to virus-infected or neoplastic cells promotes target cell recognition by natural killer cells. In the latter case, IgA and IgE antibodies directed to antigens of helminths such as *Ascaris* and *Nippostrongylus* promote killing of these parasites by eosinophils.

Two remaining effector functions of immunoglobulins involve the association of these molecules with cell membranes *before* their interaction with specific antigen. Tissue mast cells and basophils in the circulation bear high affinity surface Fc receptors for IgE. Many of these high affinity receptors are occupied by IgE in the absence of antigen. Subsequent binding of antigen through surface-bound IgE molecules initiates a series of events leading to the release of a broad array of chemical mediators with vasoactive (e.g., histamine) and inflammatory (e.g., prostaglandins, leukotrienes) activity. IgE-mediated degranulation of mast cells and basophils plays a major role in immediate hypersensitivity reactions. Resting B lymphocytes express IgD and monomeric IgM on their surface. These molecules are associated with the lymphocyte membrane through a membrane-spanning domain not found in secreted immunoglobulins. The binding of antigen to membrane IgD or IgM initiates a series of biochemical events, which promote the differentiation of B lymphocytes into plasma cells, which actively secrete immunoglobulin.

BIOLOGIC PROPERTIES OF THE HUMAN IgG SUBCLASSES

Among normal adults, IgG constitutes nearly 75 percent of the total immunoglobulins present in serum. IgG also is the predominant isotype produced during secondary (anamnestic) immune responses, where it potentially contributes to host defense through a number of diverse mechanisms (see Table 2–1). Serum IgG consists of four distinct subclasses. Although IgG subclass antibodies have comparable carbohydrate content and do not differ in their electrophoretic mobilities, they exhibit significant structural differences in the hinge region. These differences principally involve the number of amino acid residues and inter-heavy chain disulfide linkages (see Fig. 2–10) present in the hinge region. Utilization of κ and λ L chains also varies between IgG subclasses. The human IgG subclasses have been found to differ significantly with respect to a number of biologic properties, as well as in their proportional representation in serum. These differences are summarized in Table 2–3.

As evident in Table 2–3, IgG subclass antibodies differ with respect to two important effector functions, namely complement activation (via the classical pathway) and Fc-receptor binding. IgG3 antibodies are most active in fixing complement. Activation of the classical pathway is initiated through binding of complement component C1 to the C_H2 domain of the immunoglobulin molecule. It is thought that the greater activity of IgG3 in fixing complement is attributable to the fact that the extended hinge region prevents the Fab arms from sterically interfering with C1 access to the C_H2 domain. The extended hinge region of IgG3 also may be a liability, however, as IgG3 antibodies exhibit greater susceptibility to proteolysis and a shorter biologic half-life than other IgG subclasses.

IgG1 and, to a much lesser extent, IgG2 also activate the classical pathway. In contrast, IgG4 does not activate the classical pathway, and may actually interfere with the ability of other immunoglobulins to fix complement.

A second important effector function of IgG involves binding to membrane Fc receptors, particularly on mononuclear and polymorphonuclear phagocytes. Phagocyte Fc receptors exhibit preferential binding to IgG1 and IgG3. In contrast, IgG2 antibodies interact only weakly with these receptors.

IgG is the only immunoglobulin isotype capable of crossing the human placenta. It is, therefore, an important source of passive protection of newborn infants during the first weeks of life. Although all four IgG subclasses are subject to placental transport, there appears to be some degree of subclass selectivity. Notably, IgG2 is transported to a lesser extent than the other three IgG subclasses. However, the significance of this finding has not been determined.

The IgG subclasses also differ with respect to the nature of the antigens that stimulate their production. This has been demonstrated by evaluating the subclass pattern of IgG antibodies produced against polysaccharide or protein antigens following either natural infection or vaccination. Bacterial protein antigens preferentially induce IgG1 antibodies, although detectable amounts of IgG3 and IgG4 are produced. Hyperimmunization with protein antigens can, however, result in the production of substantial amounts of IgG4. Polysaccharide antigens typically induce IgG antibodies which are principally of the IgG2 subclass, although IgG1 antibodies may also be produced (particularly in children under 2 years of age).

IgA SUBCLASS ANTIBODIES

IgA consists of two distinct subclasses, IgA1 and IgA2, which differ in the amino acid composition of the hinge region and in the distribution of inter-

TABLE 2–3 ✦ Structural and Biologic Properties of the Human IgG Subclasses

CHARACTERISTIC	IgG1	IgG2	IgG3	IgG4
Concentration range in serum (mg/ml)	5–12	2–6	0.5–1	0.2–1
Number of amino acid residues in hinge region	15	12	62	12
Number of H—H disulfide bonds	2	4	11	2
Use of κ and λ L chains (κ : λ ratio)	2.4	1.1	1.4	8.0
Biologic half-life (days)	21–23	20–23	7–8	21–23
Complement activation (classical pathway)	+ +	+	+ +	None
Fc receptor binding				
Human monocytes	+ +	+	+ +	±
Human neutrophils	+ +	±	+ +	+

+ + = strong; + = intermediate; ± = weak to none.

chain disulfide linkages. Structural differences in the hinge region of these two subclasses influence their susceptibilities to proteolytic cleavage by microbial enzymes. In particular, a number of gram-positive *(Streptococcus sanguis)* and gram-negative *(Bacteroides, Porphyromonas, Capnocytophaga* and *Veillonella* sp.) mucosal organisms produce an IgA protease which selectively cleaves the hinge region of IgG1. IgA2 antibodies are resistant to degradation by this enzyme. Although the nature of the IgA subclass response pattern to protein and polysaccharide antigens is not as well-characterized as for IgG subclasses, it appears that protein antigens induce mainly IgA1 whereas carbohydrate antigens induce IgA2.

The Complement System

An important mechanism for amplification of immune responses involves a group of more than 20 proteins normally found in plasma, collectively referred to as the *complement system* (or complement cascade). Complement activation is linked to a number of events associated with inflammatory reactions, including increases in vascular permeability and recruitment of phagocytic cells. In ad-

dition, products of complement activation facilitate recognition and ingestion of infectious agents by phagocytic cells, promote direct membranolysis of susceptible gram-negative bacteria, mobilize phagocytes from the bone marrow during acute bacterial infection, and even regulate B and T lymphocyte function.

The complement cascade is subdivided into two pathways, termed the *classical* and *alternative pathways* (Fig. 2–12). These two pathways differ in the nature of the substances which trigger their activation and in the proteins involved in the initial steps in activation of each pathway. However, a recurrent pattern is observed following activation of either pathway. Thus, the initial steps in each pathway involve conversion of inactive precursors to their active forms as a consequence of limited proteolysis. These reactions are represented by the general equation: $X \rightarrow Xa + Xb$, in which X represents the native protein, Xa denotes the smaller cleavage fragment, and Xb the larger fragment generated through proteolysis. In most instances, the larger (Xb) fragment participates in the next step in complement activation, while the smaller (Xa) fragment is released into the fluid phase (often with biologic consequences). The two pathways con-

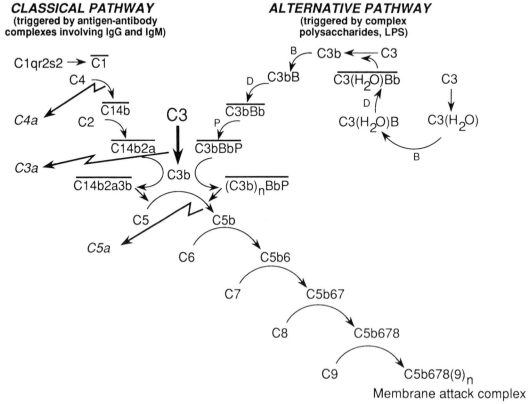

FIGURE 2–12 ✦ The complement cascade.

verge at the C5 cleavage step. Beyond this step, activation of terminal (C6 through C9) complement proteins involves assembly rather than proteolysis.

THE CLASSICAL PATHWAY

Activation of the classical pathway is typically initiated by soluble antigen-antibody complexes or by deposition of antibody on the surface of particulate targets (e.g., bacteria, viruses). Not all immunoglobulin isotypes are capable of triggering the classical pathway, however. Antigen-antibody complexes containing IgM or certain IgG subclass antibodies (IgG1, IgG2, and IgG3) are effective activators of the classical pathway, whereas complexes containing IgA, IgD, IgE, or IgG4 are not. The initial step in activation of the classical pathway involves binding of macromolecular C1 (consisting of a complex of subunits C1q, C1r, and C1s held together by calcium ions) to a single molecule of IgM or to two closely spaced molecules of IgG (termed an IgG *doublet*). C1 binding to the C_H2 domain of the antibody molecule occurs via the C1q subunit. C1q binding results in a conformational change in the associated C1r and C1s subunits, leading to activation of C1s esterase activity. C1 esterase then cleaves C4 into two fragments, C4b and C4a. Cleavage of C4 exposes a binding site on the larger C4b fragment, which can form a covalent bond on activating surfaces. Because of the reactivity of this binding site, C4b is typically deposited in close proximity to the C1 complex. C4b facilitates binding of the next component, C2, which is also cleaved by C1 esterase. The larger fragment, C2a, is deposited in the vicinity of C4b, while C2b is released into the fluid phase. The C4b2a complex possesses (via the C2a component) enzymatic activity capable of cleaving the next component in the cascade, C3. This complex is referred to as the *classical pathway C3 convertase,* which cleaves C3 into a small fragment (C3a) and a large fragment (C3b). C3b, like C4b, contains a binding site capable of mediating covalent attachment to activating surfaces. Deposition of C3b near the C4b2a complex facilitates binding of the next component, C5, which is also cleaved by this enzyme (now referred to as a C3/C5 convertase) into a small fragment (C5a) and a large fragment (C5b). C5b contains an unstable membrane-binding site, which can mediate noncovalent association of this fragment with cell surfaces. The membrane-binding site of C5b rapidly decays unless stabilized through binding of the next component, C6. Subsequent binding of C7 results in formation of a more hydrophobic complex (C5b67), which inserts into the lipid bilayer of target cell membranes. Binding of C8 to the C5b67 complex results in formation of a small pore. The final step in assem-

bly of the membrane attack complex involves polymerization of several molecules of C9 around the C5b678 complex, forming a transmembrane pore with a hydrophilic core and a hydrophobic exterior. The effective diameter of the pore increases with the number of C9 molecules polymerizing around the C5b678 complex. In the presence of these pores, through which water and small ions can freely move, the target cell is unable to maintain osmotic stability. Continued entry of water and loss of electrolytes eventually leads to osmotic lysis of susceptible cells.

C5b67 complexes can form in the fluid phase. Alternatively, these complexes can form on, and be released from, immune complexes or the surfaces of noncellular targets. Once released, the C5b67 complex can bind to nearby cells. Following assembly of C8 and C9, these can be lysed via the membrane attack complex. This phenomenon, known as *innocent bystander lysis,* appears to contribute to tissue injury seen in a number of immune complex diseases.

THE ALTERNATIVE PATHWAY

A second pathway for activation of complement exists that leads to cleavage of C3 and C5, as well as to assembly of the membrane attack complex, but bypasses the classical pathway components C1, C4, and C2. This pathway, termed the *alternative pathway,* is triggered in the absence of antibody by complex polysaccharides, lipopolysaccharides from gram-negative bacteria and teichoic acids from gram-positive bacteria, as well as by less well-characterized components on the surface of fungi and certain viruses. Although antibody is not required for alternative pathway activation, aggregated immunoglobulins as well as antigen-antibody complexes involving IgA, IgD, and IgE are capable of activating this pathway. Interestingly, alternative pathway activation by immunoglobulins involves the $F(ab')_2$ region of molecule, rather than the Fc domain involved in C1q binding and activation of the classical pathway. The alternative pathway may be particularly important in facilitating host defense during the preimmune phase of infection, during which time insufficient quantities of specific IgM and IgG are available to activate complement via the classical pathway.

Activation of the alternative pathway begins with the slow, spontaneous hydrolysis of an unstable thioester bond in the native C3 molecule, resulting in formation of the protein $C3(H_2O)$. This conformationally altered form of C3 is capable of interacting with factor B (C3 proactivator), forming a $C3(H_2O)B$ complex. Bound factor B is then cleaved by factor D (C3 proactivator convertase), resulting in formation of $C3(H_2O)Bb$ complex, which expresses C3 convertase activity. The spontaneous hydrolysis of C3, with ensuing formation of a C3 convertase, has been termed C3 "tickover" and is thought to provide the initial C3b necessary to prime the alternative pathway. Once formed, C3b binds factor B to form a C3bB complex, which is subsequently cleaved by factor D to form a second alternative pathway C3 convertase, C3bBb. Deposition of additional C3b molecules in proximity to the C3bBb complex facilitates binding and subsequent cleavage of C5. Hence, the $(C3b)_nBb$ complex displays C3/C5 convertase activity analogous to that observed with the C4b2a3b complex of the classical pathway. The C3bBb complex is quite unstable and Bb readily dissociates from C3b. However, binding of the serum protein properdin to C3bBb decreases the rate of dissociation of this complex and thereby prolongs convertase activity. As in the classical pathway, cleavage of C5 by $(C3b)_nBb$ generates a C5a and a C5b fragment, the latter of which contributes to assembly of the terminal complement proteins.

Despite the C3 tickover phenomenon, only a small percentage of the total serum C3 actually exists in the form of C3b. This is due to the presence of two regulatory proteins that coordinately act to limit C3bBb convertase formation and activity. These two proteins consist of factor H (or $\beta1H$) and factor I (or C3b inactivator). In the presence of factor I, C3b (as well as $C3[H_2O]$) is rapidly degraded to iC3b, which is unable to associate with factor B and thus no longer participates in the complement cascade. However, factor I is unable to cleave C3b when the latter is complexed with factor B. This problem is overcome through the presence of factor H, a cofactor for factor I. Factor H competitively inhibits binding of both B and Bb to C3b and enhances the rate of dissociation of C3bB and C3bBb complexes, exposing the unassociated C3b to factor I-mediated cleavage.

Deposition of C3b on a surface following C3 tickover does not necessarily lead to efficient activation of the alternative pathway. Clearly, some surfaces are potent activators of the alternative pathway, while others are relatively weak. Efficient activators of the alternative pathway appear to offer a "protected site" for C3b binding, one that minimizes the binding of factor H while permitting association of factor B with bound C3b. Under such conditions, factor I is unable to inactivate C3b and thereby limit C3 convertase activity of the C3bBb complex. On the other hand, poor activators of the alternative pathway provide a binding site for C3b, which is readily accessible to factors H and I. Some of the molecular details involved in differentiating between "activators" and "nonactivators" of the alternative pathway have been worked out. In particular, cell surface sialic acid residues have been

shown to increase the affinity of factor H for C3b, thereby limiting formation of the alternative pathway C3 convertase. Thus, the ability of factor H to interfere with the interaction between bound C3b and factor B appears to be important in defining the ability of a cell surface to activate the alternative pathway. Specifically, potent activators of the alternative pathway exhibit "restricted" factor H control, while weak activators exhibit "unrestricted" factor H-dependent control of C3 convertase formation.

BIOLOGIC EFFECTS OF COMPLEMENT ACTIVATION

Activation of complement produces a number of responses integral to the inflammatory process (Fig. 2–13). For example, enzymatic cleavage of components C3, C4, and C5 results in the generation of large fragments (C3b, C4b, and C5b), which participate in the next step in the complement cascade, and the concurrent release of smaller fragments (C3a, C4a, and C5a), which are released into the fluid phase. These smaller fragments (collectively termed *anaphylatoxins*) are able to trigger release of a variety of inflammatory mediators (including histamine) from mast cells and basophils, leading to smooth muscle contraction and increased capillary leakage. In addition to its activity as an anaphylatoxin, C5a also has a number of effects on phagocytic cells, promoting directed migration (i.e., chemotaxis), increased adherence and respiratory burst activity. The larger C3b fragment generated during cleavage of C3 has previously been discussed regarding its role in generating convertase activity in both the classical and alternative pathways. However, covalent deposition of C3b on a surface also can promote phagocytosis of the target, because phagocytes express plasma membrane receptors for C3b. This same receptor recognizes C4b fragments bound to the activating surface. The process whereby deposition of complement fragments on a target promotes receptor-mediated phagocytosis is termed *opsonization*. Although cleavage of C3b by factor I inactivates this fragment with respect to its further participation in the complement cascade, iC3b retains significant opsonic activity. Recognition of iC3b-coated particles involves a phagocyte membrane receptor distinct from that of the receptor for C3b. Finally, assembly of the terminal complement components of C5b, C6, C7, C8, and C9 on the surface of numerous species of gram-negative bacteria is sufficient to promote osmotic lysis of these organisms through formation of the membrane attack complex. Less well-characterized biologic effects of complement include (1) effects of Ba and Bb fragments on B lymphocyte proliferation and differentiation, (2) effects of C3a and C5a on T lym-

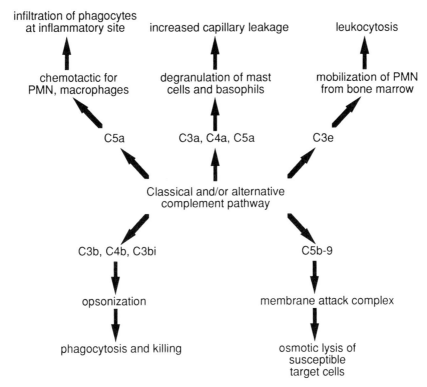

FIGURE 2–13 ✦ Biologic properties associated with activation of the complement cascade.

phocyte function, and (3) C3e-mediated mobilization of mature polymorphonuclear leukocytes from bone marrow during acute bacterial infection.

REGULATION OF THE COMPLEMENT CASCADE

Given the multiple proinflammatory effects of complement, it should be readily appreciated that excessive or prolonged generation of complement fragments can be deleterious to the host. To minimize the proinflammatory properties of complement, a number of regulatory mechanisms have evolved. These regulatory proteins are broadly subdivided into fluid phase regulatory proteins and membrane-bound regulatory proteins. An additional level of complement regulation entails the spontaneous decay of metastable membrane-binding sites (as on C3b, C4b, and C5b) and the decay-dissociation of enzyme complexes (e.g., C4b2a, C3bBb). Some regulatory proteins (e.g., C1 inhibitor) exert their effects through stoichiometric inhibition of the proteolytic activity of complement components, whereas other proteins inactivate complement fragments via enzymatic degradation (e.g., factor I-mediated inactivation of C3b and C4b). As noted above, certain membrane-bound regulatory proteins also have been identified. Two such examples are decay-accelerating factor and C8-binding protein, which appear to interfere with

effective assembly of the membrane attack complex on host cell membranes, thereby limiting complement-mediated host cell cytotoxicity.

Phagocytic Cells

Phagocytes are nonlymphoid leukocytic cells capable of engulfing and subsequently ingesting particulate matter including foreign organisms, dead or injured host cells, and cellular debris. Moreover, these cells secrete numerous cytokines involved in the initiation and regulation of immune and inflammatory responses. Various types of phagocytes are distributed throughout the body, being present in blood, tissues, and serous cavities (e.g., pleural and peritoneal cavities), where they play a major role in clearance of microorganisms.

The chief types of phagocytes found in the body include polymorphonuclear leukocytes and mononuclear phagocytes (monocytes and macrophages). As the names suggest, these cells are classified, at least in part, on the basis of cellular morphology. Polymorphonuclear leukocytes contain a segmented, multilobed (2–5) nucleus (Fig. 2–14), whereas mononuclear phagocytes contain a round or indented nucleus. Both types of phagocytes are produced in the bone marrow during hematopoiesis, and are subsequently released into the peripheral blood. Once in the bloodstream these cells

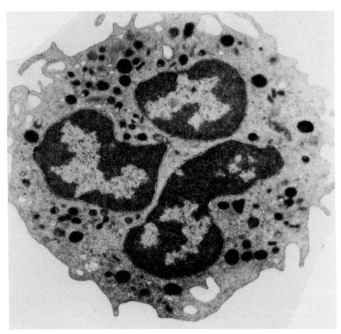

FIGURE 2–14 ✦ Transmission electron micrograph of a resting human neutrophil. Original magnification ×6000.

circulate for several hours before migrating into various tissues, either randomly or in response to specific chemical signals.

The principle phagocytic cell found in peripheral circulation is the polymorphonuclear leukocyte (PMN), comprising 50 to 70 percent of the total circulating white cell pool. PMN include neutrophils, eosinophils and basophils (collectively also known as granulocytes due to the presence of numerous granules in the cytoplasm). However, circulating neutrophils vastly outnumber both eosinophils and basophils, which represent only 1 to 3 percent and <1 percent of the total white cell pool, respectively. For this reason, the terms *PMN* and *neutrophil* often are used interchangeably. Given its numerical predominance in the circulation, the neutrophil is considered the first line of defense against infection due to extracellular bacteria.

Cells of the mononuclear phagocyte system include circulating monocytes and tissue macrophages. Although monocytes exhibit comparable phagocytic activity with that of the neutrophil, these cells comprise only 3 to 8 percent of the circulating white cell pool. Hence, the monocyte is considered to be less important in host resistance to acute bacterial infection than the neutrophil. The greater significance of circulating monocytes lies in the fact that these cells migrate into various tissues, where they undergo further differentiation into macrophages. Macrophages differ from their precursor monocytes in enzymatic, phagocytic and

microbicidal activity, as well as in cell surface membrane characteristics. In addition, macrophages in various tissues exhibit properties that are unique to the environment in which they differentiate, probably as a result of local factors. For this reason, macrophages are named according to their tissue location (Table 2–4), and may either be "fixed" in certain tissues (e.g., Kupffer cells in liver and microglia in brain) or "wandering" in serous cavities (e.g., alveolar macrophages in lung).

TABLE 2–4 ✦ Cells of the Mononuclear Phagocyte System

CELL TYPE	LOCATION
Monocytes	Bone marrow, blood
Macrophages, free	
Alveolar macrophages	Lung
Pleural macrophages	Pleural cavity
Peritoneal macrophages	Peritoneal cavity
Histiocytes	Connective tissue
Macrophages, fixed	
Kupffer cells	Liver
Osteoclasts	Bone
Microgial cells	Central nervous system
Other fixed tissue macrophages	Spleen (red pulp macrophages), lymph nodes, bone marrow, thymus, etc.

Resting macrophages possess considerable phagocytic and microbicidal activity. This activity can, however, be further enhanced as a consequence of exposure to cytokines (especially interferon-γ) produced by T lymphocytes. These activated macrophages are characterized by increased size, metabolic and phagocytic activity, and exhibit an enhanced ability to kill intracellular pathogens as well as tumor cells. Mononuclear phagocytes, like polymorphonuclear leukocytes, function as phagocytic cells in eliminating foreign bacteria and other debris. It is now clear, however, that mononuclear phagocytes contribute in other important ways to the immune response. Notably, these cells participate in immune induction by virtue of their ability to internalize, process, and present antigen, in conjunction with MHC class II molecules, to T-helper lymphocytes. In addition, mononuclear phagocytes (especially activated macrophages) elaborate a number of proteins that play a key role in the development of an immune response. These factors include (1) IL-1 (formerly referred to as lymphocyte-activating factor), which promotes activation of helper T cells and maturation of B lymphocyte precursors; (2) tumor necrosis factor (TNF), which is capable of killing certain tumor cells; (3) colony-stimulating factors, which enhance production of macrophages and neutrophils in bone marrow; and (4) interleukin-6 (IL-6), which promotes differentiation of mature B lymphocytes into antibody-secreting plasma cells and induces hepatic synthesis of acute phase proteins (involved in innate immunity).

Circulating neutrophils are rapidly mobilized to the extravascular compartment in response to acute inflammation or infection. In fact, marked neutrophil infiltration is a cardinal feature of the acute inflammatory response. Upon leaving the circulation, neutrophils must then be capable of recognizing, internalizing and degrading foreign bacteria or other noxious agents. Fortunately, neutrophils (as well as mononuclear phagocytes, which are more important in chronic inflammatory states) are well-equipped to perform these functions.

Within the peripheral blood of normal individuals, the measured neutrophil count is actually an underestimation of the total number of neutrophils in the circulation. This is due to the fact that neutrophils are distributed between two more or less distinct "pools," termed the *circulating* and *marginated pools*. Standard venipuncture techniques typically sample only the circulating pool. However, approximately one-half to two-thirds of peripheral blood neutrophils are found in a marginated pool of cells that is sequestered in postcapillary venules in loose association with vascular endothelium. It is the latter pool that provides the primary source of neutrophils exiting the circulation

during the inflammatory response. In the absence of inflammation, marginated neutrophils remain loosely, reversibly associated with the surface of vascular endothelium. In fact, neutrophils can actually be seen "rolling" on the surface of endothelial cells (Fig. 2–15*A*). However, in areas of inflammation, biochemical changes occur in both the neutrophil and endothelial cell, which result in the firm adhesion between these two cell types, followed by the movement of the leukocyte through the endothelial barrier and into the extravascular space (Fig. 2–15*B*). This latter process has been termed *transendothelial migration* or *diapedesis*. The adhesive events involved in the interaction between circulating phagocytes and vascular endothelium are quite complex. However, significant progress has been made in understanding the nature of these interactions at a molecular level. At least three major superfamilies of adhesion molecules have been found to participate in phagocyte-endothelial interactions. These include (1) integrins, (2) members of the immunoglobulin supergene family (particularly intercellular adhesion molecules, or ICAMs), and (3) selectins.

Once phagocytes have traversed the endothelial barrier, they must then move toward the target particle that is to be ingested and eliminated. This objective is met by virtue of the ability of phagocytes to migrate unidirectionally along a chemical concentration gradient generated between inflamed or infected tissues and blood vessels. The chemical substances capable of eliciting such behavior by phagocytes are termed *chemoattractants,* or *chemotaxins,* and the directed migration of phagocyte toward these agents is referred to as *chemotaxis.* A number of substances, both host-derived and bacterially-derived, have been found to promote directed migration of phagocytes (Table 2–5).

Phagocytic cells are actively motile even in the absence of chemotactic substances. Under such conditions, phagocytes exhibit random migration (i.e., movement occurring with an equal probability in all directions) (Fig. 2–16*A*). After exposure to a chemoattractant, these cells lose their typically round appearance in favor of an oriented configuration with a distinct "head" (lamellipodium) and "tail" (uropod). The process through which phagocytes adopt an orientation in the direction of a chemotactic gradient is termed *polarization.* Once this orientation has been established, the phagocyte is able to move unidirectionally toward the source of the chemical gradient (Fig. 2–16*B*). Chemotactic agents can increase the speed of migration of phagocytic cells even if a chemical gradient is not established. This effect is termed *chemokinesis* (Fig. 2–16*C*).

Chemotaxis is initiated through the interaction between chemoattractants and specific receptors on

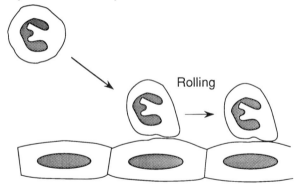

PMN (unactivated)

Rolling

Vascular Endothelium
(uninflamed)

A

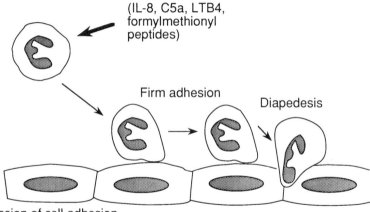

PMN (activated)

(IL-8, C5a, LTB4,
formylmethionyl
peptides)

Firm adhesion

Diapedesis

Increased expression of cell adhesion
molecules

Vascular Endothelium
(inflamed)

Endothelial cell activation by
inflammatory cytokines (IL-1β,
B   TNFα) or bacterial endotoxin

FIGURE 2–15 ✦ Interaction between circulating neutrophils and vascular endothelium in uninflamed, **A,** and inflamed, **B,** sites.

the phagocyte plasma membrane. Chemoattractant receptor expression along the cell surface is not uniform. Rather, chemoattractant receptors are present in comparatively higher density at the anterior of the cell than at the uropod, thus enabling the migrating cell to maintain its orientation. By regulating the distribution of chemoattractant receptors on the cell surface, phagocytes are able to recognize gradients as small as 1 percent across the length of the cell. It is relevant to point out that phagocytes crawl rather than swim. Phagocyte locomotion is, therefore, critically dependent upon

cell-cell or cell-substrate (e.g., connective tissue matrix protein) interactions that promote cell adhesion. Phagocytic cells of patients with congenital or acquired defects in leukocyte adhesion often exhibit impaired chemotactic activity.

A key property of phagocytic cells is their ability to recognize and ingest particulate matter. The process of ingestion involves direct contact between the phagocyte and particle, followed by formation of fingerlike projections (pseudopodia) which surround the target. The pseudopods fuse on the distal surface of the particle, which is now enveloped in

TABLE 2–5 ✦ Chemoattractants for Phagocytic Cells

CHEMOTACTIC AGENT	SOURCE(S)
C5a and C5a$_{des\ arg}$	Complement activation and cleavage of C5
Leukotriene B4 (LTB4)	Product of cellular arachidonate metabolism via the lipoxygenase pathway
Platelet-activating factors (PAF)	Platelets, leukocytes (including PMN, monocyte/macrophages, and NK cells)
Interleukin-8 (IL-8)	Mainly mononuclear phagocytes but also fibroblasts, T lymphocytes, endothelial cells, and keratinocytes
N-formylmethionyl peptides	Products of bacterial protein synthesis

NK = natural killer; PMN = polymorphonuclear leukocyte.

a membranous sac termed a *phagocytic vacuole*, or *phagosome* (Fig. 2–17). The phagosome moves to the interior of the cell, where fusion with cytoplasmic granules results in formation of a phagolysosome. It is within the phagolysosomal compartment that efficient killing of many foreign organisms occurs.

Phagocytic cells are capable of recognizing and ingesting a diverse array of particulate matter. However, their phagocytic activity is not indiscriminate. While targeting numerous species of bacteria and fungi, as well as damaged or senescent host cells, phagocytes display little interest in viable autologous cells or tissues. Particle recognition and ingestion involves specific interactions between the phagocyte membrane and one or more components on the particle surface. Efficient phagocytosis often requires that the particle be coated with one or more host serum proteins through a process termed *opsonization* (meaning "to prepare for eating"). The two principal types of serum proteins (referred to as *opsonins*) involved in this process are immunoglobulin G antibodies and cleavage fragments of complement component C3 (C3b and iC3b). Targets opsonized with IgG and/or C3 fragments are recognized through specific receptors located on the phagocyte membrane. The sequential interaction between opsonins and their corresponding receptors results in engulfment of the particle through a process termed *"zippering."*

Opsonic requirements can vary for different bacterial species or even different strains of a single

species. In general, however, there are three principal mechanisms of opsonization (Fig. 2–18).

1. Complement-dependent opsonization results from the covalent attachment of C3b and iC3b on the bacterial surface after complement activation (primarily via the alternative pathway). Phagocyte membranes possess distinct receptors for each of these fragments. Complement receptor type 1 (CR1) mediates binding of C3b-coated targets, whereas complement receptor type 3 (CR3) recognizes iC3b-coated targets. The extent to which covalently bound C3b is susceptible to cleavage by the complement regulatory proteins factor H and factor I determines whether C3b or iC3b is the predominant form presented to the phagocyte.

2. Antibody-dependent opsonization results from the binding of specific IgG antibody to bacterial surface structures via the antigen-binding domain (Fab), leaving the Fc domain exposed.

A   **Random migration**
(absence of chemotactic agent)

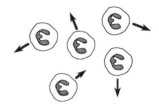

B   **Chemotaxis**
(chemotactic agent present, gradient established)

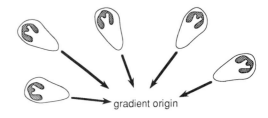

gradient origin

C   **Chemokinesis**
(chemotactic agent present, but no gradient established)

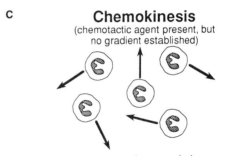

FIGURE 2–16 ✦ General types of phagocyte motility.

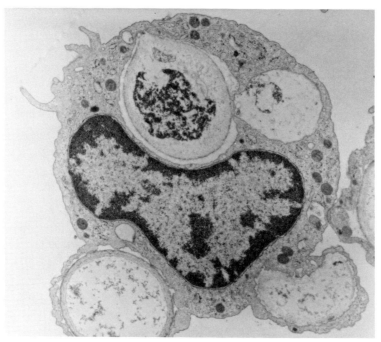

FIGURE 2–17 ✦ Transmission electron micrograph of a human neutrophil phagocytizing opsonized zymosan (yeast cell wall) particles. Original magnification ×6000.

Complement-dependent opsonization

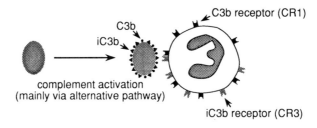

Antibody-dependent opsonization

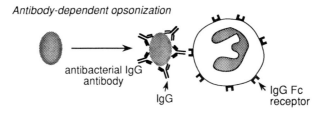

Antibody- and complement-dependent opsonization

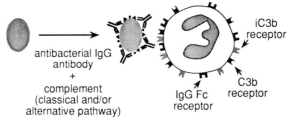

FIGURE 2–18 ✦ Mechanisms of bacterial opsonization by immunoglobulin and/or complement.

Phagocytic cells possess membrane receptors capable of binding the Fc region of IgG molecules. These receptors are distinct from C3 receptors. All four human IgG subclasses can bind to IgG Fc receptors on neutrophils, although these cells exhibit preferential binding of IgG1 and IgG3. Only IgG1 and IgG3 appear to bind to monocyte Fc receptors.

3. In many instances, antibody and complement-dependent opsonization may be required for efficient phagocytosis to occur. IgG antibodies can be particularly effective in such cases, in that they are directly opsonic (being recognized via Fc receptors) and are able to activate complement through the classical pathway (thereby enhancing C3 receptor–mediated phagocytosis). Antibodies of the IgM isotype lack direct opsonic activity, since neither PMN nor mononuclear phagocytes have Fc receptors for IgM. However, IgM deposited on a bacterial surface can be particularly effective in triggering the classical pathway of complement, thereby enhancing C3 deposition on the target surface. The opsonized target is recognized by the phagocyte solely through membrane C3 receptors. For this reason, IgM is considered an indirect opsonin.

Recent studies indicate that a number of organisms may be ingested through nonopsonic phagocytosis, that is, in the absence of antibody or C3 fragments. For example, certain organisms possess fimbriae which contain lectins (carbohydrate-binding proteins) capable of recognizing phagocyte membrane glycoproteins. One target for these bacterial lectins appears to be a glycoprotein component of the iC3b (CR3) receptor itself. Macrophages possess surface lectins capable of recognizing specific carbohydrate moieties found on bacterial surfaces. Thus, interactions between lectins on one cell and carbohydrates on the other can lead to phagocytosis in the absence of opsonization.

The process of particle uptake initiates a number of events linked to the microbicidal properties of phagocytic cells, including the fusion of cytoplasmic granules with the newly formed phagocytic vacuole and an increase in cellular oxidative metabolism. Cytoplasmic granules contain a number of proteins, both enzymatic and nonenzymatic, which are bactericidal or bacteriostatic for many organisms. There are two major classes of cytoplasmic granules present in neutrophils: the primary (azurophil) and secondary (specific) granules. The contents of these two cytoplasmic granule populations vary (Table 2–6). As a group, these antimicrobial proteins display a wide range of activity against gram-positive and gram-negative bacteria as well as fungi. Degranulation of cytoplasmic granules into the phagocytic vacuole compartment results in formation of a phagolysosome containing high concentrations of neutral and acid proteases, as well as other microbicidal constituents. This leads to effective intracellular killing with minimal damage to the host. Under conditions in which extracellular degranulation occurs, however, these enzymes also are capable of inflicting injury on host tissues. Extracellular degranulation plays a key role in the proinflammatory properties of phagocytic cells.

Stimulation of phagocytic cells by particulate agents or certain soluble factors (e.g., complement fragment C5a) leads to an increase in cellular consumption of molecular oxygen (O_2), a process termed the *respiratory burst*. This respiratory burst is associated with the generation of a number of

TABLE 2–6 ✦ Subcellular Distribution of Enzymes and Other Constituents of PMN Cytoplasmic Granules

CLASS OF CONSTITUENTS	PRIMARY GRANULES	SECONDARY GRANULES
Microbicidal enzymes	Myeloperoxidase	
	Lysozyme	Lysozyme
Neutral proteinases	Elastase	Collagenase
	Cathepsin G	
	Proteinase 3	
Acid hydrolases	N-acetyl-β-glucosaminidase	
	Cathepsin B	
	Cathepsin D	
	β-glucuronidase	
	β-glycerophosphatase	
	α-mannosidase	
Other	Defensins	Lactoferrin
	Cationic proteins	Vitamin B_{12}-binding protein
	Bactericidal/permeability-increasing	C3bi receptor (CR3)
	factor	Cytochrome b_{245}

oxygen metabolites, which are injurious to many species of microorganisms. The majority of O_2 consumed by the phagocyte is converted directly to superoxide anion (O_2^-) through the action of a membrane-bound NADPH oxidase, which catalyzes the transfer of an electron from NADPH to O_2. Superoxide radicals (O_2^-) in turn may undergo spontaneous or enzyme-catalyzed (via superoxide dismutase) conversion to hydrogen peroxide (H_2O_2), a two-electron reduction product of molecular oxygen. Alternatively, superoxide anions may react with H_2O_2 in the presence of iron to form hydroxyl radicals ($\cdot OH$). These various oxygen species appear to contribute significantly to the microbicidal activity of phagocytic cells. Additional oxidant species (hypochlorous acid, toxic aldehydes) are generated as a consequence of the interaction between H_2O_2 and the azurophil enzyme myeloperoxidase (MPO) in the presence of a suitable halide (chloride being most physiologically relevant).

Collectively, phagocyte bactericidal mechanisms are broadly categorized as being oxygen-independent and oxygen-dependent. O_2-dependent bactericidal activity is further subdivided into MPO-dependent and MPO-independent. Although these various components often work in concert to promote destruction of ingested bacteria, certain mechanisms may be relatively more important in the intracellular killing of specific microbes. Moreover, availability of O_2 may limit oxidative bactericidal activity, particularly at sites of tissue necrosis in which blood flow may be compromised. Fortunately, phagocytic cells are able to kill many species of bacteria in the complete absence of oxygen.

Polymorphonuclear leukocytes and mononuclear phagocytes constitute an important mechanism for elimination of extracellular bacteria, particularly those that engender a strong antibody response. However, these cells are less effective in the elimination of infections due to intracellular microorganisms (both viral and bacterial) or organisms, which elicit a poor humoral response. Additional host response mechanisms are called into action in such instances. These mechanisms involve stimulation of cellular immunity, in which T cell-derived cytokines (see below) induce activation of mononuclear phagocytes with enhanced microbicidal activity, as well as cytotoxic T cells (see below).

Cytokines

The interaction between various cells of the immune system often involves direct cell-to-cell contact. However, one of the principal ways in which cells communicate with each other is via the production and secretion of protein hormones termed *cytokines*. These hormones play an important role in the effector phases of both innate and acquired immune responses. A number of cytokines that contribute to innate immunity are produced by mononuclear phagocytes, and are thus referred to as *monokines*. Other cytokines are produced by antigen- or mitogen-stimulated T lymphocytes, and help orchestrate specific immune responses. These protein hormones are termed *lymphokines*. Yet other cytokines are produced by both mononuclear phagocytes and lymphocytes. A number of cytokines of this type promote growth and differentiation of immature leukocytes in bone marrow through effects on hemopoietic stem cells, and are termed *colony-stimulating factors* (CSFs). Cytokines are not stored pre-formed in cells, but rather are synthesized *de novo* following cell activation. In addition, receptors for a number of cytokines are also induced during cell stimulation. The latter feature may serve to limit the number of cells responding to specific antigen.

Cytokines exert their biologic effects through binding to specific receptors on the membrane of target cells. In some instances, the cytokine acts as an autocrine hormone, stimulating the same cell from which it was secreted. Cytokines also may stimulate cells in close proximity to the cells which secreted them (a paracrine effect). Finally, these protein hormones may enter the circulation, where they can interact with immune cells at some distance from their point of origin (an endocrine effect). Many of the cytokines share certain common features. First, cytokines often exhibit pleiotropic activity. That is, a single cytokine possesses the ability to stimulate a number of distinct cell types. For example, interleukin-1 activates T cells, induces maturation of pre-B lymphocytes, promotes osteoclast-mediated bone resorption, and induces expression of cell adhesion molecules on vascular endothelium. Second, different cytokines often evoke similar biologic responses (redundancy), as is the case with respect to the antiviral properties of interferons and tumor necrosis factors. Third, certain cytokines may influence the production of other cytokines; thus, IL-1 promotes IL-2 synthesis and secretion by T lymphocytes. Finally, cytokines may exhibit either synergy or antagonism toward other cytokines. Thus, IL-4 and IL-5 are B cell growth factors that act sequentially to promote B cell growth and differentiation, whereas interferon-γ antagonizes the ability of IL-4 to induce class switching (from IgM to IgE production) by B lymphocytes.

More than twenty cytokines have been identified to date (Table 2–7). Their biological properties may be broadly subdivided into four categories. The first group includes cytokines, which serve as mediators of innate immunity. For example, interferon-α and -β increase resistance of host cells to infection by certain viruses and also stimulate natural killer activity of large granular lymphocytes. Tumor necrosis factors also exhibit antiviral activity. In addition, these factors promote inflammation by stimulating phagocyte adherence to vascular endothelium, and cause hemorrhagic necrosis of tumors. Another cytokine, interleukin-6 (IL-6), induces synthesis of acute phase proteins that contribute to innate immunity.

A second group includes cytokines that regulate the growth and differentiation of lymphocytes. IL-2 is mainly secreted by T cells (particularly T_{helper} cells), which have been stimulated by antigen or mitogen. IL-2 induces proliferation of antigen-

primed T_{helper} and $T_{cytotoxic}$ cells. This cytokine also enhances the activity of $T_{cytotoxic}$ and NK cells. Moreover, IL-2 promotes differentiation of antigen-stimulated B cells into immunoglobulin-secreting plasma cells. Another T cell-derived cytokine, IL-4, promotes the activation, proliferation, and differentiation of B lymphocytes. B lymphocytes stimulated by this cytokine exhibit increased expression of MHC class II histocompatibility molecules, which are important in the interaction between T_{helper} cells and B cells. IL-4 also promotes class switching of B cells from IgM production to IgG1 and IgE production. Although not as potent as IL-2 as a growth factor for T cells, IL-4 does induce T cell proliferation and $T_{cytotoxic}$ activity. Another cytokine belonging to this group,

TABLE 2–7 ✦ Cytokines and Their Biologic Properties

CYTOKINE	CELL SOURCE(S)	KEY ACTIVITIES
IL-1	Mainly macrophages and keratinocytes; also fibroblasts, endothelial cells, smooth muscle, and others	Stimulates acute phase reactions; general stimulation of immune system; augments hematopoiesis
IL-2	T lymphocytes	Promotes T lymphocyte growth and activity; enhances activity of NK cells, lymphokine-activated killer cells, and macrophages; enhances Ig production by B lymphocytes
IL-3	T lymphocytes	Promotes growth of early myeloid (but not lymphoid) progenitor cells in bone marrow
IL-4	T_H lymphocytes (especially T_H2 phenotype)	B lymphocyte growth factor; induces expression of MHC class II molecules on B cells; promotes class switch to IgE; promotes growth of helper and cytotoxic T lymphocytes
IL-5	T_H lymphocytes	Stimulates growth and differentiation of eosinophils; promotes IgA production by B lymphocytes; promotes growth of activated B lymphocytes
IL-6	Lymphocytes, monocytes, fibroblasts, endothelial cells, others	Promotes final differentiation of B lymphocytes into plasma cells; induces acute phase protein synthesis in hepatocytes
IL-7	Bone marrow stromal cells	Promotes growth of early lymphoid precursors of T and B lineage
IL-8	Mononuclear phagocytes, endothelial cells, fibroblasts, T cells, keratinocytes	Chemotactic for PMN (but not mononuclear phagocytes); pan-activator of PMN
IL-9	T lymphocytes	Promotes mast cell growth; induces proliferation of some T_H lymphocytes in the absence of antigen
IL-10	T_H2 subset of T lymphocytes	Inhibits antigen presentation to T_H1 cells and release of T_H1-derived cytokines
IL-11	Bone marrow stromal cells	Potentiates IL-3 induced growth of megakaryocytes; promotes T cell-dependent IgG secretion by B cells
IL-12	B lymphocytes	Synergizes with IL-2 in generating cytotoxic T-lymphocyte and lymphokine-activated killer activity

Continued on the following page.

TABLE 2–7 ✦ **Cytokines and Their Biologic Properties** *Continued*

CYTOKINE	CELL SOURCE(S)	KEY ACTIVITIES
Granulocyte CSF	Mononuclear phagocytes, endothelial cells, fibroblasts	Promotes generation of PMN from bone marrow progenitors
Macrophage CSF	Mononuclear phagocytes, endothelial cells, fibroblasts	Promotes generation of monocytes from bone marrow progenitors
Granulocyte/ Macrophage CSF	T lymphocytes, mononuclear phagocytes, endothelial cells, fibroblasts	Promotes growth and differentiation of granulocytes and mononuclear phagocytes from bone marrow progenitors
IFN$_\alpha$	Macrophages, epithelial cells, other cell types	Inhibits viral replication in host cells; promotes NK activity; induces expression of MHC class I molecules
IFN$_\beta$	Fibroblasts	Activities similar to IFN$_\alpha$
IFN$_\gamma$	T lymphocytes	Antiviral activity; activator of macrophage function; increases expression of MHC class I and II molecules; increases activity of NK and cytotoxic T cells; antagonizes effects of IL-4
TNFα	Mononuclear phagocytes	Key mediator of endotoxic shock; induces wasting (cachexia); activates mononuclear phagocytes and PMN; increases cell adhesion molecules expression on vascular endothelium; promotes tumor necrosis; antiviral activity
TNFβ	T lymphocytes	Shares many properties with TNFα, including toxicity for tumor cells
TGFβ	T and B lymphocytes, macrophages, platelets	Increases IgA production by B lymphocytes; promotes wound healing; antagonizes action of IL-2, IL-4, and IFNγ

IFN = interferon; IL = interleukin; MHC = major histocompatibility; NK = natural killer; PMN = polymorphonuclear leukocyte; T$_H$ = T$_{helper}$; TGF = transforming growth factor; TNF = tumor necrosis factor.

transforming growth factor β (TGF-β), inhibits activation and proliferation of T lymphocytes by antagonizing the actions of other cytokines including IL-2, IL-4, and interferon-γ. The "anti-cytokine" activity of TGF-β may be important in restricting the magnitude and/or duration of immune responses, thereby facilitating the process of wound healing.

Erythrocytes and leukocytes are produced from stem cells in bone marrow at a rate sufficient to replace cells that are lost through normal attrition or consumption (particularly inflammatory cells such as PMN). The process through which the various formed elements of blood (leukocytes, erythrocytes and platelets) are produced in bone marrow from stem cells is termed *hematopoiesis*. Hematopoietic activity in bone marrow is regulated through the actions of a third group of cytokines, collectively referred to as CSFs, produced by stromal cells or by antigen-stimulated T lymphocytes. A number of CSFs have been identified, including GM-CSF, G-CSF, M-CSF, multi-CSF (IL-3), and IL-7. Whereas other cytokines (e.g., IL-2, IL-4) promote growth and differentiation of

mature leukocytes, CSFs stimulate growth and differentiation of immature leukocytes. Multi-CSF appears to act on the most primitive progenitor cells in bone marrow, possibly at the level of the pluripotent stem cell, to induce formation of all nonlymphoid cells. Other cytokines in this group, such as granulocyte CSF and macrophage CSF, act at a somewhat later stage, promoting formation of lineage-specific cells. IL-7 acts on B and T lymphoid precursors, which are at a stage of development comparable with IL-3-sensitive nonlymphoid progenitors.

A final group of cytokines share the common property of being activators of inflammatory cell function. Notable in this group is interferon-γ (also known as immune interferon), a T cell-derived cytokine that is a potent activator of mononuclear phagocyte function (phagocytic, microbicidal and tumoricidal activity, as well as antigen-presenting activity). Interferon-γ also stimulates vascular endothelial cells to increase expression of a number of cell adhesion molecules that play a major role in trafficking of inflammatory cells to sites of inflammation. Another member of this group, tumor necrosis factor β (TNFβ), also activates PMN and vascular endothelium to promote the egress of circulating leukocytes.

Cytokines influence host defensive capabilities at a number of levels. First, these peptide mediators stimulate the generation of mature leukocytes from their precursors in bone marrow. Second, they promote the growth and terminal differentiation of mature leukocytes. Further, certain cytokines are responsible for activating leukocytes. Given their influence in orchestrating immune responses, it is not surprising that cytokines can also play an important role in the pathogenesis of disease. For example, increased production of IL-1 and TNF is observed in gram-negative septic shock, and there is good evidence to suggest that these cytokines are important mediators of the hematologic and hemodynamic changes seen in septic patients. This has prompted efforts to develop effective antagonists of IL-1 and TNF in the treatment and management of septic patients. The anti-inflammatory properties of IL-1 receptor antagonist and soluble IL-1 receptor are also being evaluated in patients with rheumatoid arthritis.

The therapeutic effects of a number of recombinant human cytokines are currently under investigation, particularly in the treatment of cancer. Clinical trials involving IL-2, interferon-γ, or TNFα have met with mixed success; combination therapies capitalizing upon the often synergistic actions of these cytokines may ultimately prove more beneficial. Recombinant human colony-stimulating factors also may have therapeutic benefit. For example, G-CSF shows promise in boosting circulating granulocyte levels in cancer patients receiving cytotoxic chemotherapy. Elevation in circulating granulocyte count induced by G-CSF or GM-CSF may also be useful in preventing lethal bacterial sepsis.

Cytotoxic Effector Cells

Cell-mediated cytotoxicity (i.e., the capacity of one cell to kill another) is an important process in the elimination of intracellular parasites, as well as virus-infected and malignant host cells. Mononuclear phagocytes activated by the T cell-derived cytokine interferon-γ exhibit markedly enhanced microbicidal and tumoricidal activity. However, there are a number of other types of leukocytes that also are capable of functioning as cytotoxic effector cells. These include (1) cytotoxic T lymphocytes (CTL), (2) NK cells, and (3) lymphokine-activated killer (LAK) cells. Cytotoxic effectors differ in their expression of certain surface markers and in their antigenic specificity toward target cells.

CTLs are CD8$^+$ cells and display MHC class I restriction. That is, these cells recognize intracel-

lularly synthesized antigen (produced by virus-infected cells or tumor cells) displayed on the target cell membrane in association with MHC class I molecules. As these cells also display the T cell antigen receptor, they exhibit antigenic specificity toward target cells. NK cells belong to a subset of lymphocytes termed *large granular lymphocytes,* so named because they possess a round or indented nucleus and abundant cytoplasm containing numerous granules. These cells lack surface markers characteristic of B (surface immunoglobulin) or T (T-cell antigen receptor) lymphocytes. They do, however, express CD16, the low affinity receptor for the Fc region of IgG. NK cells participate in antibody-dependent cell-mediated cytotoxicity (ADCC) toward antibody-coated targets. A third type of cytotoxic effector, the LAK cell, is similar to the NK cell in lacking antigenic specificity. LAK activity is generated following incubation of freshly isolated lymphoid cells with high concentrations of IL-2. LAK cells display cytolytic activity toward a broader range of target cells than NK cells. Recent evidence indicates that the majority of LAK activity induced by IL-2 derives from NK cells.

CTLs develop from "pre-CTLs," which undergo maturation in the thymus. Pre-CTLs express the T cell antigen receptor/CD3 complex, as well as CD8, but are not competent for cytotoxic activity. Upon receiving appropriate signals, pre-CTLs undergo differentiation into CTLs. At least two signals are necessary for pre-CTLs to differentiate into CTLs. First, the pre-CTLs must bind specific antigen via its membrane T cell antigen receptor. This signal induces expression of IL-2 receptors on the pre-CTLs. The pre-CTL then is able to respond to a second signal provided by cytokines secreted by T$_H$ cells. These cytokines include IL-2, IL-4, IL-6, and interferon-γ. A number of changes occur as a consequence of differentiation of pre-CTL into CTL, including the emergence of cytoplasmic granules and the synthesis and secretion of cytokines, particularly interferon-γ and lymphotoxin (TNFβ). The cytoplasmic granules contain several proteins that contribute to the cytotoxic properties of CTL, including perforin (a pore-forming protein), serine esterases, and a cytotoxin (either lymphotoxin itself or a related protein).

The process of CTL-mediated killing of target cells appears to involve a number of steps (Fig. 2–19). The first phase entails the firm adhesion (termed *conjugate formation*) of the CTL to an appropriate target. Target specificity is achieved via recognition of the associated complex of antigen and MHC class I macromolecule by the T-cell antigen receptor (TCR). Cell contact is further reinforced through additional adhesive interactions that lack antigenic specificity. In the second ("lethal

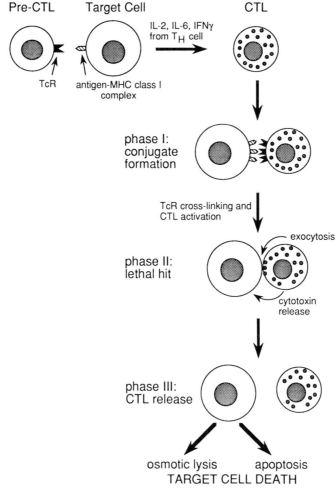

FIGURE 2–19 ✦ Stages in the activation and function of cytotoxic T lymphocytes.

hit") phase, cross-linking of TCRs leads to activation of the CTL. One consequence of CTL activation is the exocytosis of cytoplasmic granules in the region of the CTL membrane, which is in direct contact with the target cell. (This focused release of cytoplasmic granules probably accounts for the fact that CTLs typically do not kill "innocent bystander" cells with which they are not in contact.) Granule exocytosis leads to the release of perforin, a protein that polymerizes in the target cell membrane to form ion channels. These channels, if sufficient in number, allow the progressive movement of ions and water across the cell membrane, resulting in osmotic lysis. Other cytoplasmic granule constituents also contribute to the ultimate demise of the target cell. During this same period, the activated CTL secretes a cytotoxin (possibly lymphotoxin), which activates certain enzymes in the target cell that uncoil and degrade DNA through a process termed *programmed cell death,* or *apoptosis.* Under such conditions, cell death occurs

without overt lysis of the target cell. Following delivery of the lethal hit, the CTL is released from the target cell, which continues to undergo cytolysis and/or apoptosis. The CTL does not self-annihilate during the process of target cell killing. Rather, these cells recycle, and are often capable of attacking additional target cells. Although CTLs appear to participate in acute graft rejection, these cells are thought to play a significant role in the elimination of viral infections.

NK cells, unlike CTLs, do not require prior contact with target cell antigens to develop cytotoxic capability. This is not surprising, as NK cells lack surface immunoglobulins and T cell antigen receptors necessary for antigen recognition. Moreover, NK cells do not exhibit MHC restriction characteristic of CTL. NK cells emerge from bone marrow already competent for target cell killing. As is the case for CTL, however, NK activity can be increased by cytokines such as IL-2, TNF, or interferon-γ. Moreover, IL-2 induces proliferation of

NK cells. Target cell specificity of NK cells is somewhat broader than is true for CTL, but NK activity is not random (i.e., NK cells are capable of killing some tumors but not others). The nature of the target cell structure(s) recognized by NK cells has not been determined. NK activity toward target cells can be enhanced through deposition of specific IgG antibodies on the target surface. This is because NK cells possess receptors for the Fc region of IgG.

The mechanisms utilized by NK cells in target cell killing appear to be quite similar to those employed by CTLs. Like CTLs, NK cells contain numerous cytoplasmic granules (hence their morphologic features as large granular lymphocytes) and secrete a cytotoxin. The composition of the granules of CTLs and NK cells appears to be similar. It is unclear if the cytotoxin released from NK cells is identical to the protein secreted by CTLs. However, NK cells do not synthesize lymphotoxin. Although the role of NK cells in immunity is poorly understood, these cells may be important in graft-versus-host reactions seen in patients receiving bone marrow transplant.

ADVERSE IMMUNOLOGIC RESPONSES: HYPERSENSITIVITY REACTIONS

Immune responses often are able to provide protection with minimal injury to host tissues. There are, however, instances in which immune responses are associated with significant pathology. This may occur either as a result of an excessive or inappropriate response to a foreign antigen. Immune reactions that are overtly injurious to the host are termed *hypersensitivity reactions*. The clinical manifestations of hypersensitivity reactions are dependent on the host's immune response to antigen and not on the nature of the antigen itself. The mechanisms of hypersensitivity can be as diverse as the various elements of the immune system. However, all hypersensitivity reactions have one important feature in common; they occur in individuals who had previously mounted an immune response to the offending antigen.

Nearly four decades ago Gell and Coombs devised a classification scheme for describing hypersensitivity reactions on the basis of the immunologic reactions involved, rather than upon the clinical symptoms of the disease. Based upon differences in the mechanisms of initiation and chemical/cellular mediators involved, hypersensitivity reactions were divided into four types (Table 2–8). As our understanding of the organization and function of the immune system has expanded, it has become evident that many immunopathologic reactions involve both cellular and humoral immune responses and several effector mechanisms. Nevertheless, the Gell and Coombs classification scheme remains a useful tool for description of hypersensitivity reactions.

The first three types of hypersensitivity phenomena are antibody-mediated, although the immunoglobulin isotype responsible varies. Type IV hypersensitivity reactions, on the other hand, involve cell-mediated immune responses. Hypersensitivity reactions also vary with respect to the time frame in which clinical manifestations of the reaction become apparent. In type I (immediate) reactions, maximum response can occur within 5 to 15 minutes after antigen exposure, fading within 1 to 2 hours thereafter. Type II reactions develop during a period of 5 to 8 hours after antigen exposure, while type III reactions develop within 2 to 8 hours. In contrast, type IV reactions require 24 to 72 hours to develop, prompting their description as delayed hypersensitivity reactions.

Type I (Immediate Hypersensitivity) Reactions

Type I reactions are considered to be mediated by IgE antibodies. The discovery of IgE as the principal mediator of immediate hypersensitivity and allergy was made in 1966 by Kimishige and Teruko Ishizaka. Two years later, IgE was formally recognized as a distinct class of immunoglobulin. IgE produced upon initial contact with antigen binds to the surface of mast cells and basophils, which possess high affinity receptors for the Fc region of the ϵ heavy chain. IgE binding to these cells does not require the presence of specific antigen. Once bound to mast cells and basophils (which are then referred to as being "sensitized"), IgE serves as an antigen receptor. Subsequent exposure of sensitized mast cells and basophils to specific antigen results in the "cross-linking" of adjacent membrane-bound IgE molecules and their associated Fcϵ receptors. Receptor cross-linking activates a G (guanosine triphosphate-binding) protein, which in turn, stimulates the production of secondary messengers involved in mast cell and basophil activation. The consequence of this signal transduction process is mast cell (and basophil) degranulation and the *de novo* synthesis and release of other inflammatory mediators. It is the release of these pharmacologically active mediators that produces the clinical manifestations of immediate hypersensitivity. A partial list of the chemical mediators released by mast cells is provided in Table 2–9. These mediators are broadly divided into two categories: preformed (granule-associated) and newly synthesized (particularly lipid-derived) mediators.

TABLE 2–8 ✦ Classification of Immunopathologic Processes

REACTION TYPE/ DESCRIPTION	IMMUNE COMPONENT(S)	INFLAMMATORY RESPONSE	DISEASE MANIFESTATIONS
Type I			
Immediate hypersensitivity reactions	IgE	Release of pharmacologic mediators from mast cells	Anaphylaxis/atopy
Type II			
Cytolytic reactions	IgG, IgM	Binding of immunoglobulin to target cells with destruction mediated by complement or other antibody effectors	ABO incompatibility; myasthenia gravis; autoimmune hemolytic anemia
Type III			
Immune complex reactions	IgG, IgM	Formation of antigen-antibody complexes that are deposited in various tissues; leads to complement activation and recruitment of phagocytes	Rheumatoid arthritis; Arthus reaction; immune complex glomerulonephritis
Type IV			
Delayed hypersensitivity reactions	T lymphocytes (CD4$^+$)	T lymphocyte activation leads to release of cytokines, which activate macrophages and stimulate other T lymphocytes	Contact dermatitis; tuberculin-type reactions

All normal (non-atopic) individuals produce limited amounts of IgE antibody in response to various antigens. These antibodies bind to high affinity IgE receptors on mast cells and basophils as previously described. Nevertheless, non-atopic subjects are not prone to immediate hypersensitivity reactions. This is attributable to the fact that, on a given mast cell or basophil, receptor-bound IgE molecules are directed to distinct antigens. Therefore, a single antigen has a low probability of bridging two adjacent IgE molecules with specificity for that antigen. Patients with atopic disease (*atopy* refers to individuals who exhibit abnormal hypersensitivity to antigens that do not affect the general population), in contrast, produce significant amounts of antigen-specific IgE. In such individuals, the likelihood that mast cells and basophils may be sensitized with IgE antibodies with a common antigenic specificity is significantly increased (and thus, the opportunity for antigen-induced IgE cross-linking).

Clinically significant atopic disease occurs in approximately 10 percent of the U.S. population, and shows a strong familial clustering of cases. The most common form of atopic disease is *allergic rhinitis,* or hay fever, in which the hypersensitivity reactions are localized to the nasal mucosa and conjunctiva. Clinical symptoms include rhinorrhea, sneezing, and nasal obstruction. Afflicted subject often complain of itching of the eyes, nose, and throat. The disease may be seasonal (coinciding with the appearance of pollens in the environment) or perennial (house dust mites).

Other localized type I reactions include atopic dermatitis and asthma. *Atopic dermatitis* (also known as allergic eczema) is a cutaneous form of type I hypersensitivity that often accompanies allergic rhinitis and asthma. Although the cause is unknown, nearly 75 percent of patients with this disease have a personal or familial history of atopic disease. Serum IgE concentrations can be markedly elevated in these patients. The essential features of atopic dermatitis include dry, itchy skin, which results in frequent scratching and rubbing. The latter produce typical features of eczema, and may lead to secondary infection.

Asthma is a disorder characterized by reversible airway obstruction and hyperirritability of the bronchial mucosa. Nearly 10 million persons in the U.S. suffer from asthma. Clinical manifestations result from the activation and degranulation of sensitized mast cells and basophils in lung tissue. Airway obstruction results from contraction of bronchial smooth muscle induced by various chemical mediators (especially leukotrienes) and the production of a thick mucus. Approximately half of all patients with asthma have a history of atopic disease, and often have elevated serum IgE levels.

TABLE 2–9 ✦ Mast Cell-Derived Mediators of Immediate Hypersensitivity

CLASS OF MEDIATOR	PHARMACOLOGIC PROPERTIES
Preformed	
Histamine	Capillary dilatation; increased vascular permeability; constriction of bronchial smooth muscle
Eosinophil chemotactic factor of anaphylaxis (ECF-A)	Chemoattraction of eosinophils
Neutrophil chemotactic factor of anaphylaxis (NCF-A)	Chemoattraction of neutrophils
Newly Synthesized	
Platelet-activating factor (PAF)	Constriction of bronchial smooth muscle; aggregation and degranulation of platelets
Prostaglandins (especially PGD$_2$)	Constriction of central and peripheral airways; vasodilatation
Leukotrienes (LTC$_4$, LTD$_4$, and LTE$_4$)	Contraction of bronchial smooth muscle; increased vascular permeability

These patients exhibit positive skin tests toward one or more environmental allergens including pollen or house dust, and asthmatic attacks typically follow exposure to the offending allergen. This form of asthma, which often becomes apparent in infancy or childhood, is termed *extrinsic asthma* (also known as allergic or atopic asthma). A second form of asthma is found in patients with no history of atopic disease. Such patients exhibit normal serum IgE levels and are unresponsive in skin tests following challenge with the usual battery of allergens. There is no apparent relationship between airway obstruction and exposure to environmental allergens. Asthmatic attacks are typically precipitated by viral infections, inhalation of cold air, or exercise. Other triggers include irritant gases (e.g., sulfur dioxide), exposure to sensitizing chemicals, or inhalation of tobacco smoke. Clinical symptoms usually begin in adult life, although a childhood onset is not uncommon. This form of asthma is termed *intrinsic asthma* (also known as non-allergic or idiopathic asthma).

Immediate hypersensitivity reactions typically involve IgE-mediated release of chemical mediators from sensitized mast cells and basophils. Clinical symptoms typically become apparent within minutes after allergen exposure, and usually fade within 1 to 2 hours. However, in approximately 50 percent of atopic patients this immediate reaction is followed by a so-called *late phase reaction* (LPR) which develops some 3 to 4 hours after allergen challenge, peaks at 6 to 12 hours and resolves within 24 to 72 hours. The late phase reaction is an inflammatory reaction involving accumulation of several cell types including neutrophils, eosinophils, and basophils. Available evidence indicates that the LPR is caused by IgE-mediated degranulation of sensitized mast cells, which contain substances that are chemotactic for neutrophils and eosinophils. In experimental models, it has been demonstrated that mast cell granules themselves can induce an LPR, and pharmacologic agents capable of inhibiting mast cell degranulation block development of this reaction. In asthmatics, LPR-induced inflammation appears to play a significant role in destruction and remodeling of airway tissues and long-lasting bronchial hyperresponsiveness to both allergic and non-allergic stimuli.

Exposure to many allergens can also induce systemic anaphylaxis, a form of immediate hypersensitivity that affects multiple organ systems simultaneously. Allergens capable of initiating this type of response include drugs (e.g., penicillins), insect venom and certain foods (e.g., nuts). Such reactions are usually IgE-mediated. However, immunoglobulin isotypes (IgG and IgM) capable of activating complement generate anaphylatoxins (C3a, C5a), which induce degranulation of mast cells and basophils. The clinical symptoms initiated by anaphylatoxin-mediated degranulation of mast cells and basophils are indistinguishable from those triggered through the IgE receptor. Symptoms of systemic anaphylactic reactions include hypotension and shock, laryngeal edema, bronchospasm and abdominal pain. Airway obstruction and loss of blood pressure can be life-threatening, and require prompt clinical intervention.

Type II (Cytolytic) Reactions

Type II hypersensitivity reactions involve binding of antibody to target cells, which are then destroyed through the action of the membrane attack complex of complement or through cellular effectors of antibody-dependent cell-mediated cytotoxicity. Clinical manifestations of these cytolytic reactions are dependent upon the cell type(s) that are damaged. Type II reactions generally involve IgG or IgM antibodies, inasmuch as these are the isotypes capable of activating the classical pathway of complement.

Hemolysis caused by the production of anti-erythrocyte antibody, as occurs in erythroblastosis fetalis, is an example of a type II hypersensitivity reaction. This hemolytic disorder results from an Rh incompatibility between an Rh⁻ mother and an Rh⁺ fetus. An Rh⁻ mother can become "sensitized" to the Rh antigen while carrying an Rh⁺ fetus. This sensitization occurs particularly during delivery, at which time Rh⁺ fetal erythrocytes are able to enter the mother's circulation. During subsequent pregnancies involving carriage of an Rh⁺ fetus, maternal IgG antibodies cross the placenta, causing substantial lysis of fetal erythrocytes. Intravascular hemolysis can result in severe anemia and central nervous system damage caused by accumulation of bilirubin. Hemolytic reactions resulting from transfusion of ABO-incompatible erythrocytes are a similar example of type II hypersensitivity.

In other instances, inadvertent lysis of host cells occurs as a consequence of adsorption of certain drugs (especially antibiotics such as penicillins and cephalosporins) to these cells. Production of antibody against the drug-host cell complex results in antibody deposition on the target cell, which are subsequently lysed by complement. Examples of this type of hypersensitivity included drug-induced hemolytic anemia and drug-induced thrombocytopenia.

The production of autoantibodies directed against cellular components can also result in damage characteristic of type II hypersensitivity. For example, in Goodpasture's syndrome, autoantibodies are produced against the basement membrane of the lung and renal glomerular apparatus. Deposition of autoantibodies in these organs leads to tissue injury resulting from complement activation and infiltration by inflammatory cells (especially neutrophils).

Type III (Immune Complex) Reactions

Type III hypersensitivity reactions are initiated by the formation of antigen-antibody complexes that precipitate in various tissues. These immune complexes activate complement, thereby generating chemotactic factors (e.g., C5a), which promote infiltration by phagocytic cells, particularly neutrophils. The tissue pathology that ensues is principally due to the production of toxic oxygen metabolites and the release of histiolytic enzymes by neutrophils during their unsuccessful attempt to ingest the deposited immune complexes. The type of tissue damage observed is dependent on the anatomic location in which the immune complexes are deposited.

Antibodies involved in immune complex-mediated tissue injury belong to the IgG (IgG1, IgG2, and IgG3 only) or IgM class, inasmuch as these are the isotypes capable of activating complement via the classical pathway. The size of the immune complex is an important variable influencing the potential for tissue injury. Immune complexes of intermediate size (formed by one or two molecules of antigen and one or two molecules of antibody) pose the greatest threat. This is due to the fact that small complexes are relatively ineffective in activating complement, while large complexes are readily cleared by mononuclear phagocytes in the liver and spleen.

Immune complex-mediated injury may either be localized or generalized, depending on the manner in which antigen and antibody interact. A classic example of localized type III hypersensitivity is the Arthus reaction, an acute immune complex-mediated vasculitis. In this reaction, antigen is injected into the skin of an immune ("sensitized") individual who has circulating antibodies against the antigen. Immune complexes form along blood vessel walls. These complexes activate complement, liberating anaphylatoxins (C3a, C5a), which induce degranulation of mast cells and thereby enhance vascular permeability. This facilitates penetration by the immune complexes, which eventually become lodged in the basement membranes of affected blood vessels. Complement-derived chemotactic factors (C5a and C5a des arg) promote subsequent infiltration by circulating neutrophils, which migrate toward the immune complexes. The phagocytic cells are unable to ingest the entrapped immune complexes, but are able to bind the complexes via their membrane receptors for IgG and opsonic C3 fragments. Through a process termed *"frustrated phagocytosis,"* the neutrophils adhere tightly to the noningestible surface and release the contents of their cytoplasmic granules into the underlying extracellular space. Lysosomal enzymes, as well as oxygen metabolites produced during the attendant respiratory burst, cause local tissue damage. This leads to hemorrhagic necrosis and eventual vessel occlusion.

The combination of antigen and antibody within the vascular compartment can result in a more generalized form of immune complex disease, an example of which is serum sickness. Sites of deposition of these circulating immune complexes are subject to the influence of several factors, including hydrostatic pressure and turbulence. Capillaries in the renal glomeruli and synovia represent regions of increased hydrostatic pressure and turbulence, and it is in these tissues that circulating immune complexes tend to be localized. Accordingly, glomerulonephritis and arthritis are common manifestations of generalized immune complex-mediated hypersensitivity reactions. As in the Arthus reaction, tissue injury results from complement activation and subsequent infiltration by phagocytic cells. Although serum sickness was far more common when heterologous antiserum was used in the treatment of certain infectious diseases, reactions of this type are occasionally seen following intravenous administration of certain drugs (especially penicillins and sulfonamides).

Type IV (Delayed Hypersensitivity) Reactions

In contrast to the first three types of hypersensitivity, which are antibody-mediated, type IV hypersensitivity reactions are mediated by T lymphocytes. Delayed-type hypersensitivity (DTH) reactions are due to antigen-induced stimulation of CD4$^+$ T-helper cells, particularly those of the T_H1 phenotype. T helper cells of this phenotype elaborate a number of cytokines, including IL-2 and interferon-γ, which promote infiltration and activation of macrophages at the affected site. The tissue damage that ensues is a consequence of the release of lysosomal enzymes and toxic oxygen metabolites by the activated macrophages.

A common example of delayed-type hypersensitivity is contact dermatitis seen in subjects who are sensitive to cosmetics, poison ivy, poison oak, or metals such as nickel. Such substances are able to form complexes with various proteins in the skin. These complexes are subsequently internalized by antigen-presenting cells present in skin, including Langerhans cells or epidermal keratinocytes. The internalized complexes are processed and re-expressed on the surface of the antigen-presenting cell in conjunction with MHC class II macromolecules. Antigen-specific CD4$^+$ T lymphocytes present in a sensitized individual are activated by the antigen-presenting cells, resulting in the secretion of inflammatory cytokines.

The DTH reaction likely plays a significant role in the elimination of parasites and intracellular bacteria, with the activated macrophage representing a key effector cell. Persistence of the offending antigen can, however, lead to development of a chronic form of DTH that is injurious to the host. One example of a chronic DTH reaction is the granulomatous skin lesion observed in patients infected with *Mycobacterium leprae*. Because of the inability of the host to eliminate this organism, infiltrating macrophages and fibroblasts proliferate and produce collagen in an effort to "wall off" the mycobacteria. In addition, macrophages often fuse to form giant cells. The granuloma that forms as a consequence of the prolonged recruitment of macrophages can result in significant tissue destruction.

AUTOIMMUNITY

Hypersensitivity reactions produce tissue injury as a consequence of an immune response to exogenous antigens. The immune system does not typically respond to autologous (self-) antigens due to the induction of tolerance, either through clonal deletion (elimination of autoreactive T and B lymphocytes) or clonal anergy (in which autoreactive lymphocytes persist but are rendered unresponsive). Nevertheless, there are instances in which unresponsiveness to self-antigens is altered, resulting in a state termed autoimmunity. The existence of an autoimmune response is not necessarily deleterious to the host. There are instances in which autoimmune reactions are clearly beneficial in immune function and regulation. Two key examples are the recognition of MHC-encoded macromolecules by T lymphocytes and the production of anti-idiotypic antibodies. Thus, CD4$^+$ T lymphocytes recognize exogenous antigens displayed on the surface of antigen-presenting cells in association with MHC class II macromolecules. Were it not for the ability of the T lymphocyte to recognize self-MHC encoded molecules, the immune system would be unable to differentiate between self- and nonself-extracellular antigens. Anti-idiotype antibodies appear to participate in a regulatory network that can enhance or suppress immune responsiveness. Anti-idiotype antibodies are produced in response to unique variable region determinants present in immunoglobulins, including determinants involved in formation of complementarity-determining regions. These anti-idiotypic antibodies can enhance the immune response by either stimulating idiotype-bearing T helper lymphocytes or by eliminating specific T suppressor lymphocytes. Alternatively, such antibodies may stimulate T suppressor activity and thereby negatively influence production of the first (idiotypic) antibody.

A breakdown in the mechanisms controlling the proliferation and activity of auto-reactive lymphocytes can result in abnormal autoimmune reactions. The clinical manifestations of autoimmune disease may be organ-specific or systemic, depending on the distribution of the antigen responsible for stimulating the immune response. Moreover, the reaction may involve production of autoantibody, auto-reactive T lymphocytes, or both. Three principal mechanisms appear to account for the majority of autoimmune diseases in humans. In the first instance, autoantibodies are produced that are reactive toward modified or unmodified cell surface antigen. This may lead to cellular destruction through complement-mediated lysis or antibody-dependent cell-mediated cytotoxicity, or to non-cytotoxic alteration of cellular function. For example, in Graves' disease, a form of organ-specific autoimmunity, autoantibodies directed against the receptor for thyroid-stimulating hormone (TSH) are produced. These antibodies mimic normal TSH-mediated stimulation of the thyroid, resulting in overproduction of thyroid hormones.

A second pathogenetic mechanism entails the formation of autoantigen-autoantibody complexes. The antigen-antibody complexes may form in the circulation, ultimately being deposited in tissues such as the renal glomerulus, or in the intercellular spaces. Tissue pathology associated with this reaction, which is analogous to type III hypersensitivity, is mediated by complement activation and/or infiltration by phagocytic cells. A notable example of this type of systemic autoimmunity is rheumatoid arthritis, a disease characterized by the presence of antibodies (termed *rheumatoid factors*), which react with the Fc region of the patient's IgG molecules. Rheumatoid factors are usually of the IgM isotype, although IgG autoantibodies are not uncommon. Complexes formed between the rheumatoid factor and the patient's own IgG circulate for a time before being deposited in tissues such as synovial membranes. Complement activation and phagocyte infiltration produce damage associated with chronic joint inflammation.

A final mechanism of tissue injury caused by autoimmune reactions involves the generation of autoreactive T lymphocytes. Upon activation by autoantigen, these T lymphocytes secrete various cytokines which promote the infiltration and activation of mononuclear phagocytes, the products of which mediate damage to host tissues. An example of this form of autoimmunity is multiple sclerosis, a disease associated with sensory and visual motor abnormalities. The pathogenesis of this disease is associated with demyelination of nerve cells in the central nervous system. The areas of demyelination are associated with accumulations of lymphocytes and mononuclear phagocytes.

The basis for development of autoimmune disease is not completely understood but appears to be multifactorial in nature. Factors that appear to contribute to the development of autoimmune diseases include (1) release of antigens normally sequestered from immunocompetent cells (and which, therefore, do not induce tolerance); (2) molecular mimicry, such as occurs when antibodies formed in response to microbial infection cross-react with host components; (3) alterations in MHC class II molecules (possibly by drugs or infectious agents), which are recognized in a manner analo-gous to that of other allogeneic MHC molecules; and (4) polyclonal B lymphocyte activation, such as may be induced by microbial constituents (including lipopolysaccharides), certain viruses (Epstein-Barr virus), or parasites *(Plasmodium malariae)*. In general, autoantibodies induced by polyclonal B lymphocyte activators are of the IgM isotype, inasmuch as these agents bypass T-helper lymphocytes which provide signals for isotype switching. Nonimmunologic factors also appear to affect the propensity for development of autoimmune diseases. These include genetic (HLA alleles) and hormonal (sex hormone) factors. Evidence for the latter association derives from the observation that the incidence of systemic lupus erythematosus in post-pubertal women is nearly nine-fold greater than in men. On the other hand, the incidence of ankylosing spondylitis is higher among men than women.

BIBLIOGRAPHY

Abbas, A. K., Lichtman, A. H., and Pober, J. S.: Cellular and Molecular Immunology. W.B. Saunders Company, Philadelphia, 1991.

Gallin, J. I., Goldstein, I. M., and Snyderman, R.: Inflammation: Basic Principles and Clinical Correlates. Raven Press, New York, 1988.

Golub, E. S., and Green, D. R.: Immunology, A Synthesis, ed. 2. Sinauer Associates, Inc., Sunderland, Mass., 1991.

Klebanoff, S. J. and Clark R. A.: The Neutrophil: Function and Clinical Disorders. Elsevier/North-Holland Publishing Company, Amsterdam, The Netherlands, 1978.

Kuby, J.: Immunology. W. H. Freeman and Company, New York, 1992.

Monaco, J. J.: A molecular model of MHC class I-restricted antigen processing. Immunol. Today 13:173–179, 1992.

Neefjes, J. J., and Ploegh, H. L.: Intracellular transport of MHC class II molecules. Immunol. Today 13:179–183, 1992.

Paul, W. E.: Fundamental Immunology, ed. 2. Raven Press, New York, 1989.

Shakib, F.: The Human IgG Subclasses: Molecular Analysis of Structure, Function and Regulation. Pergamon Press, Oxford, England, 1990.

Stites, D. P. and Terr, A. I.: Basic and Clinical Immunology, ed. 7. Appleton and Lange, Norwalk, Conn., 1991.

von Boehmer, H., and Kisielow, P.: How the immune system learns about self. Sci. Am. October 1991, p. 74–81.

3 *General Microbiology, Metabolism, and Genetics*

Stanley C. Holt and Ann Progulske

CHAPTER OUTLINE

Macroscopic morphology
The structure and chemistry of bacterial cells
Growth and division
Physiology and metabolism
Metabolism and biosynthesis

Almost 350 years ago, the first observations of the presence of bacteria were made by Anton van Leeuwenhoek. In addition to numerous microscopic animals and plants, he also saw the three basic morphologic types of what we now call bacteria: rods, spheres, and spirals. With the development of improved light microscopic optics, techniques of staining cells, and the development of the electron microscope, bacteria were soon observed to consist of a variety of cell structures (Fig. 3–1A), including a cytoplasm containing ribosomes, nucleic acid, and, under certain physiologic conditions, storage products. Most bacteria are surrounded by a cell wall, under which lies a close-fitting cytoplasmic membrane. In addition, some bacteria contain capsules on their surface, flagella for motility, and some form of heat- and chemical-resistant endospores; others form sheaths, cysts, and specialized holdfast appendages that anchor them to surfaces in their environment.

Electron microscopy revolutionized our concepts of cell structure. In fact, this combined with intuition, suggested fundamental differences between the anatomy of bacterial cells (**prokaryotes**) and the remainder of the biologic world (**eukaryotes**). The prokaryotes such as bacteria (Fig. 3–1A), are cells that lack both a nuclear membrane and the large number of membrane-limited organelles that abound in eukaryotic cells. Eukaryotic cells (Fig. 3–1B) include plants, animal cells, protozoa, algae, and fungi. Table 3–1 describes the major differences between prokaryotes and eukaryotes. The major feature separating prokaryotes from eukaryotes is a "true" nucleus (surrounded by a nuclear membrane) in the latter. In addition, eu-

karyotes contain numerous organelles, many of which are membrane bound. These include mitochondria, Golgi bodies, and an extensive endoplasmic reticulum. Interestingly, the mitochondrion also contains genetic information similar to that of the nucleus. However, the mitochondrion is very small and contains only enough genetic information for the synthesis of up to 13 proteins. The genetic information for the other proteins required for mitochondrial function is found in the nucleus. In contrast to the complex anatomy of eukaryotic cells, the prokaryotic cell is relatively simple.

While there are significant chemical and morphologic differences between prokaryotes and eukaryotes, both have a common or universal genetic code and overall chemical composition. They also have very similar mechanisms for the replication, transcription, and translation of their genetic information into a viable and functional cell. The high degree of similarity in the genetic information suggests a common evolution of these two cell types, separating at some time in the distant past while yet maintaining a common thread to the basic mechanism for producing and transferring information into a functional cell.

MACROSCOPIC MORPHOLOGY
Size

Prokaryotic cells (i.e., bacteria) are the smallest of the unicellular organisms, usually 1 to 1.5 μm wide and 2 to 6 μm long. The most studied of the bacteria, the enteric microorganism (e.g., *Escherichia coli*), is approximately 1 μm in diameter.

47

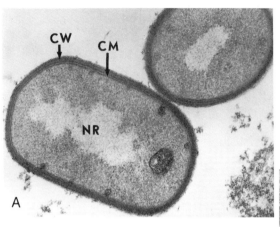
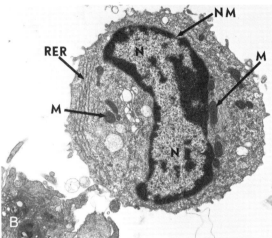

FIGURE 3–1 ✦ Electron photomicrographs of **(A)** prokaryotic cell and **(B)** eukaryotic cell. **A,** *Bacillus fastidiosus* consists of a cytoplasmic region, which contains a central fibrous nuclear region (NR), surrounded by electron dense particulate ribosome (R). The cell is surrounded by a cell wall (CW) and an inner cytoplasmic membrane (CM). **B,** In contrast, the platelet consists of numerous membrane bound organelles. The large central nucleus *(N)* is surrounded by a nuclear membrane (NM). M = mitochondria; REF = rough endoplasmic reticulum.

The smallest are the wall-less mycoplasmas, which are approximately 0.1 μm in length, while the largest are the sulfur-utilizing *Beggiatoa*, such as *Beggiatoa gigantea*, which may be as long as 26 to 60 μm.

Although it is not clear why bacteria have such a size range, it appears that the lower size limit is determined by the cytoplasmic space required to contain all of the necessary "machinery" for independent growth and development. Large bacteria have an apparent upper size limit for the necessary surface-to-volume ratios required for the efficient movement of nutrients into the cell and the products of metabolism out of the cell.

Shape

The various bacterial shapes are seen in Figure 3–2. In addition to the three basic bacterial shapes (rods, spheres, and spirals), some bacteria are square, others exist as long filaments, and a large number produce buds, similar to those of a budding tree. Others, either because of the age of the culture or environmental conditions, are very irregularly shaped, or pleomorphic. These "morphotypes" compose the general group of bacteria referred to as the *eubacteria*, or "true bacteria." The rod or cylindrical bacteria are routinely referred to as **bacilli** (distinguished from the genus *Bacillus*), the spheres are referred to as **cocci**, while spirals are referred to as **spirilla**. The spirilla are characteristic of members of the genus *Vibrio* and have a single wave form, while multiple spirillum wave forms are referred to as spirochetes. Other eubacteria are members of the actinomycetes, which are a very large group of primarily branching filaments.

COCCI

These spherical bacteria vary in diameter between 0.5 and 2 μm. The general morphology of various cocci is seen in Figure 3–3. They occur as single cells (**micrococci**), as pairs of cocci (**diplococci**), as chains (**streptococci**), or as packets of cells (**staphylococci**). Cube-shaped cellular packets are referred to as **sarcinae,** and are typical of the genus *Sarcina*. Characteristic of the cocci are the members of the genus *Streptococcus* (*i.e., S. mutans, S. sanguis, S. pneumoniae*). While these latter streptococci are spherical, they tend more toward being pear-shaped. *S. pneumoniae* is lancet shaped, while the *Neisseria* (*N. gonorrhoeae, N. meningitidis*) are bean shaped.

BACILLI

This morphotype consists of cylindrical cells, which are either large or small rods with almost parallel sides, or rods with rounded, square, or tapered ends. The bacilli are usually 0.2 to 1 μm in diameter, with lengths of approximately 10 μm being common. The majority of the bacilli are members of the genus *Bacillus* and require air for growth (**aerobic**). However, the bacilli of the genus *Clostridium* grow in the complete absence of air; that is, they are **anaerobic.** The numerous subtle variations of this morphology are discussed in later chapters.

TABLE 3–1 ✦ Distinguishing Characteristics of Prokaryotic and Eukaryotic Cells

	PROKARYOTIC CELLS	EUKARYOTIC CELLS
Major Groups	Bacteria	Algae, fungi, protozoa, plants, animals
Size (approximate)	$1 \times 3\ \mu m$	$>5\ \mu m$
Cellular Structures		
Cell wall peptidoglycan	+	−
Membrane composition	Sterols absent from most bacterial membranes	Sterols abundant
Mitochondria	−	+
Chloroplasts	−	Present in photosynthetic organisms
Gas vesicles	±	−
Nuclei		
Nuclear membrane	−	+
Chromosome number	1	1+
Mitotic apparatus	−	+
Nucleolus	−	+
Histones	±	+
Golgi apparatus	−	+
Microtubules	−	+
Ribosomes (sedimentation coefficient)	70S	Cytoplasmic ribosomes 80S; chloroplast, mitochondrial ribosomes 70S
Glycocalyx	±	±
Movement		
Cytoplasmic streaming	−	±
Amoeboid movement	−	±
Flagella	If present, simple	If present, 9 + 2
Metabolism		
Oxidative phosphorylation	Membranes	Mitochondria
Photosynthetic structure	Intracytoplasmic membranes or vesicles	Chloroplasts
Reduced inorganic compounds as energy source	±	−
Nonglycolytic anaerobic energy generation	±	−
Poly B-hydroxybutyrate reserve storage material	±	−
Nitrogen fixation	±	−
Peptidoglycan synthesis	+	−
Exo- and endocytosis	−	±
DNA base ratios (Mol% G + C)	20–70	Approx 40

+ = present; − = absent; ± = may occur in some cells.

SPIRILLA AND RELATED FORMS

In reality, the spirilla are bacilli twisted into a helix. The rigid spirilla are surrounded by a cell wall (page 57) and are represented by the genera *Spirillum* and *Vibrio*. The flexible spirilla (which also contain a cell wall) with more than one wave are typical of the spirochetes, represented by the genera *Treponema, Spirochaeta, Leptospira, Borrelia*, and *Cristispira. Treponema* are very tightly coiled, while the coils of *Borrelia* are larger and looser. *Leptospira* have very regular tight coils in the central region of the cell, with either one or both ends of the cell bent into a characteristic hook.

THE STRUCTURE AND CHEMISTRY OF BACTERIAL CELLS

Figure 3–4 depicts an idealized prokaryotic cell composed of all of its associated structures. We will describe first those components that are associated with the cell surface, that is, with the cell wall, and then those components that occupy the interior or cytoplasmic region of the cell.

Flagella and Motility

Flagella (sing. flagellum) are organelles of motility (Fig. 3–5A). The bacterial flagellum (Fig.

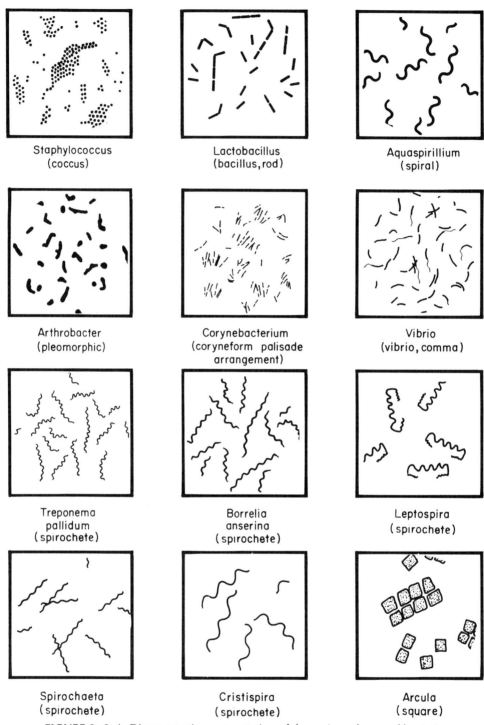

FIGURE 3–2 ✦ Diagrammatic representation of the various shapes of bacteria.

3–5B, C) is constructed of three distinct regions: a basal body, which is embedded in the cytoplasmic membrane and portions of the cell wall (or outer membrane in gram-negative bacteria; see page 53); and a hook region, which connects the basal body to the distal portion of the flagellum and filament.

The basal body itself consists of a series of discs or rings, which connect the proximal end of the filament through the hook to the cytoplasmic membrane and cell wall. The number of rings varies with the genus of bacterium and group; gram-negative cells possess four rings, while gram-positive bacteria have only two rings. The body contains the machinery for flagellar rotation, and the fact that they are embedded in the cytoplasmic membrane permits them to obtain the necessary energy (as ATP from the electron transport system in the cytoplasmic membrane; see page 73) for their rotation. Chemically, the basal bodies, hook, and filament all consist of specific polypeptides. The filament polypeptides comprise a bundle of at least three parallel or intertwined protein fibers, known as *flagellin*.

While all of the prokaryotic flagellar filament proteins belong to the same general class of flagellins, the flagellin structure of each bacterial species is sufficiently unique to confer immunologic specificity (see Chapter 2). This immunologic or "type" specificity provides the cell with its immunologic uniqueness, and is especially useful in microbiological identification of specific microorganisms and their diseases (i.e., *Vibrio cholerae,*

Pseudomonas aeruginosa). The number and arrangement of the flagella over the bacterial surface also vary among bacteria (Fig. 3–6). The genera *Pseudomonas* and *Vibrio*, for example, are unipolarly flagellated cells and hence **monotrichous,** while *Salmonella typhi, Escherichia coli,* and *Proteus vulgaris* have flagella distributed over their entire cell surface, and so are **peritrichously** flagellated.

Pili and Fimbriae

Both pili (singular pilus) and fimbriae (sing. fimbria) are attached to the outermost surface of the cell (Fig. 3–7). They are confined to the gram-negative bacteria and to selected gram-positive bacteria (i.e., *Streptococcus, Actinomyces*). They range in thickness between 0.0085 μm and 0.003 μm, and are of variable length, with lengths of 20 μm or more being common. They number ap-

A. Diplococci (double cells):

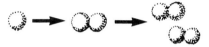

B. Streptococci: (cells in chains):

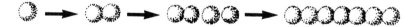

C. Tetrads: (cells in fours):

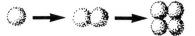

D. Staphylococci: (cells in clusters):

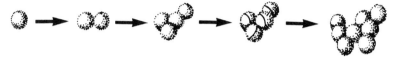

E. Sarcinae: (cells in cubes):

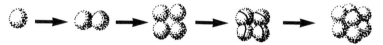

FIGURE 3–3 ✦ Various morphologies of cocci. The spherical cells can exist as single cocci, as diplococci, as arrangements of four cells (tetrads), as irregular clusters (staphylococci), or as cubes (sarcinae).

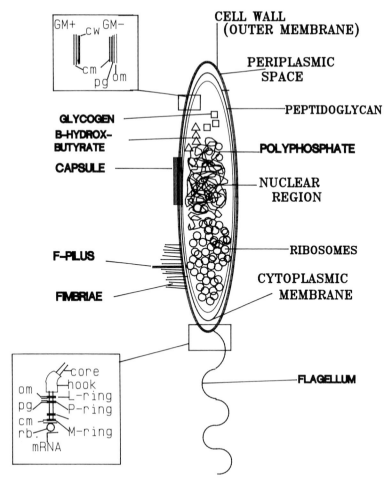

FIGURE 3–4 ✦ Diagram of a typical prokaryotic (bacterial) cell (see also Table 3–1). The structures designated in **boldface** are not found in all bacterial cells, nor are they required for cell viability. All other structures are routinely found in prokaryotes. The boxed areas are enlargements of the gram-positive cell wall and gram-negative cell envelope (see Fig. 3–9), and flagellum (see Fig. 3–5).

proximately 150 and are arranged peritrichously around the cell. The pili are distinguished from flagella in being approximately one-half their diameter as well as in being distinctively straight or "stiff" in appearance. Pili consist of essentially one protein, termed *pilin*. Small amounts of carbohydrate are also associated, suggesting that pili may be glycoproteins.

FUNCTIONS OF PILI AND FIMBRIAE

These structures function primarily in the transfer of genetic material between bacteria, as well as in adherence (i.e., **adhesins**). Pili that transfer genetic material are referred to as F or *sex* pili. The F pili form physical bridges between donor and recipient cells (see page 95), known as conjugation bridges, which permit the transfer of DNA between them. The pili are also bacteriophage (bacterial virus) receptors. Specific bacteriophage will

adsorb to the tips of the F pili, which are then retracted into the cell. This retraction brings the virus into close contact with the bacterial cell surface, where a second receptor in the outer membrane transfers the virus into the cell cytoplasm.

Pili are also adherence structures; they are referred to as either type-specific pili or fimbriae. Their adherence specificity for certain bacterial cells gives them their type-specific character. The fimbriae are irregularly distributed over the surface of the cell and are sometimes collectively referred to as a "fuzzy coat."

The type-specific fimbriae are also involved in cell-cell agglutination (type 1 fimbriae), as antigens, as well as in the agglutination of erythrocytes. The type 1 fimbriae are able to agglutinate both chicken and guinea pig erythrocytes in the absence of D-mannose; they are, however, unable to do so in the presence of this sugar. Hence, type

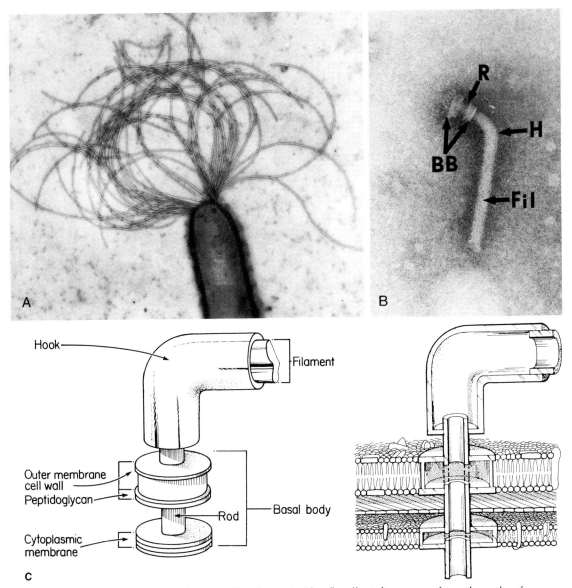

FIGURE 3–5 ✦ The prokaryotic flagellum. **A,** The flagella tuft emerges from the pole of *Aquaspirillum serpens,* strain "straight Rhodes." The central rod (R) connects the disks. **B,** The apical portion of a flagellum is seen. The filament (FiL) has been torn, and the basal body (BB) is intact. Note the hooked (H) region of the flagellum, as well as the fan disks of the basal body. **C,** The flagellum and its relationship with the cytoplasmic membrane is represented in diagrammatic form. The disks of the basal body insert into the cytoplasmic and outer membrane of the gram-negative bacterial cell envelope. (Parts **B** and **C** courtesy of Dr. R. G. E. Murray.)

1 fimbriae are "mannose-sensitive." Type 3 fimbriae are only capable of agglutinating animal red blood cells if the erythrocytes have been treated with tannic acid. Type 2 fimbriae do not hemagglutinate red blood cells, and since they resemble type 1 fimbriae structurally and antigenically, they are considered to be structural variants of the type 1 fimbriae. This hemagglutination appears to be the result of surface electrical charge interactions with specific adhesin molecules, which are firmly attached to the tips of the fimbriae.

Importantly, the ability of several of the gram-negative pathogens to express their virulence in a susceptible host is regulated by the presence or absence of fimbriae. *Neisseria gonorrhoeae,* for example, when cultured in vitro on solid agar quickly lose their fimbriae and become nonpathogenic (i.e., avirulent). These avirulent *N. gonor-*

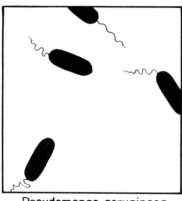

Pseudomonas aeruginosa
(Monotrichous; single
polar flagellum)

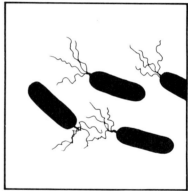

Pseudomonas fluorescens
(Lophotrichous; cluster
of polar flagella)

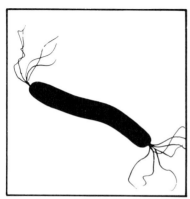

Aquaspirillum serpens
(Amphitrichous; flagella at both
poles, either single or in clusters)

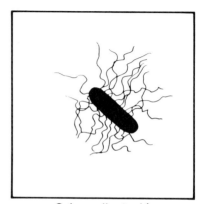

Salmonella typhi
(Peritrichous; cell
encircled by
lateral flagella)

FIGURE 3–6 ✦ Various flagella arrangements in bacterial cells.

rhoeae also are unable to infect humans since they are unable to adhere to host tissue. The adherence of *E. coli* to gastric mucosa, erythrocytes, and leukocytes, as well as the adherence of *Pseudomonas aeruginosa* to alveolar tissue, is mediated by type-specific fimbriae. *Streptococcus pyogenes* also requires fimbriae to adhere to the epithelial mucosa of the throat and to cause streptococcal sore throat.

Capsules, Slimes, and Other Surface-Associated Coverings

The outer layer is responsible for the ultimate survival and interaction of the cell with its environment, because it is this layer that is in direct contact with the influences of the environment. Bacteria, especially those that interact with cells, are usually surrounded by a slimy, gummy, or mu-

cilaginous layer, various forms of which are seen in Figure 3–8A through E. Depending upon the overall consistency of this material, this layer is referred to as either a **capsule** or a **slime layer.** The capsule is usually of uniform consistency and integrity; slime layers, on the other hand, are ill-defined and loosely formed. The oral streptococci, *Streptococcus salivarius* and *S. mutans,* form large capsules consisting of glucan (dextran) or fructan (levan), depending on the carbon source on which or in which they are grown. In the case of the streptococcal capsules, they are synthesized by specific polysaccharide synthesis enzymes at the cytoplasmic membrane and are transported to the bacterial cell surface through pores in the cell wall by specific transferases (glucosyl and fructosyl transferases) (see following section on chemical composition).

CHEMICAL COMPOSITION OF CAPSULES

Capsules are composed of either carbohydrate or protein, depending on the species, the carbon and nitrogen source, as well as the gaseous environment in which the cells are grown. Capsules have been identified that contain pectin (homopolymer of D-galacturonic acid), cellulose, and mixed carbohydrate polymers. As discussed earlier, *Streptococcus mutans* and *S. salivarius* can form dextran and levan capsules, while *S. pneumoniae*, which forms several different chemical types of capsules (see further on), forms a capsule consisting of glucose polymers and is referred to as a type 2 capsule. The type 3 capsular polymers of *S. pneumoniae* are more complex, consisting of glucose and glucuronic acid subunits. *Bacillus anthracis*, the microorganism causing anthrax, produces a polypeptide capsule of polyglutamic acid. This polyglutamyl polypeptide is produced only in the presence of CO_2 and functions as a virulence factor in anthrax.

Several of the bacterial capsules have been formulated into effective vaccines. For example, the numerous pneumoniae capsular types have been combined into a vaccine that is effective against pneumococcal diseases, while the capsular polysaccharide from *Neisseria meningitidis* is protective against meningitis for infants younger than 6 months of age. A potential capsular vaccine has been produced from *Streptococcus mutans* that may be effective against dental caries.

FUNCTION OF CAPSULES

Capsules are important in permitting bacteria to express their virulence capabilities, as well as providing them with the ability to survive the numerous host defense mechanisms with which animals and plants are endowed. Capsules also provide an immunologic specificity. Encapsulated bacteria produce smooth (S) colonies and are immunologically characterized as "S-type" colonies, while bacteria that have had their capsules removed by either genetic or chemical means produce rough (R) colonies and are termed "R-type" colonies. The S-type is associated with the virulence of pathogenic bacteria, because the capsules protect them from the host defense mechanisms, especially from phagocytosis. The immunologic specificity of the capsule is so great that even within a given bacterial species, immunologic subspecies or types may be distinguished as a result of even slight differences in the capsular composition. For example, there are nearly 15 distinct immunologic types of *Streptococcus pneumoniae*. In addition to capsules providing immunologic specificity, protection against phagocytosis, and functioning as virulence factors, capsules also serve as osmotic barriers since they themselves consist of almost 95 percent water, which prevents the too-rapid flux of water into or out of the cell.

OTHER SURFACE APPENDAGES

Several groups of bacteria secrete discernible structures, which function physically to stick or hold these cells to surfaces. These structures are referred to as holdfasts, and usually occur on bacteria existing in the aquatic environment; these are prosthecate bacteria.

A variety of bacteria, also found free-living in the natural environment—especially in environments rich in organic compounds and reduced me-

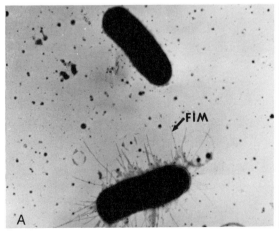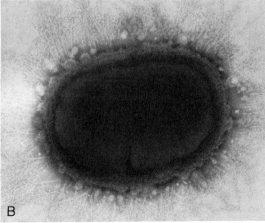

FIGURE 3–7 ✦ Electron photomicrograph of **(A)** type 1 fimbriae (FIM; pili) surrounding the surface of *Escherichia coli*. The nonfimbriated cell in **A** is representative of a cell in which fimbriae synthesis has been "switched-off." In **B**, *Porphyromonas gingivalis* numerous long fimbriae cover the cell surface and extend out of it in a tangle array of fibers.

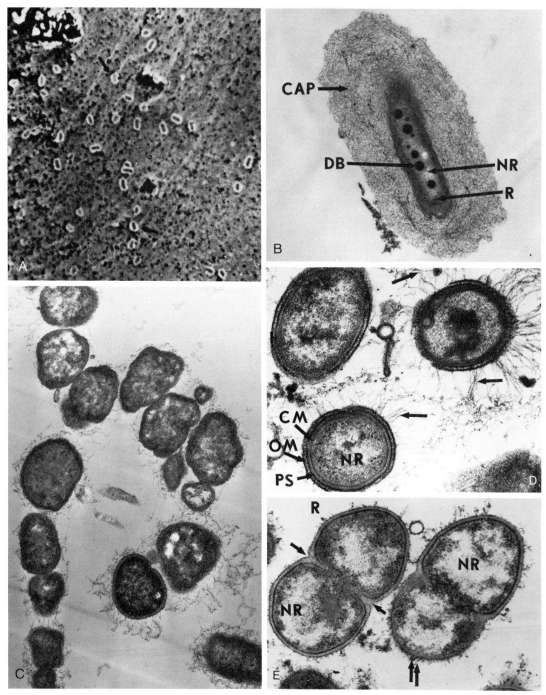

FIGURE 3–8 ✦ Electron photomicrographs of bacterial capsules. **A,** India ink smear of *Porphyromonas gingivalis* showing thick capsule. **B,** The thick alginic acid capsule of *Pseudomonas aeruginosa* surrounds the bacterial cell. **C,** The capsule of *Streptococcus mutans* is a loosely adherent structure that adheres very closely to the thick cell wall. **D,** The capsule of a *Bacillus capillus* consists of a loosely adherent fibrous layer *(arrows)*. **E,** The loosely adherent capsule of *Porphyromonas gingivalis* attaches numerous cells into an adherent cell wall. The *single arrows* in **E** indicate the ingrowing division septum, while the *double arrows* indicate loosely adherent capsular material. Note in **E** the concentration of ribosomes in the division plane of the dividing streptococci. CAP = capsular; DB = dense storage body; NR = nuclear region; R = ribosomes; PS = periplasmic space; OM = outer membrane; CM = cytoplasmic membrane.

tallic salts—form sheaths or tubes that surround and enclose these cells. In comparison to the capsule, the sheath is a very complex chemical structure.

Cell Wall

It was clear from van Leeuwenhoek's initial observations of the various shapes of bacteria, that a bacterial structure must provide and maintain these various morphotypes. Since the internal cytoplasm does not mix freely with the external environment, the existence of a rigid limiting layer, or cell wall, is required (Fig. 3–9). The cell wall (specifically its peptidoglycan; see page 60) gives the cell its shape and protects the cell cytoplasm from osmotic pressure differences between the intracellular and extracellular environments. The cell wall is also

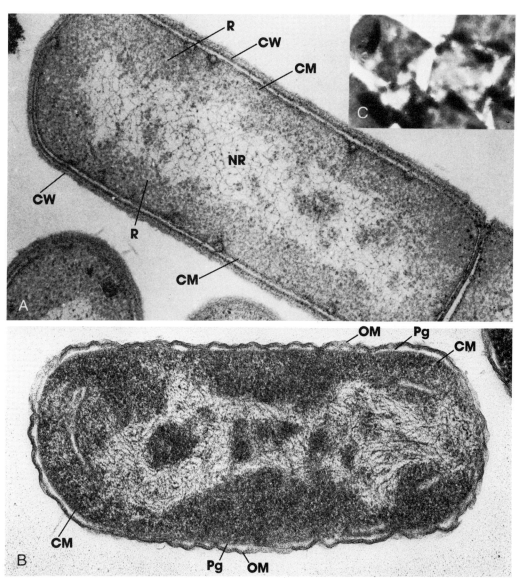

FIGURE 3–9 ✦ Electron photomicrographs of **(A)** the gram-positive bacterium, *Bacillus macroides,* and **(B)** the gram-negative, *Escherichia coli.* In **A,** the thick cell wall (CW) surrounds the thin cytoplasmic membrane (CM), which encloses the cytoplasmic region containing electron-dense ribosomes (R) and a fibrillal nucleoid (NR). **B,** The outer membrane (OM) is external to the very thin peptidoglycan (Pg), which encloses the unit cytoplasmic membrane (CM). **C,** Isolated cell wall fragments from *B. macroides.* Note that the fragments maintain their rod appearance, a result of the chemical construction of the peptidoglycan. NR = nuclear region; R = ribosomes.

the primary "sieve" in the transport of molecules into the cell. It also functions as an anchor for the capsule, as well as for pili, fimbriae, and flagella, and it is the primary receptor for the absorption of specific viruses or bacteriophages prior to their transport into the cytoplasm.

With the exception of the taxonomic group, *Mollicutes* (i.e., *Mycoplasma, Acholeplasma, Spiroplasma,* PPLO, and the archebacteria, *Halobacterium, Methanobacterium*), the rigidity and strength of the bacterial cell wall is due to a network of fibers composed of heteropolymers of the chemical class of mucopolysaccharides commonly referred to as the mucopeptide, mucocomplex, or peptidoglycan. These fibers form a tough network or **sacculus** that completely surrounds the cell.

In the *Mollicutes,* the cytoplasm is enclosed by a single, thin cell membrane, approximately 7.5 nm thick (Fig. 3–10). This membrane functions as both the cell wall and the cytoplasmic membrane (see further on). Without a cell wall to provide rigidity, these microorganisms must live in an environment where the osmotic pressure will not rupture the cells; hence, the very restricted ecologic environment in which these "wall-less" bacteria live. It is probably more useful to divide the *Mollicutes* into the wall-less *Mycoplasmas* and the peptidoglycan-less *Archebacteria.*

The ability of bacterial cells to retain or release specific dyes in the classic gram-staining technique has resulted in a clear separation of bacteria into two major groups: those that retain the blue dye crystal violet after treatment with iodine, alcohol, and counterstaining with the red dye safranin, and those that do not. Gram-positive cells retain the blue crystal violet and stain blue, while gram-negative bacteria do not retain this dye and thus stain red with safranin after alcohol treatment. The characteristic morphology of gram-positive and gram-negative cell walls is seen in Figure 3–8C, D. Immediately apparent is that the cell walls of these two major groups of bacteria are visibly different. Cell walls of gram-positive bacteria are thicker (15 to 50 nm) than those of gram-negative bacteria (7.5 to 10 nm). Some cell walls of gram-positive bacteria have been observed to reach thicknesses of 80 nm, and, depending upon the growth conditions, stage of growth, as well as C- and N-sources, the gram-positive cell wall can constitute between 20 and 40 percent of the cellular dry weight. The cytoplasmic membrane (see further on) adheres very tightly to the internal aspect of the cell wall in gram-positive bacteria.

The cell wall of gram-negative bacteria is morphologically and chemically more complex than that of gram-positive bacteria. It consists of several membranes (see page 61 for discussion of the concept of a membrane) that lay outside of the cytoplasmic membrane and enclose the electron-dense cytoplasmic region. The multilayered arrangement of the gram-negative cell wall and the fact that it cannot be separated as a unit (as can the gram-positive cell wall) have resulted in this layer being referred to as the *cell envelope.* The outermost layer of the cell envelope then is referred to as the *outer membrane.* This layer is approximately 7.5 to 10 nm thick and encloses an electron transparent space, the *periplasmic space.* The periplasmic

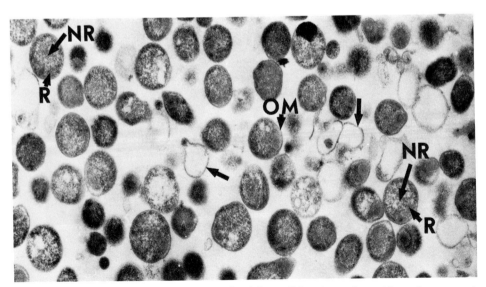

FIGURE 3–10 ✦ Electron photomicrograph of the wall-less bacterium, *Mycoplasma capricolum.* Note the absence of the cell wall. The cell is surrounded by a thin cell membrane. The *arrows* indicate the thin outer membrane. NR = nuclear region; OM = outer membrane; R = ribosomes. (Courtesy of Dr. Schlomo Rottem.)

space contains a variety of hydrolytic enzymes and chemotactic stimulants involved in the hydrolysis of large macromolecules and chemical attraction, respectively. Within the periplasmic space is a very thin peptidoglycan layer, approximately 3 to 4 nm thick. The cell wall of gram-negative bacteria consists of two layers; the outer membrane and the peptidoglycan layer enclose a periplasmic space; together they form the gram-negative cell envelope. The gram-positive bacterial cell wall consists of one thick layer.

CHEMISTRY OF THE PEPTIDOGLYCAN

The peptidoglycan is unique to the cell wall of essentially all prokaryotes (with the exceptions noted earlier); it has not been found in eukaryotes. It is responsible for the maintenance of cell shape and rigidity. The chemical composition of the cell walls of gram-positive and gram-negative bacteria is seen in Table 3–2. Gram-positive cell walls contain relatively high amounts of amino sugars (i.e., 15 to 20 percent), no lipids, and only minor amounts of amino acids. In contrast, the cell walls of gram-negative bacteria (outer membrane and peptidoglycan) are rich in lipid (10 to 20 percent), have a low amino sugar content (2 to 5 percent), and contain the full complement of amino acids that are found routinely in proteins.

The chemical structure and molecular configuration of the peptidoglycan are seen in Figure 3–11. Chemically, the peptidoglycan consists of two sugars, N-acetylglucosamine and N-acetylmuramic acid, at least four amino acids, usually glutamic acid, alanine, glycine, and lysine (Fig. 3–11B). Diaminopimelic acid can substitute for lysine (Fig. 3–12). The gram-positive cell wall consists almost entirely of peptidoglycan. The N-acetylglucosamine and N-acetylmuramic acid are chemically

TABLE 3–2 ✦ Basic Chemical Composition of Gram-Positive and Gram-Negative Cell Walls

CELL WALL COMPONENT	GRAM-POSITIVE	GRAM-NEGATIVE
Peptidoglycan	+	+
Teichoic acid and/or Teichuronic acid	+	−
Polysaccharide	+	+
Protein	±	+
Lipid	−	+
Lipopolysaccharide	−	+
Lipoprotein	−	+

+ = routinely present; − = routinely absent; ± = usually absent, but present in some genera.

linked together into a linear polymer of approximately 40 to 50 disaccharides, or glycan units. The repeating N-acetylglucosaminyl-N-acetylmuramyl dimers that form the glycan are covalently connected by random cross-links between short tetrapeptides that originate from the muramyl residues. Not all of the muramyl peptide chains are linked together through interpeptide bonding; the degree of cross-linking of the peptidoglycan will affect its rigidity as well as its strength. Therefore, the thick gram-positive cell wall has an extremely strong tensile structure, consisting of many (between 15 and 50) peptidoglycan layers, whereas the gram-negative peptidoglycan has been estimated to be only one layer thick, and consequently is a much more fragile cell wall (compare Figs. 3–9 and 3–13). To add more vertical stability to the gram-negative cell envelope, two proteins bind the outer membrane to the peptidoglycan in this group. These proteins, the **matrix proteins** and the **Braun lipoproteins,** are inserted into the outer membrane, providing this vertical stability to the outer membrane–peptidoglycan complex by providing a chemical link between these two envelope layers (see Fig. 3–18). The peptidoglycan does, however, maintain the shape and rigidity of the cell.

TEICHOIC ACIDS

In addition to the peptidoglycan, the gram-positive cell wall also contains uronic acids (Fig. 3–14). Teichoic, teichuronic, and lipoteichoic acids are the major uronic acid constituents. These amphipathic linear polyalcohol phosphate molecules are linked together as glycerol-sugar-phosphate polymers. They have not been observed in gram-negative bacteria; their formation is dependent upon growth conditions, and not all species of gram-positive bacteria form them. The predominant uronic acids are either glycerol or ribitol, and these are linked via phosphodiester bonds to the N-acetylmuramic acid of the cell wall glycan strands. The polyalcohol phosphate molecules are inserted into the pre-existing cell wall as a teichoic acid–peptidoglycan complex. Not all of the teichoic acid termini originate from the cell wall itself. The fatty acid, or acylated teichoic acid (lipoteichoic acid, or LTA), penetrates through the cell wall, with the lipid moiety intercalating the phospholipids of the cytoplasmic membrane (Fig. 3–15).

Function of the Teichoic Acids

While the exact function of these teichoic or uronic acids is unclear, since one end of the molecule probably emerges from the surface of the cell, they may contribute to the overall negative-charge density of the cell surface. This large negative surface charge and lipoteichoic acids are strong ad-

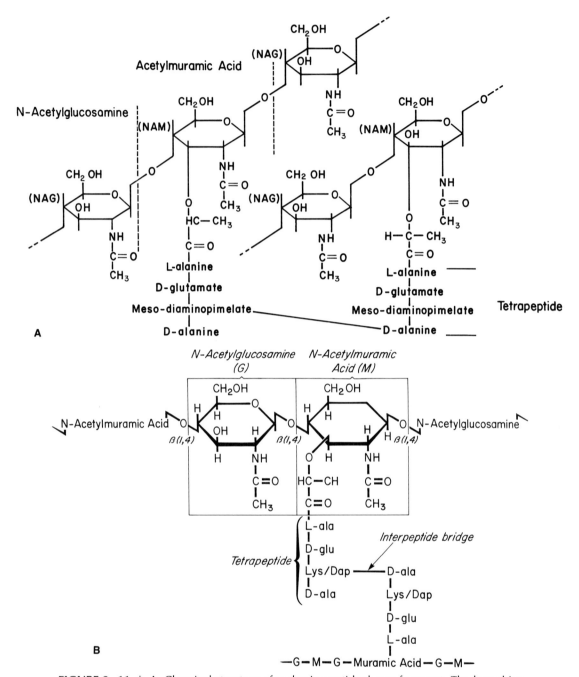

FIGURE 3–11 ✦ A, Chemical structure of a classic peptidoglycan fragment. The branching structure consists of repeating units of an *N*-acetyl-glucosamine and an *N*-acetyl-muramic acid. This glycan chain is joined to other glycan chains by tetrapeptide links consisting of L-alanine, D-glutamic acid, lysine of meso-diaminopenalic acid, and D-alanine. The interpeptide bridge between meso-diaminopenalic acid and D-alanine can consist of several different amino acids. **B,** The chemical structure of the *N*-acetyl-glucosamine-*N*-acetyl-muramic acid tetrapeptide is seen.

hesins, especially in the attachment to mammalian tissues, and adherence to red blood cells, tooth surfaces, and numerous other positively charged surfaces. The teichoic acids also are the major antigenic components of the gram-positive cell surface.

THE GRAM-NEGATIVE ENVELOPE: ITS CHEMISTRY AND FUNCTION

Chemically, the outer membrane consists of approximately 20 to 25 percent phospholipid and 45 to 50 percent protein, with the remainder (about

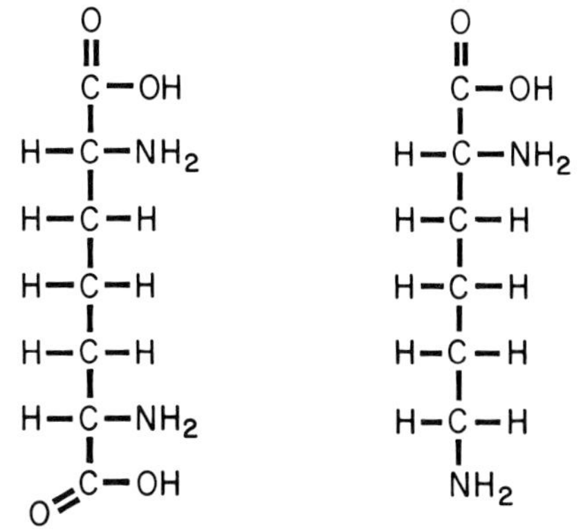

O
‖
C—OH
|
H—C—NH$_2$
|
H—C—H
|
H—C—H
|
H—C—H
|
H—C—NH$_2$
|
O≶C—OH

O
‖
C—OH
|
H—C—NH$_2$
|
H—C—H
|
H—C—H
|
H—C—H
|
H—C—H
|
NH$_2$

**Diaminopimelic   Lysine
Acid**

FIGURE 3–12 ✦ Chemical structure of diaminopimelic acid and lysine.

30 percent) consisting of the unique glycolipid, the **lipopolysaccharide,** or LPS (Fig. 3–16). The LPS is found only in gram-negative bacteria.

Structurally, the outer membrane consists of two layers arranged in the characteristic bilayer common to all biologic membranes (see page 65). The outer layer—or outer leaflet—of the outer membrane contains, in addition to phospholipids, the lipopolysaccharide. The inner leaflet of the outer membrane consists primarily of phospholipids. LPS in the outer leaflet and phospholipids in the inner leaflet produce the structural asymmetry characteristic of the gram-negative outer membrane; that is, the outer leaflet of the outer membrane is more electron-dense than the inner leaflet.

One of the primary functions of the outer membrane is as a molecular sieve, excluding molecules, with molecular weights exceeding 700, both into

and out of the cell. Molecules with a molecular weight greater than 700 enter the cell via specific proteins, referred to as *porin proteins*. The outer membrane also functions as a bacterial virus (bacteriophage) receptor and as an antigenic determinant. The outer membrane prevents the penetration of antibiotics, detergents, and other harmful molecules into the cell.

The LPS consists of three regions: the O-specific polysaccharide, the core polysaccharide, and the lipid A (Fig. 3–16). The O-specific polysaccharide, or O-somatic antigen, provides the cell with its unique antigenic makeup. The core polysaccharide joins the lipid A to the O-specific polysaccharide and consists of the unique molecule, 2-keto-3-deoxy-octanoate (KDO), and a seven-carbon heptose sugar. The lipid A is highly hydrophobic and is embedded in the outer leaflet of the outer membrane. It consists of a phosphorylated glucosamine disaccharide that is esterified with long-chain fatty acids, usually C14, C16, and C18 carbon chain lengths. In addition, lipid A contains hydroxy fatty acids thought to function as the **endotoxin.**

Functionally, the LPS protects the cell from the action of antibody and complement, is a bacteriophage receptor, and is one of the major endotoxic molecules of gram-negative bacteria; hence, it is considered an important virulence factor of these bacteria. Depending upon the lipid A type, dosage, and route of lipid A injection, it can cause hemorrhage, fever, tumor necrosis, fatal shock, septicemia, and even abortion.

Cytoplasmic Membrane

In both animal and plant cells, the cytoplasm is not readily differentiated from the outer integument, or cytoplasmic membrane. However, in pro-

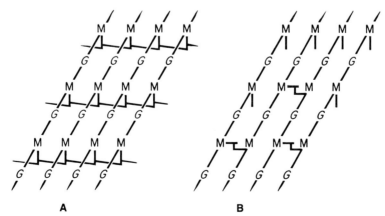

FIGURE 3–13 ✦ Diagrammatic representation of a segment of the peptidoglycan showing the cross-bridging of the molecule. This cross-bridging provides the rigidity and strength to the peptidoglycan. M = *N*-acetylmuramic acid; G = *N*-acetylglucosamine.

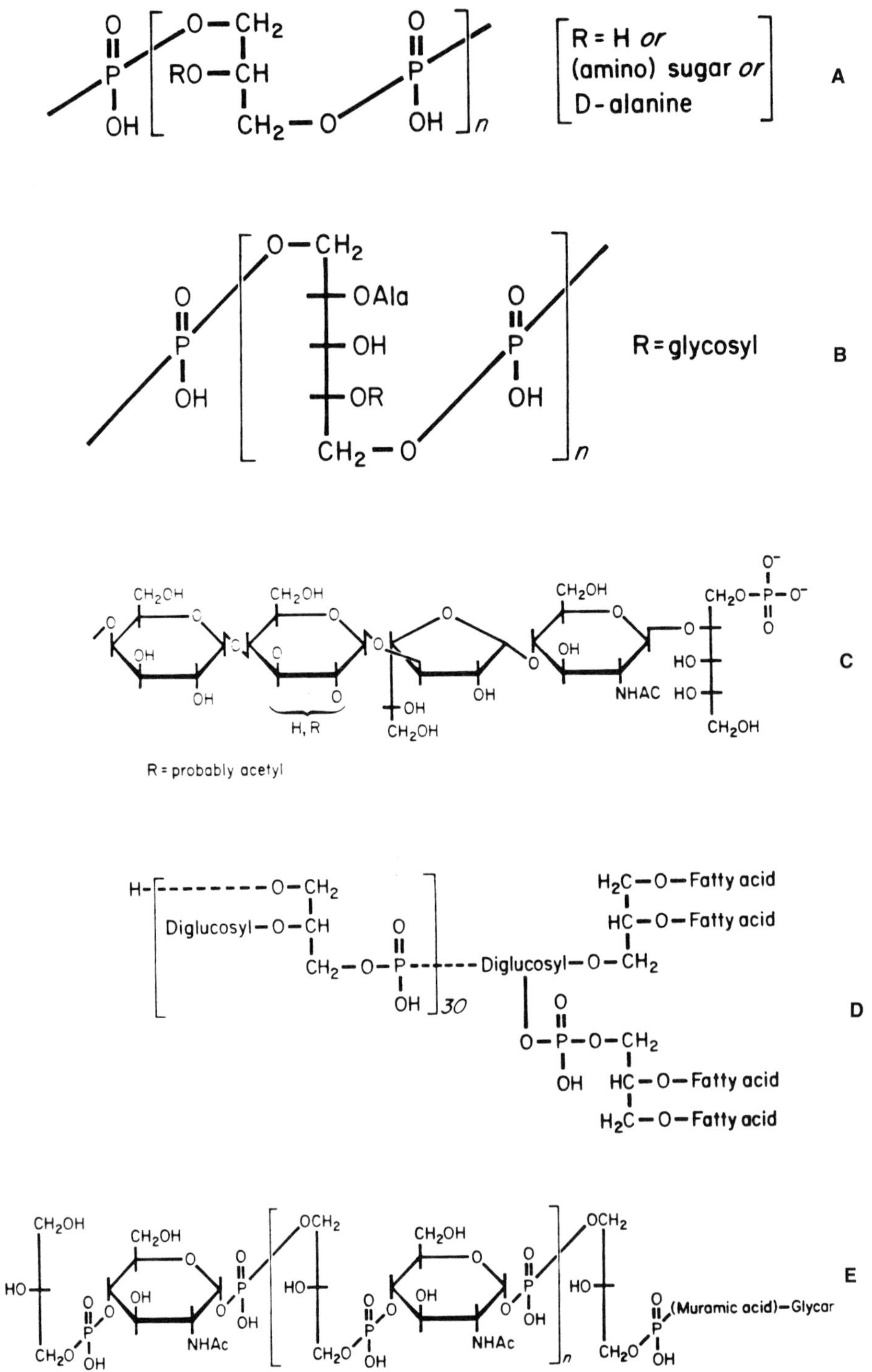

FIGURE 3–14 ✦ Chemical structure of various teichoic acids that constitute a portion of the gram-positive cell wall. **A,** Glycerol teichoic acid. **B,** Ribitol teichoic acid. **C,** Teichoic acid of *Streptococcus pneumoniae* capsule. The structure consists of oligoglycosyl ribitol units. **D,** Lipoteichoic acid of *Streptococcus faecalis*. The diglycosyl units consist of glucose a, 1– 2 glucose molecules, or sometimes referred to as kojibiose. **E,** Repeating unit of N-acetyl-glucosamine-1-phosphate-glycosyl-phosphate. These sugar molecules are present in the back-bone chain of selected peptidoglycans.

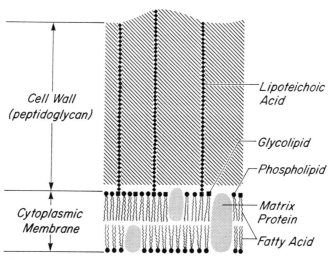

FIGURE 3–15 ✦ Diagrammatic representation of the insertion of the lipoteichoic acid into the gram-positive cell wall. The lipoteichoic acid inserts directly through the cell wall into glycolipid moieties. Teichoic acid molecules (not shown), devoid of their acyl groups, can insert directly into the matrix of the cell wall. (Redrawn from Stanier, R., et al. [eds]: The Microbial World, ed. 5. Prentice-Hall, Englewood Cliffs, NJ, 1986.)

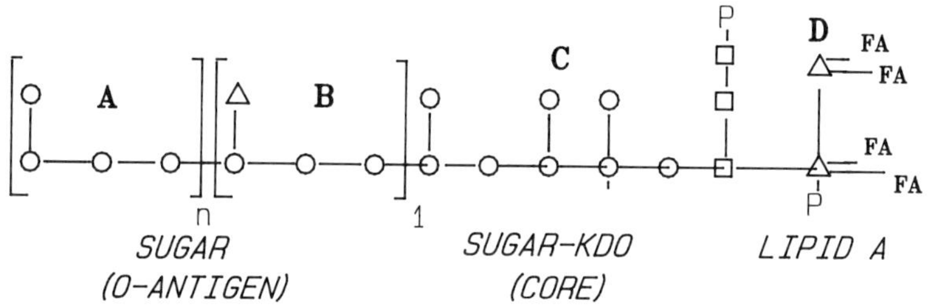

```
     ┌       ┐ ┌              ┐            P          D   FA
     │ ○  A  │ │ △     B      │     C      □          △ ─ FA
     │ │     │ │ │            │ ○    ○  ○  □
     │ ○─○─○ ├─┤ ○─○─○────────│ ○─○──○──○─○─□            FA
     │       │ │              │ │              △ ─ FA
     └       ┘n└              ┘1                P
         SUGAR                  SUGAR-KDO      LIPID A
       (O-ANTIGEN)               (CORE)
```

A=Various O-antigen sugars: i.e., rhamnose, mannose
   abequose, galactose

B=O-antigen sugar repeat

C= N-acetylglucosamine (△), glucose, galactose, heptose (○)
   2-Keto, 3-deoxy-octanoate, KDO (□)

D= b-1-6-linked N-acetylated glucosamine+
   at least 7 fatty acids (FA)

FIGURE 3–16 ✦ Schematic representation of lipopolysaccharide from *Salmonella typhimurium*. The lipid backbone (lipid A) is composed of B 1-6-linked *N*-acetylated glucosamine monosaccharides (GlcNAc). The fatty acids (Fa) vary among C-12, C-14, C-16, OH-C-16, and OH-C-12 compounds. The number and type of lipid A fatty acids vary among bacterial species. In addition, phosphate esters (P), amino groups (not shown), or both are substituted at the 1 and 4′ positions of the nonreducing and reducing glucosamines, respectively (see Fig. 3–44). An eight-carbon keto sugar 2-keto,3-deoxy-octanoic acid, KDO, links the lipid A and polysaccharide portions of the molecule. The number of KDOs is variable among species. The remainder of the core sugars include heptose, glucose, galactose, and *N*-acetylglucosamine. The O-antigen sugars in *S. typhimurim* include galactose, rhamnose, mannose, and abequose. (Reproduced with permission of Hitchcock, P. J., et al.: J. Bacteriol. 166:699, 1986.)

karyotic cells, the cytoplasmic membrane is a distinct and usually a readily separable component of the cell (see Figs. 3–1A, 3–8D, 3–9, and 3–17A). In gram-positive bacteria, the cytoplasmic membrane is in close association with the cell wall (see Figs. 3–1A, 3–8E), while in gram-negative cells it lies just below the thin peptidoglycan layer (see Figs. 3–8D, 3–9B, and 3–17A). It consists of three distinct layers, or leaflets: the outer, middle, and inner layers (Figs. 3–17B, 3–18). The cytoplasmic membrane, referred to as a **"unit membrane,"** is approximately 10 nm in diameter, consisting of 2–2.5 nm outer and inner layers and a 5 nm thick middle layer (Fig. 3–18). Chemically, both the outer and inner layers are composed of approximately 70 percent protein. The middle (hydrophobic) layer contains 30 percent lipid in addition to fatty acids, phospholipids and transmembrane proteins (e.g., permeases). The polar or hydrophilic head groups of the phospholipids are located at the outer surface of the hydrophobic region of the membrane, with the hydrophobic fatty acid "tails" extending into the central region of the membrane. The structural and permease proteins traverse the hydrophobic region. The nature of these transmembrane proteins, as well as the fact that the individual lipids within the membrane leaflets are free to exchange with each other within the leaflets, has resulted in the concept of the fluid mosaic model for biologic membranes (Fig. 3–19). This model describes a highly stable, "plastic" membrane capable of adjusting to changes in both temperature and nutritional conditions.

In summary, functionally, the cytoplasmic membrane is one of the most important components of the bacterial cell, in fact, of all cells. Without a functional cytoplasmic membrane the cell would not survive—it is the site of anabolic and catabolic metabolism and regulates the transport of molecules into and out of the cell.

The Cytoplasm and Its Inclusions

The bacterial cytoplasm consists of a central nuclear region surrounded by ribosomes mixed in a "sea" of enzymes, cofactors, amino acids, and vitamins, as well as a multitude of other ions and molecules (Figs. 3–1A; 3–8B through E; 3–9A,

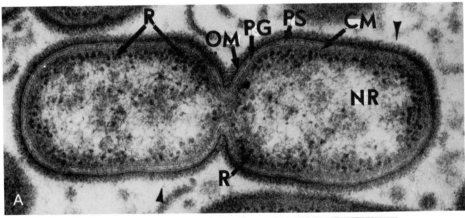

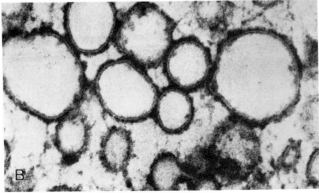

FIGURE 3–17 ✦ Electron photomicrographs of whole cells **(A)** of the gram-negative bacterium *Porphyromonas gingivalis,* and **(B)** isolated outer membrane. *Arrows* point to the thick capsule. R = ribosomes; OM = outer membrane; PG = peptidoglycan; PS = periplasmic space; CM = cytoplasmic membrane; NR = nuclear region.

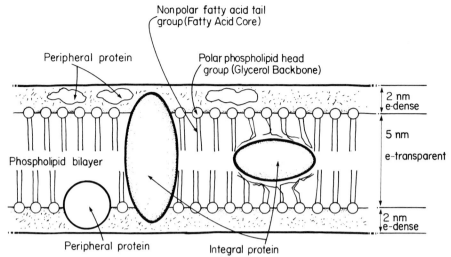

FIGURE 3–18 ✦ Diagrammatic representation of a classic unit membrane. The membrane consists of a "sandwich" of hydrophilic protein, which encloses a hydrophobic lipid layer. Proteins exist in the peripheral region of the membrane as well as traversing the membrane. The integral proteins function to transport material from the outside to the inside of the cell as well as providing structural integrity. The phospholipid head groups are embedded in the protein layers, and the fatty acid tails extend into the central region of the membrane.

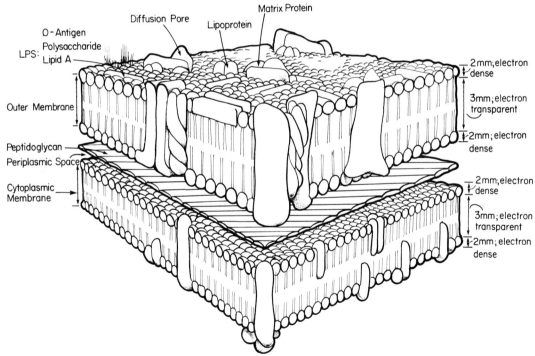

FIGURE 3–19 ✦ Three-dimensional representation of the cell envelope of a gram-negative bacterium. The cell envelope consists of a thick outer membrane, an intermediate peptido-glycan layer, and the underlying cytoplasmic membrane. Both the cytoplasmic membrane and the outer membrane are of unit construction (see Fig. 3–18). Diffusion pores, lipoprotein, and matrix proteins emerge from the surface of the membrane. Also, the O-antigen of the lipopolysaccharide emerges from the outer membrane surface as thin hairlike structures. Lipid A of the lipopolysaccharide is embedded in the outer membrane.

B; 3–10; and 3–17A). These serve as building blocks for cellular biosynthesis and energy production. The cytoplasm also contains the various RNAs and storage granules that are formed in response to the cells' chemical and physical environment.

RIBOSOMES

The ribosome is the most abundant inclusion in the bacterial cytoplasm (see Figs. 3–1A; 3–8B through E; 3–9A, B; and 3–17A). It consists of approximately 40 percent protein and 60 percent RNA. Its exclusive function is protein synthesis. The eukaryotic ribosome is larger than the bacterial ribosome. Three types of RNA exist: ribosomal RNA (rRNA), amino acid transfer RNA (tRNA), and messenger RNA (mRNA). (The reader is referred to a recent textbook of biochemistry for a description of the role of these RNA molecules in protein synthesis, as well as to pages 89 to 95 of this chapter.)

NUCLEAR REGION AND NUCLEAR ELEMENTS

Bacteria contain a nonmembrane-bound region equivalent to the eukaryotic nucleus. This fibrous region of the bacterial cell was determined to be the nucleus or nucleoid because of its non–membrane bound character (see Figs. 3–1A; 3–8B through E; 3–9A, B; 3–10; and 3–17A). The bacterial genetic material, or genome, is arranged in a linear fashion along a long circular DNA strand. This DNA strand, if laid open, would stretch almost 1400 μm (remember, the average bacterium is approximately 1 μm in diameter!). The molecular weight, or mass, of the bacterial genome varies over a wide range; for example, *Mycoplasma* species have a relatively small genome of from 0.45 to 1.1×10^9 daltons (1.2×10^6 bases, or 1000 genes), and the gram-positive cocci and rods, as well as gram-negative bacteria (i.e., *Escherichia coli* and *Bacteroides*), have very large genomes on the order of 2.8×10^9 daltons (4.2×10^9 bases, or approximately 3000 genes).

While the nuclear region contains the genetic material of the cell, many bacteria also contain DNA molecules outside the nuclear region. These small, extrachromosomal DNAs with molecular masses between 1 and 113×10^6 daltons, are referred to as *plasmids*. The plasmids are self-replicating, small, circular DNA molecules. Plasmids typically contain approximately 0.1 to 0.2 percent

TABLE 3–3 ✦ Prokaryotic Inclusions

INCLUSION	MEMBRANE-LIMITED*	SHAPE	FORMED IN PRESENCE OF	FUNCTION
Polyglycoside	−	Sphere-rod	Excess C; limiting N, S, P; cell age	Carbohydrate storage
Polyphosphate	−	Sphere	Excess PO_4	Phosphate storage
Cyanopcin	−	Undulating flattened sac	Limiting essential nutrients, N-fixation	N-reserve during N-fixation
Phycobilisome	−	Sphere-rod	Light energy receptors	Receptors of light-energy chlorophyll
Poly B-hydroxybutyrate	+	Sphere	Excess glucose or acetate	Energy and C-storage
Sulfur	+	Sphere-globular subunits	Growth in presence of H_2S	Sulfur oxidation when H_2S becomes limiting
Gas vacuole	+	Stacks-hollow cylinders with conical ends		Movement of cells in vertical plane
Carboxysome	+	Spheres, polyhedral particles paracrystalline	Ribulose-1-5-diphosphate carboxylase	CO_2-fixation
Chlorosome	+	Oblong vesicles	Light—contains chlorophyll	Storage of chlorophyll for photosynthesis
Magnetosome	+	Linear array cuboidal particles	Contains Fe_3O_4 or magnetite (lodestone)	Orientation in magnetic field

*Membrane usually consists of one-half unit membrane, 3 to 4 nm thick.

of the DNA of the cell's chromosome. While plasmids are not essential for survival of the bacterial cell, they do carry a variety of important genetic functions.

BACTERIAL STORAGE GRANULES AND INCLUSIONS

During their growth and metabolism, bacteria accumulate a variety of cytoplasmic storage products (Fig. 3–20; Table 3–3) as a result of the environment and metabolism by the cell of the large number of carbohydrates, lipids, and proteins. These inclusions include both membrane-limited and non–membrane-limited structures (Table 3–3).

GROWTH AND DIVISION

For cells to perpetuate themselves, they must grow—that is, increase in mass and size in an orderly fashion—and reproduce or divide. During physical cell separation, it must also separate all of its cellular components including RNA, DNA, and membranes into equal parts to be shared among the daughter progeny. For successful growth, division, and survival, the individual cellular components must increase prior to cell division. The cells' metabolic and biosynthetic constituents must also increase in an orderly series of events. All of these events are predetermined by the cells' genetic information. When all of these events have taken place and the cell reaches a genetically predetermined size and volume, it divides into two identical copies of itself. By definition then, *growth* is the orderly increase or synthesis of all cellular constituents from extracellular nutrients, the ultimate result of this increase being division or replication.

Transverse or Binary Cell Division

Growth of bacteria can be separated into two distinct stages: an increase in cell mass such as

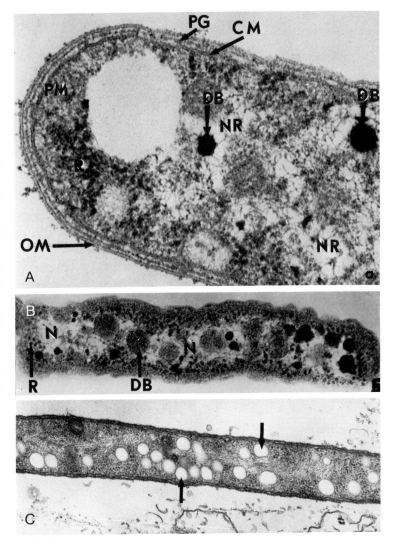

FIGURE 3–20 ✦ Electron photomicrographs of various bacterial inclusions. **A** and **B**, The small, dense, spherical bodies or dense bodies (DB) are probably polyphosphate. Note their proximity to the fibrous nucleoid (N). In **B**, the cytoplasmic region also contains electron dense ribosomes (R), and storage granules of unknown chemistry and function. **C**, Electron transparent storage granules *(arrows)* traverse the cytoplasmic region. Note that these structures are surrounded by a thin layer. R = ribosomes; OM = outer membrane; PG = peptidoglycan; CM = cytoplasmic membrane.

elongation of a bacillus, or an increase in size or volume such as in a coccus; and the division of these cells into two new daughter cells. While various modes of cell division occur in prokaryotic cells (Fig. 3–21), the most common mechanism of bacterial cell division then can be described as a binary or transverse division, or **binary fission** (Figs. 3–21 and 3–22). With only minor special differences, the majority of gram-positive and gram-negative bacteria divide in an identical fashion. Ideally, bacterial binary fission consists of at least three steps (Fig. 3–22):

1. During the initial growth or division period, bacilli increase in both length and volume, while cocci increase in volume. The nuclear material separates into two approximately equal halves, with one of the nuclear segments being attached to the cytoplasmic membrane.

2. Late in this initial division period, division septa or cross-walls develop. The septum routinely forms at the approximate center of the dividing cell as a result of the ingrowth of the cell wall. Septum formation at the approximate center of the cell is common among rods and bacilli. While gram-negative bacteria were originally thought to have a "constrictive division" (a pinching of the central region of the cell to form two identical daughter cells), the outer membrane actually is maintained as a rigid layer, with septum formation occurring as an ingrowth of the cytoplasmic membrane and peptidoglycan. Therefore, the completed septum consists of two "lamellae" of peptidoglycan that are separated by a gap.

3. In gram-positive bacteria, cell separation or binary fission occurs as the result of hydrolytic cleavage of the ingrowing peptidoglycan by specific hydrolytic enzymes, or amidases, while in gram-negative bacteria cell separation occurs by the ingrowth of the outer membrane after septum formation has been completed. This ingrowth of the outer membrane results in the physical separation of the cells into two identical daughter cells.

Other Mechanisms of Bacterial Cell Division

Bacteria such as *Hyphomicrobium, Corynebacterium,* and *Mycobacterium* divide by *budding,* a process very similar to that seen in fungi and budding yeast cells. The budding cell originates as an outgrowth of the original, or mother cell, which eventually reaches a size equal to that of the mother cell. The bud then separates to undertake an independent existence. Several of the *Actinomycetes* form filamentous cells that reproduce by the formation of spores from a chain of cells, or by a simple fragmentation of the original filament into "new" cells.

Growth and Enumeration of Bacteria

Bacterial growth, or multiplication, is measured by determining increases in cell numbers as a function of time. There are several methods for the study of bacterial growth (Table 3–4), and the reader is referred to any standard microbiology textbook for a complete description of the techniques for the measurement of this growth.

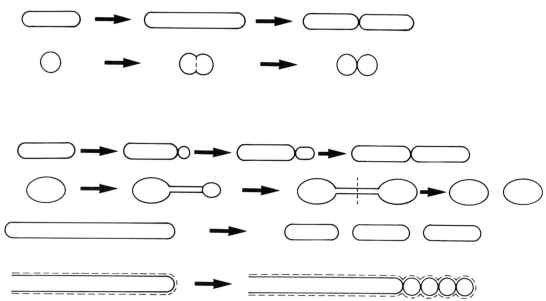

FIGURE 3–21 ✦ Diagrammatic representation of various modes of bacterial cell division. The cells routinely divide by transverse binary fission. Several cells also form budlike structures from the terminal portions of the cell.

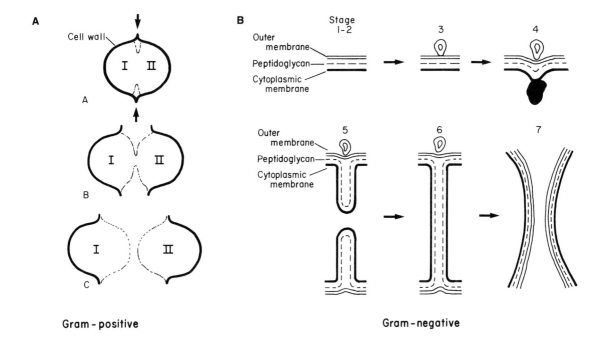

SEPTUM FORMATION

FIGURE 3−22 ✦ Diagrammatic representation of septum formation and cell division in gram-positive and gram-negative bacteria. In gram-positive division **(A)** the cell wall is seen to grow into the cell as a septum until cell division is completed. In contrast, gram-negative septum formation **(B)**, involves the constriction of the outer membrane, peptidoglycan as well as cytoplasmic membrane. The septum ingrows forming a division plane, at which time it separates to form a new outer membrane and two daughter cells. (Adapted from Burdett, I. D., and Murray, R. G.: J. Bacteriol. 119:1029, 1974.)

Mathematics of Bacterial Growth

Consider a bacterial culture growing under optimal conditions of nutrients, temperature, pH, and atmospheric conditions where all of the cells within this bacterial population are alive—that is, viable—and that they are dividing by transverse binary fission. Under these conditions, the cells in the culture are dividing at a constant and geometric rate in an exponential fashion. Thus, one cell in this culture will give rise to two cells, two to four, four to eight, and so forth. This binary series (1, 2, 4, 8, 16, 32, 64, . . .) defines exponential growth. Clearly, cells growing in this way will increase in number at a very rapid rate and will produce very large populations of cells (10^7 to 10^{11} cells per ml). This binary increase in the bacterial cell number is referred to as the *doubling time*, or *generation time*, and is defined as the time required for the cell or cells to divide, or to double itself.

The generation time can be expressed mathematically. If at specified times (i.e., 20-minute intervals) after inoculation, a sample is removed from the culture and the number of viable cells determined, one could determine the generation time. For example, if at zero time and at 20-minute intervals thereafter, the viability of the culture was determined to be 100, 200, 400, 800, 1600, and 3200 cells, the generation or doubling time would be 20 minutes. The bacterial population would also be increasing by one exponent, 2^n. Figure 3−23 plots the increase in cell number both arithmetically and in logarithmic notation. Note that by plotting the logarithms of the cell number, one can plot on one graph the results of a very large increase in cell numbers. Fortunately, cells do not grow exponentially for very long periods of time, but eventually fall prey to the vagaries of the environment (see further on). This is very important since a bacterium with a generation time of approximately 20 minutes would produce 2.2×10^{43} cells in 48 hours weighing 2.5×10^{25} tons, or almost 4000 times the mass of the earth!

The Bacterial Growth Curve

What occurs when bacteria are inoculated into a suitable growth medium and provided with all appropriate requirements for maximum growth and

TABLE 3–4 ✦ **Representative Procedure for Determining Bacterial Growth**

TECHNIQUE	APPLICATION	RESULTANT DETERMINATION
Microscopic count	Enumeration of total bacterial number	Number of cells
Electronic count	Same as for microscopic count	As for microscopic count
Plate count	Enumeration of viable bacteria in culture	Colony-forming units
Membrane filter count	As plate count	As plate count
Absorbance	Microbiologic assay. Estimation of cell increase in broth, cultures, or aqueous suspensions.	Optical density
Nitrogen determination	Measurement of cell mass	Units of nitrogen
Dry weight determination	Same as for nitrogen determination	Units of dry weight of cells
Measurements of specific biochemical parameter	Microbiologic assays	Milliequivalents of acid per ml or per culture

Modified from Pelczar, M. J., Jr., Chan, B. C. S., and Krieg, N. R.: Microbiology, ed. 5. McGraw-Hill Book Co., New York, 1986, with permission of McGraw-Hill.

division? If culture samples are taken periodically as described earlier, and either the increase in optical density (turbidity) or any other cell component is plotted as a function of time, then the result seen in Figure 3–24 occurs, which is typical of the growth of essentially all eukaryotic and prokaryotic cell populations and is referred to as the *growth curve*. The growth of cells can be divided into at least four segments or growth phases: the *lag phase*, when there is no increase in cell number; the *logarithmic* or *exponential phase*, when the cells are dividing at a constant rate per unit time; the *stationary phase*, when maximum cell numbers are reached and the cell population stops active growth; and the *death* or *decline phase*, when the number of viable cells decreases, usually at an exponential rate.

LAG PHASE

This phase of growth occurs when cells are transferred from one medium to another or from one environment to another. It is a phase of adjustment and represents the period required for the adaptation of the cells to the new environment. The cells in this phase often increase in total cell volume almost two- or threefold, but they do not divide. These cells are rapidly synthesizing DNA, new protein, and new enzymes as a prerequisite to division.

EXPONENTIAL PHASE

In this phase, cells are dividing at both a constant geometric rate, as well as at a maximum rate. Cellular components such as RNA, protein, dry weight, and cell wall polymers are also increasing at a constant rate. Because the cells in the exponential phase are dividing at this maximum rate, they are much smaller in diameter than cells in the lag phase.

The exponential growth phase usually comes to an end because of the depletion of essential nutrients, the depletion of oxygen in an aerobic culture, or the accumulation of toxic products.

STATIONARY PHASE

During this phase, there is a rapid decrease in the rate of cell division. Eventually, the total number of dividing cells will equal the number of dying

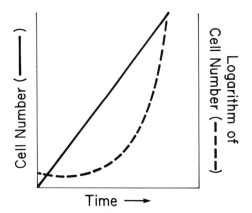

FIGURE 3–23 ✦ Mathematical representation of bacterial growth. (- - -) = logarithm of number of bacteria versus time; (—) = arithmetic number of bacteria versus time. Generation time is determined from exponential curve and equals the time required for the culture to double.

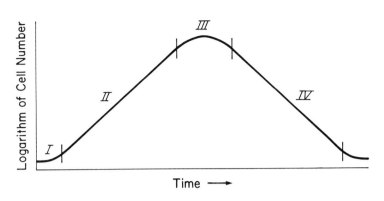

FIGURE 3–24 ✦ Typical bacterial growth curve. The various growth phases are I, Lag phase; II, Log (logarithmic), or exponential phase; III, Stationary phase; IV, Death or decline phase.

cells, and a true stationary cell population occurs. The cells then direct their resources toward survival. Energy generation is harnessed to maintain osmotic barriers, motility, and the repair and resynthesis of essential macromolecules. The energy required to maintain cells in the stationary phase is called the *maintenance energy* and is obtained from the degradation of cellular storage products (i.e., glycogen, starch, lipids). After all of the storage products are exhausted, the cells then degrade their own cellular components, which ultimately leads to the death phase.

DEATH PHASE

As conditions become increasingly inimical, the cells reproduce more slowly, and death overtakes them in increasing numbers. The cells eventually enter the logarithmic death phase, during which the decrease in the number of viable cells occurs at a regular, unchanging rate, a rate that approximates that of the exponential growth phase but is of negative slope.

Finally, the rate of cell death and the increase in cell numbers tend to balance each other at a very low population level, and a phase of readjustment and final dormant phase are reached. The cells can exist in this condition for weeks or months, and complete sterility of the culture may not occur for a considerable length of time.

PHYSIOLOGY AND METABOLISM

Cell growth and division require that the environment provide all the chemical constituents required for metabolism and the generation of energy (i.e., ATP; see page 73). The specific requirements are dependent on the genetic make-up of the particular bacterial species. Some species with diverse nutritional flexibility (i.e., *Pseudomonas*) are capable of synthesizing many of their metabolites from simple precursors, whereas others are more demanding (i.e., *Bacteroides*, *Treponema*, and

Porphyromonas) and require the input of more complex nutrients for growth and reproduction.

For purposes of this discussion of bacterial physiology, we assume the reader has some familiarity with the basic metabolic pathways for the utilization of sugars, amino acids, and lipids, as well as for the generation of energy by electron transport and anaerobic respiration.

Carbohydrate Utilization

The physiology of a cell can be considered under the general heading of *metabolism,* a process that denotes the chemical changes occurring in living cells. Metabolism can be divided into catabolism and anabolism, two interdependent processes.

Catabolism is the degradation (breakdown) of chemical compounds (substrates) into their constituent atoms, molecules, or molecular groups. Catabolism also includes the formation of the necessary energy for the cell to carry out its macromolecular syntheses (i.e., cell wall formation, protein synthesis), as well as all of the other activities required of growing and metabolizing cells (motility, reproduction, taxis).

Anabolism is the conversion or synthesis of catabolically generated carbon skeletons into the macromolecules that constitute the physical and chemical make-up of the cell. It comprises all of the cell-building activities of the cell. Anabolic events occur to constantly replace cellular constituents that either have been used by the cell or need to be replaced.

Basic Nutritional Requirements

The basic constituents of all cells are water, solids, and trace elements, with water accounting for 80 to 90 percent of the total cell weight. For a cell to grow, it must either obtain from the environment or synthesize itself, all required basic cellular constituents. For example, oxygen and hydrogen are obtained from the hydrolysis of water, while essential carbon, nitrogen, phosphorus, and other essential elements are provided from the environment (i.e., from the growth medium). Trace elements, such as magnesium (Mg), calcium (Ca), iron (Fe), manganese (Mn), and others, which are essential for a multitude of enzymatic cellular reactions, are usually supplied from **trace elements** in the water, growth vessels, etc.

Carbon, the essential structural cellular element, is provided either by the dark reactions of photosynthesis through the Calvin cycle and the oxidation (loss of electrons or hydrogen) of inorganic carbon compounds, such as CO_2, or by the oxidation of organic compounds. Both mechanisms not only generate the needed carbon for the growth of the cell, but also generate a large amount of the energy. Nitrogen, required for protein synthesis, is usually supplied from amino acids as well as from the degradation of proteins in peptones or tryptones, which are constituents of many bacterial growth media. Several bacteria can utilize nitrogen in the form of NO_3^-, which is reduced to NH_3, and then used in biosynthetic reactions. Some bacteria utilize atmospheric dinitrogen (nitrogen fixation) from the atmosphere and reduce it to NH_3.

Sulfur, another important element, is usually supplied by direct metabolism of the sulfur-containing amino acids. For example, the sulfhydryl group ($-SH$) of methionine or cysteine is released by the oxidation of the amino acid with the formation of sulfate ($SO_4^=$), which like NO_3^- can be reduced to H_2S (or NH_3). The H_2S (NH_3) can then be used in further amino acid biosynthesis.

Autotrophs and Heterotrophs

Bacteria can be divided into two broad metabolic groups on the basis of their distinctive nutritional requirements: heterotrophs or organotrophs that use organic compounds as a source of electrons and autotrophs or lithotrophs that use an inorganic electron source. It also is possible to categorize bacteria in terms of the source of electrons in energy generation for ATP synthesis. Thus, photoautotrophs utilize light as an inorganic electron donor, while chemoautotrophs utilize inorganic molecules as sources of energy and electrons.

Sources of Energy

To survive, all organisms must have an energy source such as solar energy (phototrophs) and chemical energy (chemotrophs). Among the large number of metabolically diverse bacteria, there also is a great diversity in chemotrophic energy metabolism. The three major mechanisms of energy generation in bacteria are respiration, fermentation, and anaerobic respiration. Aerobic bacteria use oxygen as a terminal electron acceptor, reduce it to water, and, in this process of *aerobic respiration,* form large amounts of energy as ATP (adenosine triphosphate). The oxidation of organic compounds (i.e., sugars) by respiratory means provides an enormous number and variety of bacteria with their ATP. Some bacteria are capable of using organic compounds in the complete absence of oxygen, that is, under anaerobic conditions. This metabolic process, *fermentation,* produces not only ATP but also a variety of organic end products (i.e., alcohol from glucose in the yeast fermentation, or lactic acid in streptococci, depending on the fermentative pathway used). Other bacteria also are capable of obtaining energy while growing anaerobically if using inorganic molecules such as NO_3^- or $SO_4^=$ as electron acceptors in the absence of oxygen. This anaerobic process of energy generation is referred to as *anaerobic respiration.*

METABOLISM AND BIOSYNTHESIS

From this brief introduction to the nutrition of bacteria, it should be clear that prokaryotic cells have a diverse ability to metabolize an extraordinarily large number of organic and inorganic compounds. In fact, it is probably correct to assume that for essentially every natural compound in our environment, as well as for many manufactured compounds, there is a microorganism that can metabolize it. The metabolism of all of these compounds serves one purpose—to provide the cell with the necessary carbon and energy for growth and reproduction. Even with this remarkable diversity in metabolism, there is a surprising degree of unity of the biochemical mechanisms for the overall metabolic processes. Therefore, no matter what the organism, the same building materials and essentially identical metabolic mechanisms exist—truly a "unity of biochemistry."

Energy Requirements of Bacteria

The formation of simple compounds or complex macromolecules require energy; that is, they are endergonic reactions. The energy required to chemically "drive" these biosynthetic processes is routinely provided to the cell as ATP. ATP is the major energy currency of cells and is formed by a variety of catabolic reactions that are not only capable of producing this unique molecule but importantly, transferring it to other energy-yielding exergonic reactions. It is the coupling of endergonic reactions with exergonic ones that permits the multitude of chemical reactions to proceed and the cell to grow and synthesize its numerous macromolecular components.

ATP FORMATION

The production of ATP is a function of the degree to which any organic compound is degraded; in fact, all energy-yielding reactions are the result of aerobic and anaerobic oxidation reactions. *In all cases, however, it is the production of ATP in exergonic reactions and its transfer and use in endergonic reactions that link metabolism into a unified process.*

How is ATP produced in biologic reactions of a bacterial cell? For the most part, the oxidation reactions required for the generation of ATP result from a series of interdependent electron transfer reactions in which electrons are reversibly oxidized and reduced. These reactions constitute the electron transfer chain (see page 75 for an in-depth discussion of electron transport). At specific points along this electron transfer chain, energy as ATP is produced (Fig. 3–25A). The aerobic generation of ATP through this electron transport chain is referred to as *oxidative phosphorylation* (see further on for more discussion). Note in Figure 3–25A that simple examination of the electron transport chain does not provide any useful information as to how the passage of electrons through this series of electron carriers is capable of producing energy as ATP. Peter Mitchell in 1961 provided the most plausible hypothesis for how ATP generation could occur when electrons flow through the electron transport system (Fig. 3–25B). He proposed the *chemiosmotic hypothesis (proton motive force potential),* in which ATP was formed by a change in electrical potential between the outside and inside of a membrane-bound organelle such as the eukaryotic mitochondrion or chloroplast or the prokaryotic cytoplasmic membrane. The flow of electrons through the electron transport system functions to release energy in such a way as to push positively charged hydrogen ions (i.e., H^+, protons) across the boundaries of the membrane. In the process of this proton flow there is the production of both a pH gradient and an electrical potential gradient because of the positive charge carried by the proton. The flow of hydrogen ions back across the membrane results in the production of ATP through this **proton motive force potential.** The flow of these electrons at specific sites within the membrane, known as the *ATPase enzyme complex,* results in the production of ATP.

Embden-Meyerhof-Parnas Pathway — Glycolysis

Bacteria, as well as many animals and some plants, metabolize or degrade carbohydrates such as starch, cellulose, dextrans, levans, glycogen, sucrose, and lactose, to pyruvic acid (pyruvate). This degradation is routinely carried out by the Embden-Meyerhof-Parnas (EMP) glycolysis, or glycolytic, pathway (Fig. 3–26). Both humans and bacteria have common intermediates to pyruvic acid, and beyond pyruvate, metabolic specialization occurs. For example, pyruvate is metabolized to lactic acid in muscle glycolysis of humans while in yeasts, the pyruvate is converted to CO_2 and acetaldehyde, with the latter being converted to ethanol in yeast fermentation. These latter reactions constitute the **alcoholic fermentation.** Note that while ATP is required for the carbohydrate (i.e., glucose) to enter the pathway, it must first be "activated" by being phosphorylated. The result is a net gain of two ATPs per mole of glucose degraded. Notice that the electron transfer molecule, pyridine nucleotide in its oxidized form (nicotinic acid adenine dinucleotide, NAD^+), which is reduced ($NADH_2$) in the upper portion of the EMP pathway, is reoxidized ($NADH + H^+ \rightarrow NAD^+$) in the conversion of pyruvate to reduced end products. It is essential that reduced pyridine nucleotide be regenerated so that the EMP pathway continues to function in the utilization of carbohydrates.

In the EMP pathway, glucose is first phosphorylated to produce an activated glucose-6-phosphate, which is ultimately split into two trioses, glyceraldehyde-3-phosphate (three-carbon units), which are subsequently oxidized to pyruvate. The oxidation of glyceraldehyde-3-phosphate results in the release of a pair of electrons (two H atoms), which under anaerobic conditions reduce the pyruvate to lactic acid or ethanol (Fig. 3–26). Under aerobic conditions, the electrons enter the respiratory chain (see Fig. 3–25A and below).

Respiration

While the EMP pathway is the central pathway for carbohydrate metabolism, the conversion of glucose to pyruvic acid can be considered in reality to be an anaerobic process in that it can occur either in the presence or in the absence of oxygen. However, the majority of eukaryotes and prokaryotes (as well as humans) do not live in an anaerobic environment, and the carbohydrate that is metabolized to pyruvate in glycolysis is usually metabolized further under aerobic mechanisms involving oxygen. Thus, in humans and in higher animals, although lactic acid is produced from the reduction of pyruvate by NADH (for the regeneration of NAD for further glycolysis), it is not the final end product. Instead, lactic acid is partly converted to the storage product, glycogen, and a portion of it is completely oxidized to CO_2 and water. This latter oxidation is the result of the process of **aerobic respiration** and is accomplished by the further oxidation of pyruvate through the **tricarboxylic acid cycle** (Krebs cycle, TCA cycle, citric acid cycle).

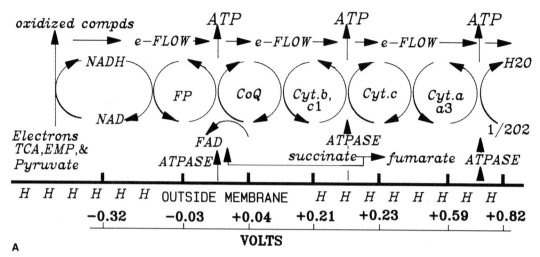

oxidized compds

ATP   ATP   ATP

e—FLOW   e—FLOW   e—FLOW   H2O

NADH

FP   CoQ   Cyt.b,   Cyt.c   Cyt.a
                c1   a3

NAD

1/2O2

Electrons
TCA,EMP,&
Pyruvate

FAD   ATPASE

ATPASE   succinate   fumarate   ATPASE

H H H H H H   OUTSIDE MEMBRANE   H H H H H H H H

−0.32   −0.03   +0.04   +0.21   +0.23   +0.59   +0.82

VOLTS

A

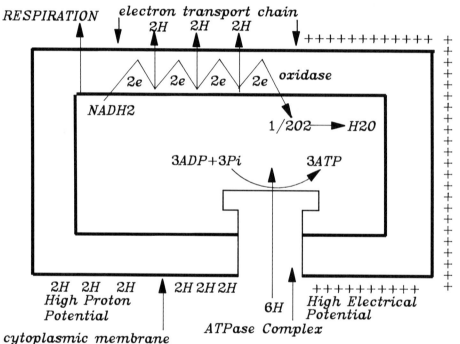

RESPIRATION   electron transport chain
            2H   2H   2H
                                    +++++++++++ +
2e   2e   2e   2e   oxidase

NADH2

1/2O2 ⟶ H2O

3ADP+3Pi   3ATP

2H 2H   2H   2H 2H 2H   ++++++++++ +
High Proton   High Electrical
Potential   6H   Potential
        ATPase Complex

B *cytoplasmic membrane*

FIGURE 3–25 ✦ A, Electron transport system (ETS) produces ATP by oxidative phosphory-lation. Electrons from various electron generating cycles (TCA, EMP, pyruvate), are passed to NAD^+ and then to the electron acceptors such as flavoprotein (FP), coenzyme Q (CoQ), cytochromes b and c_1, cytochrome c, and cytochromes a and a_3. Each electron acceptor is reduced and reoxidized when it passes the electrons on to the next acceptor. Oxygen is ultimately reduced to form water in aerobic respiration; NO_3^-, and $SO_4^=$ are reduced to NH_3, and H_2S, respectively, in anaerobic respiration. Flow of electrons through ETS results in high H-ion concentration outside cytoplasmic membrane, and low concentration inside. The re-sultant pH and electrochemical gradient results in H ions being drawn back into the cell at ATPase sites in the membrane. The electrons that are transported down this voltage gradient liberate their energy, with the resultant formation of ATP at ATPase sites (see also Fig. 3–28B). **B,** Diagrammatic representation of the Mitchell or chemiosmotic hypothesis of energy generation. Electrons and protons (a hydrogen atom), which are generated by fatty acid and carbohydrate oxidation (i.e., respiration; see Fig. 3–28), are carried by electron carriers to an electron acceptor (i.e., O_2, NO_3^-, $SO_4^=$), which is reduced. The transport of electrons across the membrane results in the transport of protons to the outside of the membrane. This electron flow produces both a proton gradient and a gradient in electric potential, which functions to push protons back across the membrane at specific sites (ATPase complex) where ATP is generated by the process of oxidative phosphorylation.

Tricarboxylic Acid Cycle—Citric Acid Cycle

The TCA cycle (Fig. 3–27) is a true cycle (compared with the EMP pathway), in that the end product of the cycle, oxalacetic acid, is regenerated so as to react continuously with the acetyl-CoA that is supplied from glycolysis. Citric acid, the result of the condensation of oxalacetic acid and acetyl-CoA, are considered to be the start of the cycle. The energy-rich acetyl-coenzyme-A (acetyl-CoA) is formed from pyruvate by an activation with coenzyme A. The citric acid is converted in a true cyclic fashion to a series of important intermediates, which can be used in a variety of other essential biosynthetic reactions. Therefore, the TCA cycle can be considered to be an **amphibolic cycle,** in that it functions in both catabolic as well as anabolic reactions. Basically, then, the TCA cycle has two major functions: (1) to supply carbon skeletons for cell structure and (2) to generate large numbers of

electrons. It is these electrons that enter the aerobic or anaerobic **electron transport system** (Figs. 3–25A, 3–28) and are used for the generation of ATP.

Electron Transport Chain—Cytochrome Pathway

The electron transport system exists in the eukaryotic mitochondrion and in the cytoplasmic membrane of prokaryotes. Its primary function is the transfer of the electrons generated in the TCA cycle by a reversible series of oxidation-reduction reactions involving specific enzymes and cofactors. These enzymes and cofactors function as an internal oxidation/reduction system, transferring electrons in stepwise fashion through the electron transport chain to an ultimate electron acceptor: oxygen in aerobic respiration (Fig. 3–25A) and an inorganic molecule (NO_3^- or $SO_4^=$) in anaerobic respiration (Fig. 3–28). Several important enzymes

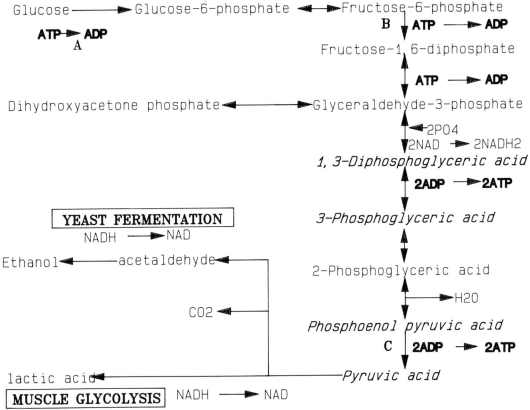

FIGURE 3–26 ✦ The Embden-Meyerhof-Parnas (glycolytic) pathway of glucose catabolism. Enyzmes (A, B, C) are for those steps which are not freely reversible. In the absence of oxygen, there is the formation of lactic acid (muscle) or CO_2 plus ethanol in the yeast (alcoholic) fermentation. Pyruvic acid is also the central compound in the formation of a large number of dissimilatory end-products of carbohydrates (see p. 80). The reactions of substrate-level phosphorylation are described in boldface italics. A = Hexokinase (glucose-6-phosphatase). B = Phosphofructokinase (fructose-1,6-diphosphatase). C = Pyruvate kinase (phosphoenol pyruvate synthase).

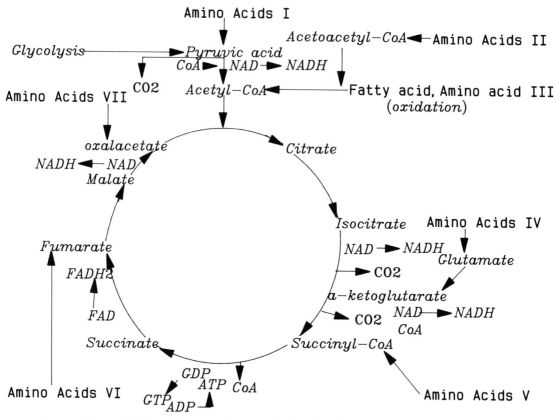

FIGURE 3–27 ✦ The Krebs (tricarboxylic acid) cycle oxidizes pyruvic acid to three CO_2 molecules and transfers electrons to NAD^+ or FAD. The GTP formed is the only high-energy triphosphate formed directly. The four-carbon oxaloacetic acid is regenerated and can start another cycle by picking up another molecule of acetyl-CoA. The nucleotide reactions function to transfer electrons to the electron transport chain. Amino acids and fatty acids are oxidized at various points in the cycle. The CO_2 generated is utilized in CO_2-fixation via the Calvin cycle (see Fig. 3–36). Amino acids I, ala, cyst, gly, ser, threo; II, ala, tyros, leu, lys, trypt; III, isoleu, leu, trypt; IV, arg, hist, gluNH$_2$, prol; V, isoleu, met, val; VI, tyr, ala; VII, asp.ac, aspNH$_2$.

are involved in the initial steps of electron transport. These enzymes are the dehydrogenases, which have NAD or NADP (a phosphorylated pyridine nucleotide) as their coenzyme. A second dehydrogenase, the flavoproteins, is linked to NAD in the respiratory chain. These flavoproteins contain either flavin adenine dinucleotide (FAD) or its mononucleotide (FMN) as their prosthetic group. The vitamin, riboflavin, is the major part of the coenzyme, and it functions in the reversible transfer of electron pairs through the chain. The third enzyme in the electron transport system is the coenzyme, coenzyme Q, or ubiquinone, so named because of its ubiquitous nature in all cells. The other major class of oxidation/reduction compounds in the electron transport chain is the cytochromes (Fig. 3–29). The cytochromes are heme or iron (Fe) derivatives, which contain a single Fe atom. It is the Fe atom that is reversibly oxidized and

reduced by the passage of an electron through the chain. Interestingly, the initial electron transfer compounds, NAD, FAD, and coenzyme Q of the electron transport chain, all function in the transfer of two hydrogen atoms (i.e., $2H^+ + 2e^-$), while the cytochromes transfer only electrons. The proton portion of the hydrogen atom is associated with $-NH_2$ groups or $-COOH$ groups; however, they are also transferred to oxygen. The terminal cytochrome, cytochrome oxidase (cytochrome a/a$_3$) contains copper; however, it is only cytochrome a$_3$ that reacts with oxygen to produce water in aerobic respiration; NO_3^- or $SO_4^=$ produces NH_3 or H_2S, respectively, in anaerobic respiration (Fig. 3–28). Thus, the electron transport chain permits the flow of electrons (a pair of electrons or hydrogen atoms), resulting in a stepwise release of energy, a portion of which is conserved as ATP. Remember, ATP is formed by way of proton motive force (see page

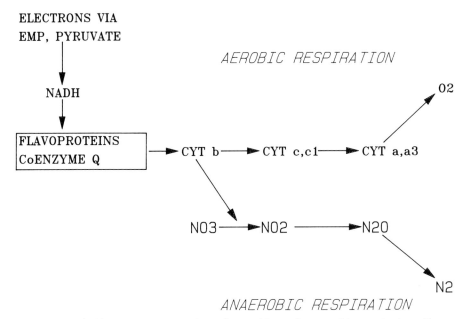

ELECTRONS VIA
EMP, PYRUVATE

AEROBIC RESPIRATION

NADH

FLAVOPROTEINS
CoENZYME Q ⟶ CYT b ⟶ CYT c,c1 ⟶ CYT a,a3 ⟶ O2

NO3 ⟶ NO2 ⟶ N2O ⟶ N2

ANAEROBIC RESPIRATION

FIGURE 3–28 ✦ Electron transport through aerobic and anaerobic respiration. Electrons generated from glycolysis pyruvate, TCA, are transferred to nucleotides and flavoproteins to the electron transport cytochromes. In aerobic respiration (see also Fig. 3–25), the electrons are passed to oxygen to form water, or are passed via anaerobic respiration to NO_3^- or $SO_4^=$ to generate N_2, NH_3, or H_2S.

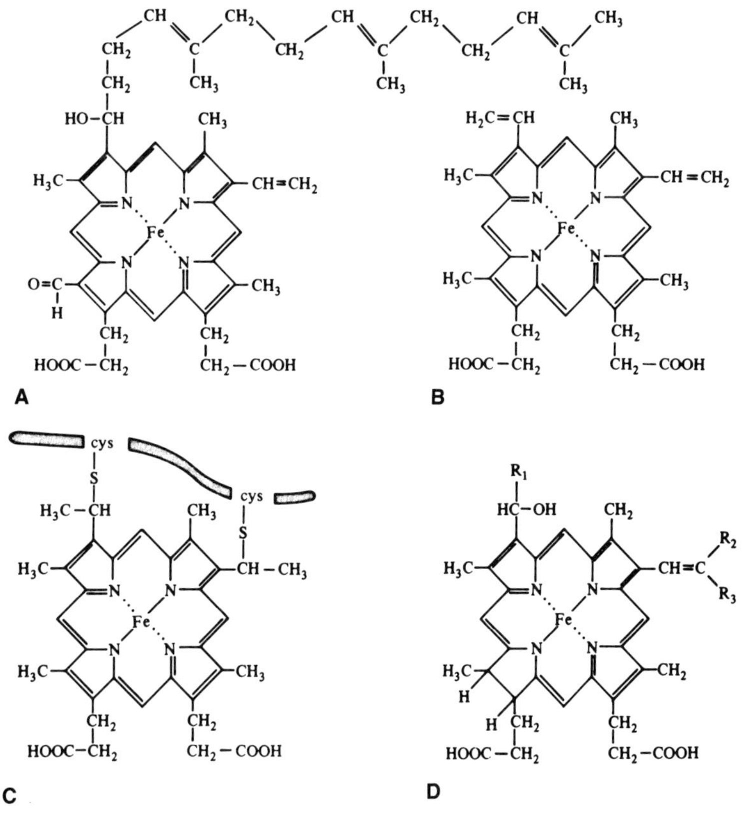

FIGURE 3–29 ✦ The basic structure of various types of cytochromes showing their specific prosthetic groups. In the a-type cytochrome **(A)** the cytochromes contain a formyl group as the side chain. In **B**, the b-type cytochrome, the prosthetic group is a heme. In the c-type cytochrome **(C)** the prosthetic group is linked to a protein by way of cysteine (cys) bridges. In **D**, the d-type cytochrome has as its prosthetic group a derivative of dihydroporphyrin. (From Gottschalk: Bacterial Metabolism, ed. 2, Springer Verlag, New York, 1986, with permission.)

A

B

C

D

73), in which proton and electrical gradients are established so that there is a flow of electrons across a membrane with the generation of ATP (Fig. 3–25B). The remainder of the energy is released as heat.

Generation of Energy as ATP: A Summary

Energy as ATP is generated at several places in the metabolism of a carbohydrate such as glucose to water, or other inorganic end products. ATP is formed in the EMP pathway from the transition between the EMP pathway and the TCA cycle, from the electrons that are released from the TCA cycle, and through the electron transport chain. The ATP yields from each of these metabolic pathways are seen in Figures 3–30 and 3–31. For each mole of glucose that enters the EMP pathway, eight ATPs are produced; the electrons that enter the electron transport chain from the TCA cycle function to oxidize 12 coenzymes, two $FADH_2$ (1 from each turn of the TCA cycle), and 10 $NADH_2$ (two from glycolysis, two from the transition between glycolysis and TCA, and six from the required two turns of the TCA cycle for each mole of glucose). Three ATPs are produced from each $NADH_2$, two ATPs from each $FADH_2$, and 34 ATPs from oxidative phosphorylation through the cytochrome system. The total yield of energy from the complete oxidation of one mole of glucose to $CO_2 + H_2O$ is therefore 38 ATPs; 34 ATPs are produced from oxidative phosphorylation, two ATPs from glycolysis, and two additional ATPs are produced from a guanosine triphosphate (GTP) reaction in the TCA cycle. Note that in glycolysis alone (that is, in the anaerobic oxidation of glucose to lactate or ethanol) only two ATPs per mole of glucose are produced. Clearly then, aerobic oxidation of glucose is a far more efficient energy-generating process than anaerobic metabolism.

Fermentation

Since anaerobic bacteria, as well as some facultative anaerobes, do not possess the cytochromes of the aerobic electron transport system, they cannot obtain energy through oxidative phosphorylation. Bacteria growing in an anaerobic environment obtain their energy directly from glycolysis and from the process of substrate level phosphorylation (Fig. 3–26), or from anaerobic respiration (Fig. 3–28). Since substrate level phosphorylation is essentially the only mechanism of energy generation available to anaerobic bacteria, the energy obtained in these anaerobic processes is far less than obtained from aerobic respiration. Rather than pyruvate being converted to acetyl-CoA, and eventually metabolized through the TCA cycle, the pyruvate that is formed is reduced to a large number of end products characteristic of the specific bacterial species (Table 3–5 and Fig. 3–32). These

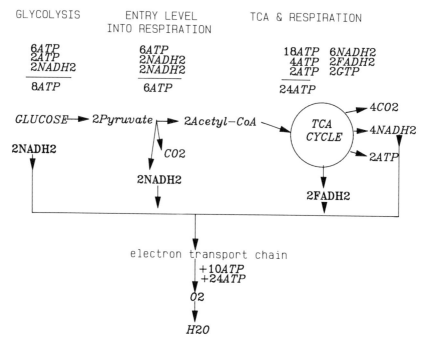

FIGURE 3–30 ✦ Summary of energy yields of ATP in glycolysis, entry into respiration, and TCA and respiration. Note the dramatic differences in energy yield between aerobic respiration and glycolysis.

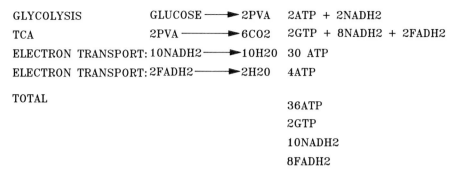

FIGURE 3–31 ✦ Summary of maximum energy yield per mole of glucose metabolized by glycolysis and respiration.

specific anaerobic reactions are referred to as fermentation chemical reactions in which organic compounds serve as ultimate electron acceptors.

Several groups of bacteria including oral *Prevotella* and *Porphyromonas* are even capable of fermenting amino acids; however, they do so in very complicated and specific ways and will not be considered here.

Pentose-Phosphate Pathway—Hexose Monophosphate Shunt

This catabolic pathway for carbohydrates is similar to that of EMP. The pentose-phosphate pathway (Fig. 3–33), or hexose monophosphate shunt, possesses several reactions of glycolysis and therefore can be considered as a "shunt" pathway of glycolysis. In this pathway, while electrons are

generated from the oxidation of glucose, not much energy is produced as ATP; in fact, the major function of this pathway is to provide reducing power (NADPH) for the multitude of biosynthetic reactions of the cell that require this pyridine nucleotide, as well as pentose phosphates required for nucleotide biosynthesis.

Entner-Doudoroff Pathway

The Entner-Doudoroff pathway (Fig. 3–34) is confined to aerobic and anaerobic bacteria and absent from eukaryotic cells. Identical to glycolysis and the hexose monophosphate shunt, glucose is phosphorylated by ATP. The glucose-6-phosphate formed in the Entner-Doudoroff pathway is converted to a gluconic acid, which is dehydrated, and then cleaved to the two trioses, pyruvic acid and

TABLE 3–5 ✦ **Major End Products of Glucose Dissimilation by Representative Prokaryotes***

GENERA	REPRESENTATIVE PRODUCTS	REPRESENTATIVE GENERA*

Lactic acid bacteria
  Streptococcus
  Lactobacillus
  Leuconostoc
	Lactic acid, acetic acid, formic acid, and ethyl alcohol; only lactic acid homofermentative; lactic acid plus other compounds homofermentative	A, C

Propionic acid bacteria
  Propionibacterium
  Veillonella
	Propionic acid, acetic acid, carbon dioxide	H

Enterobacter group
  Escherichia
  Enterobacter
  Salmonella
	Formic acid, acetic acid, lactic acid, succinic acid, ethyl alcohol, carbon dioxide, hydrogen, 2,3-butylene glycol	B, G

Acetone, butyl alcohol group
  Clostridium
  Eubacterium
  Bacillus
	Butyric acid, butyl alcohol, acetone, isopropyl alcohol, acetic acid, formic acid, ethyl alcohol, hydrogen, and carbon dioxide	C, D, E, F

Acetic acid bacteria *Acetobacter*	Acetic acid, gluconic acid, kojic acid	

*See Figure 3–32.

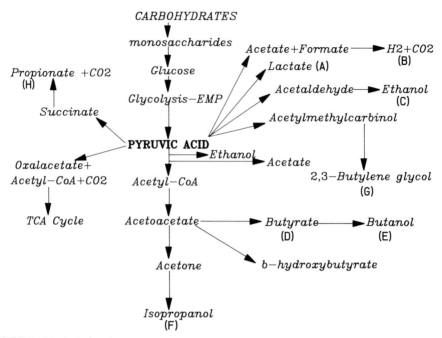

FIGURE 3–32 ✦ Role of pyruvic acid in the formation of a variety of reduced end products from the dissimilation of glucose. The letters indicate representative groups of bacteria that dissimilate glucose to the end product in Table 3–5. (Adapted from Pelczar, M-J, Chan, E. C. S., Krieg, NR [eds]: Microbiology, ed. 5. McGraw Hill, New York, 1986, with permission from McGraw-Hill.)

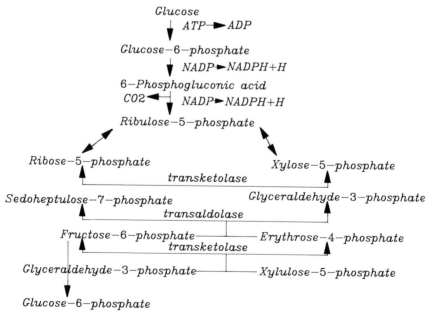

FIGURE 3–33 ✦ The pentose phosphate pathway of glucose catabolism. This pathway functions to produce ribose-5-phosphate and NADPH + H$^+$. The pyridine nucleotide serves as an important source of reducing power for fatty acid biosynthesis, while the ribose-5-phosphate functions in nucleotide biosynthesis.

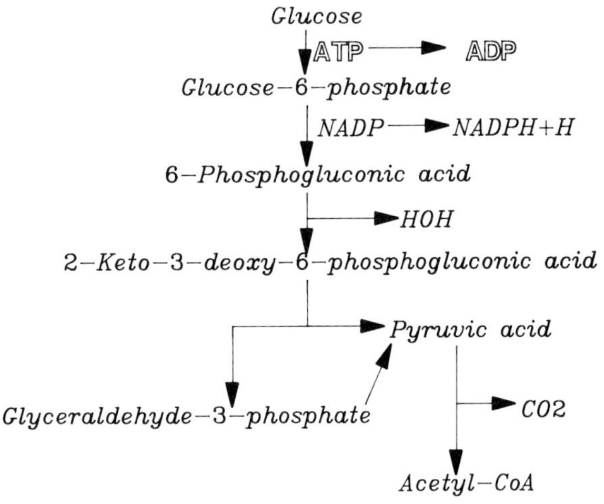

Glucose
$$\downarrow ATP \longrightarrow ADP$$
Glucose$-6-$phosphate
$$\downarrow NADP \longrightarrow NADPH+H$$
$6-$Phosphogluconic acid
$$\downarrow \longrightarrow HOH$$
$2-Keto-3-deoxy-6-$phosphogluconic acid

Glyceraldehyde$-3-$phosphate $\longrightarrow$ Pyruvic acid $\longrightarrow CO2$

Acetyl$-CoA$

FIGURE 3–34 ✦ The Entner-Doudoroff pathway of glucose catabolism. This metabolic pathway, for the dissimilation of glucose, occurs in selected gram-negative bacteria, especially *Pseudomonas* and *Azotobacter*.

glyceraldehyde-3-phosphate. These trioses are activated by coenzyme A, and the acetyl-CoA produced is catabolized via the TCA cycle. Energy and carbon skeletons are then produced as described for the TCA cycle and electron transport.

Glyoxylate Cycle

Several bacteria, notably members of the genus *Pseudomonas*, are capable of metabolizing acetic acid, as well as other higher fatty acids. Since eukaryotic cells are not required to metabolize acetate alone, the glyoxylic acid (or glyoxylate) cycle is limited to bacteria. In the glyoxylate cycle (Fig. 3–35), acetete is activated with coenzyme A to acetyl-CoA; however, there is no formation of pyruvate as an intermediate. The acetyl-CoA enters the glyoxylate cycle at two places by condensation reactions; the first is with oxalacetate to produce citrate identical to that found in the TCA cycle, and the second involves a condensation of the acetyl-CoA molecule with glyoxylate to produce malate. Both malate and citrate enter the TCA cycle. The two critical enzymes responsible for the functioning of the glyoxylate cycle are isocitrate lyase and malate synthase. Both enzymes function to replenish the pool of carbon for the TCA cycle, and are therefore known as *anapleurotic enzymes*,

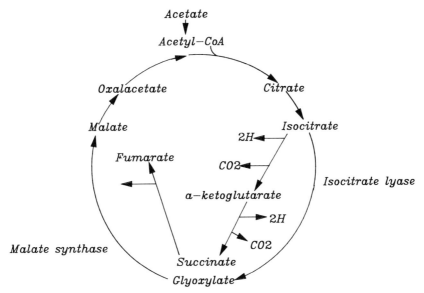

FIGURE 3–35 ✦ The glyoxylic acid cycle or bypass. It functions to replenish the pool of intermediates of the TCA cycle. Isocitrate lyase and malate synthase are enzymes specific to the cycle. Note the reactions common to the TCA cycle. (Adapted from Pelczar et al. See Fig. 3–32, ed. 5; and from J. Mandelstam, K. McQuillen, and I. Dawes [eds.]: Biochemistry of Bacterial Growth, ed. 3. John Wiley & Sons, New York, 1982.)

in that they maintain the necessary levels (pool) of intermediates for biosynthesis.

Photosynthesis

Plants, algae, and selected microorganisms can use light as a source of energy; that is by the process of *photosynthesis*. Plants, blue-green bacteria (cyanobacteria), and algae carry out an aerobic, or *oxygenic, photosynthesis* in which the CO_2 generated in other metabolic reactions (i.e., TCA) is reduced to carbohydrate or cell material (CH_2O) in the presence of the chemical reductant, water:

$$2H_2O + CO_2 \xrightarrow[\text{light}]{} (CH_2O) + O_2 + H_2O$$

In contrast, selected photosynthetic bacteria, while using light as an energy source, cannot do so in the presence of oxygen. Further, they cannot use water as a reductant, and consequently do not produce oxygen as one of the end products of metabolism. They carry out an *anoxygenic photosynthesis* in which compounds other than water function as the chemical reductant. Hence,

$$2H_2A + CO_2 \xrightarrow{\text{light}} (CH_2O) + 2A + H_2O$$

Since the chemical reductant in the anoxygenic photosynthetic bacteria can be a variety of compounds, it is designated as H_2A. Inorganic compounds such as H_2, H_2S, and even S_2O_3, as well as organic compounds such as acetate, lactate, or succinate, can function as chemical reductants. The cell mass (CH_2O), which was formed from the CO_2 generated as a product of the TCA cycle (see Fig. 3–27), is "fixed" from the "dark reactions" of photosynthesis, or the Calvin cycle (Fig. 3–36).

Synthesis of Major Cellular Macromolecules

It should now be clear that the generation of energy as ATP, and reducing power as pyridine nucleotide through the various catabolic cycles, functions to provide the cell with the ATP and pyridine nucleotides to drive the biosynthetic reactions necessary for the growth and anabolic reactions of the cell. Approximately 150 different small organic molecules are used for the biosynthesis of the basic cellular macromolecules (i.e., polysaccharides, lipids, proteins, and nucleic acids). In fact, these small organic molecules are synthesized from only 12 key precursor metabolites.

The biosynthesis of several selected macromolecules and their organization into functional units are common to most bacteria. We will assume that the reader is familiar with the synthesis of the amino acids and lipids. Both are synthesized from the end products of the metabolic pathways that have already been discussed. Figure 3–37 provides a basic summary of the interrelationships among

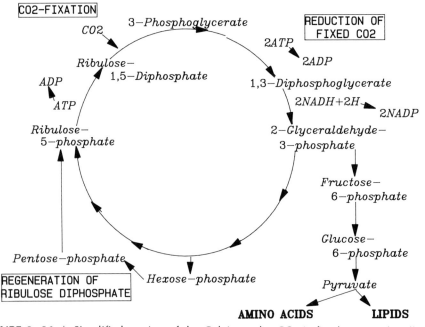

FIGURE 3–36 ✦ Simplified version of the Calvin cycle. CO_2 is fixed autotrophically into organic molecules. These are the "dark reactions" of photosynthesis because no light is directly required for the reactions to proceed. However, light energy is required for the production of ATP and NADPH.

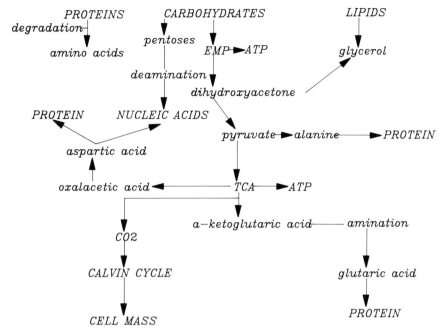

FIGURE 3–37 ✦ Interrelationships among carbohydrates, lipids, and proteins leading to the synthesis of macromolecules.

carbohydrates, lipids, and proteins, which lead to the synthesis of macromolecules.

PURINE AND PYRIMIDINE BIOSYNTHESIS

The purines and pyrimidines (Fig. 3–38) are nucleic acid (DNA, RNA) precursors and are synthesized from several amino acids and CO_2 in a stepwise process that involves at least 12 different enzymes and at least five different compounds (Fig. 3–39).

The purine and pyrimidine nucleotides (base-sugar-phosphate) are essential to a large number of critical biosynthetic functions of the cell. They are, for example, central components of several vitamins and coenzymes, and are essential compounds in cell wall molecules (peptidoglycan, lipopolysaccharide), as well as being involved in the formation of amino acids and complex lipids. Figure 3–40 describes the basic biosynthetic pathways for the formation of the purine and pyrimidine ribonucleotide triphosphates.

The ribonucleotides (ribose-containing nucleotides) are precursors for the synthesis of RNA (ribose nucleic acid), while the deoxyribonucleotides (deoxyribose-containing nucleotides) function in the synthesis of DNA (deoxyribose nucleic acid). The ribonucleotides are synthesized by the action of the phosphorylated pyridine nucleotide, NADP, and the enzyme thioredoxin reductase (Fig. 3–41). The nucleotides are reduced to the triphosphates,

while the cofactor is reduced to the deoxyribose of the DNA. Energy is supplied as ATP.

POLYSACCHARIDE BIOSYNTHESIS

Activation may be required for some simple sugars to be able to pass through, or be transported across, bacterial membranes and cell walls. This activation usually entails a phosphorylation, in which a nucleotide phosphate in the presence of a specific enzyme (kinase) produces a sugar-phosphate. This sugar-phosphate is easily transported into the cell, as well as functioning as a precursor of polysaccharide formation. The nucleotide, uridine triphosphate (UTP), for example, activates glucose to UDP-glucose. This activated glucose (the glucose phosphate is a high-energy molecule) now has sufficient energy for the subsequent linkages of additional glucose molecules to form a polysaccharide, a glucose polymer.

The type of sugar polymer formed, as well as its linkage, is also determined by its monosaccharide composition and the chemical interactions required for linkage. The homopolysaccharide (one sugar type) glycogen, for example, consists of poly-1,4-glucose units, and the glucose-glucose bonding occurs under the control of UDPG → UDP. The heteropolysaccharides (several different sugars) are composed of more than one sugar, and separate enzymes are required. These enzymes function to catalyze the addition of each sugar to the developing chain. Interestingly, in the forma-

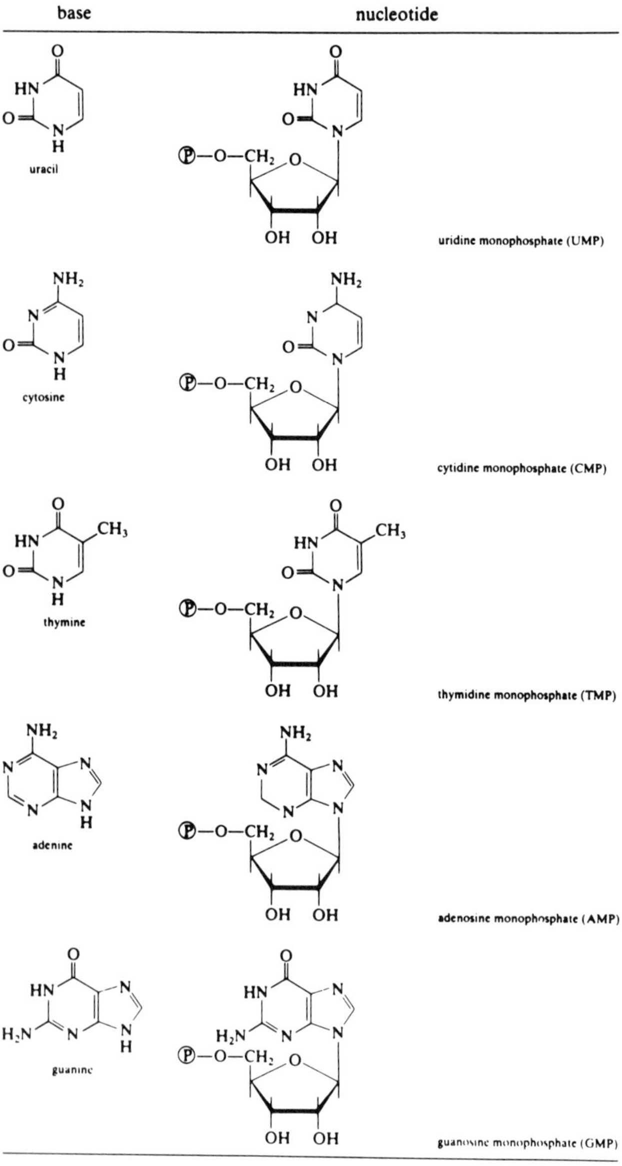

base | nucleotide
---

uracil

uridine monophosphate (UMP)

cytosine

cytidine monophosphate (CMP)

thymine

thymidine monophosphate (TMP)

adenine

adenosine monophosphate (AMP)

guanine

guanosine monophosphate (GMP)

FIGURE 3–38 ✦ Important pyrimidines, purines, and corresponding nucleotides.

tion of the important polysaccharides dextran, levan, and fructan, the nucleotide sugars (sugar + UTP sugar − PO_4 + UDP) are not involved in polymer formation, but these polymers are synthesized under the control of specific enzymes (i.e., dextransucrase):

Sucrose + dextransucrase→dextran + fructose

The energy required for the synthesis of the polymer is obtained by hydrolysis of the glycosydic bond of the sugar molecules.

PEPTIDOGLYCAN BIOSYNTHESIS

The peptidoglycan maintains the shape and structural integrity of bacteria. It consists of repeating glycan polymer of *N*-acetylglucosamine and *N*-acetylmuramic acid to which peptide sub-

units are attached (see Fig. 3–11). The biosynthesis of the peptidoglycan takes place in four distinct stages and at distinct locations within the bacterial cell (Fig. 3–42):

Stages 1 and 2. Both stage 1 and stage 2 are carried out in the cell cytoplasm and involve the formation of UDP-sugars. UDP-*N*-acetylglucosamine and UDP-*N*-acetylmuramic acid are formed as a result of ATP-requiring reactions. The specific amino acids are then sequentially added to form the UDP-sugar-pentapeptide, and after elimination of one terminal amino acid the tetrapeptide is attached to a lactylcarboxyl group of *N*-acetylmuramic acid. An amino acid bridge connects the terminal carboxyl group of each side chain with the free amino group of lysine or diaminopimelic acid.

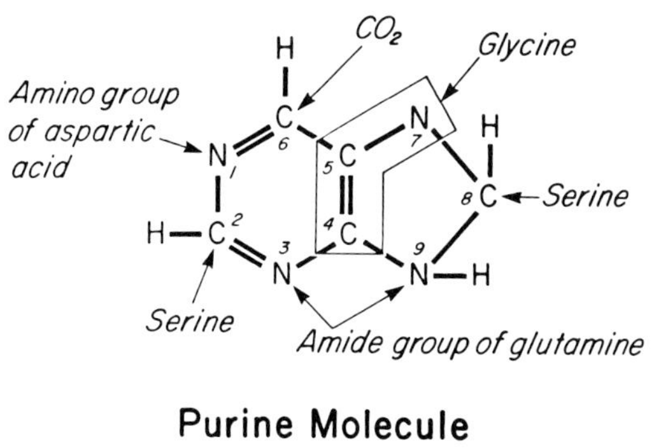

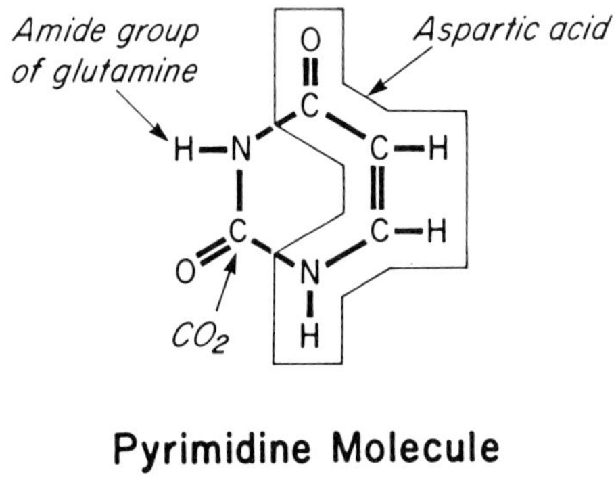

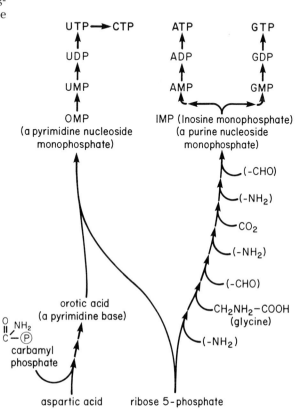

Purine Molecule

Pyrimidine Molecule

FIGURE 3–39 ✦ Representation of the precursor molecules that are involved in the formation of purine **(A)** and pyrimidine **(B)** molecules. Each of the fragments of these two molecules are formed from the indicated amino acids or carbon dioxide.

Stage 3. The nucleotide-sugar pentapeptide formed in the cytoplasm is then transported to the cell surface by a specific carrier molecule, an isoprenoid c_{55}-carrier lipid, **bactoprenol** or **undecaprenol.** After linkage of this carrier to the UDP-sugar-pentapeptide, N-acetylglucosamine molecules are added to it in the periplasm and the entire repeating unit is then transported across the cytoplasmic membrane where it is chemically linked to an "acceptor" of partially completed polymer in the developing cell wall. The isoprenoid carrier is regenerated by the removal of an inorganic phosphate by the action of a phosphatase enzyme.

Stage 4. The final stage in the formation of the peptidoglycan is the cross-linking of the polypeptide chains in the cell wall matrix itself. Cross-linking occurs either directly, as an amide bond between diaminopimelic acid or lysine and the penultimate D-alanine of an adjacent peptidoglycan chain, or indirectly, by the addition of a pentaglycine bridge between the penultimate D-alanine. In both cases the D-alanine is released into the bacterial cytoplasm to be utilized in other chemical reactions.

LIPOPOLYSACCHARIDE BIOSYNTHESIS

The basic structure of the lipopolysaccharide is seen in Figure 3–16, and its mechanism of syn-

FIGURE 3–40 ✦ Simplified generalized scheme for the formation of the various nucleotide phosphates. Aspartic acid ribose-5-phosphate undergoes a series of addition and deletion reactions to eventually form the purine and pyrimidine nucleotide monophosphates. These in turn are converted to the four purine and pyrimidine bases: uridine triphosphate, cytidine triphosphate, adenosine triphosphate, and guanosine triphosphate, respectively.

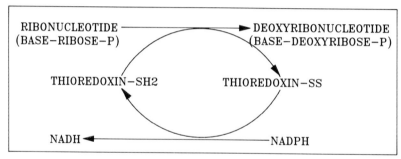

FIGURE 3–41 ✦ Formation of deoxyribonucleotides from ribonucleotides. Pyridine nucleotide and the enzyme thioredoxin reductase function in the reduction of the ribonucleotide to the deoxyribonucleotide.

thesis and transport in Figure 3–43. The lipid A is the endotoxic portion of the LPS and is covalently linked to the polysaccharide core. The O-antigen contains a variety of sugar residues, which provide it with the immunologic specificity characteristic of the large number of gram-negative bacteria.

Core Polysaccharide

The core polysaccharides routinely are heptose phosphate residues, which are linked to a unique

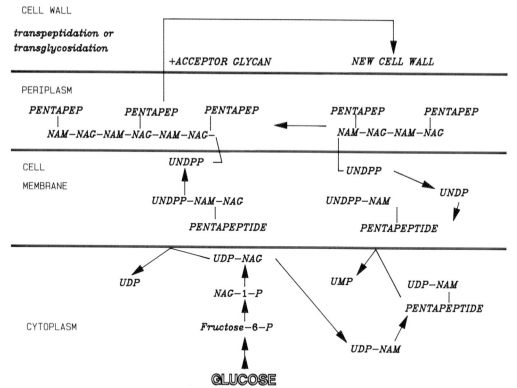

FIGURE 3–42 ✦ Diagrammatic representation of the formation of a new cell wall. New cell wall synthesis occurs in three regions of the cell: in the cytoplasm, in the periplasm and cell membrane, and on the cell wall. Glucose is utilized in the cytoplasmic region to form uridine, dinucleotide phosphates (see Fig. 3–40), which "carry" muramic acid pentapeptides to the cell membrane. The UDP-pentapeptide is covalently linked to an N-acetylglucosamine. This unit, formed in the cell membrane is then carried by an undecaprenol C55 lipid carrier (UND) through the cell membrane, where it is further linked to additional N-acetylmuramic acid and N-acetylglucosamine repeating units. This entire unit then is transferred from the periplasm to the growing cell wall. The peptide-linked and sugar-linked cell wall is formed at the outer surface by transpeptidation and transglycosidation reactions.

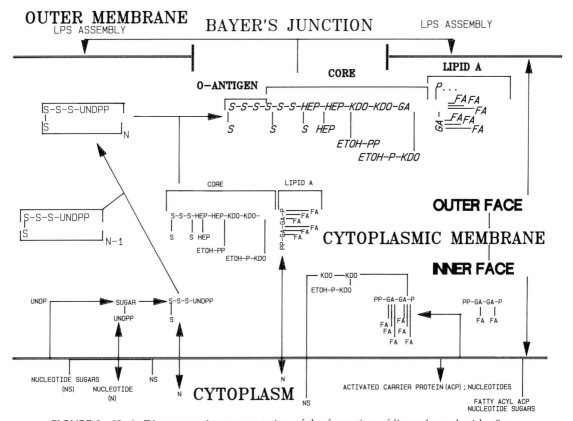

FIGURE 3–43 ✦ Diagrammatic representation of the formation of lipopolysaccharide. Synthesis of the lipopolysaccharide occurs in the cell cytoplasm, on the membrane surfaces of the cytoplasmic membrane, and on the surface of the outer membrane. The lipopolysaccharide is formed from nucleotide sugars (NS) and fatty acyl nucleotide sugars, which are formed in the cytoplasm. These two units are transported to the interface of the cytoplasmic membrane by C55-undecaprenol lipid carriers (UND), as well as by activated carrier proteins (ACP). These two units, the sugars and fatty acyl units, are elongated on the inner face of the cytoplasmic membrane. The three components of the lipopolysaccharide molecule—the core, lipid A, and O-antigen—are then transferred to the outer face of the outer membrane where they are linked by covalent linkage into small O-antigen, core, and lipid A complexes. These complexes are then transferred through the Bayer's junction in the outer membrane, where they are assembled along the outer membrane surface into the completed lipopolysaccharide structure.

8-carbon sugar acid, 2-keto-3-deoxyoctanoate, or KDO. It is the KDO that links the O-antigen and core polysaccharide to the lipid A. Initial synthesis of the LPS occurs in the bacterial cytoplasm where the O-antigenic sugars are attached to the polysaccharide backbone. The UDP-activated sugar precursors are then transferred from the cytoplasm to undecaprenyl phosphate, a lipid carrier similar to that involved in peptidoglycan synthesis. In LPS synthesis, the undecaprenyl phosphate exists in the cytoplasmic membrane. The soluble sugar precursors are first polymerized into the O-antigen subunits, which then attach to the lipid A core polysaccharide to form the complete LPS molecule. The entire completed LPS molecule is then trans-located to the outer membrane by an unknown mechanism.

O-Antigen

The O-antigen is covalently linked to the core polysaccharide through heptose and KDO. Two important characteristics of this linkage are: (1) the disaccharides are linked together by pyrophosphate (P-P) bridges rather than by glycosidic ones, and (2) the free (open) positions of the disaccharides are esterified with fatty acyl residues. These fatty acyl residues are exceedingly important in stabilizing the LPS in the outer membrane by penetrating into the hydrophobic portion of the membrane where they are held securely.

Lipid A

Mild acetic acid hydrolysis of the entire molecule easily removes the lipid A from the O-polysaccharide and KDO-heptose. Chemically, the lipid A consists of D-glucosamine-4-phosphate, which is linked to several long-chain fatty acids and to the phospholipid ethanolamine (Fig. 3–44). Its synthesis is identical to that for phospholipids. However, one major difference between the lipid A and the membrane phospholipids is that in the lipid A, hydroxy fatty acids predominate. The hydroxy fatty acids are linked to the glucosamine disaccharides through either ether or amide linkages. The disaccharide also carries a phosphate group as well as a pyrophosphorylethanolamine residue. Intramuscular or intravenous injection into animals (such as mice, hamsters, and guinea pigs) with small amounts of lipid A result in endotoxemia. *The lipid A is therefore considered to be the endotoxic portion of the LPS.* Injection of large amounts of lipid A into animals can result in fatal shock.

Nucleic Acid Biosynthesis
REPLICATION OF DNA
Structure of DNA

For a cell to perpetuate itself unchanged, it must be able to provide its "daughters" with a complete

and accurate copy of its genetic material. In order to do this correctly, the cell's genetic material, DNA (deoxyribose nucleic acid), must be faithfully duplicated without errors (mutation). In Figure 3–45 a portion of the DNA (molecular weight, 10^6 daltons) is shown. Chemically, the DNA molecule consists of a repeating nucleic acid monomer or nucleotide of the four bases—adenine, cytosine, guanine, and thymine—and the five-carbon sugar (pentose) deoxyribose arranged in a double helix. The bases are chemically linked together as base pairs of adenine-thymine and guanine-cytosine, which are themselves linked together through a backbone of covalently linked sugars that alternate with phosphate groups. The process of DNA duplication (replication) begins by the breaking of the H-bonds between the adenosine-thymine (A-T) and guanine-cytosine (G-C) base pairs at specific points in the double helix. This results in the separation of the two individual helices at those points. Each of the separate strands is then used as a template for the synthesis from the 5' end of the molecule to the 3' end of a new strand of DNA that is **complementary** to the original strand (Fig. 3–46). This results in formation of two new DNA strands identical to the parent molecule. Note that the nucleotide pairs in the new strand are in the same

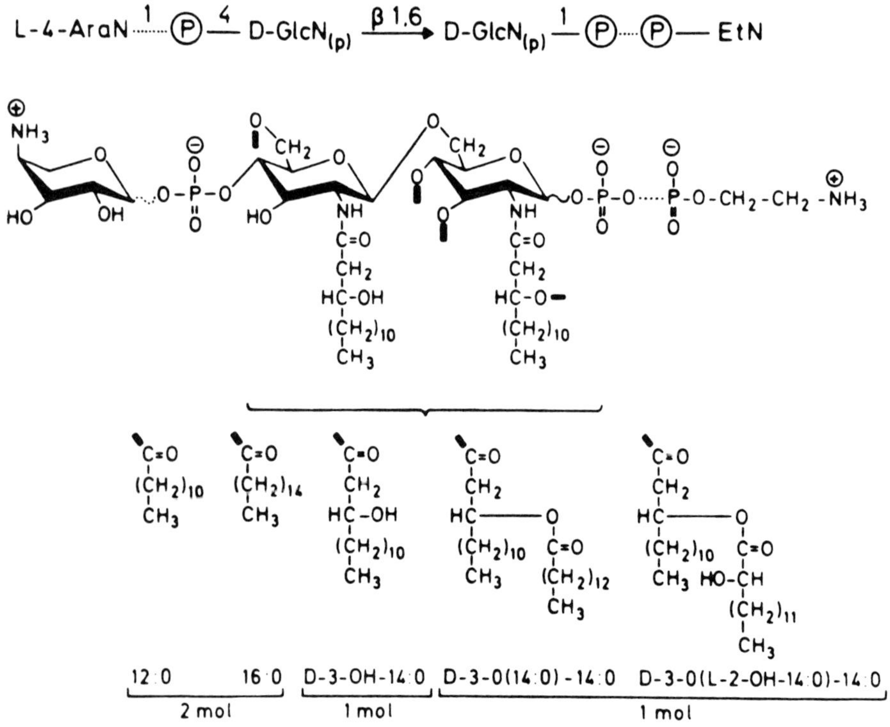

FIGURE 3–44 ✦ Chemical structure of the lipid A from *Salmonella* species. The structure consists of a central backbone of B-1, 6-linked, d-glycosamine disaccharide units which have at positions 4' and 1 phosphomonoester residues. Long-chain fatty acids of 10, 12, 14, and 16 carbons are linked to the amino and hydroxyl groups of the glucosamine disaccharides. The molar ratios of the various fatty acids are indicated in the lower portion of the figure. (From Lüderitz, O., et al.: Naturwissenschaften 65:578, 1978, with permission.)

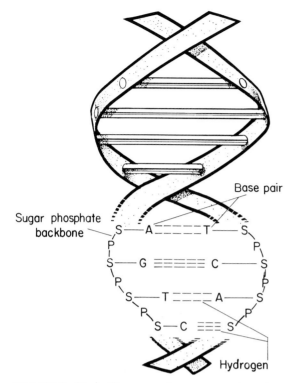

FIGURE 3–45 ✦ Diagrammatic representation of a portion of the helical DNA molecule. The alpha-helix consists of repeating units of a sugar phosphate backbone. The two helices are connected by complementary base pairs consisting of adenine (A)–thymine (T), and guanine (G)–cytosine (C). The base pairs are connected by hydrogen bonding.

order and arrangement as they were in the original strand. This occurs because the order and arrangement of the nucleotides in the "old half" of the newly formed double helix was conserved in its original form. Thus, the original double helix has now produced two complete double helices, each an exact replica of the original. Since each of the two new double helices consists of one chain of the old double helix, plus a new complementary chain, this mode of replication is referred to as *semiconservative replication.*

How does a bacterial chromosome replicate and "know" where to begin the replication of the DNA molecule? When the bacterial chromosome duplicates itself during cell division, there is a unique "point of origin," where replication is initiated. Although there are many points of origin in the eukaryotic chromosome, there is only one such point in the bacterial chromosome. During this replication from the point of origin, the bacterial chromosome replicates in a bidirectional fashion, with replication beginning at the point of origin and proceeding in both directions at an equal rate (Fig. 3–47). Replication is completed 180 degrees from its origin. The replication process is very complex genetically and biochemically with a number of replication proteins associated in a multienzyme complex, or replication apparatus.

REPLICATION OF RNA
Structure of RNA

The RNA molecule consists of the sugar, ribose, and the bases adenine, guanine, cytosine, and uracil, which substitute for thymine. In contrast to the double stranded–helix DNA molecule, RNA is usually single stranded. There are three unique forms of RNA: messenger RNA (mRNA), transfer RNA (tRNA), and ribosomal RNA (rRNA). The mRNA is the "messenger" for the genes of the DNA molecule and is a true linear copy of that molecule. As such, it consists of nucleotide triplets, or **triplet codons,** which carry the genetic information for the synthesis of the 20 naturally occurring amino acids within a developing polypeptide chain (Table 3–6). The tRNA carries specific amino acids to the ribosomes for their incorporation into the growing polypeptide chain, which will eventually make the specific protein that was dictated by mRNA. The rRNAs also carry triplet codons; however, these codons indicate the starting

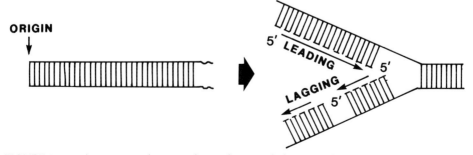

FIGURE 3–46 ✦ DNA synthesis at the replication fork proceeds *continuously* in the 5' to 3' direction along only one strand of DNA, called the leading strand. Because DNA polymerases can synthesize from d NMPs only in the 5' to 3' direction, as portions of the lagging strand are exposed, complementary DNA is synthesized *discontinuously* as fragments of DNA. As a final step the fragments are linked together by the enzyme DNA ligase.

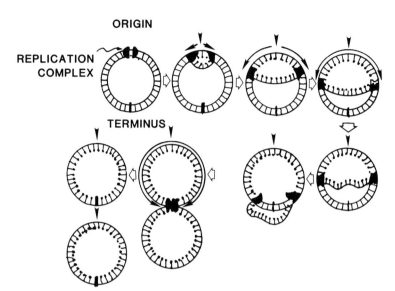

ORIGIN

REPLICATION COMPLEX

TERMINUS

FIGURE 3–47 ✦ Replications of the bacterial chromosome occur in a bidirectional manner. Replication is initiated by binding of the replication complex at the origin, designated *ori*, and terminated at a point opposite *ori* on the circular chromosome. The replication rate is 800 nucleotides per second per replication fork and is independent of the growth rate. Since there are two replication forks per chromosome, a bacterial chromosome of 3.8×10^6 base pairs will be replicated in 40 minutes.

and stopping points of polypeptide in the protein synthetic process. Genetically, they carry the requisite information to signal chemically for a stop in protein synthesis; the "stop" codons are sometimes referred to as "nonsense codons," in that they do not carry information for the production of an amino acid. The tRNAs also function with the ribosomal protein in the physical structure of the ribosome, the site of protein synthesis.

RNA SYNTHESIS (TRANSCRIPTION)

The synthesis of the RNA molecule is very similar to that previously described for DNA synthesis; however, new RNA strands are synthesized on a

TABLE 3–6 ✦ **The Genetic Code***

5'-OH TERMINAL BASE		MIDDLE BASE				3'-OH TERMINAL BASE
		U	*C*	*A*	*G*	
	UUU	Phe(F)	UCU Ser(S)	UAU Tyr(Y)	UGU Cys(C)	U
	UUC	Phe(F)	UCC Ser(S)	UAC Tyr(Y)	UGC Cys(C)	C
U						
	UUA	Leu(L)	UCA Ser(S)	UAA Termination	UGA Termination	A
	UUG	Leu(L)	UCG Ser(S)	UAG Termination	UGG Trp	G
	CUU	Leu(L)	CCU Pro(P)	CAU His(H)	CGU Arg(R)	U
	CUC	Leu(L)	CCC Pro(P)	CAC His(H)	CGC Arg(R)	C
C						
	CUA	Leu(L)	CGA Pro(P)	CAA Gin(O)	CGA Arg(R)	A
	CUG	Leu(L)	CCG Pro(P)	CAG Gin(O)	CGG Arg(R)	G
	AUU	Ile(I)	ACU Thr(T)	AAU Asn(N)	AGU Ser(S)	U
	AUC	Ile(I)	ACC Thr(T)	AAC Asn(N)	AGC Ser(S)	C
A						
	AUA	Ile(I)	ACA Thr(T)	AAA Lys(K)	AGA Arg(R)	A
	AUG	Met(M)	ACG Thr(T)	AAG Lys(K)	AGG Arg(R)	G
	GUU	Val(V)	GCU Ala(A)	GAU Asp(D)	GGU Gly(G)	U
	GUC	Val(V)	GCC Ala(A)	GAC Asp(D)	GGC Gly(G)	C
G						
	GUA	Val(V)	GCA Ala(A)	GAA Glu(E)	GGA Gly(G)	A
	GUG	Val(V)	GCG Ala(A)	GAG Glu(E)	GGG Gly(G)	G

*All but four of the triplets of nucleotides are allocated to specific amino acids. UAA, UAG, and UGA indicate chain termination, while AUG represents the chain-initiating N-formyl-methionine. Both three-letter and one-letter abbreviations are shown for the amino acids; e.g., phenylalanine, PHE(F).

DNA template, and specific base pairing occurs by complementary bonding (Fig. 3–48). The major difference between DNA synthesis and RNA synthesis is that in the latter the phosphodiester bonds between adjacent bases are formed by the enzyme DNA-dependent RNA polymerase. RNA synthesis also differs from DNA synthesis in that newly formed RNAs are synthesized from short segments of DNA, and therefore require a much finer degree of control. Control is effected by genetic "signals" in the DNA molecule that indicate to the DNA-dependent RNA polymerase exactly which portions of it are to be copied. Importantly, since only one DNA strand is used in the synthesis of an RNA molecule, and since the two DNA strands are complementary, there must be a mechanism for choosing the correct strand for RNA synthesis—that is, the strand that carries the appropriate genetic information. The mechanism distinguishes the correct strand, *sense strand,* from its complementary strand, so only this sense strand is copied (Fig. 3–48).

Finally, for RNA synthesis to occur, the RNA polymerase must bind to a segment of DNA molecule, the *promoter region,* which consists of a sequence of bases (recognized by the RNA polymerase) that precedes the gene(s) that is to be transcribed. The RNA polymerase then travels down the sense strands of DNA, transcribing a series of genes until it recognizes a *"stop" codon* (also known as a *termination codon,* or *terminator*) and falls off the DNA, releasing a strand of mRNA into the cytoplasm (Fig. 3–49). This mRNA molecule is a **polycistronic message** (or transcript) of RNA since it contains the sequence of more than one gene.

Protein Synthesis (Translation)

It should be clear that all essential biochemical reactions that occur in a cell are catalyzed by specific enzymes (proteins), and that the structure of all proteins is determined by the nucleotide sequence in the DNA molecule (see Table 3–1). The specific piece of DNA that designates a specific protein is the *structural gene.* How does it do so? The information in the DNA molecule is transferred to various RNAs that arrange amino acids in their unique order on the ribosome to produce a polypeptide, which eventually forms a functional protein (Figs. 3–50 and 3–51). This sequence from conversion of the information in the DNA molecule to formation of a functional protein comprises *transcription* and *translation.* All three classes of RNA participate in the protein-forming reactions of translation (see earlier). In one sense, translation (protein synthesis) involves a different alphabet from replication and transcription. In translation, the alphabet consists of amino acids instead of nucleotides. A sequence of nucleotides results in DNA or RNA molecules, whereas an orderly sequence of amino acids results in a protein, just as sequences of letters result in a word.

The process of protein synthesis involves the **activation** of a specific amino acid and its attachment to the tRNA molecule that contains the codon for that particular amino acid (Fig. 3–52). This tRNA molecule then "passes on" the amino acid to a specific site on another molecule of RNA, the mRNA, which is recognized by the complementarity of the triplet codons on the RNA molecules. The genetic information for production of specific tRNA-amino acid complex is carried by the mRNA. Subsequent to the attachment of the first

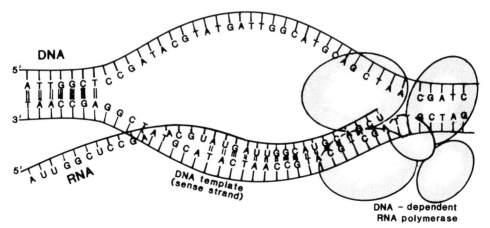

FIGURE 3–48 ✦ Transcription is the synthesis of RNA on a DNA template. The strands of the DNA molecule are unwound for a short distance. Then the enzyme complex, DNA-dependent RNA polymerase, uses ribonucleotide triphosphates (ATP, CTP, GTP, or UTP) and the sense strand of the unwound DNA as a template for the synthesis of a single strand of RNA complementary to the DNA. Note the complementary pairing G to C and A to U (rather than A to T as in DNA).

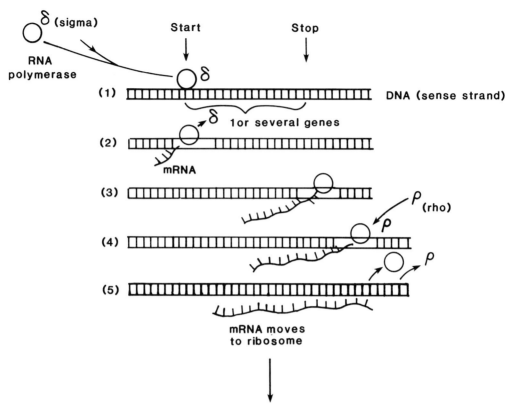

FIGURE 3–49 ✦ DNA transcription. A gene or group of sequentially transcribed genes (operon) has a start signal (promoter) sequence where the DNA-dependent RNA polymerase binds with the help of the sigma factor. The helix unwinds and the RNA polymerase begins the synthesis of complementary RNA to one strand, the sense strand (see also Fig. 3–48) of DNA (2 and 3). One or several genes may be encoded for on a single mRNA molecule, or RNA transcript. Once the RNA polymerase reaches the stop signal, which may or may not require the binding of an additional protein called *rho (4)*, it falls off the DNA strand, releasing the mRNA *(5)*, which then moves onto ribosomal complex formation for protein synthesis.

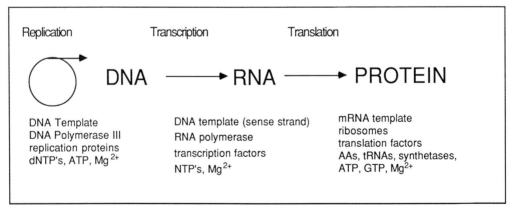

FIGURE 3–50 ✦ The flow of genetic information in prokaryotes is undirectional: from DNA to RNA to protein. Reverse transcription, the production of DNA on RNA templates, occurs in eukaryotic cells. (Adapted from Glass, R. E.: Gene Function.)

DNA

FIGURE 3–51 ✦ mRNA is transcribed into protein in a continuous manner in which mRNA synthesis (transcription) and protein synthesis (translation) can actually occur simultaneously. As the mRNA is elongated (3) ribosomes can bind (4 and 5) and begin translation. Several ribosomes translate one mRNA molecule at a time, forming a complex known as a polyribosome (6).

amino acid on the RNA molecule, a second amino acid, again designated by a specific mRNA, is transferred to the ribosome (by tRNA), with formation of a peptide bond and initiation of a large polypeptide and eventually a functional protein. When the polypeptide is a specific length (as designated by the DNA molecule and molecular information for the formation of that protein), the polypeptide synthesis is terminated and the protein is liberated from the mRNA-ribosome complex by a termination signal, again from a specific codon. Remember, these codons constitute the "start" and "stop" codons.

The events of protein synthesis can be summarized in the following way (Fig. 3–52):

1. The amino acids to be used in the synthesis of a specific protein are activated by an amino acyl-tRNA synthetase plus ATP.
2. The activated amino acid next binds to a tRNA molecule, a reaction catalyzed by the enzyme that was originally bound to the amino acid. The amino acid to be carried to

the ribosome for polypeptide formation is linked to the terminal nucleotide of the tRNA molecule.

3. The tRNA-amino acid complex is carried to the surface of the ribosome, where it (the amino acid) is added to the growing polypeptide chain (initiation).
4. On the surface of the ribosome one end of an mRNA molecule binds at a specific site, such that the reading or translation of the mRNA codon occurs in the correct sequence.
5. The first tRNA-amino acid complex attaches to the chain-initiating codon of the mRNA molecule.
6. A second tRNA-amino acid complex is transported to the ribosome and binds at the first codon site (step 1, elongation).
7. A dipeptide bond is formed between the carboxyl group of tRNA-amino acid complex 2 and the amino group of tRNA-amino acid complex 1. The formation of this initial dipeptide bond results in the release of tRNA1.

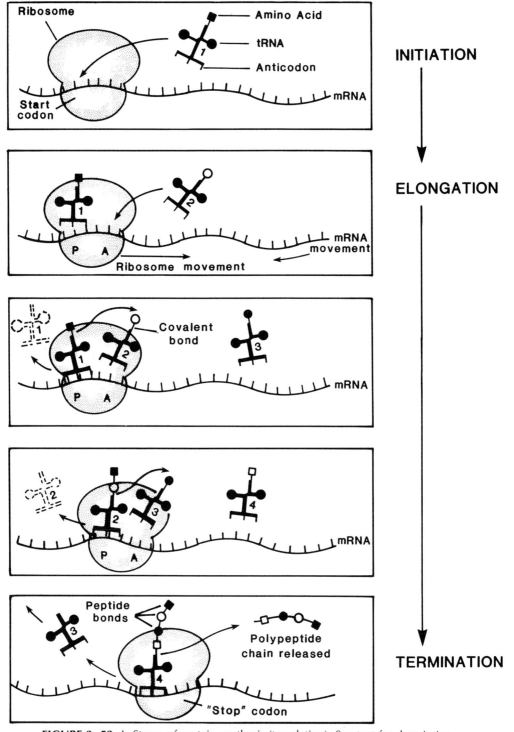

FIGURE 3–52 ✦ Stages of protein synthesis (translation). See text for description.

The mRNA is then moved along the ribosome to a position adjacent to the next codon, so as to be ready for the next tRNA-amino acid complex (step 2, elongation).

8. Peptide formation continues until the peptide chain is of the appropriate length. The termination of the amino acid addition process results from interaction of a nonsense or termination codon.

9. The completed polypeptide chain dissociates

from the terminal tRNA molecule and is organized into a functional protein by the appropriate folding and bending of the polypeptide.

Regulation of Cellular Activities

Bacteria need to be extremely economical with their energy supply and synthesize only cellular materials they require. The control of protein synthesis, that is, regulation of gene expression, can be accomplished either by regulating DNA transcription (mRNA synthesis) or by regulating RNA translation (protein synthesis). Although regulating translation is effective for regulation of enzyme levels, it is also wasteful. Transcription regulation is not only more energy efficient, it also allows the **coordinate regulation** of linked as well as unlinked genes. For example, several enzymes are necessary for the metabolism of lactose by bacteria. If lactose is not present or available to the bacterial cell, then it would be wasteful for the cell to synthesize the lactose-utilizing enzymes. If the synthesis of each of the enzymes required for lactose utilization is regulated by the same promoter sequence on the DNA, then either all the enzymes are synthesized or none of them are synthesized (i.e., they are under *coordinate regulation*). Consequently, most gene regulation in prokaryotes occurs via transcription, by controlling initiation and termination rates of the synthesis of mRNA. This regulation requires the interaction of certain regulatory molecules and specific DNA sequences in the promoter region of the DNA.

The *regulatory molecules* are small, diffusible proteins or organic molecules that can interact with the regulatory regions (see further on). The activity of regulatory proteins often is modified by **effector** molecules such as sugars or RNA. The regulatory proteins are multimeric, allosteric proteins with recognition sites for both DNA and the particular effector molecule. These effector proteins are *constitutive* (i.e., synthesized at a constant rate independent of the genes they control) and may either prevent or promote transcription. Regulatory proteins that prevent transcription are called *repressors* and function by **negative control,** whereas those that promote transcription are called *activators* and function by **positive control.**

The DNA regulatory region where these molecules function contains three main elements: a **promoter** (P), in which transcription is initiated (where the RNA polymerase binds); a repressor binding region, or **operator** (O); and a promoter-potentiation site where the activator interacts. These sites are not necessarily physically distinct and, although a promoter is necessary, only one of the other two sites may be present in any regulatory region.

The lac operon (Fig. 3–53) is an example of an operon regulated by **negative control** or **negative repression.** Regulation of this *operon* (a series of structural genes under control of the same promoter and regulatory region) is mediated by the protein encoded by the lac I regulatory gene, a gene not contained in the lac operon itself. The regulatory protein is produced constitutively and binds to the operator site of the lac operon, preventing passage of RNA polymerase, and thus, transcription. When lactose or an analogue of lactose enters the cell, it binds to the allosteric regulatory protein, changes its conformation, and inhibits its binding to the operator. Thus, the RNA polymerase is free to move down the DNA and transcribe the rest of the operon (which contains gene-encoding enzymes needed for the utilization of lactose).

Some operons are regulated in an opposite manner from the lac operon. Examples of these are the operons encoding enzymes involved in the catabolism of maltose and arabinose (Fig. 3–54). The regulatory proteins for these operons form a complex with each specific sugar and this complex then binds near the promoter, allowing RNA polymerase binding and transcription of the operon. These operons are under **positive control** or **regulation.**

EXTRACHROMOSOMAL DNA

Some bacteria contain extrachromosomal DNA molecules that are distinct **replicons,** that is, they are not covalently linked to the chromosome. These covalently closed circular molecules of DNA, called *plasmids* (Fig. 3–55), range in size from less than 1 kb (1000 bases) to well over 100 kb, exist in the cytoplasm, and reproduce independently of the chromosome. Many, but not all, bacteria contain plasmids, and some bacteria contain more than one type of plasmid. Because plasmids replicate independently of the bacterial chromosome, there are often several identical copies of a plasmid per cell; these are called *multicopy plasmids.* Plasmids code for genes not essential for growth of the cell but for properties that might be advantageous in certain environments. For example, plasmids called *R factors* carry genes that confer resistance to antibiotics. Other plasmids may encode genes for surface structures, resistance to heavy metals, toxins, and a variety of other proteins and virulence factors. Plasmids have been found in oral gram-positive organisms such as *Streptococcus* sp., but evidence indicates that they occur less frequently in oral gram-negative species such as *Porphyromonas.*

CONJUGATION

Certain plasmids may be transferred from cell to cell in a process called *conjugation* (explained later). One of these **conjugative plasmids** is the F

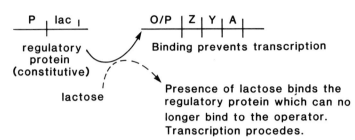

structural genes

P | lac | O/P | Z | Y | A |

regulatory
protein
(constitutive)

Binding prevents transcription

lactose

Presence of lactose binds the
regulatory protein which can no
longer bind to the operator.
Transcription procedes.

FIGURE 3–53 ✦ The lactose operon of *E. coli* is under negative control.

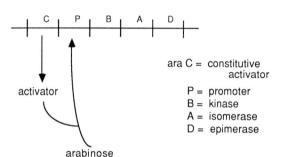

| C | P | B | A | D |

activator

arabinose

ara C = constitutive
           activator
P = promoter
B = kinase
A = isomerase
D = epimerase

FIGURE 3–54 ✦ The arabinose operon of *E. coli* is under positive control. Unless the activator is coupled to arabinose, it cannot bind to the regulatory sequence and RNA polymerase cannot bind to the promoter. When arabinose is present, it combines with the activator, and this complex binds to the regulatoy region, thereby promoting the binding of RNA polymerase, and transcription occurs.

plasmid of *Escherichia coli*. This plasmid is 94.5 kb in size (2 percent the size of the *E. coli* chromosome) and approximately one third of the plasmid DNA encodes for genes involved in the transfer of DNA. Cells that carry an F plasmid, F^+ *bacteria* (also called male cells), produce long, thin pili (F or sex pili) that are hollow, protein appendages several microns in length and 8 nm in diameter. When F^+ cells and F^- cells (those lacking an F plasmid, or female cells) are mixed, *conjugal pairs* (or *mating pairs*) form by the attachment of a male sex F pilus to the surface of a female cell (Fig. 3–56). By an unknown mechanism, a single linear strand of the F plasmid is transferred to the recipient cell (Fig. 3–56), probably through the hollow pilus, or *mating tube*. This transfer is always initiated at a unique site on the plasmid called *ori T* (origin of transfer) and occurs at a rate of 10^4 nucleotides (bases) per minute. At 37°C the transfer of the entire F plasmid is thus complete in 2 minutes. After the transfer of the F plasmid is

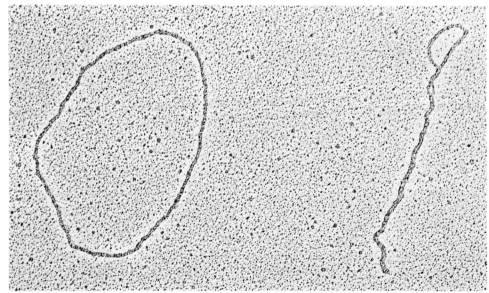

FIGURE 3–55 ✦ Electron micrograph of two molecules of plasmid col E1. The molecule on the left is relaxed and the one on the right, supertwisted. (Courtesy of Dr. D. Lang.)

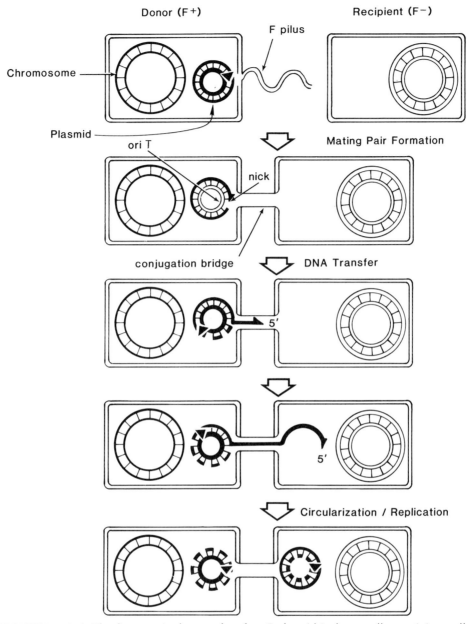

Donor (F$^+$)   Recipient (F$^-$)

F pilus

Chromosome

Plasmid

ori T

nick

Mating Pair Formation

conjugation bridge

DNA Transfer

5′

5′

Circularization / Replication

FIGURE 3–56 ✦ The first step in the transfer of an F plasmid is donor cell-to-recipient cell contact, mediated by the F pilus of the donor cell, resulting in mating pair formation. Once the conjugation bridge has been formed, possibly utilizing the hollow F pilus itself, a nick at the origin of transfer site (*ori* T) generates a 5′ end of single-stranded DNA, which is transferred to the recipient cell. In order for the transferred DNA to become an autonomously replicating DNA element, a complementary strand of DNA must be produced in the recipient cell to form a double-stranded DNA molecule and this double-stranded molecule must circularize. This is, thus, a rolling-circle mode of replication.

complete, the recipient (female) cell is then an F$^+$ (male) cell, since the F plasmid contains the genes that encode for pilus expression.

F plasmids may at times *integrate* (insert themselves) into the bacterial chromosome. This occurs at frequencies of 10^{-5} (1 in 100,000) to 10^{-7} (1

in 10,000,000) per generation of bacteria. Bacteria that contain an F plasmid integrated into their chromosome are called *Hfr* cells since they give a *high*(H) *fr*equency(fr) of transfer and recombination of their genes into a recipient (F$^-$) cell. This high rate of recombination occurs when the F plasmid is transferred as described earlier for F⁺ cells, but because the leading edge of the F⁺ factor is now attached to the chromosome, transfer of the chromosome also occurs. The transfer of the *cointegrate* DNA (F factor and chromosomal DNA) occurs at the same rate as the F plasmid alone, and thus requires approximately 100 minutes for transfer of the entire chromosome. However, transfer of the entire chromosome rarely occurs, since any minute disruption of mating pairs breaks the cell-to-cell contact and shears the donor DNA, terminating DNA transfer. The transfer of chromosomal genes during *Hfr*-mediated pairing occurs in a highly reproducible order since the transfer always begins at the point of origin and proceeds in one direction. The time of entry of donor genes (the time required for each particular gene to be transferred) is a measure of relative (molecular) distances on the chromosome. This is why distances between genes on genetic maps of bacterial chromosomes are expressed in minutes.

In addition to F plasmids, R plasmids (plasmids that confer resistance to antibiotics) are also conjugative plasmids. Many R plasmids carry genes that confer resistances to several classes of antibiotics. The presence of transmissible plasmids that carry multiple genes encoding resistance factors for several antibiotics explains the occurrence and rapid spread of multiple resistant microorganisms.

Some multiple resistant plasmids may even be transferred from one bacterial species to another. To make matters worse, plasmid-mediated drug resistance can be somewhat nonspecific, conferring resistance not only to a certain antibiotic but also to its synthetic derivatives. Since conjugation commonly occurs in nature, it is probably the most frequent mechanism of transfer of antibiotic resistance in vivo.

Some bacteria are able to transfer their genetic material in the absence of pili (see further on). In gram-positive bacteria such as *Enterococcus faecalis,* it has been postulated that a "sex phenome" may be present on the bacterial cell surface, which induces the cells to mate. However, it is not clear whether such a substance actually exists.

TRANSFORMATION

Conjugative as well as nonconjugative plasmids and pieces of bacterial chromosomes can be transferred from cell to cell by a process called *transformation*. During transformation, naked DNA is taken up by "competent" cells. A state of **competency** is induced when certain bacterial species are treated with calcium and magnesium chloride. This treatment induces some unknown state in the bacterial cell that allows the transport of a DNA molecule through the cell membrane(s) and peptidoglycan into the cytoplasm. Transforma-

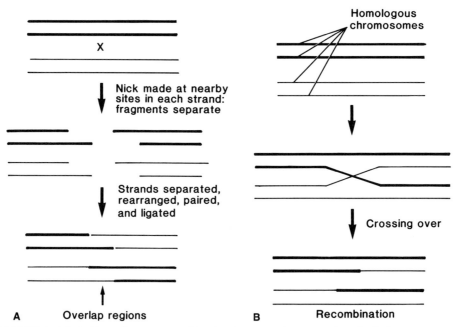

FIGURE 3–57 ✦ Homologous recombination is a complex event for which the mechanisms are not yet fully understood. The recombination process can be simplistically diagrammed as in **A** or **B**, in which two double-stranded DNA molecules are broken and rejoined. Experiments have determined that the joining requires homologous base-pairing and that overlap regions are present at many stages in the recombination process. DNA replication does not appear to be required for recombination to occur.

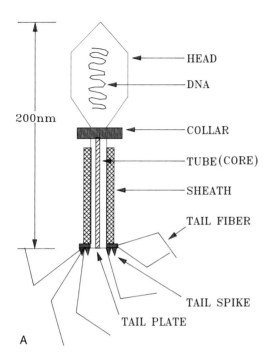

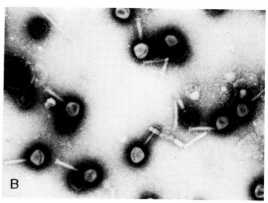

A

B

FIGURE 3–58 ✦ Schematic representation **(A)** and electron photomicrograph **(B)** of T-2 bacteriophage of the bacterial virus T-2. This bacteriophage consists of a large diamond-shaped head, which encloses double-stranded DNA. The head is attached to a long thin tail by a collar. The tail fibers attach to the tail plate.

HEAD
DNA
200nm
COLLAR
TUBE(CORE)
SHEATH
TAIL FIBER
TAIL SPIKE
TAIL PLATE

tion of gram-negative bacteria usually requires closed circular DNA, whereas gram-positive *Bacillus* sp. are transformed more efficiently by linear (cut) DNA.

As soon as a plasmid has been introduced into a cell via transformation, it can replicate and its genes will be expressed by the recipient cell. However, pieces of a chromosome that are introduced into a recipient cell by transformation must first *recombine* with (insert into) the recipient chromosome before the genes are expressed. This process of inserting into the chromosome, *homologous recombination* (Fig. 3–57), occurs when two sequences of DNA that are identical or nearly identical to one another align and form complementary base-pairing between strands of DNA unwound from two different DNA molecules. This puts the identical (or *homologous*) sequences in exact register. Subsequent to this, the two internal strands of homologous DNA break and are religated (recombined), but the ligation occurs between the broken ends of the two opposing strands, which results in a cross-over product. This crossing over must occur at two sites in order for a new sequence to be inserted into the chromosome during transformation. Transformation is commonly used in the laboratory for purposes of genetic analysis and for DNA cloning (see later discussion of cloning) and also may occur in nature.

Bacterial Viruses

Viruses that infect and grow in bacteria are called *bacteriophages* (Fig. 3–58) and may be con-

sidered as specialized extrachromosomal DNA elements that have the added capabilities to encode a (viral) protein coat and kill the host cell. Bacteriophages have no metabolic or synthetic capabilities of their own and must rely entirely on the host for these functions, so they are unable to multiply in the absence of a sensitive host. Bacteriophages consist of a replicon of genetic material (DNA or RNA) encapsulated by a protein coat (head *capsid*) (Table 3–7), which acts as a vehicle for transfer of the replicon. In addition, some bacteriophages have a protein tail through which the phage particles attach to the host cell surface as an initial step of infection. There are two types of phages: (1) *virulent* phages, which multiply within a susceptible host cell, giving rise to progeny phage and resulting in host cell lysis and death (Fig. 3–59); and (2) *temperate* phages, which have the ability to either enter the lytic cycle as virulent phages or **lysogenize** the host cell (Fig. 3–60). While in the lysogenic state, the phage nucleic acid integrates into the chromosome and thus undergoes controlled replication within the cell without causing host cell lysis.

Phage genomes (DNA) vary from a few kilobases (encoding three proteins) to well over 100 kilobases, encoding 135 genes (see Table 3–7), or 4 percent of the size of a bacterial chromosome.

Bacteriophages can mediate the transfer of small segments of chromosomal (or even plasmid) DNA between cells, by a process called *transduction*. This phage-mediated gene transfer results in either movement of random regions of DNA *(generalized transduction)* or transfer of certain limited portions

TABLE 3–7 ✦ Comparison of Bacteriophage Characteristics

| PHAGE | CLASS* | INFECTIVE CYCLE | VIRION CHARACTERISTICS | | VIRAL GENOME | |
			HEAD SIZE (nm)	TAIL (nm)	SIZE (kb)	FORM
	Lambdoid	Temperate	60	135 × 15	48.6	ds, linear
P1	—	Temperate	65	150 × 12	91.5	ds, linear
P2	—	Temperate	60	135 × 10	33	ds, linear
Mu	—	Temperate	54	135 × 18	38	ds, linear
T4	T-even	Virulent	80 × 110	98 × 20	166	ds, linear
T7	T-odd	Virulent	58	20 × 19	40	ds, linear
O × 174	Isometric	Virulent	25	—	5.4	ss, circular
M13	Filamentous	Virulent	—	900 × 9	6.4	ss, circular
MS2	RNA phage	Virulent	26	—	3.6	ss, linear, RNA

Data from Bukhari et al. (1977), Luria et al. (1978), and *Gene Function,* R. Glass (1982).
*Abbreviations: kb, 10^3 nucleotides.

of the bacterial chromosome *(specialized transduction)*. Some phages can facilitate either type of transduction while others are limited to one type or the other.

GENERALIZED TRANSDUCTION

Occasionally, during maturation of phage particles in the cytoplasm of the bacterial cell, a small amount of the bacterial DNA will be erroneously packaged by the phage capsid. This erroneous packaging is random and can include any part of the bacterial DNA. The phage particle containing bacterial host DNA then continues the maturation cycle as normal and is able to infect another cell, eventually injecting the bacterial DNA along with the rest of the viral DNA. In order for this transferred (injected) donor chromosomal DNA fragment to be expressed and maintained stably by the recipient cell, it must be recombined (via homologous recombination) into the recipient host cell genome.

SPECIALIZED TRANSDUCTION

Upon phage infection with specialized transducing phages, the viral DNA inserts into the host cell's chromosome at a specific site. For the temperate bacteriophage *lambda*, the site is designated *att B* and lies between the bacterial *gal* and *bio* genes. Integration of the circular phage genome occurs through homologous recombination (analogous to insertion of the F plasmid at specific sites on the bacterial chromosome to form an *Hfr*). Upon

FIGURE 3–59 ✦ The lytic life cycle of a bacteriophage begins when the phage attaches to the surface of the bacterial host. After injection of the phage genome into the host, the host's metabolism is controlled by the phage genome, which encodes and directs the synthesis of phage progeny and finally lysis of the host cell. (Typically, 50 to 200 bacteriophages are produced per infected cell.) The released progeny phages are then able to attach and infect other susceptible bacterial hosts.

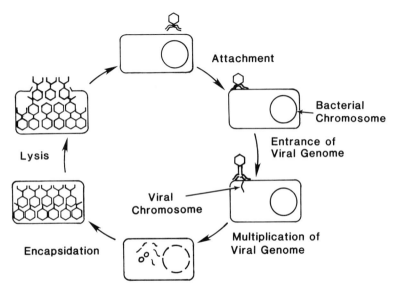

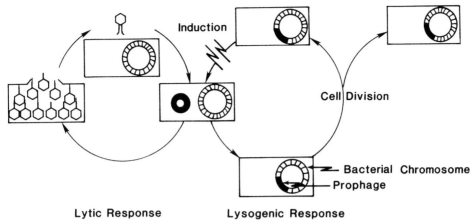

Lytic Response   Lysogenic Response

FIGURE 3–60 ✦ A temperate bacteriophage can enter into one of two life cycles. Upon infection of the bacterial host, it can continue through the lytic cycle, resulting in the production of numerous infective viral particles and lysis of the host (see Fig. 3–13). Alternatively, it may enter the lysogenic cycle, in which the bacteriophage genome is integrated into the bacterial chromosome as a prophage or the genome may be present as a stably inherited autonomous genetic element, identical to a plasmid. The lysogenic cycle may continue through numerous cell divisions until interference with the host's cell metabolism or DNA synthesis induces a change from the lysogenic cycle to the lytic cycle.

excision of the phage DNA, some adjacent chromosomal DNA may be accidentally excised and packaged in the viral capsid along with the viral DNA. (When this happens with lambda phage, *gal* or *bio* genes are excised along with the phage DNA.) This bacterial DNA is then injected into the next bacterial host. This type of transduction is "specialized" since only specific regions of the chromosomal DNA (that which is directly adjacent to the integrated viral DNA) are transduced. Both types of transduction occur in nature and have been used for many years by scientists studying gene expression and for genetic mapping.

The properties of transformation, conjugation, and transduction are summarized in Table 3–8.

Mutation

The DNA of an organism may be damaged or changed during cell growth by its internal or external environment. If the change is permanent (i.e., one that is heritable), the change is called a *mutation* and the organism whose DNA is mutated is called a *mutant* organism. Mutations may inactivate a gene product, modify its activity, or, very infrequently, create a new property of the gene

TABLE 3–8 ✦ Characteristics of Gene Transfer in Bacteria

CHARACTERISTIC	TRANSFORMATION	CONJUGATION	TRANSDUCTION
Mode of DNA transfer	Across the cell membrane of the recipient	Through pili after cell-to-cell contact	Within the protein coat of a bacteriophage
Bacteria involved	Both gram + and gram −	Almost only gram −	Both gram + and gram −
Amount of donor DNA transferred	About 20 genes	From 20 genes to entire chromosome	About 20 genes
Plasmid transfer	Yes	Yes	Yes
Resistance to deoxyribonuclease (degrades DNA)	No	Yes	Yes
Unidirectional transfer	No	Yes	No
Important as exchange mechanism in nature	Probably	Yes	Yes

product. Mutations that inactivate essential genes are, of course, lethal to the cell. Nonlethal mutations affecting dispensable gene products may result in such things as a change in growth requirements, the ability to survive in the presence of cidal (lethal) agents, resistance to bacteriophages, or no phenotypic change at all.

MUTATION CLASSIFICATION

A mutation that affects just one nucleotide is a *point mutation*. Examples include *base pair substitutions* (the replacement of one base by another) and *frameshift mutations* (the addition or deletion of one or more base pairs), which alter the translational reading frame. Base pair substitutions may result in a *missense mutation,* which results in the encoding of a different amino acid from the wild type protein, or a *nonsense mutation,* which results in a codon (UAG, UAA, or UGA) that codes for termination of polypeptide synthesis. In this case termination occurs too soon, resulting in a *truncated* (or shortened) protein that is inactive.

Spontaneous mutations occur naturally at a rate of 10^{-8} per generation and are the result of DNA replication errors within the bacterium. *Induced mutations* are caused by external factors such as irradiation, chemical substances, or heat. Induced mutations occur at a variable but greater frequency than spontaneous mutations.

CHEMICAL MUTAGENS

Several chemical compounds originally thought to be safe are now known to be mutagenic agents, causing chromosomal damage in a wide range of organisms in both prokaryotes and humans (Table 3–9). These chemical mutagens can be divided into three main groups according to their mode of action: *base analogues,* compounds that alter the structure of nucleic acids *(base modifiers),* and DNA-binding or *intercalating agents.* The base analogues such as 5-bromouracil and 2-amino-purine have structures similar to thymine and adenine, respectively. Introduction of these base analogues instead of the normal base into the DNA during DNA synthesis results in mispairing at the site of the modified base during replication.

Some chemical mutagens directly modify template DNA in situ. Nitrous acid and hydroxylamine behave in this manner, resulting in incorrect base pairing in daughter cells. Alkylating agents (the largest class of mutagens) alkylate several components of DNA and induce mutations both directly through mispairing and indirectly by error-prone repair (as described for thymine-thymine dimers further on).

Compounds that intercalate (insert) between stacked nucleotide bases, such as acridine orange and ethidium bromide, cause frameshift mutations by an as yet unknown mechanism.

TABLE 3–9 ✦ Mutagenic Agents and Their Specificities

MUTAGENIC AGENT	SPECIFICITY	MECHANISM*
Spontaneous	Substitution	Mispairing
	Frameshift	Slipping
	Multisite	Recombination
	All types	Misrepair
UV radiation	All types	Misrepair
Base analogue		
5′-bromour-acil	A·T↔G·C†	Mispairing
2′-amino-purine	G·C↔A·T	Mispairing
Base modifiers		
nitrous acid	A·T↔G·C	Mispairing
hydroxyl-amine	G·C↔A·T	Mispairing
alkylating agents	Mainly transi-tions§	Mispairing
	All types	Mispairing
Intercalators	Frameshift	Slipping
	All types‖	Misrepair

*Mispairing (nonstandard base pairing) may arise spontaneously or through the presence of nucleotide derivatives. Slipping refers to imperfect pairing between complementary strands due to base sequence redundancy. All types of mutations may be induced indirectly by faulty repair mechanisms (misrepair).

†G·C↔A·T is most common.

‡A·T↔G·C transitions occur 10- to 20-fold more frequently.

§EMS and MNNG are highly specific for G·C↔A·T transitions (though other mutations are induced by error-prone repair).

‖The wide range of lesions induced by international chemical reference (ICR) compounds may stem from their alkylating side chain.

Exposure of bacteria to ultraviolet irradiation (254 nm) generates pyrimidine dimers (usually thymine-thymine) in the DNA. Thymine dimers are unable to form hydrogen bonds (base pair) so bacterial repair mechanisms are called upon to excise and repair the affected bases. During this repair, mistakes may be made in the insertion of bases, resulting in a mutated gene.

Transposons

Transposons (TN) (Table 3–10) are *genetic elements* (short sequences of DNA) that translocate between DNA sequences of no apparent homology; that is, they "jump" from one site to another in no apparent pattern. There appear to be no specific sequences that transposons recognize; they can even transpose between a plasmid and a chromosome.

Transposons vary in size from 4 to 21 kb and contain coding regions that confer resistance to one

TABLE 3–10 ✦ Properties of Transposable Genetic Elements*

GENETIC ELEMENTS	SIZE (bp)*	TERMINAL REPETITION ELEMENT†	DRUG RESISTANCE‡
Tn1 (Tn2, Tn3)§	4,957	38 bp inverted	Ampicillin
Tn5	5,400	1,450 bp inverted	Kanamycin
Tn9	2,638	ISI direct	Chloramphenicol
Tn10	9,300	1,400 bp inverted	Tetracycline
Bacteriophages			
Mu	38,000	11 bp inverted	—

After Calos and Miller (1980) and *Gene Function,* R. E. Glass (1982).
*bp = base pairs.
†Refers to direct repetitions flanking inserting element. The 15 bp terminal repeat associated with prophage lambda represents the common core 0 present in both att B and att P.
‡Refers to antibiotic resistance encoded by transposon.
§Tn1, Tn2, and Tn3 are very similar (the complete DNA sequence of Tn3 is known).

or more antibiotics or even to toxin genes. One striking characteristic of transposons is that they have terminal inverted or direct repeats (see Table 3–10), which are required for transposition activity.

Transposons are ubiquitous in prokaryotic cells. For example, the antibiotic resistance genes of several R plasmids are transposon-like structures. The frequency of transposon transposition varies from 10^{-3} to 10^{-6}, depending on the particular transposon. Transposition is relatively nonspecific, yet is not entirely random because insertion can occur in any gene; however, there are certain "hot spots" on the chromosome where insertions occur more frequently. The location of these "hot spots" depends on the particular transposon.

The insertion of a transposon in a gene interrupts that gene, resulting in gene inactivation, or mutation. This type of *insertional inactivation* has frequently been used to generate mutations in specific genes for genetic studies. Just as a transposon jumps into a gene, it can as easily jump out.

This "jumping out," or *excision,* may reactivate the mutated (target) gene if the excision is precise, or may result in a deletion of adjoining chromosomal or plasmid DNA when excision is not precise (i.e., some of the adjoining DNA is removed with the transposon excision). Regardless of whether or not the excision is precise, the transposon remains intact and can subsequently insert into another gene and begin the process once again.

Genetic Engineering

The discovery and isolation of (bacterial) enzymes that cut and paste (*restrict* and *ligate,* respectively) pieces of DNA in a test tube has allowed the combining of fragments of DNA from different organisms in order to produce new combinations or sequences of DNA, or *recombinant DNA.* The

application of this technology has already resulted in the production of quantities of highly purified vital proteins such as human insulin, interferon, interleukin II, and human growth hormones. A multitude of bacterial genes also have been cloned. Figure 3–61 outlines a general procedure for cloning antigens of any bacterial cell, in this case genes of *Bacteroides* sp. Initially, chromosomal DNA is isolated from the donor bacterium and is restricted by an *endonuclease* (an enzyme that cuts DNA), which recognizes a certain DNA sequence (usually 4 to 6 bases in length) and makes a staggered cut in that particular sequence (see Fig. 3–18), wherever that sequence occurs in the chromosome. The *vector* DNA, which is either a plasmid or bacteriophage genome (in this case the multicopy plasmid, pUC9), is also restricted with the same enzyme and thus has staggered (*sticky*) ends complementary to those of the chromosomal DNA pieces. Upon mixing these two DNA species in the presence of the enzyme ligase (a DNA pasting-together enzyme), the complementary ends recombine in a random fashion. When both ends of the plasmid vector are ligated to the opposite ends of a piece of the chromosomal DNA (Fig. 3–62), a covalently closed circular (CCC) piece of recombinant DNA is formed. Under appropriate laboratory-induced conditions (salt washes and heat shock, see *transformation*), *E. coli* bacteria will take up CCC DNA into their cytoplasm. Like a naturally occurring plasmid, this recombinant plasmid will then be replicated and its genes will transcribe the formation of proteins by the host cell. Since the plasmid encodes (in this case) for ampicillin resistance, cells that have taken up a plasmid can be selected on medium containing ampicillin. Because each gene on the recombinant plasmid may be expressed, the donor bacterial DNA that is ligated into the plasmid vector will also be transcribed into RNA, and the RNA will be translated into the ap-

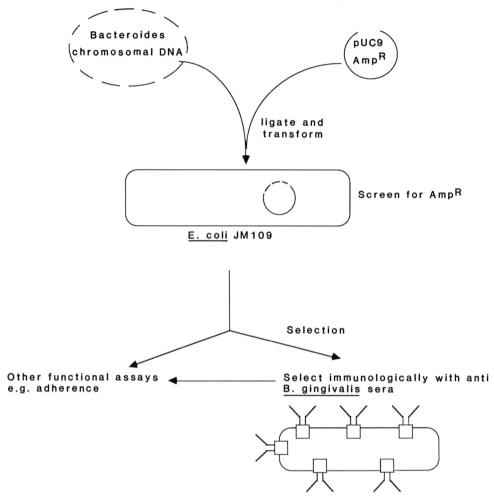

FIGURE 3–61 ✦ Protocol for cloning a *Bacteroides* antigen gene in *E. coli*.

propriate protein(s) by the *E. coli* host. Suppose, for instance, that a piece of *Bacteroides* DNA that encodes a *Bacteroides* surface protein (or antigen) is ligated into the plasmid vector, and the resulting recombinant plasmid is used to transform an *E. coli* cell. This *E. coli* cell will then synthesize the *Bacteroides* surface antigen. The transformed *E. coli* cell is thus a kind of hybrid cell that can be identified in the midst of thousands of other *E. coli* transformants (which contain other pieces of the *Bacteroides* chromosome) by the fact that this particular transformant, or clone, will react with anti-*Bacteroides* antisera. In this way, one gene and its product (the antigen) can be isolated and studied independently of other *Bacteroides* genes. In addition, once a gene is cloned into *E. coli*, it may be produced in large quantities by the *E. coli* cell.

Because of the universal genetic code, virtually any DNA can be used as donor DNA, and bacteriophages, in addition to certain plasmids, can be

used as cloning vectors. Genes can be cloned into several gram-positive species of bacteria as well as other gram-negative species besides *E. coli*. Depending on the gene to be cloned, a variety of clone selection techniques can also be used.

Several genes of dentally important bacteria have been cloned. These include virulence genes of *Streptococcus mutans* (including glucosyl-transferase) and *S. sanguis;* a gene encoding *Porphyromonas gingivalis* pili; a fimbrial gene of *Actinomyces viscosus;* a gene encoding a protease of *P. gingivalis;* and surface antigen genes of *A. actinomycetemcomitans, P. gingivalis, Prevotella (Bacteroides) intermedia,* and *Eikenella corrodens*. Several of these cloned proteins are likely candidates for vaccines.

DNA Probes

Recognizing the principle that a single-stranded piece of DNA will voraciously bind to a complementary single strand of DNA, researchers have created DNA probes. The probes are used to detect the presence of a particular gene or sequence of DNA in a particular DNA preparation (Fig. 3–63). These probes are selected fragments of DNA that contain specific gene sequences. Almost any DNA segment can be selected as a probe. If a desired DNA sequence is known, the probe can even be synthesized. To make it possible to visualize the probe, either radioactive or enzymatic labels are attached.

Several DNA probes are already used in clinical diagnostic laboratories to rapidly detect the presence of specific viruses and bacteria, as well as a variety of human genes and mutations. The great advantages of DNA-probe diagnostic tests are their specificity and speed. Among the DNA probes currently in use are those for (1) the screening for the presence of the AIDS virus in donated blood; (2) testing for bacterial meningitis, yielding results in 10 minutes; (3) testing for streptococcal throat infection requiring 1 hour; and (4) testing for the presence of *Neisseria gonorrhoeae*, genital herpes, or *Chlamydia*.

Several DNA probes have recently been developed for the detection of various periodontopathic species of bacteria. These are now commercially available. Since these tests are relatively simple and specific, coupled with the development of non-

radioactive techniques for labeling probes, it may be possible in the near future to detect the presence of these bacteria during a routine dental examination. This information would undoubtedly be helpful in identifying potential disease sites before tissue breakdown occurs and the bacteria associated with periodontal treatment resistant sites.

The Nature of Bacterial Virulence

A *pathogenic microorganism* is capable of producing disease in a susceptible host. Some bacteria are extremely pathogenic. For example, *Treponema pallidum*, the infectious agent of syphilis, has a minimal infectious dose estimated at 1 to 3 microorganisms. Other bacteria, such as *Vibrio cholerae*, which have a minimal infectious dose of 1×10^8 bacteria, are much less pathogenic. Bacteria that cause disease are *virulent* microorganisms. Virulence is actually the product of many interacting variables, involving both the microorganism and the host. A *virulence factor* is a property or characteristic of a pathogenic microorganism that allows it to cause disease. The sum total of virulence factors of a pathogenic bacterium includes the mechanisms by which the bacterium evades the host's defensive mechanisms, establishes an infection, and damages host cells. *Infection*, as defined here is an invasion or colonization

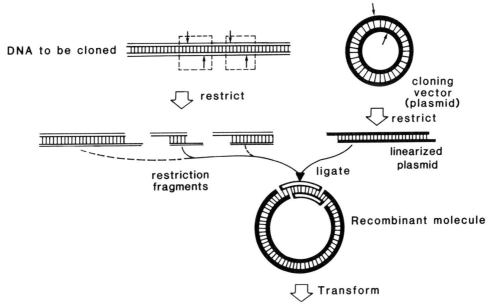

FIGURE 3–62 ✦ The DNA to be cloned *(white)* and the cloning vector *(solid)* are restricted with the same endonuclease to generate fragments of DNA with "sticky" or complementary ends. The recombinant molecule is formed in vitro when the "sticky" ends from one source of DNA anneal (in the presence of the enzyme ligase) with the complementary ends of the vector DNA. The recombinant DNA molecule is then used to transform a suitable host, often an *E. coli* strain.

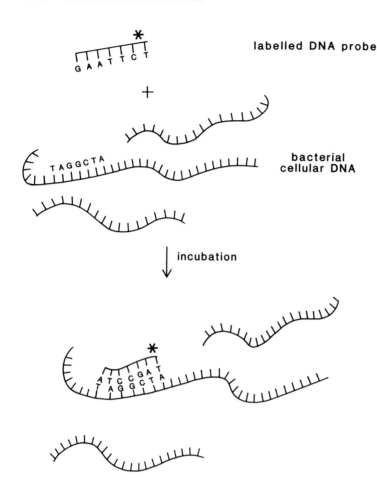

labelled DNA probe

FIGURE 3–63 ✦ DNA probes allow the defection of specific genes or DNA sequences. In the hypothetical case depicted here, the probe DNA contains a sequence specific for a certain species of bacteria. The target (bacterial cellular DNA) could be from a plaque sample. If the particular species for which the DNA probe is specific is present in the plaque, then that complementary DNA sequence will be present in the bacterial cellular DNA and the probe will bind to the target DNA. This type of assay only works with single-stranded DNA, so that prior to incubation of the target DNA with the probe, the DNA is denatured by heat to generate single strands of the DNA.

of the host by a pathogenic microorganism or its products, resulting in disease in the host. Bacteria may establish an infection by two mechanisms: (1) colonization and invasion of tissues of the host, and (2) the production of toxins that may disseminate and produce cytotoxic effects on tissues distant from the initial site of infection. Therefore, for an infection to occur, the infecting organism *(etiologic agent)* must be able to (1) gain access to host tissue, (2) multiply on or in host tissue, (3) resist host defense mechanisms, and (4) damage host tissues. The last part of this chapter will discuss the microbial (virulence) factors involved in the establishment of an infection.

Bacterial Adherence

For bacteria to cause disease, they must first enter and establish themselves in the host tissue. The initial mechanism is adherence to host tissue. In a vast majority of diseases, an individual becomes infected by colonization of mucosal surfaces of the upper respiratory tract, the intestinal tract, and/or the genitourinary tract. Because secretions (including saliva), ciliary action, peristalsis, des-

quamation, excretion, coughing, sneezing, swallowing, and blood flow wash away or remove unattached bacteria, attachment to host cells is a requirement of all pathogens of mucosal surfaces, including the oral cavity. It has been estimated that each person swallows approximately 1 liter of saliva a day! It is thus not surprising that unattached bacteria are washed away faster than they multiply (divide).

The requirement for the attachment of bacteria to host tissues prior to infection is founded on the following evidence:

1. In vitro experiments have indicated a propensity for certain bacteria to infect specific tissues that is comparable with the ability of these bacteria to adhere to the tissue (Table 3–11). It has not been demonstrated that a high incidence of infection by a specific pathogen is associated with poor adherence of that pathogen to the isolated tissue in vivo. For example, several streptococcal species colonize the oral cavity but with differing site predilections. *S. salivarius* is primarily found on the dorsum of the tongue and on the buccal mucosa, while *S. mutans* and *S. mitis* are found abundantly in dental plaque *(S. mutans* is recovered in high numbers

TABLE 3–11 ✦ Relationship Between Site of Infection and In Vitro Adherence

SITE OF INFECTION	SOURCE OF TARGET CELL	ORGANISM	RELATIVE ADHERENCE TO TARGET CELL (IN VITRO)	RELATIVE INCIDENCE OF INFECTION
Endocarditis	Heart-valve endothelium	Streptococci (viridans group), staphylococci	Good	High
		Escherichia coli	Poor	Low
		Pseudomonas	Good	High (in heroin-using adults)
Mucosal colonization	Buccal mucosa	*Streptococcus mitis*	Poor	Low
		S. salivarius	Good	High
		E. coli	Good	Low
Pyoderma	Skin epithelium	*Streptococcus pyogenes*		
		Skin strain	Good	High
		Pharyngeal strain	Low	Moderate
Pharyngitis	Buccal cells	*S. pyogenes*		
		Skin strain	Moderate	Low
		Pharyngeal strains	Good	High
Cervicitis	Vaginal cells	Anaerobic bacteria	Poor	Low
		Neisseria gonorrhoeae	Good	High
		Streptococcus agalactiae (group B)	Moderate	None
		C. vaginale	Moderate	Intermediate
Pyelonephritis	Uroepithelial cells	*E. coli*		
		Pyelonephritis strains	Good	High
		Nonpyelonephritis strains	?	?

from supragingival plaque), but in low numbers on mucosal surfaces. In vitro, these species are found to adhere to tissue cells of the tissue type that they colonize but not to other cells or other dental surfaces.

2. Bacterial variants that are found to have a reduced capacity to adhere in vitro have decreased infectivity in vivo (see Table 3–12). For instance, certain colony types of *Neisseria gonorrhoeae* that have a very limited ability to adhere to genital epithelial cells are unable to cause human infection in vivo, whereas colony types that adhere well in vitro have a high infectivity rate in vivo. The same is true for variants of several other pathogens including *Salmonella, E. coli, Proteus mirabilis,* streptococci, and *Actinomyces viscosus.*

3. The bacterial binding capacity of epithelial cells from individuals prone to certain bacterial infections is sometimes higher than those tissues from uninfected individuals (Table 3–13). For example, greater numbers of uropathogenic *E. coli* bind to urinary tract epithelial cells of women who have recurrent urinary tract infections than to urinary tract epithelial cells of normal women; cells of individuals with virus infections bind more *Streptococcus sanguis* than cells from uninfected individuals; and certain strains of piglets that are susceptible to diarrhea caused by *E. coli* (which

have the K88 adhesin) bind more *E. coli* than do other piglets.

Bacterial adherence is mediated by bacterial cell surface structures called *adhesins,* which recognize specific receptors on the particular host cell surface (Fig. 3–64). The occurrence and distribution of host cell receptors for particular (bacterial) adhesins determines the tissue and species *tropisms* (specificities) of bacteria.

Because both bacterial and tissue cell surfaces are net negatively charged, bacteria must overcome this repulsion by charge and hydrophobicity localization. To this end, bacterial adhesins are commonly located on surface appendages such as fimbriae (Table 3–14).

There are several pathogens for which adherence mechanisms are known in detail (Table 3–14). *Actinomyces viscosus* strain T14V, an etiologic agent of root caries in rats, mice, and probably humans, synthesizes at least two antigenically distinct types of fimbriae, designated type 1 and type 2. Type 2 fimbriae mediate lactose-sensitive adherence of *A. viscosus* to several species of streptococci and to neuraminidase-treated erythrocytes. Type 1 fimbriae, on the other hand, mediate the adsorption of strain T14V to saliva-treated hydroxyapatite (SHA), a surface that mimics the saliva-coated tooth surface. This adsorption is not inhibited by

TABLE 3–12 ✦ Relationship Between Epithelial Cell Adherence In Vitro and Bacterial Infectivity In Vivo

BACTERIA	BACTERIAL VARIANTS	RELATIVE ADHERENCE IN VITRO	RELATIVE INFECTIVITY IN VIVO
Actinomyces viscosus	Fimbriate	Good	High
	Nonfimbriate	Poor	Low
Gonococci	T_1 (fimbriate)	Good	High
	T_4 (nonfimbriate)	Poor	Low
Escherichia coli (enterotoxigenic)	CF +	Good	High
	CF −	Poor	Low
Streptococci	Dextran +	Good	High
	Dextran −	Poor	Low
Salmonella	Fimbriate	Good	High
	Nonfimbriate	Poor	Moderate
E. coli	K88 +	Good	High
	K88 −	Poor	Low
Proteus mirabilis	Fimbriate	Good	High
	Nonfimbriate	Poor	Low
Bordetella pertussis	Fimbriate	Good	High
	Nonfimbriate	Poor	Low

TABLE 3–13 ✦ Correlation Between In Vitro Adherence to Target Host Cells and Predisposition to Acquire Infection

SUBJECTS	BACTERIA	TARGET CELLS	TARGET CELLS FROM	RELATIVE IN VITRO ADHERENCE
Females with recurrent urinary tract infections	*Escherichia coli*	Vaginal periurethral epithelial cells	Subject	High
			Normal	Low
Individuals with damaged heart valves (i.e., rheumatic heart disease)	Streptococci	Endothelium of heart valves	Damaged	High
			Normal	Low
Individuals with viral infections	*Streptococcus sanguis, S. agalactiae*	Tissue culture cells	Virus-infected culture	High
			Uninfected culture	Low
Staphylococcal carriers	*Staphlococcus aureus*	Nasal epithelium	Carrier	High
			Noncarrier	Low
Genetic variants of pigs	*E. coli* K88	Intestinal epithelium	K88-resistant phenotype	Low
			K88-susceptible phenotype	High
Primates	*Neisseria gonorrhoeae*	Organ cultures of oviducts	Human	High
			Nonprimate	Low

lactose. The receptors on the SHA surface for the *Actinomyces* type 1 fimbriae are a specific class of salivary proteins, proline-rich-proteins (PRPs). Since these proteins are a component of saliva that preferentially adsorb to the tooth surface, it is thought that the type 1 fimbriae are the principal adhesins involved in the adherence of *A. viscosus* to tooth surfaces in vivo.

Group A streptococci (i.e., *S. pyogenes,* the etiologic agent of pharyngitis, rheumatic fever, and glomerulonephritis) bind to epithelial cells by M-protein lipoteichoic acid (LTA) complexes present on the surface of the streptococci. The LTA molecules, which consist entirely of glycerol-PO_4, are anchored to the cytoplasmic membrane by covalent binding to the membrane glycolipids. The host ep-

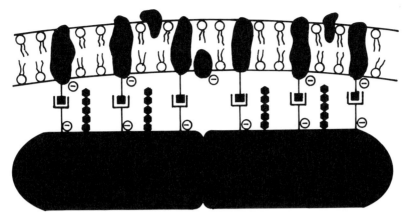

FIGURE 3–64 ✦ Attachment of a bacterial cell to a host cell membrane or surface usually occurs by *specific* binding of bacterial cell structures (adhesins Ψ) to target host cell receptors (∎). Because there is a net negative charge on both cell surfaces, the bacterial cell may contain hydrophobic molecules (⊝), which are attracted toward phospholipid molecules (hydrophobic) in the host cell membrane. Several different types of bacterial cell surface structures may act as adhesins, see Table 3–14. (From Beachey, Bacterial Adherence. Chapman and Hall, London, 1980, p.p. 1–29, with permission.)

ithelial receptor for the LTA adhesin is probably the membrane protein, fibronectin. Both purified LTA and antibodies to LTA (but not those to other surface antigens) block adherence of streptococci to cell membranes.

Type 1 fimbriae are one of several adhesins that mediate the binding of *E. coli* to host epithelial cells. Since the binding of type 1 fimbriae to epithelial cells can be inhibited by the presence of mannose, it appears that the epithelial cell receptor

TABLE 3–14 ✦ Specific Adhesins and Receptors of Various Bacteria

BACTERIA	ADHESIN	RECEPTOR
Streptococcus pyogenes	LTA-M protein fibrillae	Fibronectin
Escherichia coli	Type 1 fimbriae	D-mannose
Klebsiella aerogenes		
K. pneumoniae		
Serratia marcescens		
Shigella flexneri		
Enterobacter cloacae		
Salmonella typhi		
S. paratyphi A		
S. paratyphi B		
S. typhimurium		
Citrobacter freundii		
E. coli (uropathogenic)	MR fimbriae	GalNacoal-3GalNacbl-3-Galal-4Galbl-4GlcCer (Globotetraosylceramide and Globotriosyl-ceramide)
	MR and type 1 fimbriae	Same as above plus D-mannose
E. coli CFA 1	MR fimbriae	?Gal Nacbl-4-Galal-4GlcCer (GM_2 ganglioside)
CFA 11		
E. coli K88	MR fimbriae	?b-D-Gal or GalNac and GlcNac
Actinomyces viscosus	Type 1 fibrillae	Proline-rich protein or glycoprotein
Vibrio cholera	Fimbriae	Fucose and mannose
Mycoplasma	Membrane protein	Sialic acid, glycophorin
Neisseria gonorrhoeae	Fimbriae	Galbl-3GalNac-bl-4Gal
Proteus species	Fimbriae (type 4)	?
Bordetella pertussis	Fimbriae	? Sterol
Pseudomonas aeruginosa	Fimbriae	?
Chlamydia	?	N-acetylglucosamine

contains mannose since cells treated with concanavalin A, a plant lectin that binds to mannose residues, also prevents adherence of *E. coli* to the epithelial cells.

Once bacteria have colonized a target tissue, fimbriae may be detrimental to the bacterial cells since their presence may increase the chance of phagocytosis. Consequently, after the initial colonization bacteria may undergo phenotypic changes and no longer synthesize fimbriae. This appears to be the case with pyelonephritic *E. coli*. While the *E. coli* are infecting the lower urinary tract and bladder, they contain high numbers of type 1 fimbriae. However, once the infection progresses to the kidneys, the cells contain very few, if any, fimbriae.

It should now be obvious that the adherence of bacteria to host tissues promotes colonization and facilitates penetration of target tissues by virulent bacteria. This adherence of bacteria to host tissue cells, may, in certain cases, permit a close association between the toxigenic bacteria and their target tissues. This close association may enhance the activity of the toxins by delivering the toxin directly to the target tissue. For example, *Vibrio cholerae* (the causative agent of cholera) adherence to the intestinal mucosa facilitates the local delivery of the cholera toxin (choleragen) to the intestinal cells. In a similar fashion, attachment of enteropathogenic *E. coli* to intestinal epithelial cells allows local delivery of the enterotoxin to the intestinal mucosal cells, resulting in traveler's diarrhea. *S. mutans* cells use sucrose to produce extracellular capsular polysaccharides, or *glucans,* which allow the cells to adhere to the tooth surface, primarily in protected fissures and indentations. As a byproduct of their metabolism, *S. mutans* cells produce lactic acid, a toxic end product, since a sufficient buildup of this acid causes demineralization of the tooth surface and, thus, ultimately caries. If the streptococci were not closely attached to the tooth surface, the acid would be quickly diluted and neutralized by saliva.

Virulence Factors

During the infection process, not only must microbial components or products adhere to host tissues and resist host defense mechanisms, but they must also damage tissue directly by production of toxins or indirectly by induction of an immunopathologic response. The following section will discuss in more detail the bacterial components that are determinants of disease.

SURFACE APPENDAGES

Bacterial pili (fimbriae) commonly function as adhesins (see Table 3–14). Several pathogenic bacteria contain more than one type of fimbriae and thus more than one type of adhesin. As discussed earlier, the F pili of gram-negative bacteria attach to neighboring cells and facilitate the transfer of DNA from cell to cell. This DNA exchange mechanism mediates the transfer of antibiotic resistance genes as well as virulence genes (including genes encoding various types of fimbriae) between cells.

EXTRACELLULAR CAPSULES AND SLIME

The capsule of *S. mutans* is required for adherence and virulence, but a capsule that functions as an adhesin is relatively unusual for pathogenic bacteria. Recent evidence suggests that capsules of some pathogens such as *A. viscosus, Neisseria meningitidis,* and *S. pneumoniae* may actually reduce adherence. However, the overall effect of the presence of extracellular polysaccharides is a substantial increase in virulence. This is due primarily to the antiphagocytic properties of capsules. Several pathogens for which capsules decrease **opsonization** and have antiphagocytic properties are listed in Table 3–15. In mixed infections, the presence of a capsule of one bacterial species may protect neighboring unrelated bacteria from phagocytosis. Polysaccharide capsules may also hinder the effects of antibiotics in vivo by preventing the antibiotic from coming into direct contact with the bacterial outer membrane or cell wall.

A detailed series of studies of *Bacteroides fragilis* has shown that strains producing a capsule are virulent (able to cause abscess formation), whereas strains without a capsule are avirulent. The virulent property of the capsule was further substantiated in rat experiments where implantation of purified capsular polysaccharide uniformly produced abscesses.

LIPOPOLYSACCHARIDES

Lipopolysaccharides (endotoxin; LPS) elicit a broad spectrum of pathophysiologic properties (Table 3–16), and depending on the amount of host exposure, can result in cardiovascular collapse and even death within an hour or two. Experimental findings indicate that irreversible hemorrhagic shock primarily results from adsorption of LPS from the bowel. Most of the endotoxic biologic properties are directly attributable to the lipid A portion of the molecule; however, the polysaccharide moiety confers resistance to neutrophils, is a major antigen for many bacterial species, and also functions to neutralize serum components.

The direct role of LPS in many chronic human diseases is ill defined, but several characteristics of typhoid fever and meningococcal septicemia are compatible with the known effects of LPS. Endotoxins are incompletely neutralized by antibodies

TABLE 3–15 ✦ Invasive Factors of Microbial Species Pathogenic to Mankind

INVASIVE FACTOR	BACTERIAL SOURCE	ACTIVITY
Capsule	*Streptococcus pneumoniae* *Klebsiella pneumoniae* *Hemophilus influenzae* *Bacillus anthracis* *Yersinia pestis*	Inhibits phagocytosis
M protein of cell wall	Group A streptococci	Inhibits phagocytosis
Extracellular enzymes	*Clostridium perfringens*	
Collagenase	*Porphyromonas gingivalis*	Hydrolyzes collagen
Hyaluronidase	Staphylococci, streptococci, Clostridia	Hydrolyzes hyaluronic acid
Lecithinase	*Clostridium perfringens*	Hydrolyzes lecithin
Coagulase	*Staphylococcus aureus*	Clots fibrin
Fibrinolysin (kinase)	Staphylococci, streptococci	Lysis of fibrin clots
Proteases, nucleases and lipases	Staphylococci, streptococci, *Bacteroides* species	Depolymerization of proteins, nucleic acids, and fats
Leukocidin	Staphylococci, streptococci	Lysis of red blood cells
Hemolysin	*Actinobacillus actinomycetemcomitans*	Lysis of PMNs
IgA protease	*Porphyromonas gingivalis* *Prevotella intermedius* Oral streptococci *Neisseria gonorrhoeae*	Cleavage/inactivation of IgA

TABLE 3–16 ✦ Biologic Properties of Lipopolysaccharides

ACTIVITY	EFFECT/ MECHANISM
Pyrogenicity	Causes fever by release of pyrogen from phagocytic cells
Mitogenic for T-cells	Stimulates T-cells, independent of B cells
Irreversible shock	Death
Cardiovascular collapse	Death
Necrosis of tumors	Stimulates macrophages
Cytotoxic to fibroblasts	Kills fibroblast in vitro
Chemotactic to PMNs	Altered resistance to bacterial infections
Activates complement	Alternate pathway, independent of Ab
Platelet aggregation	Thrombosis in vitro?
Bone resorption	Loss of periodontal bone
Intravascular coagulation	Activation of clotting factors
Leukopenia and leukocytosis	Decrease in number of circulating lymphocytes, granulocytes
Interferes with gluconeogenesis and glycogenesis	Loss of hepatic glycogen

(against the O-antigen component) and are stable to heat and even autoclaving. It should be noted that medical apparatus, especially that used for intravenous administrations, which may become contaminated by gram-negative organisms, is not detoxified by autoclaving and should not be used.

There is evidence that LPS may contribute to much of the tissue damage, especially bone resorption, in periodontal diseases. Several LPSs from putative periodontopathogenic species have been purified and the biologic effects studied. The chemical composition of the LPSs of *Bacteroides* sp., *Porphyromonas* sp., *Eikenella corrodens*, and *Capnocytophaga* differs from that of the classic or enteric *(E. coli* and *Salmonella typhimurium)* LPS, while that of *A. actinomycetemcomitans* appears to be similar to *S. typhimurium* LPS. The LPSs of *Eikenella* and *A. actinomycetemcomitans* are stimulatory to bone resorption when tested in in vitro assays, and purified *E. corrodens* LPS by itself causes loss of periapical bone in vivo. The mechanisms by which these LPSs cause bone resorption are unknown, but the uptake of Ca^{++} is inhibited. Therefore, the resorption is probably not via stimulation of osteoclastic activity. In addition to their effects on bone, these same LPSs are also mitogenic to B cells (independent of T cells) and *A. actinomycetemcomitans* LPS aggregates platelets and is toxic to macrophages.

Several pathogenic bacteria, including suspected periodontal pathogens (i.e., *Bacteroides* and *Porphyromonas* species and *A. actinomycetemcomitans*), produce copious amounts of membrane blebs, which may be a mechanism for delivery of membrane-bound LPS to distant sites in the absence of lysis of the bacteria. This blebbing may have important implications in periodontal diseases, especially since it has been demonstrated that LPS can be found in periodontal tissues in the absence of penetration by bacteria.

Cell Wall Components

In addition to maintaining the shape of bacterial cells and serving as a protective barrier, peptidoglycan (see earlier discussion) may also have virulence-associated properties. For instance, it activates complement, has pyrogenic activity, interferes with phagocytosis, and may contribute to damage of fallopian tubes during gonococcal infections. Streptococcal peptidoglycan contributes to the development of a chronic inflammatory response in a rheumatoid arthritis model system. The peptidoglycans of oral species of bacteria have been shown to be mitogenic and to stimulate bone loss in an in vitro assay. Purified preparations of peptidoglycans from oral isolates of *Bacteroides, Porphyromonas, Eikenella,* and *Actinomyces* are toxic to macrophages at high concentrations (greater than 50 μg/ml), and at lower concentrations significantly inhibit lysozyme activity.

Exotoxins

Both gram-negative and gram-positive bacteria produce diffusible protein molecules, or exotoxins, that injure tissue directly. These toxins are usually heat labile, have a direct necrotic effect on tissues they come in contact with and are among the most powerful poisons known to humans (Table 3–17). For example, 1 mg of tetanus toxin is enough to kill 1 million guinea pigs. The potency of these toxins is often expressed as the LD_{50}, which is the amount required to kill 50 percent of a test population. Most exotoxins can be inactivated by chemical treatment, which results in retention of the antigenic properties of the active toxin molecule. These chemically detoxified proteins, or *toxoids,* are often used to stimulate a protective immune response (i.e., diphtheria and pertussis toxoids). The pharmacologic actions of most exotoxins are known and are generally quite slow, often requiring several days of full activity (Table 3–17). Many exotoxins are plasmid-encoded, and several have been cloned. Few exotoxins from oral isolates have been identified. However, *A. actinomycetemcomitans* isolates produce a leukotoxin that is released in blebs from the bacterial cell surface. This heat-labile, soluble toxin destroys human and monkey blood PMNs and gingival crevice PMNs but not other human cells or PMNs from a variety of other species. The leukotoxic activity does not require phagocytosis of the bacteria, but binding of the leukotoxin to the target cell membrane is an initial and prerequisite step in the cytotoxic reaction. Leu-

kotoxic activity can be inhibited by sera from patients with juvenile periodontitis.

Hydrolytic Enzymes

Most pathogenic species of bacteria synthesize a variety of enzymes that are useful in the host-parasite confrontation. Many gram-negative bacteria contain proteolytic and hydrolytic enzymes in their periplasmic space. In addition, both gram-negative and gram-positive organisms may produce extracellular lytic enzymes that increase the virulence of certain pathogenic species (see Table 3–15). These enzymes, for the most part, function to provide nutrients for growth and contribute to the invasiveness of the organism. For instance, *Porphyromonas gingivalis* produces a collagenase as well as high levels of peptidases. These peptidases are active on glycine-proline peptides, peptides that are major components of collagen of the periodontal ligament. *Capnocytophaga* species possess peptidase as well as acid and alkaline phosphatases, which may degrade bone proteins.

Several pathogenic bacteria produce proteolytic enzymes that degrade human serum proteins. IgG, IgM, C3, and C5 are degraded by *P. gingivalis* isolates, whereas strains of *Prevotella intermedia* degrade IgG and C3. The degradation of serum components may cause reduced phagocytosis and a subsequent reduction of bactericidal activity by PMNs. This may explain why *P. gingivalis* promotes the survival of avirulent bacteria in polymicrobial infections in guinea pigs and inhibits phagocytosis of other bacteria present in in vitro assays.

IgA protease is an important virulence factor in some bacterial infections of the mucous membranes, particularly gonorrhea. Since IgA is the primary antibody present in mucous membrane secretions and is a potent host defensive mechanism that can prevent bacterial adherence to the host cells, it is not surprising that the ability to produce an IgA protease would be clearly advantageous to a mucosal surface pathogen. Of 21 bacterial species found to produce an IgA-cleaving enzyme (out of 800 tested), more than half are oral streptococci and species associated with destructive periodontal disease. The remaining positive isolates include respiratory tract pathogens and *Neisseria gonorrhoeae.* The periodontal disease-associated isolates that were found to produce an IgA protease included several species of *Bacteroides* and *Capnocytophaga.* Interestingly, nonoral *Bacteroides* species were unable to cause degradation of IgA. The *Porphyromonas* IgA protease is different from all other IgA proteases in that it results in total destruction of the IgA molecule, whereas the others cleave the immunoglobulin at only one site.

TABLE 3–17 ✦ Exotoxins Produced by Various Toxigenic Bacteria

MICROBIAL SPECIES	DISEASE	TOXIN DESIGNATION	ACTIVITY OR EFFECT OF TOXIN
Bacillus anthracis	Anthrax	Factors 1, 2, and 3	Pulmonary edema, capillary thrombosis
Yersinia pestis (Pasteurella pestis)	Plague	Plague toxin	Lethality in mice related to anti-cAMP effects and shift in hormone balance
Corynebacterium diphtheriae	Diphtheria	Diphtheria toxin	An inhibitor of protein synthesis; causes necrosis of tissue
Streptococcus pyogenes	Pyogenic infections	Streptolysin O	Hemolysin
		Streptolysin S	Hemolysin; cytotoxic for many subcelluar organelles
	Scarlet fever	Erythrogenic toxin	Rash
Staphylococcus aureus	Pyogenic infections	Alpha toxin	Hemolytic, dermonecrotic; paralysis of smooth muscle
		Delta toxin	Hemolytic and dermonecrotic
		Leukocidin	Leukolytic
	Food poisoning	Enterotoxin	Vomiting and diarrhea
	Scalded skin syndrome	Exfoliatin	Exfoliation
Vibrio cholerae	Cholera	Enterotoxin (choleragen)	Activates adenyl cyclase with increased hypersecretion of Cl^-, HCO_3^-, and H_2O
Escherichia coli	Infant diarrhea Traveler's diarrhea	Enterotoxin	Activates adenyl cyclase (?)
Pseudomonas aeruginosa	Opportunistic pathogen in burn patients, the immunosuppressed, and those with cystic fibrosis	Exotoxin	Possible effects on liver (?)
Clostridium tetani	Tetanus	Tetanospasmin	Blocks nerve transmission in CNS, resulting in spastic paralysis
Clostridium botulinum	Botulism	Types A, B, E, and F principal cause of botulism in humans	Acts on peripheral nervous system: blocks release of acteylcholine, resulting in flaccid paralysis
Clostridium perfringens	Gas gangrene	Alpha toxin	A lecithinase: lyses RBCs and leukocytes
		Kappa toxin	A collagenase: attacks connective tissue
		Theta toxin	Hemolysin
	Food poisoning	Enterotoxin	Vomiting, diarrhea
Clostridium novyi, C. septicum, and *C. sporogenes*	Gas gangrene	Alpha toxin	Lecithinase: lyses RBCs and leukocytes
Shigella dysenteriae	Bacillary dysentery	Enterotoxin	May be involved in diarrhea
Actinobacillus actinomycetemcomitans	Juvenile periodontitis	Leukotoxin	Leukolytic

BIBLIOGRAPHY*
Structure

Bayer, M. E.: Areas of adhesion between wall and membrane of *Escherichia coli*. J. Gen. Microbiol. 53:345, 1968.

Costerton, J. W.: How bacteria stick. Sci. Am. 238:86, 1978.

Costerton, J. W.: The role of electron microscopy in the elucidation of bacterial structure and function. Ann. Rev. Microbiol. 33:459, 1979.

Leive, L. (ed.): Bacterial Membranes and Walls. Marcel Dekker, New York, 1973.

Nikaido, H., and Nakae, T.: The outer membrane of gram-negative bacteria. Adv. Microbiol. Physiol. 20:163, 1979.

Nikaido, H., and Vaara, M.: Molecular basis of the permeability of bacterial outer membrane. Microbiol. Rev. 49:1, 1985.

Osborn, M. J., and Wu, H. C. P.: Proteins of the outer membrane of gram-negative bacteria. Ann. Rev. Microbiol. 34:369, 1980.

Pettijohn, D. E.: Prokaryotic DNA in nucleoid structure. CRC Crit. Rev. Biochem. 4:175, 1976.

Salton, M. R. J., and Owen, P.: Bacterial membrane structure. Ann. Rev. Microbiol. 30:451, 1976.

Schleifer, K. H., and Kandler, O.: Peptidoglycan types of bacterial cell walls and their taxonomic implications. Bacteriol. Rev. 36:407, 1972.

Shiveley, J. M.: Inclusion bodies of procaryotes. Ann. Rev. Microbiol. 28:167, 1974.

Shockman, G. D., and Barrett, J. F.: Structure, function and assembly of cell walls of gram-positive bacteria. Ann. Rev. Microbiol. 37:501, 1983.

Silverman, M., and Simon, M. I.: Bacterial flagella. Ann. Rev. Microbiol. 31:397, 1977.

Ward, J. B.: Teichoic and teichuronic acids: Biosynthesis, assembly, and location. Microbiol. Rev. 45:211, 1981.

Wittmann, H. G.: Components of bacterial ribosomes. Ann. Rev. Biochem. 51:155, 1982.

Wittmann, H. G.: Architecture of prokaryotic ribosomes. Ann. Rev. Biochem. 52:35, 1983.

Metabolism

Dagley, S., and Nicholson, D. E.: An Introduction to Metabolic Pathways. Blackwell Scientific, Oxford and Edinburgh, 1970.

Gottschalk, G.: Bacterial Metabolism. Springer-Verlag, New York, 1979.

Gottschalk, G., and Andreesen, J. R.: Energy metabolism in anaerobes. In Quayle, J. R. (ed.): International Review of Biochemistry, Vol. 21. Springer-Verlag, New York, 1979, pp. 5-115.

Haddock, B. A., and Jones, C. W.: Bacterial respiration. Bacteriol. Rev. 41:47, 1977.

Ingeledew, W. J., and Poole, R. K.: The respiratory chains of *Escherichia coli*. Microbiol. Rev. 48:181, 1984.

Jones, C. W.: Bacterial respiration and photosynthesis. Thomas Nelson and Sons, Walton-on-Thames, Surrey, England, 1982.

Moat, A. G.: Microbial Physiology. John Wiley and Sons, New York, 1979.

Racker, E.: From Pasteur to Mitchell; a hundred years of bioenergetics. Fed. Proc. 39:210, 1980.

Rose, A. H.: Chemical Microbiology, ed. 3. Plenum, New York, 1976.

Zeikus, I. G.: Chemical and fuel production by anaerobic bacteria. Ann. Rev. Microbiol. 34:423, 1980.

Biosynthesis

Caskey, C. T.: Peptide chain termination. Trends Biochem. Sci. 5:234, 1980.

Clark, B.: The elongation step of protein biosynthesis. Trends Biochem. Sci. 5:207, 1980.

Hunt, T.: The initiation of protein synthesis. Trends Biochem. Sci. 5:178, 1980.

Kozak, M.: Comparison of initiation of protein synthesis in prokaryotes, eukaryotes and organelles. Microbiol. Rev. 47:1, 1983.

Preiss, J.: Bacterial glycogen synthesis and its regulation. Ann. Rev. Microbiol. 38:419, 1984.

Troy, F. A., II: The chemistry and biosynthesis of selected bacterial capsular polymers. Ann. Rev. Microbiol. 33:519, 1979.

Growth

Bauchop, T., and Elsden, S. R.: The growth of microorganisms in relation to their energy supply. J. Gen. Microbiol. 23:457, 1960.

Cole, R. M., and Hahn, J. J.: Cell wall replication in *Streptococcus pyogenes*. Science 135:722, 1962.

Ingraham, J. L., Maaloe, O., and Neidhardt, F. C.: Growth of the Bacterial Cell. Sinauer Assoc., Sunderland, Mass., 1983.

Pooley, H. M.: Localized insertion of new cell wall in *Bacillus subtilis*. Nature 274:264, 1978.

Genetics

Alberts, B., Bray, D., Lewis, J., Raff, M., Roberts, K., and Watson, J. D.: Molecular Biology of the Cell. Garland Publishing, New York, 1983.

Clewell, D. B.: Plasmids, drug resistance and gene transfer in the genus *Streptococcus*. Microbiol. Rev. 45:409, 1981.

Lewin, B.: Genes III, ed. 3. John Wiley and Sons, New York, 1987.

Nossal, N. G.: Prokaryotic DNA replication systems. Ann. Rev. Biochem. 52:581, 1983.

Smith, H. O., and Danner, D. B.: Genetic transformation. Ann. Rev. Biochem. 50:41, 1981.

*The references listed here represent an assortment of articles and books that will be useful to the reader in extending and interpreting this chapter. The titles have been listed under major subject headings for ease of locating useful information.

4 *Bacterial Classification*

Violet Haraszthy and Joseph J. Zambon

Microbiologists have always been confronted with the problem of making comparisons between microorganisms. Thus a classification system is needed, first, to provide an orderly framework to catalogue microbial lifeforms that can assume an almost limitless variety of shapes and growth requirements and, second, to communicate with one another and to answer the question: Is the microorganism isolated by scientist A the same as the microorganism isolated by scientist B? Finally, and most important for the health-related professions, a system of bacterial classification is necessary for the diagnosis of infectious diseases and to answer the question: What is the microorganism responsible for this patient's illness?

For all of these reasons, bacterial classification is an essential component of modern microbiology. It is also a constantly evolving process. As more is learned of certain microorganisms, old groupings are changed and new taxonomies are formulated. A classic example is that of the black-pigmented *Bacteroides* species (Fig. 4–1). Originally, these microorganisms were classified as *Bacterium melaninogenicum*. As these microorganisms were more intensively studied, it became clear that there were significant differences among strains of *Bacteroides melaninogenicus* in their ability to ferment sugars. Based on these sugar fermentations and other biochemical characteristics, the species *Bacteroides melaninogenicus* was divided into three subspecies. The strongly fermentative strains were categorized as *Bacteroides melaninogenicus*, subspecies *melaninogenicus*, while the nonfermentative strains were categorized as *Bacteroides melaninogenicus*, subspecies *asaccharolyticus*. Strains that were intermediate in their ability to ferment sugars were categorized as *Bacteroides melaninogenicus*, subspecies *intermedius*. Subsequent examination of these same species using newly developed molecular biology techniques revealed significant differences in the sequence of deoxyribonucleic acid bases. Based on these data, each of the subspecies was elevated to species status as *Prevotella melaninogenicus*, *Porphyromonas asaccharolyticus*, and *Prevotella intermedia*, respectively. Each of these changes may appear trivial or even deliberately confusing to those unfamiliar with bacterial taxonomy, but each change is made only after consideration of appropriate data.

Dating back to the work *Species Plantarum* by the Swedish taxonomist Linnaeus, published in 1753, bacteria have been categorized into a taxonomic hierarchy (Table 4–1), and in this hierarchy, they have been named using a two-part **epithet.** This is the same convention used to name animal or plant species. In zoology and botany, however, a species can be defined in more precise terms than is possible in microbiology. In these disciplines, species are the smallest group that can sexually interact to produce fertile offspring. This definition is inappropriate for bacterial species, which most often reproduce asexually and which are not so clearly delineated as plant and animal species. Bacterial species are considered to represent a group of strains that share a number of common features. A bacterial strain is defined as the descendant of a single pure (**axenic**) culture.

The first part of a bacterial name is the *genus* name, which, by convention, is a latinized, usually descriptive word, spelled with a capital letter. The second part of this binomial name, or *binonem,* is the *specific* epithet, which is, by convention, spelled with a lower case letter. Some species, as in the example of *Prevotella melaninogenicus* described earlier, may also make use of a *subspecies epithet,* for example, *Bacteroides melaninogenicus,* subsp. *intermedius.* Many species names are descriptive. *Actinobacillus actinomycetemcomitans* is such a descriptive species name. "*Actinobacillus*" refers to the fact that microorganisms in this genus exhibit a star-shaped formation (hence, "actino" for star) in the center of the colonies on agar surfaces and the bacterial cells are short rods ("bacillus"). The specific epithet "actinomycetemcomitans" refers to the fact that this microorganism was first isolated together with *Actinomyces israelii* from lesions of cervicofocial actinomycosis. Hence, "actinomycetemcomitans" means "together with *Actinomyces.*"

Since bacterial species are not defined in relation to reproductive ability as are species of whales, for example, microbiologists use other features of the microorganism to make groupings or **taxa.** The earliest groupings, and those still commonly used in clinical microbiology today, are based on relatively easy to define properties (Table 4–2). These include the size and shape of the bacterial cells seen under the light microscope, the ability to hold

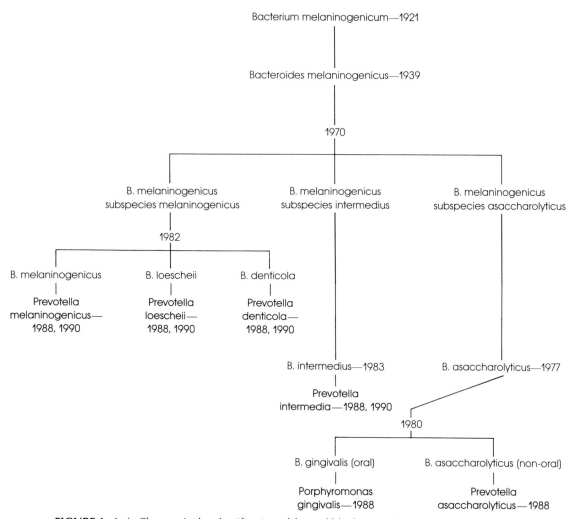

FIGURE 4–1 ✦ Changes in the classification of the oral black-pigmented *Bacteroides* species.

TABLE 4–1 ✦ **Hierarchy of Bacteria Taxa**

RANK
Kingdom
Division
Class
Order
Family
Genus
Species

certain stains such as the Giemsa and Gram stains, evidence of cellular motility as seen using phase contrast or darkfield microscopy, ability to grow at different temperatures and in different gaseous environments, the size and shape of the bacterial colony on certain types of media—there are literally hundreds of properties that can characterize a bacterium and can be used in categorization. As our knowledge and methods have improved, additional properties have been examined and incorporated into these schemes. The analysis of metabolic acid end products by gas-liquid chromatography is one such development that is now standard practice in the identification and taxonomy of bacteria.

The most basic analysis in taxonomy is an examination of the bacterial genome, which generally range from 1 to 8 $\times$ 10^9 daltons (Table 4–3). All other phenotypic properties such as bacterial size, shape, and metabolism are based on the kind and arrangement of nucleotides in the bacterial DNA. Several techniques have been developed for use in bacterial taxonomy, based on characterization of the bacterial genome. First is the determination of deoxyribonucleic acid base composition or the mole percent guanine plus cytosine content (**mol% G + C).** As the name implies, this method gives information on the amount of the specific nucleotide bases, guanine and cytosine, in bacterial DNA.

TABLE 4–2 ✦ Typical Features for the Phenotypic Classification of Bacteria

1. Cellular characteristics
   a. Gram stain
   b. Size
   c. Shape
   d. Presence of flagella, fimbria
   e. Motility
2. Colony characteristics
   a. Size
   b. Shape
   c. Color
   d. Consistency
   e. Edge
3. Physiologic characteristics
   a. Temperature for optimum growth
   b. Growth environment
      1. Aerobic
      2. CO_2 enriched air
      3. Anaerobic
      4. Facultative
   c. Biochemical reactions
      1. Indole
      2. Nitrate/nitrite reduction
      3. H_2S production
      4. Gas production
   d. Fermentation of specific sugars
   e. Pattern of metabolic acids as determined by gas-liquid chromatography

TABLE 4–3 ✦ Methods for the Classification of Bacteria

I. Phenotypic
II. Genetic—Based on DNA analysis
   1. Percent guanine plus cytosine
      a. Thermal denaturation
      b. Buoyant density centrifugation
   2. DNA base sequence
III. Chemotaxonomy
   1. Lipids
   2. Cell wall polymers
   3. Isoprenoid quinones
   4. Cytochromes
   5. Bacterial enzymes
IV. Serology

In eukaryotic cells this percentage varies within a very small range, but in prokaryotic cells it can vary from 25 to 75 percent. The mol% G + C gives information only on the composition of the bacterial genome, and even distantly related bacterial species can have the same mol% G + C.

In zoology and botany, evolutionary relationships between species can be derived by examination of fossil records. However, there is very little available in the way of microbial fossil data and the evolution of bacterial species has been very difficult to examine.

All of the available molecular methods for evaluating phylogenetic relationships (DNA-DNA and DNA-rRNA hybridization, 5S rRNA and protein sequencing, 16S rRNA oligonucleotide cataloging, and enzymological patterning) have advantages and limitations. In general, macromolecular sequencing is preferred because it permits quantitative interpretation of relationships. Of the macromolecules used for phylogenetic analysis, the ribosomal RNAs (rRNA) have proven the most useful because of their high information content, conserved nature, and universal distribution. The high homology between sequences of rRNAs from phylogenetically diverse sources is, by itself, persuasive evidence that all ribosomes are related through a common ancestral ribosome.

Ribosomal RNA sequencing is a powerful technique for examining both distant and close phylogenetic relationships among bacteria. The small subunit of rDNA (16S) evolves slowly and is useful for studying distantly related organisms. The internal transcribed spacer region and intergenic spacer of the rDNA repeat units evolve fastest and may vary among species within a genus or among a population. The 16S and the larger 23S subunit vary in their nucleotide sequences but they contain regions that are conserved almost perfectly among different organisms.

Several methods have been developed to examine DNA base sequence homology, including DNA-DNA hybridization. These same techniques are also being used in the diagnosis of bacterial infections by means of species-specific "DNA probes." DNA-DNA hybridization techniques involve the purification of bacterial DNA from one species and breaking the double-stranded DNA helix into single strands using either thermal denaturation or alkali treatment. These single DNA strands are immobilized onto a substrate such as a nitrocellulose filter and are then reacted with radiolabeled, single-stranded DNA from another bacterial strain. At points on the DNA strands where there are complementary bases, a heteroduplex will form. For identical microorganisms, there should be 100 percent hybridization (see Chapter 2). Between less closely related microorganisms, there is less heteroduplex formation and more areas of single-strandedness. Following the hybridization reaction between strands, the mixture is treated with an enzyme, DNAase, which cleaves the unpaired, single-stranded DNA but leaves the heteroduplexes untouched. The degree of DNA hybridization is then measured by determining the amount of radioactivity bound to the substrate.

Since DNA base content and base sequence reflect the entire basis for other phenotypic properties expressed by the microorganism, these assays are thought to reflect bacterial relationships, and hence bacterial taxonomy, more accurately than other tests. However, even the bacterial genome within a single species can change. It can vary over time, for example, as genetic elements are transferred between microorganisms by means of transduction and conjugation (see Chapter 2). Bacterial taxonomy, whether based on phenotypic traits or on the bacterial genome, can also be expected to change.

One specialized area of research in bacterial taxonomy is known as **numeric (phenetic)** taxonomy. Using this approach, a large number of traits (usually 100 to 200) such as Gram stain characteristics, motility, sugar fermentations, and biochemical reactions are determined in a group of microorganisms. Each trait or character is assigned a value of 1; that is, no more weight is assigned to one feature as compared with any other feature. Thus, in numeric taxonomy, gram-positivity or negativity, which is generally considered to be an "important" trait, is weighted the same as fermentation of individual sugars. By compiling the number of similar features among different strains, referred to as "operational taxonomic units," the degree of relatedness can be calculated and expressed as a simple matching coefficient or percent similarity. By means of statistical calculations including "cluster analysis" or "ordination" which are often derived through the use of computers, similar strains can be grouped together. The relationships among strains can be plotted as a **dendogram** (Fig. 4–2) for data derived by cluster analysis or as a **taxonomic map** for data derived from ordination.

Prior to January 1, 1980, the complete list of bacterial names contained microorganisms for which **type strains**—the standard reference bacteria strain which is used to define a bacterial species—did not exist. Some of these strains dated back to the 1800s and had undergone numerous reclassifications. Starting on January 1, 1980, however, all accepted bacterial names were listed in a publication, "Approved Lists of Bacterial Names." In order for a bacterial name to be accepted, that is, to have scientific standing, it must appear on this list. New species or reclassifications of existing species must be published in the *International Journal of Systematic Bacteriology.* Subsequent questions on the validity of a bacterial species are reviewed by the Judicial Commission of the International Union of Microbiological Societies.

In addition to the methods described earlier for the classification of bacteria, there are two other methods that have been useful. These are chemotaxonomy and serology. **Chemotaxonomy** makes use of physical and chemical characteristics for the classification of bacteria. There are a number of factors that can be measured, including lipids, cell wall polymers, isoprenoid quinones (which are a special class of cell membrane lipids), cytochromes, and bacterial enzymes. In addition, the pattern of soluble proteins extracted from bacterial cells can be "finger-printed" by the use of two-dimensional electrophoresis.

Serotaxonomy involves the use of antigen-antibody reactions for bacterial classification. Special serodiagnostic reagents are developed to detect the presence of particular antigens. A group of bacterial strains can then be distinguished based on the presence of these antigens. For example, the causative microorganism of juvenile periodontitis, *Actinobacillus actinomycetemcomitans,* has been divided into five serologic groups, or serogroups.

BIBLIOGRAPHY

Johnson, J. L.: Use of nucleic acid homologies in the taxonomy of anaerobic bacteria. Int. J. Syst. Bacteriol. 28:308, 1973.

Shah, H. N. and Collins, M. D.: Proposal for reclassification of *Bacteroides asaccharolyticus, Bacte-*

Percent similarity

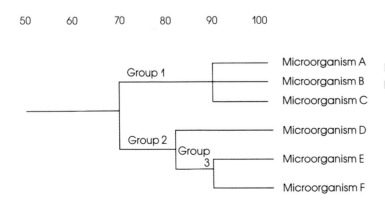

FIGURE 4–2 ✦ Dendogram of a hypothetical microorganism.

roides gingivalis, and *Bacteroides endodontolis* in a new genus, *Porphyromonas.* Int. J Syst. Bacteriol 38:128, 1988.

Skerman, V. B. D., McGowan, V., and Sneath, P. H. A. (eds.): Approved lists of bacterial names. Int. J. Syst. Bacteriol. 30:225, 1980.

Sneath, P. H. A.: Classification of microorganisms. In Norris, J. R., and Richmond, M. H. (eds.): Essays in Microbiology. John Wiley, Chichester, UK, 1978.

Willcox, W. R., Lapage, S. P., and Holmes, B.: A review of numerical methods in bacterial identification. Antonie van Leeuwenhoek Journal of Microbiology and Serology 46:233, 1980.

5 *Normal Microbial Flora of the Human Body*

William F. Liljemark and Cynthia G. Bloomquist

CHAPTER OUTLINE

Is the normal oral flora necessary to the human host?
The normal flora of the human host
Concepts and terms for the study of normal microbial flora
The normal flora's significance in the human host
The normal microbial flora of the body by anatomic region

IS THE NORMAL ORAL FLORA NECESSARY TO THE HUMAN HOST?

Pasteur hypothesized that the normal bacterial flora was essential to life. *Germ-free* animals aseptically delivered from their mothers and raised in a sterile environment with sterilized water and food have been extensively studied in contrast to their conventional counterparts. *Germ-free* animals develop an enormously enlarged cecum, and have greatly diminished peristalsis, a thinner alimentary lamina propria, shallower crypts of Lieberkuhn, a more regular epithelium, and shorter-lived enterocytes. Further, the intestinal epithelium renewal rate is half that of conventional animals. The immune system of the germ-free animal also is markedly underdeveloped, such that the reticuloendothelial system, lymph nodes, and immunoglobulin levels are greatly decreased, and exhibit weak, delayed hypersensitivity. These immune system differences probably result from a lack of stimulation of their immune systems. Germ-free animals live almost twice as long as conventional animals, and they eventually die of intestinal atonia, whereas conventional animals frequently die of infections. Thus, although the indigenous flora is not essential for life, and indeed, may even shorten it, the normal flora profoundly affects the host in many ways.

THE NORMAL FLORA OF HUMANS

Human beings have diverse microbial flora associated with their skin and mucous membranes from shortly after birth until death. The normal adult is composed of over 10^{14} cells, of which about 10 percent or 10^{13} are human cells. The various body surfaces and the gastrointestinal tract of humans contain about 10^{14} prokaryotic and eukaryotic microbial cells, including one arthropod, numerous protozoans, several dozen fungi, and over 700 distinct species of bacteria. These high cell numbers are due to the great density of microbes found on or in the various body surfaces (Table 5–1). There are from 10^3 cells/cm^2 of skin to greater than 10^{11} cells/gm of dental plaque or feces. Considering that a gram of water occupies 10^{12} cubic microns, that same gram could contain, at most, 10^{12} bacteria, supposing the organisms were 1 micron in diameter. In reality, for example, packed cells of streptococci contain about 2.3×10^{11} cells/gm.

CONCEPTS AND TERMS FOR THE STUDY OF NORMAL MICROBIAL FLORA

The fields of medical microbiology, microbial ecology, and epidemiology have evolved as separate disciplines. Because of this, many synonyms are used to describe the normal flora.

The term *normal flora* collectively describes the various microbial types frequently found by culture or microscopy on the skin or mucous membranes and in certain body cavities in normal, healthy individuals. The species and numbers of the flora vary in different areas of the body and sometimes at different ages. Normal flora is used as a synonym for *indigenous microflora* and *endogenous flora*. Indigenous species are **amphibiotic** in humans and are defined as (1) frequently encountered in one or more typical human anatomic regions, (2) found at least as often in the absence of disease as in its

TABLE 5–1 ✦ Distribution of Flora in the Healthy Human Body

BODY SITE	FLORA	NUMBER OF ORGANISMS
Blood	Sterile, occasional transient low-level bacteremia from trauma	—
Cerebrospinal fluid, tissues, uterus and fallopian tubes, middle ear, paranasal sinuses	Sterile	—
Skin, external ear	*Staphylococcus epidermidis, Corynebacterium* sp., *Propionibacterium* acnes, *Lactobacillus* sp., *Micrococcus* sp., fungi	10^3–10^4/cm^2 (10^6 axilla and groin)
Conjunctiva	*Staphylococcus epidermidis, Corynebacterium* and *Propionibacterium* sp.	Few (17–46% sterile)
Nose and nasopharynx	*Staphylococcus epidermidis, Corynebacterium* sp., *Staphylococcus aureus, Propionibacterium* acnes (nares), *Hemophilus parainfluenzae*	10^5/ml
Oropharynx	Alpha and nonhemolytic *Streptococcus* sp., *Neisseria* and *Branhamella* sp., enterococci, *Corynebacterium* sp., *Bacteroides* and *Fusobacterium* sp., *Staphylococcus* sp.	10^7/ml
Oral cavity	See Chapter 25	10^8/ml saliva and 10^{11}/g plaque
Esophagus	Transient oral flora	—
Stomach	Transient oral flora and organisms from food	0–10^3/ml normal fasting individual, dependent on pH
Small intestine		0–10^4/ml
upper	*Streptococcus* sp., *Lactobacillus* sp., *Staphylococcus* sp., yeasts	
distal	*Bacteriodes* sp., coliforms, enterococci, *Streptococcus* sp.	~10^4/ml
Colon		
Breastfed infant	*Bifidobacterium* sp., *Lactobacillus* sp., enterococci	?
After weaning	*Bacteroides* sp., *Bifidobacterium* sp., *Eubacterium* sp., *Lactobacillus* sp., *Peptostreptococcus* sp., *Ruminococcus* sp., *Streptococcus* sp., coliforms	10^{11}/g feces
Kidneys and urinary bladder	Usually sterile except for anterior urethra	—
Anterior urethra	*Staphylococcus epidermidis, Corynebacterium* sp., *Streptococcus faecalis*	—
Urine, midstream	Same as anterior urethra	0–10^3/ml
Vagina		
Prepubertal and postmenopausal	Skin and colonic species	?
Childbearing years	*Peptococcus* sp., anaerobic and facultative *Lactobacillus* sp., *Staphylococcus epidermidis, Neisseria* sp., *Bacteroides* sp.	10^9/g secretions

presence, and (3) having as their primary habitat the human species.

The term *amphibiotic* also describes the relationship between two organisms. Thus the amphibiont, in relation to its host, can be assigned a space between *symbiosis* (that is, the living together of two dissimilar organisms, with both organisms benefiting, which is not the case for the normal flora and the human host) and pathogenicity (see definition further on). The typical amphibiont that constitutes the normal flora is obligately parasitic (nonsaprophytic) and not overtly, actively, or obligately pathogenic in a particular host. The amphibionts that compose the normal flora would, when disturbed, promptly re-establish themselves in a stable ecosystem.

Some members of the normal flora are found at a low frequency in the human population and are not pathogenic for their particular host, but are potentially pathogenic for other members of the population. These hosts are commonly called *carriers*. The *pathogenicity* of any microorganism denotes the ability to cause disease. *Virulence* introduces the concept of degree—that is, virulent organisms exhibit pathogenicity when introduced into the host in very small numbers. It frequently is measured by the number of microorganisms necessary to kill 50 percent of a given host and is termed the LD_{50} *(median lethal dose)*. Different strains of a bacterial species vary in their ability to cause disease. For example, type 3 *Streptococcus pneumoniae* strains are more virulent than other polysaccharide types. Similarly, one strain of *Salmonella typhimurium* may have an LD_{50} for mice of 100 cells, and another strain an LD_{50} of 1000 cells. The median lethal dose is bacterial strain-specific, as well as host animal species-specific. The virulence of members of the normal flora usually is low in an uncompromised host.

Infection refers to the presence and multiplication of a microorganism in or on body tissues. *Infectious disease* is the clinical expression of an infection that disrupts the host while producing a characteristic group of symptoms. Infections caused by the normal flora are sometimes called *endogenous infections*. Specifically, these occur from traumatic disruptions to skin or mucous membrane by outside forces (broken bones, cuts, burns, bullets, and so forth) or by health care personnel (e.g., nasogastric and endotracheal tubes, IVs, catheters, or scalpels). Endogenous infections usually result when an indigenous microbe is thrust into an unusual anatomic region (e.g., a human bite). Infections caused by endogenous microbes, called *opportunistic infections,* also occur at a microbe's usual anatomic habitat following a disease or other predisposing factor (such as debilitating chronic conditions such as diabetes mellitus or alcoholism, stomach ulcers, colon and other invasive cancers, antibiotics, immune and nutritional deficiencies, stresses), which compromise the host. Both endogenous and opportunistic infections can be *iatrogenic* or "healer induced." When infections arise in a hospital they are called *nosocomial* or "hospital acquired."

Many of today's serious nosocomial infections are caused by *Escherichia coli, Klebsiella pneumoniae, Staphylococcus aureus,* and *Proteus mirabilis*. These organisms frequently are members of the normal human flora. Inasmuch as these bacteria are not considered to be highly virulent in their usual habitat in a human, they are considered "nonpathogens." However, when the health of a host is compromised, or a microbe is inserted into a new environment, a relatively less virulent "nonpathogen" may quickly become a pathogen.

Prevalence describes the percent of a particular site of the population sampled that contains a certain organism, at a certain time or age. For example, approximately 40 percent of the anterior nares of adults contain *S. aureus*. A synonym is *frequency,* as it also refers to a percent at a given time. These terms should *not* be confused with *incidence,* which refers to the *rate* at which a certain event occurs, as in the number of new cases of a specific disease occurring during a certain period.

THE NORMAL FLORA'S SIGNIFICANCE TO THE HUMAN HOST

Knowledge of the specific habitats and diverse roles of the normal flora is necessary for dental health care providers. The normal flora serves both as a defense mechanism against infection from exogenous microbes and as a source of potentially virulent organisms. The study of the normal flora is important for a number of reasons:

1. In countries with active public health programs, infections are more often a result of indigenous bacteria rather than of exogenous pathogenic microorganisms. For example, one in 20 people admitted to hospitals develops a nosocomial infection. In 1984, 40 percent of such infections were urinary tract infections, usually caused by indigenous bacteria introduced through catheterization. This represents 600,000 infections per year in the United States.

2. There are increasing numbers of people surviving in an immune compromised state, either from medical treatment for cancer, or due to AIDS or AIDS-related diseases. *Candida albicans* is a normal, albeit not ubiquitous, microbial member of the mouth, pharynx, small intestine, and colon. An opportunistic infection by *C. albicans* in the oral cavity or vagina (thrush or candidiasis) is often seen in conjunction with broad-spectrum antimicrobial therapy; overgrowth can also occur in the colon in conjunction with neomycin therapy, which causes a diarrhea consisting of almost a pure growth of *C. albicans*. Oral candidiasis is of prognostic significance as it is a frequent indicator of progressive disease among patients not yet diagnosed with AIDS (WR-5 adults, in the Walter Reed AIDS Staging System for adults).

3. The normal microbial flora may provide protection from similar but more pathogenic species. For example, bacteriocidal antibodies to *Neisseria meningitidis,* a common causative agent of spinal

meningitis, have been found in children colonized with a normal resident, *N. lactamicus*. These provide at least partial protection against all capsular types of *N. meningitidis*.

This example suggests the significant contribution made by the indigenous microflora to the general immunity of the host. It is apparent, teleologically, that many of the indigenous microbes are closely related to their more virulent relatives and often possess common antigens. Humans have frequent transient bacteremias from chewing and from breaks in the skin and mucous membranes. We have thus acquired low-level circulating antibody titers against most of our indigenous flora which may cross-react, thus elevating the host's immunity to exogenous pathogens.

4. The normal microflora provides a barrier to *colonization* (see definition later) by exogenous bacteria via the spatial inhibition of potential adhesion sites, by physiologic competition for limited nutrients, or by inhibitory substances produced by the normal species. A widely studied bovine and porcine example is the exquisite sensitivity of newborn calves or piglets to colonization by the piliated enterotoxigenic strains of *Escherichia coli*, which causes a potentially fatal diarrhea. This susceptibility to enteropathic *E. coli* decreases sharply with age, and disappears 4 to 6 days after birth, as the intestinal epithelia of these animals are then sufficiently colonized with bacteria. This protection is termed *bacterial interference*.

Alternately, in certain cases, the indigenous microflora actually assists exogenous pathogens. A prime example is that of *Entamoeba histolytica*, the causative agent of amebic dysentery, which colonizes a germ-free animal, but will not cause disease unless the animal is subsequently conventionalized with one or more of the normal gastrointestinal microorganisms.

5. Dental plaque (as with the rest of the oral flora on other oral sites, presumably) exists in a remarkable state of homeostasis under conditions of rigorous oral cleansing, general good health of the host, and low-sugar diet. Healthy dental plaque is predominantly *Streptococcus sanguis* and the maintenance of these species contributes to healthy teeth.

6. Lastly, the normal flora has been suggested to have an affect on the nutrition of the host. It is well established in rodents, via coprophagy, that quantities of vitamins are absorbed from the feces. The dependence of the microbial intestinal flora to aid digestion in ruminants also is essential. Similarly, the production of vitamin B_{12} by certain intestinal bacteria has been suggested as a nutritional source for humans. However, the human colon has little absorptive capacity, and any significant contribution to host nutrition or aid in digestion is unlikely.

Factors Influencing the Composition of Normal Flora
ACQUISITION OF THE NORMAL FLORA

The healthy full-term neonate has a fairly gentle introduction to the microbial world. Cultures of the nose, nasopharynx, oropharynx, umbilicus, rectum, and feces are often negative on the first day of life. The skin is colonized during vaginal births and contains a sparse population of cocci and corynebacteria. The nasopharynx of the newborn is sterile, but within 2 or 3 days the infant acquires the normal flora of the mother or caregiver. The newborn's mouth is sometimes sterile or contains the same organisms as the mother's vagina. These organisms diminish in number, and a few days after birth are replaced largely by the caretaker's flora. Within 4 to 12 hours after birth, alpha and nonhemolytic streptococci become established as the prominent members of the mucous membranes of the mouth and oropharynx, and remain so for life.

The gastrointestinal tract of the newborn is usually sterile. Under normal conditions, intestinal flora are established during the first 24 hours. The stool of the breastfed infant is soft, light yellow-brown, with a faint, acidic odor. *Lactobacillus bifidus* is prominent, as are enterococci, coliforms, and streptococci. In contrast, artificially fed infants have hard, dark, foul-smelling stools that contain *L. acidophilus*, coliforms, enterococci, and anaerobic species. *L. bifidus* may again predominate following the addition of 12 percent lactose to formula. Remarkably, by 5 to 7 days, the intestinal flora of the formula-fed infant contains the same complexity of anaerobes as the adult.

The vulva of the newborn is also sterile. After 24 hours it gradually acquires a rich and varied flora of corynebacteria, micrococci, and nonhemolytic streptococci. Two or 3 days after birth, estrogen from the maternal circulation induces the deposition of glycogen in the vaginal epithelium, which facilitates the growth of lactobacilli. These organisms produce acid from glycogen, and a flora like that of the adult female develops. After the passively transferred estrogen is gone, the glycogen, lactobacilli, and acid disappear, and the pH again becomes alkaline. At puberty the glycogen again appears and an adult flora with lactobacilli reappears.

SPECIFICITY OF MICROBIAL ADHERENCE MECHANISMS AND FACTORS AFFECTING COLONIZATION

In vitro and in vivo studies of the interactions between bacteria and the human host have led to an understanding of the role of colonization in the ecological development and maintenance of a characteristic flora. The relative ability to adhere (**av-**

idity) of a number of bacterial species and their natural distribution despite the moving streams that bathe the different epithelial surfaces have been found to correlate positively with their in vitro adherence to different epithelial cell lines. An example of this tissue tropism is the difference between the adherence of *Streptococcus pyogenes* (group A streptococci) and *Escherichia coli*. Both of these bacteria adhere avidly to human epithelial cells; however, *S. pyogenes* is virtually limited to the pharynges and skin epithelial cells, whereas *E. coli* is rarely found at these sites but adheres avidly to periurethral epithelial cells.

Bacterial adherence is thus remarkably cell- and surface-specific, which appears to be mediated by the attraction of species-specific microbial *adhesins* (some of which are *lectins*) to complementary host cell-specific receptors. The bacterial adhesins are sometimes, but not always, found on the surface appendages of bacteria, termed *pili* in gram-negative species and *fimbriae* in gram-positive species (see Chapter 3). Clearly, the extent to which an organism can attach to a particular surface will influence the extent to which it can colonize. Adherence is not the only prerequisite for colonization. The ability to survive the local environmental conditions (that is, the amount of oxygen, pH, nutritional sources, bacterial antagonists and symbionts, the unidirectional flow of fluids over epithelial surfaces, mucociliary clearing systems, epithelial cell turnover, local immune systems, and nonspecific host antimicrobial agents) is necessary for colonization. Obviously, the ability to grow under these environmental conditions is also essential.

THE NORMAL MICROBIAL FLORA OF THE BODY BY ANATOMIC REGION
Skin

The composition of the skin's microbial flora (Table 5–2) varies according to age and the environment due to different levels of moisture, body temperature, and concentration of skin surface lipids. For example, the perineum and toe webs are higher in moisture and are more frequently colonized by gram-negative bacilli than are drier areas of skin.

Staphylococcus epidermidis (biotype I) constitutes a major proportion of the flora, constituting more than 90 percent of the resident flora in some areas. *S. epidermidis* frequently causes an endogenous infection following the insertion of a ventriculoatrial shunt in the treatment of hydrocephalus. *S. aureus* is found on the skin of the arms and trunk of 5 to 25 percent of the population and

TABLE 5–2 ✦ Cultivable Microflora of the Human Skin

SPECIES	PREVALENCE (%)
Staphylococcus epidermidis	85–100
Staphylococcus aureus	5–25
Propionibacterium acnes	100
Corynebacterium sp.	55
Lactobacillus sp.	55
Micrococcus luteus	20–80
Acinetobacter calcoaceticus	20–30
Fungi* (especially lipophilic yeasts but not *C. albicans*)	40–80
Candida parapsilosis	1–15
Pityosporum sp.*	Common
Dermatophytic fungi† (*Epidermophyton floccosum, Microsporum* sp., *Trichophyton* sp.)	Common

*Especially in areas rich in sebaceous glands.
†Found on nonliving surfaces (hair, nails, keratinized skin).

reflects the density of colonization in the nose. The perianal skin is more frequently colonized and can be considered the major habitat of this species. The nonlipophilic *Corynebacterium* species are frequently found on glabrous skin, while *Propionibacterium acnes* is ubiquitous and more common in areas rich in sebaceous glands, such as the axilla and face. Consequently, children younger than age 10 are rarely colonized with *P. acnes* because of the lack of sebum secretion before puberty. Gramnegative bacteria usually are found only in the moist intertrigenous areas and include *Acinetobacter* sp. and occasionally others such as *Klebsiella pneumoniae* (as well as enterococci, *E. coli,* and *Proteus* sp.). Two lipophilic yeasts, *Pityosporum ovale* and *P. obiculare,* are present on the scalp or chest and back. Nonlipophilic yeasts, such as *Torulopsis glabrata,* are variably present. *Candida albicans* is not considered a normal resident of the skin. Other fungi and yeasts are sometimes present in skin folds. Dermatophytic fungi, which only grow on nonliving body structures (hair, keratinized skin, and nails), are often found. *Demodex folliculorum,* or the follicle mite, resides in and around the eyelashes and the hair follicles of the outer nose folds and chin.

Although the skin is constantly contaminated with organisms from exogenous and endogenous sources, it normally supports the growth of only three major types of bacteria. This is remarkably apparent, especially in the perianal area, which is in regular contact with the concentrated and varied fecal flora, but which, within an hour or so of defecation, retains only the resident staphylococci and corynebacteria. The external skin is highly acidic and dry and is constantly shedding, making it unfavorable for colonization by exogenous species. The metabolic activity of the normal gram-positive flora also contributes to the stable ecosystem of the skin by breaking down the complex lipids in sebum, produced by the sebaceous glands, producing a fatty acid coating that inhibits the growth of many pathogenic bacteria and fungi. Further, sweat glands secrete lysozyme, which interferes with cell wall synthesis and keeps the numbers of the resident gram-positive species in check.

The microbial flora of the external ear is similar to the flora on skin rich in sebaceous glands. *Staphylococcus epidermidis* and *Propionibacterium* sp. predominate. Acid-fast nonpathogenic *Mycobacterium* sp. are also found.

Conjunctiva (Eye)

The flora of the conjunctival sac is sparse (Table 5–3). Approximately 17 to 49 percent of culture samples are negative. The predominant microorganisms are *Corynebacterium* sp., *Propionibacterium* sp., and *Staphylococcus epidermidis*. These species presumably arise from the skinlike flora of the eyelids. A gram-negative species resembling hemophilus, called *Moraxella,* is also found here. Conjunctival flora is held in check by the mechanical flow of tears, the presence of the antibacterial enzyme lysozyme, and the production of other inhibitors by the normal eye flora (see subsequent section on the oropharynx).

Nose and Nasopharynx

The anterior nares have a flora somewhat similar to that of the skin (Table 5–4). The posterior nares, nasopharynx, and sinuses are more difficult to culture, and studies of the flora in these areas are limited. In health the sinuses are considered to be sterile. The anterior nares and nasopharynx share many similar species with the oropharynx, but

TABLE 5–3 ✦ **Cultivable Microflora of the Conjunctiva**

SPECIES	PREVALENCE (%)
Staphylococcus epidermidis	32–68
Staphylococcus aureus	6–28
Corynebacterium and *Propionibacterium* sp.	27–58
Moraxella sp.	Frequent
Hemophilus parainfluenzae	25
Fungi (often airborne *Aspergillus* sp.)	6–24
Pseudomonas aeruginosa	1–7

TABLE 5–4 ✦ **Cultivable Microflora of the Nose and Nasopharynx**

SPECIES	PREVALENCE (%)
*Staphylococcus epidermidis**	90
*Staphylococcus aureus**	30–40
Corynebacterium sp.	55
Propionibacterium acnes*	30–40
Hemophilus parainfluenzae	35–65
Hemophilus influenzae	12
Branhamella catarrhalis	12
Streptococcus pneumoniae	0–17
Streptococcus pyogenes (Group A)	1–5
Alpha hemolytic or nonhemolytic streptococci	Uncommon
Moraxella nonliquefaciens	5–10
Neisseria meningitidis	0–10

*Especially anterior nares.

there are notable exceptions. Especially apparent is the presence of staphylococci, and the absence of alpha or nonhemolytic streptococci, in the nose and nasopharynx. The opposite occurs in the oropharynx. The anterior nares are especially associated with staphylococci; either *S. epidermidis* or *S. aureus* predominate. *Corynebacterium* sp., *Propionibacterium* sp., and *Haemophilus parainfluenzae* are also frequently found in the nose and nasopharynx. *Streptococcus pneumoniae, Haemophilus influenzae, Corynebacterium diphtheriae* and *Bordetella pertussis* are also found in some individuals.

Some species of the normal nasal flora are not ubiquitous but are commonly found in a small fixed percentage of the healthy population. These "carriers" provide a reservoir of potentially virulent species for other members of the population, especially those in a compromised state. Although the perineum could be considered its major residence, *S. aureus* is estimated to be found in 20 to 85 percent of the anterior nares in a healthy population, with a figure of 30 to 40 percent probably being most accurate, half being permanent carriers and half transient carriers of several weeks or less. Although the nose and nasopharynx flora is the most probable source of the microbes associated with sinusitis and otitis media, a diagnosis based on its flora correlates poorly with these diseases and does not aid diagnosis. The adult nasopharyngeal carrier is also important in the transmission of spinal meningitidis by *Neisseria meningitidis* and provides a reservoir for infection of individuals living in close quarters. An interepidemic carriage rate of 5 to 30 percent can be compared with meningococcal disease in military populations, which is associated with carriage rates as high as 90 percent.

Oropharynx

The most important group of microorganisms native to the oropharynx, uniquely different than the nasopharynx, is the predominant alpha and non-hemolytic streptococci (Table 5–5). Often erroneously called *viridans streptococci,* this group contains a wide variety of species with unique colonization patterns. These species are frequent members of the oral cavity (see Chapter 25). It is more than possible that the species present on the buccal mucosa also are present on the oropharyngeal mucosa, especially those species shed from the various oral surfaces present in high numbers in saliva. However, the oropharyngeal flora is not identical to the salivary flora. For example, *Streptococcus mutans* has been suggested to be a member of the normal oropharyngeal flora. It is not known to adhere with any degree of avidity to epithelial cells; rather, it colonizes the hard surfaces of teeth. Consequently, *S. mutans* may be just a transitory member of the salivary flora, not a resident of the oropharynx.

Other than the predominant alpha and nonhaemolytic streptococci, *Neisseria* sp. and *Branhamella catarrhalis,* frequently are found. *B. catarrhalis* is an occasional serious causative agent of pneumonia, suppurative sinusitis, and otitis media. *Corynebacterium* sp., *Propionibacterium* sp., *Hemophilus parainfluenzae,* and *H. influenzae* also are present, as are staphylococci, lactobacilli, *Acinetobacter* sp., *Mycoplasma* sp., and spirochetes.

The oropharynx also contains a number of anaerobes, but studies of the anaerobic species have been limited. *Bacteroides* sp., *Fusobacterium necrophorum,* and certain anaerobic cocci have been cited. Similar to the nasopharynx, the oropharynx also is the site of carriage of a number of potentially virulent organisms, such as the only pathogenic member of the corynebacteria, *C. diphtheriae.* Although asymptomatic carriage of this microbe is not found in an adequately immunized population, depressed urban areas and the native population of Alaska constitute a current reservoir of this disease. In tropical areas, the skin is also a reservoir. Other potential pathogens carried in the normal oropharyngeal flora are *Klebsiella pneumoniae, Pseudomonas aeruginosa, Streptococcus pneumoniae, Neisseria meningitidis,* and *Proteus mirabilis.*

One of the best examples of the normal flora's positive role in host defense can be seen in seriously ill patients. There is a markedly increased susceptibility of the respiratory tract of seriously ill patients to colonization by gram-negative bacilli. Gram-negative colonization has been positively

TABLE 5–5 ✦ Cultivable Microflora of the Oropharynx

SPECIES	PREVALENCE (%)
Alpha and nonhemolytic *Streptococcus,* sp.	93–99
S. salivarius	50–75
S. sanguis	25–75
S. mitis	25–75
S. milleri	25–75
S. mutans	25–75
Streptococcus sp. (Group D)	90–100
Streptococcus pneumoniae	1–50
Streptococcus pyogenes (group A)	1–6
Neisseria sp. and *Branhamella catarrhalis*	81–97
Neisseria meningitidis	5–15
Corynebacterium sp.	15–90
Propionibacterium acnes	11–12
Staphylococcus epidermidis	3–70
Staphylococcus aureus	35–40
Hemophilus parainfluenzae	20–35
Hemophilus influenzae	5–20
Lactobacillus sp.	1–37
Bacteroides sp.	Common
Fusobacterium necrophorum	Common
Anaerobic *Micrococcus* sp.	11–12
Acinetobacter calcoaceticus	5–30
Peptostreptococcus sp.	10
Klebsiella pneumoniae	5
Pseudomonas aeruginosa	5
Candida albicans	3–6
Actinomyces sp.	Common
Mycoplasma sp.	Common

correlated with the loss of fibronectin, a high molecular weight protein, present on the surface of normal oropharyngeal epithelial cells. Fibronectin is thought to promote the attachment of the indigenous gram-positive species, which normally interfere with the attachment of potential gram-negative bacterial pathogens such as *Pseudomonas aeruginosa.* The sequelae following the eradication of the predominant streptococci with high doses of penicillin can cause a similar gram-negative overgrowth.

The healthy climax community of the oropharynx is maintained by several species. Alpha hemolytic streptococci and nonpathogenic *Neisseria* sp. (and *Staphylococcus epidermidis,* found most often in the nose) are known to inhibit the colonization of *S. aureus, Neisseria meningitidis,* and *Streptococcus pyogenes* (group A streptococci). Children with high numbers of alpha-hemolytic streptococci are not colonized following exposure to Group A streptococci. Further, strains of *S. salivarius* and *S. mitis* have been shown to produce a cell-free filtrate called *enocin,* which is capable of inhibiting *S. pyogenes* by interference with pantothenate utilization.

Gastrointestinal Tract

The intraluminal environment of the stomach is usually sterile. Studies have shown low counts of alpha-hemolytic streptococci, anaerobic cocci, lactobacilli, *Staphylococcus epidermidis,* and *Candida albicans* that tend toward zero several hours after meals. These are transitory species from saliva and ingested materials. Gastric pH is the major factor controlling microbial growth in the stomach.

The flora of the small intestine is highly dependent on the location of sampling. The upper small intestine is usually sterile or has similar species and counts as the stomach. Coliforms and *Bacteroides* species are rarely present. The lower small intestine contains a flora that closely approximates the colon but with much lower counts of approximately 10^5 versus 10^{11}. The nature of the streptococci change from primarily alpha-hemolytic in the upper small intestine to enterococci (or group D streptococci) in the lower small intestine. The lower intestine also has some coliforms and the beginning of an anaerobic flora.

The normal colonic microbial flora appears to be the same as in the feces because of the difficulties associated with sampling the intestinal epithelium. Microbial counts in the transverse colon are two to three logarithmic values lower than fecal samples. The "holding" function of the colon allows certain organisms to multiply. Although there are substantial quantitative differences at various locations of the colon versus fecal flora, there are no marked qualitative differences in the major groups of bacteria.

Bacteroides thetaiotaomicron is the most prevalent and numerically predominant fecal species (Table 5–6). Other *Bacteroides* sp. are common, especially *B. vulgatus, B. distonis,* and *B. fragilis* (these species were formerly classified as subspecies of *B. fragilis*). *Eubacterium* species and anaerobic cocci are found in high numbers (*Peptostreptococcus* sp., *Veillonella* sp., *Acidaminococcus* sp., and facultative-anaerobic streptococci, especially *Streptococcus intermedius*). *Lactobacillus* sp., especially *L. acidophilus,* are also prevalent. The facultative streptococci, *Bacillus* sp., and *Clostridium* sp. are prevalent, and probably represent species arising from oral secretions and ingested materials, respectively. More than 450 bacterial species are found, including those associated with the skin (staphylococci) and pharynges (gramnegative species). Some fungi and yeasts, such as *Candida albicans,* also occur. Various protozoa, *Mycoplasma* sp. and spirochetes, are often found.

TABLE 5–6 ✦ Cultivable Microflora of the Colon (Feces)

SPECIES	PREVALENCE (%)
Bacteroides sp.*	99
B. thetaiotaomicron	87
B. vulgatus	70
B. distasonis	53
B. fragilis	49
Eubacterium sp.*	94
E. aerofaciens	49
E. lentum	43
Bifidobacterium sp.*	74
B. adolescentis	55
Lactobacillus sp*	78
L. acidophilus	45
Peptostreptococcus sp.*	45
P. productus	30
Ruminococcus sp.*	45
Anaerobic *Streptococcus* sp.*	34
S. intermedius	28
Facultative *Streptococcus* sp.	99
S. faecalis	80
S. faecium group	31
S. mitis	31
S. lactis	28
S. bovis	18
Escherichia coli	93
Fusobacterium sp.*	18
Bacillus sp.*	82
Clostridium sp.*	100
Propionibacterium acnes	9
Actinomyces naeslundii	6
Veillonella sp.	34
Klebsiella pneumoniae	20
Staphylococcus epidermidis	31
Staphylococcus aureus	11
Pseudomonas aeruginosa	11
Candida albicans	14
Other yeasts	36
Spirochetes	Common
Various protozoa	?
Mycoplasma sp.	Common

*Numerous other species in the genera occur as well.

Spirochetes, fusiform bacilli, and cocci have been seen attached to the epithelial surfaces of the colon when examined by electron microscopy.

Genitourinary Tract

Secretions around the female urethra and uncircumsized male contain a flora similar to that of the skin, as well as *Mycobacterium smegmatis,* a harmless microbe sometimes confused with *Mycobacterium tuberculosis.* The skin flora frequently present in the distal urethra of both sexes contains *Corynebacterium* sp., nonhemolytic streptococci, and *Staphylococcus epidermis,* as well as *Streptococcus faecalis.* The internal urethra, bladder, urine, and kidneys are usually sterile.

The adult female genitourinary tract has a microbial flora constantly changing with the variation of the menstrual cycle. Although complex, fewer species are present than in the oral or colonic flora. The major aerobic and facultative strains are *Streptococcus epidermidis,* staphylococci, lactobacilli, and corynebacteria. Lactobacilli, combining both facultative and aerobic species, are the species most commonly associated with vaginal flora, and constitute a large portion of the bacteria present (Table 5–7). They are so named because they produce lactic acid and help maintain the pH of the vagina and external cervical os at approximately 4.4 to 4.6.

Anaerobic bacteria predominate over aerobic bacteria 10-fold. Peptococci are the most frequently found and are numerically predominant. Peptostreptococci, anaerobic lactobacilli, eubacteria, anaerobic gram-negative bacteria, *Mycoplasma* sp. and spirochetes are also found. *Staphylococcus aureus* has been found in 15 percent of healthy women, and is correlated positively with nasal carriage. Further, 60 percent of the women with vaginal *S. aureus* also had nasal *S. aureus,* versus 23 percent of women without vaginal *S. aureus.*

TABLE 5–7 ✦ Cultivable Microflora of the Vagina

SPECIES	PREVALENCE (%)
Peptococcus sp.	64
Anaerobic *Lactobacillus* sp., *L. fermentum*	45
Facultative *Lactobacillus* sp.	50
Staphylococcus epidermidis	28–94
Staphylococcus aureus	5–15
Branhamella catarrhalis and *Neisseria* sp.	60–80
Bacteroides sp.	60–80
Corynebacterium sp.	38–76
Peptostreptococcus sp.	30–40
Eubacterium sp.	5–23
Enterobacteriaceae sp.	18–40
Candida albicans	30–50
Streptococcus sp.	
Alpha hemolytic	14
Group B (*S. agalactiae*)	20–40
Enterococci (group D)	30–80
Nonhemolytic (not B or D)	36
Torulopsis glabrata	Common
Escherichia coli	9–27
Trichomonas vaginalis	10–25
Mycoplasma sp.	Common

BIBLIOGRAPHY

Beachey, E. H.: Bacterial adherence: Adhesin-receptor interactions mediating the attachment of bacteria to mucosal surfaces. J. Infect. Dis. 143:325, 1981.

Cottone, J. A., Terezhalmy, G., and Molinari, J.: Practical Infection Control in Dentistry. Lea and Febiger, Malvern, Penn., 1991.

Gibbons, R. J.: Adherence of bacteria to host tissue. In Schlessinger, D. (ed.): Microbiology 1977. American Society for Microbiology, Washington, DC, p. 395, 1977.

Goldmann, D. A., Leclair, J., and Macone, A.: Bacterial colonization of neonates admitted to an intensive care environment. J. Pediatrics 93:288, 1978.

Hentges, D. J.: Human Intestinal Microflora in Health and Disease. Academic Press, New York, 1983.

Johnston, D. A., and Bodey, G. P.: Semiquantitative oropharyngeal culture technique. Appl. Microbiol. 20:218, 1970.

Mackowiak, P. A.: The normal microbial flora. N. Engl. J. Med. 307:83, 1982.

Marples, M. J.: Life on the human skin. Sci. Am. 220:108, 1969.

Marsh, P. D.: The significance of maintaining the stability of the natural microflora of the mouth. Br. Dent. J. 171:174, 1991.

Martin, R. R., Buttram, V., Besch, P., Kirkland, J. J., and Petty, G. P.: Nasal and vaginal *Staphylococcus aureus* in young women: Quantitative studies. Ann. Intern. Med. 96:951, 1982.

Onderdonk, A. B., Zamardhi, G. R., Walsh, J. A., Mellor, R. D., Munoz, A., and Kass, E. H.: Methods for quantitative and qualitative evaluation of vaginal microflora during menstruation. Appl. Environ. Microbiol. 51:333, 1986.

Redfield, R. R., Wright, D. C., and Tramont, E. C.: The Walter Reed staging classification for HTLV-III/LAV infection. N. Engl. J. Med. 314:131, 1986.

Rosebury, T.: Microorganisms Indigenous to Man. McGraw-Hill, New York, 1962.

Savage, D. C.: Microbial ecology of the gastrointestinal tract. Ann. Rev. Microbiol. 31:1781, 1977.

Savage, D. C., and Fletcher, M. (eds.): Bacterial Adhesion: Mechanisms and Physiological Significance. Plenum Press, New York, 1985.

Woods, D. E., Straus, D. C., Johanson, W. G., and Bass, J. A.: Role of fibronectin in the prevention of adherence of *Pseudomonas aeruginosa* to buccal cells. J. Infect. Dis. 143:784, 1981.

6 *The Streptococci*

Burton Rosan

CHAPTER OUTLINE

*The pyogenic streptococci (*Streptococcus pyogenes, *The "Lancefield Group Streptococci")*

Streptococcus pneumoniae

The oral streptococci

THE PYOGENIC STREPTOCOCCI (*STREPTOCOCCUS PYOGENES,* THE "LANCEFIELD GROUP STREPTOCOCCI")

The streptococci are gram-positive coccal bacteria that divide in one plane. Since they do not separate easily after division, they tend to form chains and thus can be distinguished from staphylococci, which usually divide in different planes leading to bunches, or grapelike clusters, of cocci (Fig. 6–1). The streptococci, which are catalase negative, also differ from the staphylococci that are catalase positive. The streptococci constitute a major population in the oral cavity with several different species associated with the different ecologic niches in the mouth. Thus, *Streptococcus sanguis* and *S. mutans* are found in dental plaque, whereas *S. salivarius* is found primarily on the tongue and *S. mitis* on other mucosal tissues. It is also clear that these species are associated with different diseases (e.g., *S. mutans* causes dental caries, whereas *S. sanguis* is frequently involved in subacute bacterial endocarditis). Therefore, an understanding of the taxonomy of these bacteria provides information about the factors involved in the virulence of these organisms. This is not an easy task because taxonomic schemes were developed long before bacterial genetics were understood, at a time when the relationship between structure and function among bacteria was generally based on speculation rather than fact. Much of the knowledge of these relationships of streptococci stems from studies of *S. pyogenes,* an or-

ganism involved in systemic diseases (e.g., streptococcal pharyngitis, scarlet fever, rheumatic fever, and various types of skin infections). Since patients with a history of rheumatic fever often pose special problems in dental therapy, it is important to study the pyogenic cocci as etiologic agents in these diseases and to establish the appropriate background for the study of the oral streptococci.

Hemolysis and the Streptococci

Blood and blood products have been used as a constituent of bacterial media from the earliest days of bacteriology when it was observed that the streptococci isolated from purulent throat and skin infections often caused complete lysis of red blood cells ("*hemo*-lysis"). This was easily recognized in a blood agar medium as a zone of complete clearing around the colonies. Other streptococci also found in the oropharynx that did not appear associated with local disease caused a type of "incomplete lysis," in which the red blood cells shrink and take on a greenish tinge. The latter phenomenon occurs only in the presence of oxygen and is due to the reduction of hemoglobin. This incomplete hemolysis was called alpha hemolysis (α-hemolysis) and the streptococci that produced it were designated *Streptococcus viridans,* whereas the complete lysis of the red blood cells was called beta hemolysis (β-hemolysis) and the organisms causing it were called *Streptococcus hemolyticus.* We now know that both names are misnomers and that there are many species that cause α hemolysis, many others that cause β hemolysis, and some species that pro-

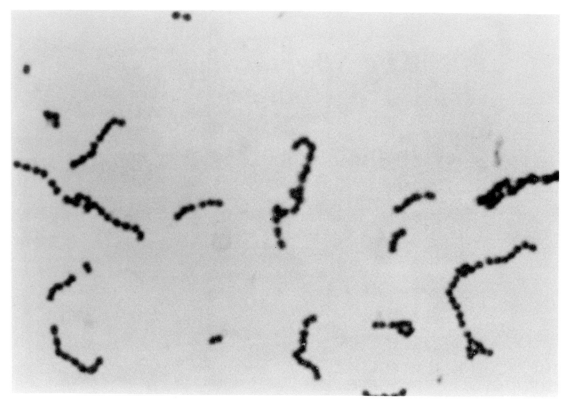

FIGURE 6–1 ✦ Gram stain of group A streptococci. (From Schneierson, S. S.: Atlas of Diagnostic Microbiology. North Chicago, Ill., Abbot Laboratories, 1965, with permission.)

duce both types of hemolysis, depending on strain and growth conditions. There are also many streptococci that are anhemolytic; the latter are often referred to as the gamma (γ) streptococci. The story of the hemolysis and the α-streptococci will unfold in discussing the oral streptococci but for the moment let us concentrate on unraveling the tale of the β-hemolytic streptococci and the diseases associated with these organisms.

The Lancefield Serologic Grouping Scheme

It soon became clear that hemolysis was not sufficient to distinguish among the streptococci causing disease. Attempts to distinguish organisms by the usual biochemical methods—that is, fermentation of sugars—were not very fruitful. Thus, attention was focused on developing a serologic method of distinguishing among the β-hemolytic streptococci. Rebecca Lancefield found that heating the streptococci at 100°C for 10 minutes at pH 2 extracted components from the streptococci. Extracts from the human β-hemolytic streptococci reacted with rabbit antisera prepared against the human isolates but not against the bovine isolates. These isolates were called the Lancefield serologic

group A and were given the species designation of *S. pyogenes* (Greek *pyon*, pus; *genan*, to produce). In contrast, extracts from bovine strains reacted with homologous antisera (antisera prepared against the bovine strain) but not with antisera prepared against the human strains. These strains were called the Lancefield group C and actually were found to contain several different species based on biochemical differences (*S. equisimalis*, *S. zooepidemicus*, and *S. dysgalactiae*). Because of its simplicity and accuracy, the Lancefield extraction procedure became the basis for establishing the serologic grouping scheme, which is still employed to identify many streptococci (Table 6–1). There are now about 20 groups (A–H; K–V) recognized. In addition to its importance in differentiating among the streptococci, the Lancefield extraction was an important milestone in developing methods to determine the composition and structure of the bacterial cell wall.

THE GROUP ANTIGENS ("C" CARBOHYDRATE)

Although earlier studies suggested that the antigen in the Lancefield extract responsible for the reaction was a protein, or "nucleoprotein," subsequent studies proved conclusively that the anti-

TABLE 6−1 ✦ Diseases Caused by Streptococci

SEROLOGIC GROUP	SPECIES	DISEASES
Group A	*Streptococcus pyogenes*	**Acute**
		Pharyngitis, pyoderma (impetigo), erysipelas, scarlet fever, pneumonia, otitis media, sinusitis, puerperal fever, septicemia
		Post-Streptococcal
		Rheumatic fever, glomerulonephritis
Group B	*S. agalactiae*	Neonatal sepsis, meningitis, puerperal sepsis
Group C	*S. equisimilis, S. equi, S. dysgalactiae, S. zooepidemicus*	Bovine mastitis, mild pharyngitis in humans
Group D	*Enterococcus faecalis, E. faecium, E. durans*	Genitourinary infections, wound infections, root canal infections, endocarditis
Group H	*S. sanguis*	Dental plaque, endocarditis

gens responsible for distinguishing between the Lancefield groups A and C were carbohydrates (polysaccharides). The localization of these poly-saccharides and other wall polymers is shown diagrammatically in Figure 6–2. The cell wall is composed of the peptidoglycan to which is linked the polysaccharide and the outer surface proteins. An early generic term for the streptococcal polysaccharides, regardless of source, was *C carbohydrate*. The backbone of the C carbohydrate from both groups A and C streptococci is composed of rhamnose and *N*-acetyl-glucosamine. Branches of *N*-acetyl-glucosamine are responsible for the serologic specificity of the group A polysaccharide, whereas the group C polysaccharide contains *N*-acetyl-galactosamine branches. Thus, it appears that subtle differences in composition determine the serologic specificity of some of the Lancefield

groups and may be related to the normal habitat of the streptococci. (These concepts will appear again in discussing the exquisite specificity in the ecology of the oral streptococci.) As more C carbohydrates from other serologic groups were examined, it was found that not all were true carbohydrates. Some (e.g., Groups D, H, and N) were composed of teichoic acids (see page 136), components also associated with the cell surface. One of the functions of teichoic acid may be the attachment of streptococci to tissue cells.

THE TYPE ANTIGENS: THE M PROTEINS

It soon became clear that not all group A streptococci were equally virulent. In an attempt to define the basis of virulence, Lancefield and her co-workers found that only cells containing a trypsin-

FIGURE 6–2 ✦ Diagrammatic representation of the cell wall of a *Streptococcus*. The fimbriae are shown as if they are separated from the T and R proteins; however, these proteins may also be fimbrial. The separation between the proteins and carbohydrate is for illustrative purposes, and there is no clear evidence to support a distinctly layered appearance for these surface components. The teichoic acids are not shown but would be found attached to cell membrane (see Fig. 6–11).

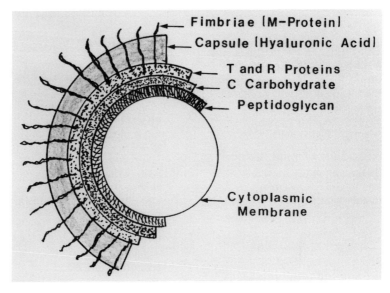

Fimbriae (M−Protein)
Capsule (Hyaluronic Acid)
T and R Proteins
C Carbohydrate
Peptidoglycan
Cytoplasmic Membrane

sensitive protein, called *the "M" protein*, were virulent. This name was chosen because the protein was present only in cells from "matt"-like rough colonies, which characterized the more virulent strains. Subsequent studies showed that these rough colonies resulted from the digestion of the capsular hyaluronic acid present on the group A streptococci by the organism's own hyaluronidase (see further on). More than 70 different M types have been identified; some (such as M type 3) are more closely associated with throat infections and rheumatic fever, whereas others (such as M type 12) are more closely associated with skin infections and nephritis. Antibodies against M proteins are opsonic (i.e., they stimulate phagocytosis) and protect the animals and humans against infection by the same M type strain. The antibody can also be used diagnostically to characterize the M type of an isolated strain; this is very important epidemiologically for identifying the source of the organism in an epidemic. The fact that the antibody against the M protein completely protects against the infection indicates this protein is a major virulence factor of the group A streptococci. Subsequent studies showed that the group A streptococci contained other proteins in their cell wall (e.g., T and R), which also were useful in their classification.

The Virulence Factors
SOMATIC

Although the M protein is the principal virulence factor in the group A streptococci, these organisms contain a number of other components associated with virulence. These may be divided into three categories: (1) the **somatic** virulence factors, which are associated with structural components of the cell surfaces; (2) **spreading factors**; and (3) **erythrogenic toxin(s),** which causes scarlet fever. Table 6–2 lists these factors, their pathogenic activity, and whether they are immunogenic. At the top of the list is, of course, the M protein, which, as indicated previously is both antiphagocytic and immunogenic (induces an antibody response). The antiphagocytic activity may be associated with an inhibition of complement binding. The hyaluronic acid capsule, which also appears to be antiphagocytic, does not induce antibody, because its composition is nearly the same as the hyaluronic acid found in human connective tissues. An extract containing the group A polysaccharide and fragments of peptidoglycan (group A polysaccharide complex) produces recurrent inflammatory lesions in rabbits resembling the joint and skin lesions seen in patients with rheumatic disease. Although no direct etiologic connection has been made between these diseases and the group A polysaccharide complex, there is a direct connection between infection with group A streptococci and rheumatic fever. Most theories postulate a cross-reaction between streptococcal wall and/or protoplast membrane antigens and heart tissues. One of these components may be an actinlike protein that induces an Arthus-like reaction in the heart valves. This **autoimmune** reaction results in an inflammatory lesion closely associated with rheumatic heart disease.

SPREADING FACTORS
(EXTRACELLULAR ENZYMES)

In addition to the somatic components that appear to be involved in the virulence of the group

TABLE 6–2 ✦ Virulence Factors of the Group A Streptococci

STRUCTURAL COMPONENTS	BIOLOGIC ACTIVITY	ANTIGENICITY
Hyaluronic acid capsule	Antiphagocytic	No
M protein	Antiphagocytic, attachment to cells	Yes
Peptidoglycan–C polysaccharide complex	Recurrent inflammation of joints and skin	Yes
Lipoteichoic acid	Attachment to cells	Yes
Protoplast membranes	Antigenically similar to heart tissues	Yes
Extracellular Enzymes (spreading factors)		
Streptolysin O (O$_2$ sensitive)	Hemolysin, cardiotoxic	Yes
Streptolysin S (O$_2$ stable)	Hemolysin, leukotoxic	No
Hyaluronidase	Hyaluronic acid depolymerase	Yes
Streptokinase	Digests fibrin	Yes
DNAse	Hydrolyzes DNA	Yes
NADase	Hydrolyzes nicotinamide adenine dinucleotide	Yes
Proteases	Hydrolyzes protein	Yes

A streptococci, these bacteria produce a number of extracellular enzymes—some that lyse host cells and others that can hydrolyze a number of macromolecules found in host tissues. These properties enable these streptococci to cause infections characterized by suppurative exudates, which often spread along fascial planes. These spreading infections contrast with the localized suppurative swellings usually associated with staphylococcal infections (see Chapter 7). Although the actual degree to which these spreading factors contribute to the virulence of the group A streptococci has never been established, these enzymes have become important both diagnostically and, paradoxically, in the treatment of postoperative swellings, and recently for dissolving clots in coronary arteries.

Streptolysin O. This oxygen-labile hemolysin is a potent immunogen, and antibodies against this component are produced during active streptococcal infection. These antibodies form the basis for the **antistreptolysin O** (ASO titer) assay for streptococcal infection. This hemolysin has been reported to have cardiotoxic properties. The importance of such observations is based on there still being some conjecture about the etiology of rheumatic carditis, although most investigators now consider it to be an autoimmune disease. However, despite its cardiotoxicity, no one has satisfactorily explained how this hemolysin affects heart tissue in the presence of high ASO titers generally present in patients with rheumatic fever.

Streptolysin S. This is the oxygen-stable hemolysin responsible for the hemolysis seen on blood agar plates. It also appears to have leukotoxic effects, although its relationship to disease is not understood; unlike most proteins, it is a poor antigen.

Hyaluronidase. As indicated previously, the group A streptococci produce both hyaluronic acid and the enzyme hyaluronidase, which removes the capsule. Presumably, the hyaluronidase functions in disease by breaking down the ground substance (hyaluronic acid) of connective tissue and allowing the organisms to spread. Although the streptococcal strains possessing this enzyme appear to be more virulent, the contribution of hyaluronidase and other spreading factors has not been quantitated. However, it is clear that these enzymes are produced during infection because increased antibody titers to them occur in patients with group A streptococcal disease. Thus, even if these enzymes do not play a crucial role in the disease process, they are diagnostically important since there are several clinical tests for streptococcal infection based on combinations of these antigens.

Streptokinase. This enzyme converts serum plasminogen to plasmin, an enzyme that digests fibrin. Presumably, dissolving fibrin clots can aid in the spread of the streptococci and thus intensify an infection. However, the major importance of this fibrinolysin as well as several other streptococcal enzymes is their use in chemotherapeutic preparations that dissolve the blood clots and emboli found in many thrombocytic diseases. (The actual enzyme is obtained commercially from the group C streptococci.)

Streptodornase. This enzyme hydrolyzes DNA which is found in large amounts in purulent exudates as a result of lysis of the phagocytic cells. The lysis leads to decreased viscosity of the exudate and enhanced spread of organisms. However, many other inflammatory diseases, including those which result in thrombi, have exudates containing DNA. The viscosity of these exudates reduces the effectiveness of the phagocytic mechanisms necessary to "clean up" these exudates. In some types of infections, the combination of the fibrin clot and the viscosity prevents antibiotics from efficiently reaching the bacteria. Again, combinations of the streptococcal enzymes have been developed for therapeutic use to reduce the viscosity of exudates. These enzymes have been employed to loosen the "mucus" such as found in patients with cystic fibrosis. Perhaps it is the ultimate paradox that the bacterial virulence factors become the agents used to reduce the severity of certain infections.

Other Spreading Factors. There are many other streptococcal enzymes that hydrolyze host components. Among them are nicotinamide adenine diphosphorylase (NADase) and various proteases.

Erythogenic Toxin

Some strains of *Streptococcus pyogenes* carry a lysogenic phage; when the phage DNA is incorporated into the streptococcal chromosome, the organism produces a toxin responsible for the scarlet fever rash. Before the antibiotic era, scarlet fever was feared because it often preceded symptoms of rheumatic fever and a prolonged illness. It is now considered a symptom in some cases of streptococcal pharyngitis and not essential for development of rheumatic fever. Indeed, the rash may have the beneficial effect of alerting both the patient and the physician to the seriousness of the "sore throat."

Pathogenesis of Streptococcal Pharyngitis

The local streptococcal lesion can be divided into three stages: attachment, spreading, and recovery.

ATTACHMENT

It has been estimated that approximately 2×10^6 organisms are necessary to initiate a lesion. A number of studies suggest bacterial attachment is mediated by lipoteichoic acid, which binds to the epithelial cell surface via their lipid ends. There is also some evidence that M protein and perhaps also the C polysaccharide take part in attachment. Regardless of the exact molecular mechanism of attachment, the bacteria proliferate and probably gain access to the underlying connective tissues via microscopic breaks in the epithelium. As in most infectious diseases, there is a prompt and vigorous inflammatory response mounted by the host to eliminate the bacteria. This response is characterized by a fluid exudate (edema) and primarily a polymorphonuclear (PMN) cellular infiltrate.

SPREADING

The PMNs cannot phagocytize the organisms efficiently because of the M protein. The streptococci multiply rapidly in the connective tissue. The PMNs die, releasing their intracellular components (proteins, nucleic acids, and so on). The viscosity of this suppurative exudate might ordinarily confine this infection locally, but *S. pyogenes* produces the DNAses, proteases, and streptokinases that hydrolyze these components and allow the organisms to spread. In addition, they produce hyaluronidase, which breaks down the ground substance, allowing even further spread of the bacteria. If unchecked by the administration of appropriate antibiotics or the production of sufficient M protein antibodies, the organisms may gain entrance to the cervical lymph nodes or the sinuses, draining the ear and nasal pharynx to cause septicemia, that is, circulation of virulent bacteria in the blood, or blood poisoning.

RECOVERY

Even if untreated, most patients with streptococcal sore throat eventually recover because of the production of antibodies to M protein. These antibodies are opsonic and enhance phagocytosis but are specific for the M type antigen that induced them. However, recovery from the local disease does not necessarily mean that all is well. Approximately 3 percent of the patients will develop a *poststreptococcal* disease called *rheumatic fever,* which can be more life-threatening than the local infection. It is the danger of rheumatic fever that necessitates the rapid and accurate diagnosis of all pharyngitis patients.

Clinical Signs and Symptoms of Streptococcal Pharyngitis

Streptococcal pharyngitis is characterized by a short incubation period (2 to 3 days), a high fever (103°F to 104°F), pain, chills, headache, and often stomach cramps. The throat, particularly the tonsils or the tonsillar fauces, may appear "beefy red," a suppurative exudate may be present, and the cervical lymph nodes are enlarged and painful. A comparison of the incidence of antibodies to streptococcal products with the number of known cases of streptococcal disease suggests that perhaps as many as 20 percent may be asymptomatic (subclinical). In addition to pharyngitis, the group A streptococci cause a number of other serious diseases; for example, puerperal fever (a septicemia originating from an infected uterus following delivery or abortion), skin infections, and occasionally acute endocarditis.

Diagnosis

Because of the seriousness of poststreptococcal diseases and the similarity of symptoms of streptococcal sore throat and other upper respiratory diseases—for example, mononucleosis, adenovirus infection, influenza, diphtheria, and furospirochetal infection (this is just an abbreviated list)—a differential diagnosis is essential. As in most infectious diseases, diagnosis is based first on the clinical signs and symptoms and then on the appropriate laboratory tests.

THROAT CULTURE

The throat swab is plated on blood agar and also placed in an enrichment broth, in case the numbers of group A streptococci in the sample might be low. The sample from the broth is also plated on blood agar. The presence of β-hemolytic, bacitracin-sensitive streptococci is diagnostic for streptococcal pharyngitis. Bacitracin discs are used because group A streptococci are particularly sensitive to this antibiotic. A catalase test should also be performed but cannot be done on blood agar plates because the erythrocytes are rich in this enzyme. Once the organism has been isolated, it should be screened for antibiotic sensitivity and it may be serotyped if necessary.

THROAT SAMPLES

Rapid tests for identification of group A streptococci are commercially available as latex agglutination and ELISA tests for bacterial antigen.

SEROLOGIC TESTS

Although these tests are not necessary for the diagnosis of the local infection, it is often prudent to take a sample of the so-called acute phase serum from the patient with a diagnosed group A streptococcal infection. If complications develop, an increased titer of the "convalescent phase serum" compared with the "acute phase serum" is important in the diagnosis of poststreptococcal disease.

Antistreptolysin O (ASO) (Titer). This test has already been described briefly in connection with the virulence of streptolysin O. In this test, the patient's sera, usually both acute and convalescent samples, are mixed with streptolysin prior to adding the erythrocytes. The reduction of hemolysis in the sample compared with a normal serum control, which allows complete hemolysis to occur, is used as a measure of the amount of antibody present. Patients who have had a streptococcal infection show significantly less hemolysis in the convalescent serum compared with the acute serum. This indicates that more antibody (i.e., an increase in ASO titer) is present.

Antihyaluronidase Titer. This test measures the antibody to streptococcal hyaluronidase. This test, as well as the anti-DNAse titer, is used primarily when the infection is suspected but the ASO test is inconclusive.

Streptozyme Test. This is a patented test kit in which the erythrocytes have been coated with several streptococcal enzymes (e.g., streptolysin, hyaluronidase, DNAse, and protease). Addition of patient's serum containing antibody against any one of these enzymes will cause hemagglutination. A number of similar commercial tests for group A streptococcal infection are now available.

Epidemiology

Streptococcal sore throat usually is spread by aerosol droplets from carriers, often asymptomatic children. As in many other infectious diseases, "lowered resistance" of the patient—because of an antecedent respiratory infection, crowded housing (socioeconomic factors), or seasonal factors—appears to be an important factor in the individual's susceptibility to infection. Indeed, during periods of rapid army mobilization, the barracks were often sources of streptococcal epidemics, and it was common practice to give recruits prophylactic antibiotic therapy. The mortality rate prior to antibiotic therapy was 1 to 3 percent. Although antibiotics seem to have diminished the severity of poststreptococcal complications such as rheumatic fever and glomerulonephritis, the actual incidence of these diseases is about the same.

Treatment

Penicillin is still the antibiotic of choice, since few of the group A streptococci have developed resistance to it. In patients allergic to penicillin, erythromycin is used. The physician will usually maintain therapy for at least 10 days in cases of proven group A infection. Sulphonamides are not used, because they do not prevent the poststreptococcal complications. Tetracyclines also are not used, because many streptococci are resistant to these drugs.

Prevention

Although type-specific immunity to M protein has been demonstrated, there are too many M types to make a vaccine feasible. Moreover, purification of the proteins is difficult. There are also some antigenic substances in purified M proteins that may immunologically cross-react with heart tissues. Techniques of gene cloning may provide a highly purified M protein or active fractions of M protein suitable for vaccines in the future.

Rheumatic Fever

As indicated previously, rheumatic fever is not an active infection but usually results from a previous group A streptococcal pharyngitis. Indeed, the diagnosis is based on a set of signs and symptoms known as the Ducket-Jones criteria, shown in Table 6–3. A combination of major and minor criteria is necessary to establish the diagnosis of rheumatic fever. Some understanding of the pathogenesis of this disease is necessary for the dental health care personnel because patients with histories of rheumatic carditis have a predilection for endocarditis following dental therapy.

It is generally agreed that no streptococcal toxin is responsible for the scarring and subsequent stenosis of the coronary valves associated with rheumatic fever. Rather it appears to be some component of the streptococci that has antigenic deter-

TABLE 6–3 ✦ Criteria for Diagnosis of Rheumatic Fever (Duckett-Jones)

MAJOR SIGNS OR SYMPTOMS	MINOR SIGNS OR SYMPTOMS
Cardiac	Fever
Murmurs	Arthralgia (joint pain)
Pericarditis	Previous rheumatic
Congestive heart failure	fever or rheumatic
Polyarthritis	heart disease
Chorea (uncoordinated	Increase in erythro-
movements)	cyte sedimentation
Erythema marginatum	rate
Subcutaneous nodules	Positive C-reactive
Evidence of previous	protein
streptococcal infection	Leukocytosis
Scarlet fever	
Positive group A strep-	
tococcal culture	
Rise in ASO titer or	
titer against other	
streptococcal pro-	
teins	

minants similar to the proteins in the coronary valves. These components are different enough to be recognized as foreign by the patient's immune system and thus antibodies are produced against them. The antibodies cross-react with the proteins in the valves, which results in complement-fixation and initiates an Arthus-like reaction in the valves. The inflammatory reaction in the valves may result in scarring, subsequent stenosis, and the inability of the valves to function properly. Because of the mechanics of blood flow, the mitral valve seems to be more frequently affected than other cardiac valves. It also is, at least partially, the fluid mechanics that concentrate the bacteria resulting from bacteremia at the site of the damaged valve. These bacteria, commonly oral streptococci, appear to attach readily to damaged valves and initiate infective endocarditis, which is a potentially fatal disease. This infection is described in more detail in the section on oral streptococci.

STREPTOCOCCUS PNEUMONIAE

Pneumococcal pneumonia is still among the most frequent causes of death associated with infectious disease, particularly in people with lowered resistance (i.e., geriatric populations, patients receiving cancer chemotherapy or immunosuppressive therapy, and patients with diabetes or influenza). The epithet "Captain of the Men of Death" is still appropriately applied to this disease. In addition to its importance clinically, much of our knowledge of the molecular basis of virulence and microbial genetics stems from studies of *Streptococcus pneumoniae*. Thus, the organism and the diseases it causes provide an excellent model for studying the molecular basis of infectious disease.

PHYSIOLOGY

As with all streptococci, the organism is gram-positive and catalase-negative. It is α hemolytic under aerobic conditions but does produce an oxygen-labile hemolysin. This results in β hemolysis under anaerobic conditions and thus it differs from most of the α hemolytic streptococci found in the oral pharynx, in which no hemolysis is observed under anaerobic conditions. Another useful property that distinguishes *S. pneumoniae* from other viridans streptococci is its sensitivity to a chemical called Optochin (ethyl cuprin hydrochloride). Thus, a simple diagnostic test for pneumococcal pneumonia is to plate a sputum sample on blood agar and place an Optochin disc over the streak. After incubation, the presence of α hemolytic colonies containing ovoid pairs of gram-positive cocci (diplococci, Fig. 6–3A), which are sensitive to Optochin, is confirmatory evidence for the presence of *S. pneumoniae*.

Serology
CAPSULAR POLYSACCHARIDES

The most distinctive feature of *S. pneumoniae* is a capsule composed of a polysaccharide that can be visualized by several special staining techniques (Fig. 6–3B). The polysaccharide is not only shed from the surface during growth, but because the organism tends to lyse spontaneously as it ages (autolyze), relatively large quantities of the polysaccharide are found in the spent medium. The lysis is due to a specific enzyme that cleaves the peptidoglycan of the pneumococcus. This *pneumococcal autolysin* is activated by bile salts such as desoxycholate. Indeed, a bile solubility test was once used to diagnose pneumococcal infections. The polysaccharide can be easily recovered from the spent medium and autolyzed cell cultures by relatively simple procedures. Figure 6–4 is a diagrammatic representation of the structure of the serotype III polysaccharide. This polysaccharide is composed of alternating units of glucose and glucuronic acid. There are some 80 different serologically distinct types of pneumococcal polysaccharides, many with markedly different compositions. As suggested by their name, these polysaccharides are strongly immunogenic and form the basis for a serologic classification scheme used to distinguish the various strains. Fortunately, only about 14 of these serotypes are responsible for over 90 percent of the infectious disease caused by this species.

TRANSFORMATION OF SEROTYPES

You may recall from Chapter 3 that the molecular biology revolution originated with the observation that the capsular type of pneumococcus could be transformed by adding an extract of smooth cells of one type to rough cells derived from another type (rough cells are those that have lost their capsular polysaccharide, generally as a result of being cultured in vitro). The discovery by Avery and his colleagues that the transforming agent was DNA is responsible for this revolution.

SPECIES-SPECIFIC ANTIGEN

A component of the cell wall originally called the "C" substance (not to be confused with the "C" carbohydrate of the β-hemolysis streptococci), but now known to be a specific type of ribitol teichoic acid containing choline, appears to be common to most strains of *S. pneumoniae*. Thus, this is one of the rare bacterial antigens that are species specific. However, it is the type-specific polysaccharide antigens that are clinically important. (The "C" substance is used clinically for testing for the presence of a blood component with which it reacts. This is called the *C-reactive protein* [CRP] test.) This is a nonspecific test for the presence of acute inflammatory diseases.

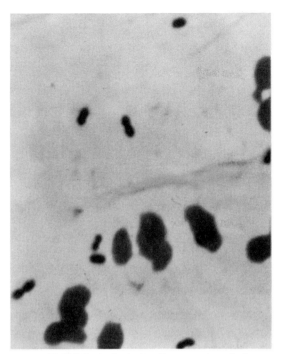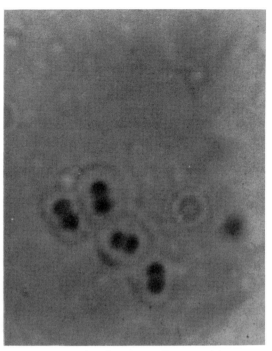

FIGURE 6–3 ✦ A, Gram stain of *Streptococcus pneumoniae* in suppurative exudate. **B,** Quellung reaction (capsular swelling test). (From Schneierson, S. S.: Atlas of Diagnostic Microbiology. Abbot Laboratories, North Chicago, Ill., 1965, with permission.)

THE CAPSULAR SWELLING TEST

Antisera against the specific pneumococcal polysaccharide will precipitate the molecule from solutions, agglutinate cells containing the polysaccharide capsule, or cause the capsule to "swell." The **Quellung** (German for swelling) **reaction,** or capsular swelling test, is most frequently used for diagnosis because of its simplicity and specificity. It consists of incubating a wet mount containing pneumococcal cells with antisera. The antibodies react with the polysaccharide in the capsule, perhaps changing its refractive index. When viewed in a microscope it appears that the capsule has swollen (see Fig. 6–3B). This test can often be carried out directly on fresh sputum samples of patients with suspected pneumococcal pneumonia, thereby speeding the diagnosis significantly. This test was especially important in the pre-antibiotic era when the only specific treatment for pneumococcal pneumonia was administration of antisera produced in horses. It was obviously important to choose the right horse (sic). Since death from pneumococcal pneumonia can occur within 6 days, rapid diagnosis was and still is essential. The antibodies against the capsular polysaccharide are both diagnostic and therapeutic, indicating that the capsule functions as the major virulence component of this species.

VIRULENCE FACTORS

Capsular Polysaccharides. The capsular polysaccharides are not only the major antigens of *S. pneumoniae* but also the most important virulence factors. It has been suggested that the hy-

Glucuronic Acid   Glucose

FIGURE 6–4 ✦ Structure of pneumococcal serotype 3 capsular polysaccharide.

drophilic nature of the capsule prevents their phagocytosis by polymorphonuclear leukocytes. Thus, the capsules of the pneumococci are said to be *antiphagocytic*, and despite their completely different nature, they perform the same function as the M protein of the group A streptococci. When coated with specific antibody, the bacteria are readily phagocytized. (As mentioned previously, the process of antibody-enhanced phagocytosis is called opsonization.) Indeed, the resolution of pneumococcal pneumonia occurs by a process called "crisis," which is associated with the production of opsonizing antibody by the patient (see further on).

Toxins. The beta (β) hemolysin has already been described; this component is said to have leukocidin properties (i.e., it can destroy human leukocytes). In addition, in many cases of pneumococcal pneumonia, in which the bacterial infection appears to be eliminated with effective antibiotic therapy, the patients still die with symptoms resembling a true toxemia (circulating toxin). An intensive search for such a toxin, however, has still not been completely successful.

PATHOGENESIS OF LOBAR PNEUMONIA

The disease is generally divided into four stages: (1) proliferation, (2) early consolidation, (3) advanced consolidation, and (4) resolution by crisis or death by complication. The beginning of the disease is often associated with an upper respiratory infection such as influenza. This results in reduced ciliary and epiglottal reflexes and a thick, copious mucous secretion. The pneumococci, which become trapped in this viscous mucous, are aspirated into the alveoli where they resist phagocytosis and multiply (proliferation). The bacteria induce an inflammatory reaction initially characterized by increased fluid (edema—early consolidation). This is followed by the cellular portion of the inflammatory response—the polymorphonuclear leukocytes attempt to phagocytose the bacteria, die, and lyse. Death of phagocytes results in a thick, purulent exudate, or pus (advanced consolidation). All this occurs in the relatively short time of 2 to 6 days and is characterized by sudden high fever, coughing, pain on breathing, and hypoxia (lack of oxygen). Resolution is associated with a sudden, copious perspiration ("sweats") and a drop in fever. It is due to the production of opsinizing antibodies. However, in many cases, particularly in older patients ("old man's friend") or in those with lowered resistance, the organisms enter the bloodstream (bacteremia) and are distributed to other vital organs such as the meninges, where their multiplication often leads to rapid death (death by complication). Indeed, prior to the antibiotic era 36 percent of patients died of this disease.

DIAGNOSIS

In addition to the clinical signs and symptoms, radiographs, sputum cultures, and blood cultures are taken. As indicated previously, before the advent of antibiotics it was routine to perform a Quellung test on the sputum sample. The presence of α-hemolytic, Optochin-sensitive, gram-positive diplococci is diagnostic for infection with *S. pneumoniae*. A positive blood culture portends very serious consequences.

TREATMENT

Penicillin is still the antibiotic of choice, with erythromycin being used in patients allergic to penicillin. In recent years there have been strains reported that are resistant to multiple antibiotics, suggesting a plasmid mediated transfer. Because of the appearance of such strains and the inability to control the disease in some patients, a vaccine has been developed.

PREVENTION

Since this is a disease with lowered resistance, maintenance of good health is clearly one preventive method. However, the vaccine contains 14 capsular polysaccharides which represent the most common disease-producing strains. The vaccine is particularly valuable for compromised patients such as those with Hodgkin's disease or sickle cell anemia, splenectomized patients, and miners exposed to various dusts. It also has been effective in reducing the frequency of middle ear infection in children particularly subject to this infection.

THE ORAL STREPTOCOCCI

The oral streptococci constitute one of the most populous groups of bacteria in the mouth. Recent studies have divided these organisms into ever more numerous species. *S. mutans* has now been partitioned into several species: *S. mutans and S. sobrinus* (human strains) and *S. rattus, S. cricetus,* and *S. ferus* (usually found in rodents). More recently, there has been a rather extensive revamping of the speciation of the other α-hemolytic streptococci of the oral cavity. In this chapter rather then trying to describe all the variations among the individual species that constitute the groups, the organisms will be "lumped" together under the most common species designation. Thus, we take the point of view of the lumper rather than splitter to provide the reader with a basic grasp of the properties of the streptococcal groups found in the mouth. With the exception of *S. salivarius,* most of the strains of these species produce a greenish zone of α hemolysis around colonies on blood agar. Because of this, they have previously been referred to as *S. viridans,* and indeed even today one sees this term used in some articles. However, this is the ultimate in "lumping" and truly is a misnomer. Its use makes it difficult to understand the relationship of each of the major streptococcal groups to its ecologic niche within the oral cavity and to disease. Thus, although *S. salivarius* is often considered a member of this group, it rarely if ever produces α hemolysis. Its normal habitat is the tongue, from which large numbers are shed, and it is the predominant organism in saliva. For this reason, the detection of *S. salivarius* is an indication of salivary contamination, just as *Escherichia coli* is an indicator of fecal contamination. Although all the data are not yet in, it appears that members of the *S. mitis* group are more commonly found on the buccal mucous membranes (nonkeratinized), whereas the *S. sanguis* and *S. mutans* group are the quintessential tooth organisms; moreover, the latter species appears to be the most cariogenic of the oral streptococci. Obviously, such differences in ecologic distribution and disease potential suggest not only specific attachment of each species to the tissues but also metabolic differences which provide selective advantages for each species to exist in its distinct ecologic niche. The remainder of this section will deal with exploring the nature of these selective advantages and particularly the enhanced cariogenicity of *S. mutans*.

Streptococcus salivarius

PHYSIOLOGY

This species is the most easily identified oral streptococcus because it forms "gumdrop" colonies on agar medium containing sucrose. Typical colonies of this organism grown on mitis-salivarius agar (MSA) are highly convex in shape and look like gumdrop candies. The component responsible for this type of colony is an extracellular levan produced from sucrose in the medium. As shown in Figure 6–5, a levan is a linear polymer of fructose, which is synthesized by an enzyme on the surface of *S. salivarius* called a fructosyltransferase or a levan-sucrase. This enzyme cleaves the high energy glycosidic bond between glucose and fructose in sucrose and uses part of the energy released during hydrolysis to link the fructose units together to form the levan. The residual glucose that results

from this hydrolysis is converted to lactate via the Embden-Meyerhof pathway (Chapter 3). It is important to remember that only a small amount of the sucrose is used to form the levan. Most is converted to fructose and glucose by the enzyme invertase (see further on); these monosaccharides are then metabolized by the usual glycolytic pathways. It should also be noted that the disaccharide sucrose is unusual in possessing the high-energy glycosidic bond between glucose and fructose, thus making it the only dietary substrate usually available for this type of polymer formation. Similar kinds of reactions take place among the other oral streptococci, but they result in the formation of dextrans, polymers of glucose. Table 6–4 lists the biochemical reactions of the oral streptococci, which are commonly employed to identify them; however, adequate identification for most clinical purposes can often be achieved using just a few of these tests. Thus, the minimum properties that would identify the majority of *S. salivarius* are grampositive cocci in chains that are catalase-negative, show no hemolysis, and form gumdrop colonies on MSA. However, commercial testing is now available that uses as many as 20 different tests to identify the streptococci precisely. The simplicity and accuracy of these tests have led to the replacement of the more cumbersome tube fermentation tests.

SEROLOGY

Although serology is probably less important in the taxonomy of *S. salivarius* than in the β-hemolytic streptococci, it has great potential as a tool for probing the relationship of the bacterial surface to the ecology of these organisms. Most strains of *S. salivarius* belong to Lancefield group K, although some contain the group F or O antigens. The antigens defining these groups are either cell wall or capsular polysaccharides distinct from the levans produced by this species. It appears that those strains containing the K antigen adhere more strongly to human buccal epithelial cells in vitro than the K-negative strains. However, many strains, regardless of antigenic composition, aggregate with strains of *Veillonella* sp., which are gram-negative anaerobic cocci that are major res-

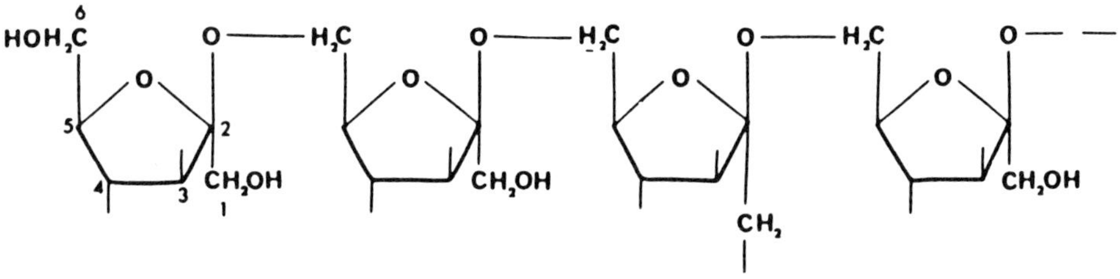

FIGURE 6–5 ✦ Structure of levan from *Streptococcus salivarius*.

TABLE 6–4 ✦ Biochemical Identification of Oral Streptococci

TESTS	*S. SALIVARIUS*	*S. SANGUIS*	*S. MITIS*	*S. MUTANS*
Hemolysis	Nonhemolytic	Alpha	Alpha	Alpha
Catalase	Neg.	Neg.	Neg.	Neg.
Arginine hydrolysis	Neg.	Pos.	Neg.	Neg.*
Esculin hydrolysis	Neg.	Pos.	Neg./pos.	Pos.
Levan ("gumdrop" colonies)	Pos.	Neg.	Neg.	Neg.
Dextran	Neg.	Pos.†	Pos.†	Pos.†
Mannitol	Neg.	Neg.	Neg.	Pos.
Sorbitol	Neg.	Neg.	Neg.	Pos.
Inulin	Pos.	Pos.	Neg.	Pos.
Peroxide production	Neg.	Pos.	Pos.	Var.‡

*The serotype b strains *(S. rattus)* do hydrolyze arginine.
†Some strains do produce small amounts of levan but do not form "gumdrop" colonies.
‡Var. = variable.

idents of the human tongue. *S. salivarius* is rarely found in dental plaque and, correspondingly, generally does not adhere well to saliva-coated hydroxyapatite, an in vitro model for dental plaque formation. Thus, the surface of this species seems to contain one or more components that favor its attachment to the tongue or bacteria associated with the tongue, and perhaps it is not surprising that this organ is its major habitat in the human oral cavity.

FIMBRIAE

In Chapter 3 (p. 51) the structure and functions of fimbriae (pili) found in gram-negative bacteria were described. Although the oral streptococci have analogous structures that presumably also function in attachment (adhesin), less is known of their structure, composition and functionality as adhesins. What is evident (Fig. 6–6) is that the oral streptococci differ in both the quantity and quality of their fimbriae. Thus, *S. salivarius* contains numerous long fimbriae, whereas the fimbriae in some strains of *S. sanguis* are shorter and less dense. Other strains of *S. sanguis* (*S. crista*) have large, dense fimbriae localized to only one area of the cell wall. Strains possessing these polarized fimbriae often adhere to strains of *Bacterionema matruchotii* in aggregates known as "corncobs," found on the surface of supragingival plaque (see Fig. 26–11, Chapter 26). Another type of corncob is formed with *Fusobacterium nucleatum* and may be responsible for the ability of these organisms to take up residence in subgingival plaque. *S. mutans* does not appear to have a significant amount of fimbriae compared with the other oral streptococci. The fimbriae of *S. mitis* appears similar to *S. sanguis* but the antigenic composition of the surface as well as the chemical composition of the cell walls of *S. mitis* and *S. sanguis* differ. In the final analysis, it is the molecular composition of the

fimbriae, not their appearance, which governs where the bacterium will reside. Although the fimbriae appear to be delicate in thin sections from which water has been removed following fixation, negative staining of the whole organism as seen in Figure 6–7, suggests they may be more substantial and firmly bound into the cell wall. Efforts directed at dental plaque prevention are attempting to identify the fimbrial structure and composition and develop specific biological or chemotherapeutic reagents that will inhibit their activity.

Streptococcus sanguis

The name of this organism is descriptive of its isolation from blood cultures of patients with subacute bacterial endocarditis ("sanguine" is Latin for blood). It is still among the most frequent species isolated from patients with this disease and also is among the most frequent organisms isolated from dental plaque. Since endocarditis often results from a bacteremia following dental treatment, a simple deduction leads to the conclusion that these dental plaque bacteria may enter the circulation during dental treatment to cause this very serious and often fatal disease. Thus, an appreciation of the structure-function relationships of this organism is essential for understanding plaque formation and maturation as well as the pathogenesis of endocarditis.

PHYSIOLOGY

It has only been within the last 20 years that an acceptable physiologic classification of the "viridans streptococci" has been developed (note that the latter descriptive terminology is acceptable, whereas *S. viridans* is not). In any event a comparison of some of the physiologic characteristics of these organisms is provided in Table 6–4 (see

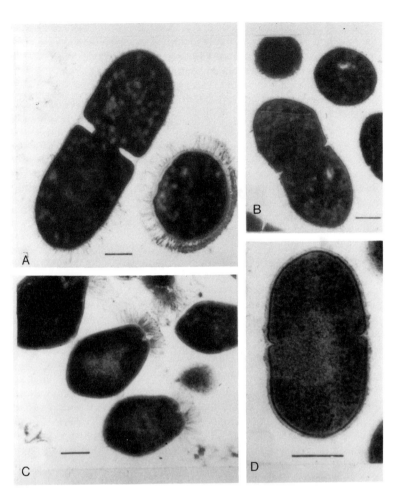

FIGURE 6–6 ✦ Transmission electron micrographs of oral streptococci. **A,** *S. salivarius.* **B,** *S. sanguis* (typical plaque isolate). **C,** *S. sanguis* (corncob-forming strain with localized fimbriae). **D,** *Streptococcus mutans.*

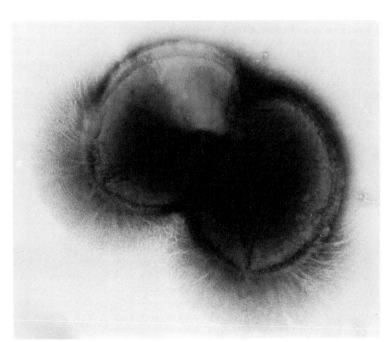

FIGURE 6–7 ✦ Negative stain of corncob-forming strain. (Courtesy of Dr. Pauline Handley.)

also Fig. 6–6). Examination of this table suggests that *S. sanguis* may be reasonably identified by its failure to ferment either mannitol or sorbitol and its ability to produce ammonia and carbon dioxide from arginine. (Since *S. milleri* resembles *S. sanguis* in many respects, no separate discussion of this species will be included here.)

Arginine Hydrolase. The arginine hydrolase pathway results in the breakdown of arginine into urea and finally into ammonia and carbon dioxide. This can provide energy for bacterial growth in the absence of fermentable carbohydrate and enables *S. sanguis* to exist in plaque in the absence of fermentable carbohydrates. Moreover, production of ammonia may neutralize acids produced by bacterial fermentation, providing an environment more suitable for bacterial growth. It has been suggested that this pathway may be the reason *S. sanguis* is less cariogenic than most strains of *S. mutans*, which do not possess this pathway. Indeed, the possibility that one could reduce the acidity of plaque by the formation of ammonia from metabolizable urea was the basis of an earlier anticariogenic toothpaste. More recently, a tetrapeptide called Sialin containing arginine and other basic amino acids was developed; this peptide is metabolized by dental plaque and salivary sediments to yield ammonia. Measurements of plaque pH using *Stephan Curves* (see Chapter 27) indicated that plaque or salivary sediment (an in vitro model for plaque) treated with Sialin did not show the usual dramatic fall in pH after a sugar rinse. This approach to caries prevention was based on the idea that organisms like *S. sanguis* can increase plaque pH if given the appropriate substrate. Unfortunately, this approach to caries prevention was not cost effective.

Dextran Formation. Another property of ecologic interest in *S. sanguis* is the production of dextrans. These glucose polymers, like the polymers of fructose, are produced enzymatically from sucrose by dextransucrase or glucosyltransferase. These enzymes are associated with the surface of this organism, although their exact mode of attachment to the cell wall is still unknown. Most dextran produced by *S. sanguis* is "soluble," which means it is predominantly a linear polymer of α-1,6 glucosyl pyranose (Fig. 6–8). The dextran accumulates in the spent medium and can be readily precipitated by addition of an equal volume of ethanol. The aqueous solubility of α-1,6 dextrans makes their contribution to the attachment process questionable; however, the *S. sanguis* enzymes may bind the more insoluble dextrans produced by *S. mutans*, providing a mechanism of attachment of this more cariogenic organism to dental plaque. Although more cariogenic, this latter species generally has a much lower ability to adhere to tooth surface than does *S. sanguis*.

Glycogen Storage. Many oral streptococci are capable of producing internal stores of glycogen (intracellular polysaccharide, or IPS), which can be metabolized and used as energy source during periods when external sugars are not available.

Perioxide Production. Although classically it has been stated that streptococci possess no direct pathway to oxygen, it is clear that several species do produce small amounts of H_2O_2. Presumably this is due to the direct transfer of hydrogen from reduced flavoprotein to molecular oxygen; however, the exact pathway is still unknown. Since these organisms do not possess a catalase or peroxidase, the perioxide accumulates and may become toxic. This is one reason anaerobic incuba-

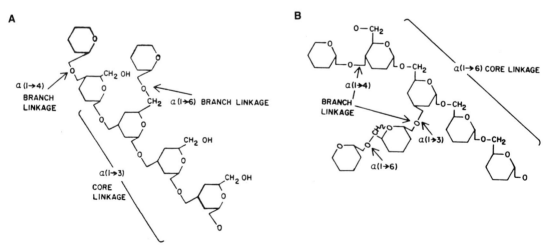

FIGURE 6–8 ✦ A, Dextran containing α(1,6)-glucose backbone and side chain typical of soluble dextrans. **B,** Dextran with α(1,3)-glucose side chains. The extent of these α(1,3) linkages determines the solubility of the dextran. (From Loesche, J. W.: Dental Caries, A Treatable Infection. Charles C Thomas, Springfield, Ill., 1982, with permission.)

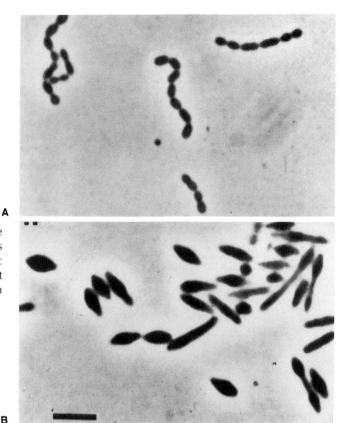

FIGURE 6–9 ✦ Effects of oxygen on the shape of *S. sanguis* cells. **A,** Normal cells grown under anaerobic or microaerophilic conditions. **B,** Cells grown in cultures that have been shaken to increase concentration of dissolved oxygen.

tion is often used to grow these bacteria. Indeed, even small amounts of dissolved oxygen in the medium can result in quite marked cytotoxic effects, as shown in Figure 6–9. *S. sanguis* cells form large pleomorphic rods when grown in flasks that permit a large surface area of the medium to be exposed to the air and absorb oxygen. The viability of these rod-shaped forms is low compared with the usual coccal forms (Fig. 6–9A). The peroxide not only is autotoxic, but also can inhibit other bacteria. This may explain why the presence of *S. sanguis* in plaque has been suggested to be beneficial. (In addition, a bacteriocin produced by *S. sanguis* inhibits certain gram-negative plaque bacteria.) An additional role for streptococcal H_2O_2 may be as a substrate for the lactoperoxidase in saliva. This enzyme catalyzed the oxidation of thiocyanate (SCN^-) ion to hypothiocyanate ($OSCN^-$) in the presence of H_2O_2. The hypothiocyanate is also toxic to many streptococci and lactobacilli, although an exact role for this reaction in vivo has not been described. In any case, it is clear that *S. sanguis,* by both its numbers in plaque and its range of metabolic activities, can play an important role in oral ecology.

SEROLOGY

Group H Antigen. If confusion exists in the physiologic classification of oral streptococci, then

"chaos" would be a mild description for the serologic classification. Indeed, the two problems were interrelated because the inadequate physiologic classification led to using strains not properly speciated for immunization. Even today, one of the largest commercial suppliers still uses an antiserum that probably does not detect the true group H antigen (the most common antigen in *S. sanguis*) for its serologic identification. Thus, many strains being used for oral ecologic studies are often actually a different streptococcal species than the one the author thought he or she was investigating. This has led to confusion in deciding which organisms live in which place.

Recent studies have shown that the group H antigen is a membrane lipoteichoic acid (LTA) containing a small number of α-glucosyl units, which form the antigenic determinant. Thus, it is homologous with the group D and group N antigens, which are also membrane LTAs but of different serologic specificity. Since some teichoic acid is present on the surface of the organism, this component may be responsible for the adherence of *S. sanguis* to salivary pellicle. These speculations were stimulated by the observation that LTA is believed to play an important role in the adhesion of group A streptococci to epithelial cells, presumably via the lipid end of the molecule. As shown in Figure 6–10, LTA is an amphipathic molecule,

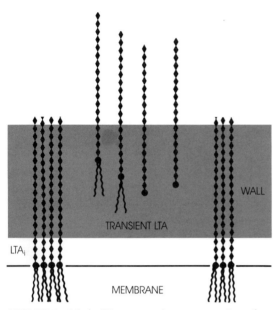

FIGURE 6–10 ✦ Diagrammatic representation of attachment and secretion of teichoic acids. The LTA_i is the lipoteichoic attached to the cell membrane via the lipid *(wavy line)* end. Some of the lipid may be lost during passage through the wall (deacylation); the deacylated teichoic acid accumulates in the wall and is also found in the spent medium. Note that the proposed orientation of the LTA in the cell wall would make it difficult for the molecule's lipid end to function in attachment. (From Wilken and Knox: Prog. Immunol. 3:135–143, 1977, with permission.)

of which one end is a hydrophobic lipid and the other end a hydrophilic lipid. Several studies suggested that salivary pellicle attachment is mediated by hydrophobic interactions, which could involve LTA. Others have suggested the hydrophilic portion of the molecule interacts with the phosphate or calcium ion in the hydroxyapatite or sulfate groups in the salivary pellicle. However, the evidence to support any of these hypotheses is not yet convincing. Indeed, the major biologic function of LTA is still unknown, possibly because no LTA-negative mutant has been isolated. However, *S. mitis* strains do not contain LTA yet appear to adhere well, particularly to buccal epithelial cells.

Type Antigens. In contrast to the group A streptococci, the antigen that separates the group H streptococci into two serotypes is a polysaccharide that is similar in some respects to the polysaccharide that forms the group-specific antigen in the β-hemolytic streptococci. These paradoxes serve to illustrate that in discussing serologic groups and types, operational definitions are used (i.e., a group contains the largest number of strains, whereas a serotype is a smaller part of the group).

There is no theoretic significance in the concept of serologic group or type; it is merely a convenient means allowing us to categorize bacteria. Group antigens may be polysaccharides, teichoic acids, or proteins. The same spectrum of molecules can be associated with type specificity. (The group A streptococci are defined by a polysaccharide and typed by protein; the pneumococci are typed by polysaccharides.) The importance of type specificity among strains of *S. sanguis* is that the type 1 strains appear to adhere better to salivary pellicles than the type 2 strains. However, it is not clear whether differences in the type-specific polysaccharides or other surface components are responsible for differences in adhesion.

Other Surface Antigens. The importance of microbial adhesion as a virulence factor was first pointed out by dental researchers who have been studying the molecular basis for the specificity of bacterial attachment to various surfaces. The oral streptococci have been important models because of the clear ecologic differences among the various species. Although these investigations are still ongoing, they have shown that the picture of a simple surface composed of only a few different antigenic polymers is inaccurate (see Fig. 6–2). Indeed, it appears that in addition to the peptidoglycan, *S. sanguis* contains one or more polysaccharides, several forms of teichoic acids, and perhaps nine or more different proteins or glycoproteins. A major goal of current investigations is to determine which components function as adhesins.

Streptococcus mitis (S. mitior, miteor, S. sanguis–Biotype II, S. oralis)

Although placed in parentheses, the other names listed have been used to describe similar organisms. Indeed, it has been proposed that only *S. oralis* is correct for some of these species. This surfeit of names for what are at the very least similar organisms illustrates one of the major problems in trying to study the relationship between structure and biologic activity among oral streptococci. The difficulty in defining this species is that they do little physiologically and are antigenically heterogeneous. Thus, there are few positive characteristics for defining them. Indeed, they are classically defined by exclusion (i.e., if an oral streptococcus is not *S. salivarius, S. sanguis,* or *S. mutans,* then it must be *S. mitis*).

PHYSIOLOGY

Table 6–4 illustrates the difficulty in identifying *S. mitis;* very few characteristics are positive and these do not differentiate this species from other oral streptococci. The distinction between *S. mitis* and *S. oralis* is that the latter species produces both an IgA protease and a neuraminidase, whereas the former is negative for these properties. These characteristics appear to be important in governing the ecological niche occupied by each of the organisms.

SEROLOGY

The difficulties in identifying *S. mitis* are not eased by serology. Antisera prepared against an individual strain often are strain specific and only react with antigens from the strain that induced them. When cross-reactions are present, they do not appear to define any large groups, but react rather haphazardly with various strains. Although *S. mitis* is often called *S. sanguis II*, not only does it lack the group H antigen, but also no LTA has been found in any of the strains tested. Thus, it appears to be the only group of streptococci and indeed perhaps the only species among the *Lactobacillaceae* that does not contain LTA. Indeed, *S. mitis* is one of the few gram-positive bacteria that do not contain LTA. It is interesting to speculate that the absence of this molecule may be related to the minimal metabolic capabilities of this species. Many strains of this species react with Lancefield groups K and O antisera, but the exact nature of these reactions is not known. Thus, for the most part *S. mitis* is still identified after all the other possibilities have been eliminated.

Streptococcus mutans

As indicated previously, there is good genetic evidence that the species previously called *S. mutans* really consists of several different species. The latter epithet has been reserved primarily for strains of serotypes c, e, and f that reside in human hosts. Other species that are physiologically very similar to *S. mutans* are found in rodents (e.g., *S. rattus, S. cricetus,* and *S. ferus*). The physiology of these organisms, particularly their carbohydrate metabolism, is so similar that it is logical to consider them as the "mutans" group. Moreover, these metabolic properties are intimately related to their ability to cause dental caries.

PHYSIOLOGY

Fermentation. In contrast to many other oral streptococci that ferment only a small variety of carbohydrates, the *S. mutans* group ferments many sugars. In particular, their ability to ferment *mannitol* and *sorbitol,* sugar alcohols derived from mannose and glucose, respectively, distinguishes them from other oral streptococci. Indeed, so consistent are these properties that attempts have been made to use them as rapid screening methods for the identification of these organisms. With the exception of some strains of *S. rattus,* the mutans

group does not hydrolyze arginine. Thus, a working definition of *S. mutans* would be α-hemolytic streptococci, which ferment mannitol and sorbitol but do not hydrolyze arginine. In addition to fermenting a wider variety of sugars, these organisms show quantitative differences in the amount of acid produced from glucose. *S. mutans* accumulates more acid and causes a larger drop in pH on solid media than do *S. sanguis* strains.

Sucrose Metabolism

DEXTRAN.   As indicated previously, many oral streptococci can synthesize carbohydrate polymers from sucrose utilizing the cleavage of the high-energy glycosidic bond in sucrose as an energy source. In the *S. mutans* group of organisms the glucosyltransferase predominates and the major carbohydrate produced is a dextran (glucan). In contrast to the linear α-1,6 dextran produced by *S. sanguis,* the polymer produced by *S. mutans* contains up to 40 percent α(1,3)-branches, as shown in Figure 6–9. This renders the polymer much less soluble and so distinctly different in properties from the usual dextran that it has been called a *mutan*. The mutan is relatively insoluble and its presence on the bacterial surface causes it to become "sticky" so that the bacteria do not separate easily. At one time, this property was believed important in bacterial adherence to tooth surfaces but now it is believed to be more important in holding plaque together (cohesion) rather than initiating attachment via the salivary pellicle. The importance of mutan production in dental caries has been established by examining mutants, which have a reduced capacity or have lost the ability to produce insoluble dextrans and are no longer as cariogenic as the parent strains. The importance of glucosyltransferase in relationship to dental caries has resulted in attempts to develop vaccines or other chemotherapeutic agents, which would interfere with its activity and thereby possibly reduce dental caries (see Chapter 27). Although the fructose released during the formation of the mutan is utilized to produce acid and potentiates the cariogenic capacity of these organisms, only a small part of the total dietary sucrose is needed to produce even relatively large amounts of the mutan associated with these organisms. Most sucrose is metabolized via another pathway.

INVERTASE.   The hydrolysis of sucrose to glucose and fructose by the enzyme invertase represents the dominant pathway of sucrose metabolism in *S. mutans* and other oral streptococci. These monosaccharides are transported into the cell via a proton motor force (PMF) or through the phosphotransferase system (PTS). The latter involves the phosphorylation of the monosaccharide before transport across the cell membrane. The phosphate donor is phosphoenolpyruvate (PEP), a product of the Embden-Meyerhof pathway (Chapter 3). The contribution of each of these transport systems is dependent upon the growth rate of the bacteria and the concentration of the sucrose in the medium. In the presence of sugar limitation, PTS is favored, whereas the PMF transport system is favored when there is excess carbohydrate. Perhaps more important, these factors also determine the amounts and types of end products produced. Thus, sugar excess also factors lactate formation, as opposed to sugar limitation in which larger quantities of acetate, formate, and ethanol are produced. These findings explain the special relationship between sucrose metabolism and dental caries.

SELECTIVITY OF SUCROSE FOR *S. MUTANS.* The special relationship between sucrose and *S. mutans* has been used to formulate media containing high concentrations of the sugar (20 percent), which inhibit other streptococci but permit *S. mutans* to grow. Further selectivity is provided by adding bacitracin to the medium (MSB), since *S. mutans* is more resistant to this antibiotic than are other oral streptococci.

SEROLOGY

Serotypes.   The differentiation of *S. mutans* into serotypes antedates the division of the group into different species. Indeed, as previously indicated, there is a close association between the serotype and the species. The serotype antigens are cell wall polysaccharides composed of rhamnose, glucose, and, in some serotypes, galactose. The serologic specificity resides in terminal sugar linkages, which are sometimes similar enough to result in cross-reactions among some types. These can often be removed by absorbing the antibody with cells of the cross-reacting species, resulting in a type-specific antiserum. However, in serotypes a and d, the polysaccharides do carry two distinct antigenic determinants. The presence of these type-specific antigens has provided a means of rapid identification of the species and their localization in human dental plaque. The exact biologic role for these polymers is not completely understood nor is it known if they play some role in virulence. Table 6–5 lists the relationship between species, serotypes, and specific antigenic determinants of the cell wall polysaccharides among the *S. mutans* group.

Protein Antigens.   In addition to the polysaccharide type-specific antigens, an important protein

TABLE 6–5 ✦ Species and Serotypes and the Mutans Streptococci

SPECIES	SEROTYPES	ANTIGENIC DETERMINANTS*
S. mutans	c	Glucose-α(1,4)-glucose
S. ferus	c	
S. mutans		Glucose-β(1,6)-glucose and Glucose-β(1,4)-glucose
S. mutans	f	Glucose-α(1,6)-glucose
S. rattus	b	Galactose
S. cricetus	a	Glucose-β(1,6)-glucose
S. sobrinus	d	Galactose-β(1,6)-glucose
S. sobrinus	g	β-galactose

*The backbones of these polysaccharides are composed predominantly of rhamnose.

antigen has been identified in *S. mutans*. This antigen—variously identified as antigen I/II, B, P1, and SPaA—is important because antibodies that react with this protein appear to be protective against dental caries. The antigen has been purified to homogeneity from culture supernatants of *S. mutans,* where it accumulates in relatively large amounts in certain strains. The exact biologic role for this protein remains unknown, although it has been shown to act as an adhesin for the initial attachment of these organisms to the salivary pedicle. Attempts are being made to prepare large quantities of this antigen by gene-cloning methods so that its role in the carious process can be assessed. The availability of this protein will also enable studies of its usefulness as a caries vaccine. Unfortunately, some investigators have found that antibodies against this protein appear to cross-react with human heart tissues. Since it has been suggested that cross-reactions between streptococcal antibodies and heart tissues could be a factor in rheumatic heart disease, it is hardly likely that such a vaccine will be permitted to be used until its cross-reactive properties can be eliminated. In this case, the skills of the microbial geneticist are called on to dissect and clone the portion of the gene that produces proteins for protective vaccines and to eliminate those portions responsible for cardiac cross-reactions.

7 *The Staphylococci*

Burton Rosan

CHAPTER OUTLINE

Physiology

Antibiotic resistance

Bacteriophage typing

Somatic antigens

Virulence factors

Pathogenesis of staphylococcal disease

Treatment

Although similar to the streptococci in shape, smears of staphylococci reveal bunches of gram-positive cocci similar to clusters of grapes. Indeed, the name derives from the Greek *staphyle,* a bunch of grapes. These bunches result from the division of this species in different planes rather than in a single plane, as streptococci divide (Table 7–1). However, the novice often confuses the two genera in Gram stains. This confusion can easily be eliminated by placing a couple of drops of 3 percent H_2O_2 on a colony (as long as it is not on blood agar). If bubbles of O_2 are detected, catalase is present and the organism must be a *Staphylococcus;* no bubbles indicates the organism is probably a *Streptococcus*. The two species of staphylococci most commonly found in humans are *S. aureus* and *S. epidermidis*. As the latter name indicates, this species is found primarily residing on the skin and is generally considered to be nonpathogenic. In contrast, *S. aureus* is a potential pathogen and may be carried asymptomatically in the nasopharynx of up to 40 percent of individuals. It is probably from this site that it finds its way to the oral cavity where it is occasionally found in low numbers (i.e., 350 organisms per milliliter saliva). Thus, it does not usually play a significant role in intraoral infections but may cause serious infections associated with accidental or surgically induced wounds, including those around the head and neck. In addition there are strains that produce an enterotoxin that causes a type of food poisoning.

PHYSIOLOGY

The staphylococci prefer aerobic conditions, although they will grow anaerobically. They produce much larger colonies than the streptococci (1 to 4 mm in diameter), and *S. aureus* may be golden yellow because of carotenoid pigments. However, pigment production is variable and cannot be used as a valid guide to speciation. The two most important characteristics distinguishing the nonpathogenic *S. epidermidis* from the pathogenic *S. aureus* are coagulase production and mannitol fermentation (Table 7–2). Coagulase is an extracellular enzyme produced by pathogenic strains of staphylococci, which activates either prothrombin or a similar substance that induces the conversion of fibrinogen to fibrin. In addition, most pathogenic strains produce DNAse. The staphylococci are among the hardiest of all non-spore-forming bacteria and are resistant to heating at 60°C for 30 minutes and may be stored at 4°C for long periods without affecting viability. They are also resistant to high concentrations of NaCl. These properties have been utilized to prepare a selective and differential medium called mannitol salt agar, which contains 7.5 percent NaCl, 1 percent mannitol, and phenol red, an acid-base indicator. The presence of *S. aureus* in a clinical sample is assumed if growth occurs and mannitol is fermented.

ANTIBIOTIC RESISTANCE

Perhaps no other species symbolizes the success—as well as the major weakness—of the "antibiotic revolution." Thus, the initial success in the treatment of staphylococcal infections with penicillin was followed very shortly by the realization that these organisms become resistant to this antibiotic. It soon became apparent that almost as rapidly as new antibiotics against *S. aureus* were

147

TABLE 7–1 ✦ Comparison of Staphylococci and Streptococci

STAPHYLOCOCCI	STREPTOCOCCI
Cocci arranged in bunches	Cocci arranged in chains
Catalase-positive	Catalase negative
Salt tolerant	Sensitive to high salt*
Facultative aerobe	Facultative anaerobe
Localized-type infection	Spreading-type infection
Coagulase-positive	Coagulase-negative (usually)
Antibiotic resistance	Most are sensitive to penicillin†

*Except *Enterococcus faecalis,* which is tolerant of salt at concentrations up to 6.5%.
†Except *E. faecalis,* which tends to be resistant to high concentrations of penicillin and other antibiotics.

TABLE 7–2 ✦ Comparison of the Human Staphylococci

S. AUREUS	S. EPIDERMIDIS
Coagulase-positive	Coagulase-negative
Ferments mannitol	Does not ferment mannitol
DNAse-positive	DNAse-negative
Found in upper nasal pharynx	Found on skin
Pathogenic	Nonpathogenic

developed, resistant organisms appeared. It is now known that penicillin resistance often is associated with an enzyme, penicillinase, which is coded for by a gene on a plasmid. These plasmids may carry several antibiotic resistant genes and thus have been called resistance transfer factors (RTFs). In staphylococci, these factors may be transferred rapidly among strains by a bacteriophage vector through the process of transduction (see Chapter 3). Thus, development of resistance to penicillin has helped our understanding of microbial genetics, which may aid in controlling bacterial infections, cancer, and other diseases in which genetic changes or anomalies occur.

BACTERIOPHAGE TYPING

The patterns of lytic specificity between the phage and host have been used as a means of typing the staphylococci. It is generally not necessary to phage type an infection due to *S. aureus,* but every so often there is an outbreak of staphylococcal infection following surgery or in a hospital nursery. These outbreaks can have tragic consequences, and it is essential to determine if the same phage type is causing all the infections. Once this is determined, the carrier is sought by matching the phage types carried by patients or hospital personnel with the types isolated from the infections. (It usually is the hospital personnel who become carriers.) In this way, the carrier can be identified and appropriate isolation procedures taken.

SOMATIC ANTIGENS
Capsules

Polysaccharide capsules that appear to be antiphagocytic have been identified. This slime layer may be associated with the ability of some pathogenic strains to adhere to catheters and other materials and thus to provide a nidus for infection.

Teichoic Acids
RIBITOL TEICHOIC ACID

Staphylococci have ribitol teichoic acid in their cell walls. The antigenic determinant of these teichoic acids is usually a hexosamine residue. Such hexosamine residues are widely distributed among other bacteria and in eukaryotic cells and thus may be responsible for the large number of serologic cross-reactions often observed with staphylococcal antisera.

GLYCEROL TEICHOIC ACID

The glycerol teichoic acids have the same structure and cytoplasmic membrane association as those found in streptococci. The antigenic determinant is often the same hexosamine that determines the specificity of the cell wall ribitol teichoic acid and this results in some confusion between the two. In strains of *S. epidermidis,* the antigenic determinant of the teichoic acid is glucose.

Protein A

The surface of many staphylococcal strains contains a protein that binds to the Fc region of most IgG subclasses of mammalian species. In humans, all IgG subclasses except IgG3 bind, while most IgM and IgA subclasses are not bound. In addition to these immunochemical interactions, protein A–Fc interactions associated with cell surface can lead to a variety of biologic effects. These include both systemic and local anaphylactic reactions; the latter

show the typical wheal and erythema reaction associated with histamine release. Arthus reactions
associated with complement activation by both the
classic and alternate pathways are also produced
by protein A–Fc interactions. Opsonic antibody
may be blocked because of competition of protein
A for the Fc receptors on phagocytes. It has also
been observed that protein A activates B lymphocytes but not T lymphocytes.

Clumping Factor

If plasma is mixed with staphylococci on a slide,
the organisms will agglutinate. This is due to a
component in the cell wall of coagulase-positive
strains, which causes clumping of the bacteria.
This can be used as a rapid screening test for coagulase-positive strains. However, other organisms,
such as *Streptococcus faecalis,* can also clump in
the presence of plasma and therefore the test must
be interpreted with caution.

VIRULENCE FACTORS
Coagulase

As indicated previously, this enzyme is found
in most pathogenic strains of *S. aureus* and causes
plasma to clot.

Other Enzymes

These organisms produce hyaluronidase and a
fibrinolysin called staphylokinase, which, like its
streptococcal counterpart, causes dissolution of fibrin clots. It also produces DNAses and RNAses.

Hemolysins

The staphylococci produce at least four distinct
hemolysins, which unfortunately have been labeled
with Greek letters and are often confused with the
types of hemolysins found in the streptococci. All
the hemolysins in the staphylococci cause complete
lysis of erythrocytes. The major differences among
them involve the kind of erythrocytes they lyse and
the conditions under which lysis occurs. These
hemolysins cause lysis of various human and animal cells and, thus, have been called "cytolytic toxins."

α-HEMOLYSIN

This is the major hemolysin produced by this
organism. It does not lyse human red blood cells
but will lyse rabbit erythrocytes; it does damage
human platelets and macrophages. The gene for α
toxin is believed to be carried on a transposon and
expressed as a water soluble protein.

β-HEMOLYSIN

This is the so-called hot-cold hemolysin and is
more commonly found in *S. aureus* strains isolated
from animals. It is best observed by placing sheep
blood agar plates at 4°C after growth has occurred.
After overnight incubation in the cold, the plates
are transferred to 37°C for several hours. Zones of
hemolysis will often be seen surrounding the
golden colonies of staphylococci. This hemolysin
functions as a sphingomyelinase.

OTHER HEMOLYSINS

Two other hemolysins, the δ and γ, have been
described. In addition, a leukocidin is found in
most *S. aureus* strains.

Epidermolytic Toxin

This toxin causes a number of skin lesions. Its
activity is associated with cleavage of desmo-
somes, which connect cells in the lower layers of
the epidermis.

Enterotoxins

These are relatively heat-stable and trypsin-re-
sistant toxins produced by 50 percent of *S. aureus*
strains. They are one of the major causes of food
poisonings associated with the "church picnic" type
of syndrome in which pre-prepared foods, such as
salads, whipped creams, and so forth, become contaminated with staphylococci that grow and produce toxins if the foods are not kept cold. Within
4 to 6 hours following ingestion of these preformed
toxins, the patient exhibits symptoms of diarrhea
and nausea, which may last up to 24 hours.

Toxic Shock Syndrome
Toxin 1 (TSST-1)

Toxic shock syndrome was first reported in 1978
in menstruating women using a particular kind of
extra-absorbent tampon. The etiology was determined to be *S. aureus* strains producing a toxin
eventually named toxic shock syndrome toxin 1
(TSST-1). In many respects, the toxin resembled
one of the types of enterotoxin produced by this
species and indeed had originally been named
staphylococcal enterotoxin F. Although the exact
pathogenesis of the disease is still not clear, it appears that the tampons allowed a more aerobic environment than the less absorbent older variety
tampons. This favored the overgrowth of the staphylococci. If TSST-1 is produced, it gives rise to a
toxemia that may enhance the activity of endotoxin
several thousand times. Since small amounts of
endotoxin are nearly always available from the

large number of indigenous gram-negative organisms, it is possible that this enhancement may lead to the profound shock and death associated with endotoxin.

PATHOGENESIS OF STAPHYLOCOCCAL DISEASE

Although much remains to be known about diseases associated with the staphylococcal toxins, many common staphylococcal diseases appear to be associated with the multiplication and spread of the organism at local sites. Occasionally, if the local infection is particularly severe or if the patient is in poor health, the organism may invade other tissues or enter the bloodstream, leading to a septicemia. The most common local infection is the boil or furuncle, which is associated with the blockage of a sebaceous gland and the overgrowth of the staphylococci in this location. In this small lesion many of the characteristics of the more serious staphylococcal lesions are observed. First and most characteristic of staphylococcal infection is the suppuration which often localizes to form an abscess. The pus consists of necrotic cells that have released their cytoplasmic proteins and of nucleic acids, which cause a viscous consistency and give the exudate its yellowish green color. The wall of fibrin that surrounds the abscess may be due to the release of coagulase from the bacteria. It is noteworthy that in streptococcal infections, in which spreading factors are dominant extracellular products, the infections spread rather than remaining localized. In general, these small boils heal without consequence, but occasionally several boils may coalesce to form a carbuncle, which can be more serious. Sometimes the bacteria spread to bone where they may set up an osteomyelitis (a "furuncle of the osseous medulla"). However, osteomyelitis usually occurs following traumatic wounds—for example, fractures, particularly those of the compound type in which bone is exposed. Staphylococcal wound infections have signs and symptoms similar to those of the local abscess, except that the initiating factor may be a traumatic or a surgically created wound.

The exact role of the various virulence factors (i.e., hemolysins, enzymes, coagulase, and toxins) in these infections is not clear, so that it has not been possible to develop a specific vaccine against this disease. Indeed, it appears that most of us have relatively high antibody titers against many of the components found in staphylococci, yet few of us appear immune to the various diseases caused by this organism. Herein lies the danger and the challenge, since it is most discouraging to observe patients developing a staphylococcal infection following what appears to be successful surgery.

TREATMENT

As indicated previously, laboratory diagnosis is relatively easy, since the presence of gram-positive, catalase-positive cocci, in bunches, that ferment mannitol and produce coagulase, establishes the diagnosis of an *S. aureus* wound infection. It is obviously essential to establish antibiotic susceptibility of the strain, as this may be the key aspect of successful therapy. Antibiotic resistant strains are ubiquitous, particularly in hospitals because of widespread use of antibiotics. In general until the exact antibiotic sensitivities are established, the synthetic penicillins (i.e., methicillin or oxacillin), which are not hydrolyzed by penicillinase, may be used. Alternatively, many clinicians start with a cephalosporin type of antibiotic. Whatever the final choice, therapy must be intensive. Drainage should be established as soon as the suppuration is evident, since these lesions do not respond to antibiotic therapy alone.

8 Genus Actinomyces and Other Filamentous Bacteria

Richard P. Ellen

CHAPTER OUTLINE

Taxonomy

Pathogenicity

Ecology of Actinomyces viscosus *and* A. naeslundii

Members of the genus *Actinomyces* and other gram-positive filamentous bacteria in the family Actinomycetaceae are common within the indigenous microbiota colonizing the mouths of humans and various other animals. They are commensals that usually coexist peacefully with their hosts, but, under some conditions, they emerge as opportunistic pathogens involved in infections of both soft tissues and teeth. Of the oral Actinomycetaceae, the genus *Actinomyces* has been studied the most thoroughly in terms of taxonomy, pathogenicity, natural ecology, and interbacterial relationships within the oral microbial community.

TAXONOMY

The oral gram-positive filamentous bacteria have an entangled history in all three interrelated areas of taxonomy: classification, nomenclature, and identification. The inclusion in the family *Actinomycetaceae* of major genera and species has changed considerably over the years, depending on the criteria used for clustering or separating clinical isolates. Attempts will be made in this chapter to present a simplified taxonomy. Emphasis will be placed on the genus *Actinomyces* when examples and illustrations are presented.

Classification and Nomenclature

Members of the family Actinomycetaceae have many features in common. They are all gram-positive, nonmotile, nonacid-fast, nonspore-forming bacilli with a tendency to grow as branched filaments in tissues and under some laboratory conditions. They often demonstrate polymorphism; one gram-stained smear may contain cells of different shapes—filaments mixed with diphtheroids,

short rods, or even coccobacilli. Actinomycetaceae genera all ferment carbohydrates. A rather obvious common trait is that all members of Actinomycetaceae are true bacteria with the following characteristics distinguishing them from fungi:

1. They are prokaryotic.
2. They have typical bacterial cell wall composition, lacking chitin.
3. Although they may branch, branching cells have a similar diameter; they do not produce aerial hyphae.
4. They are sensitive to antibiotics that are active against bacteria.

Why, then, the name "Actinomyces," which means "ray fungus"? The name was chosen more than 100 years ago as a metaphor describing the histopathologic appearance of debris from soft tissue lesions caused by these infectious agents. Regulations governing microbial nomenclature honor precedent; thus, the name "Actinomyces" remains, even though it is literally inaccurate.

The current classification scheme reflects a composite that evolved mostly from a dizzying array of microbiologic tests of physiologic traits, serology, and acid end-product analysis. Recently, analysis of cell wall chemistry, total protein profiles, DNA homology, and the use of computer-assisted numerical taxonomy to cluster the findings for isolates into a manageable expression of degree of similarity has greatly influenced classification. Currently, Actinomycetaceae is composed of the five genera listed in Table 8–1: *Actinomyces, Arachnia, Bifidobacterium, Bacterionema,* and *Rothia.* Only two of these genera, *Actinomyces* and *Bifidobacterium,* currently contain more than one species (Table 8–2).

Including recently proposed additions, genus *Actinomyces* contains 11 species (see Table 8–1).

151

TABLE 8–1 ✦ Classification and Identification of Genera in Actinomycetaceae

GENUS	SPECIES	GROWTH ENVIRONMENT	ACID END PRODUCTS
*Actinomyces**	*bovis* *israelii* *meyeri* *gerencseriae*	Anaerobic	Acetic Lactic Succinic
	naeslundii *viscosus* *odontolyticus* *pyogenes* *hordeovulneris* *howellii* *georgiae*	Facultatively anaerobic	
Arachnia†	*propionica*	Anaerobic	Acetic Propionic Succinic
Bifidobacterium†	>25 species	Anaerobic	Acetic Lactic
Bacterionema†	*matruchotii*	Facultatively anaerobic	Acetic Propionic Lactic Formic
Rothia	*dentocariosa*	Aerobic	Acetic Lactic Succinic

* Actinomyces species listed include species described in J. G. Holt (ed.): Bergey's Manual of Systematic Bacteriology, 1984–89, and new species subsequently proposed in the International Journal of Systematic Bacteriology.

†These genera are classified in Actinomycetaceae because they demonstrate branching during laboratory cultivation. Proposals have been raised to move them to other families:

Arachnia → Propionibacteriaceae
Bifidobacterium → Lactobacillaceae
Bacterionema → Corynebacteriaceae or Mycobacteriaceae

They are either strict anaerobic or facultative anaerobes that often grow better on primary isolation under anaerobic conditions. *Actinomyces naeslundii* and human isolates of *A. viscosus* are so similar by standard tests (except for catalase activity, for which *A. viscosus* is positive) and by virtue of their similar cell wall structure and serologic cross-reactivity that a merger into one species or into two "genospecies" of *A. naeslundii* has been suggested. The most recent classification proposal recognizes immunofluorescence serotype 1 of *A. naeslundii* as distinct genospecies 1, and groups serotypes II and III of *A. naeslundii* with serotype II of *A. viscosus* as genospecies 2 of *A. naeslundii* (Fig. 8–1). It is interesting to note that by the criteria of serology, DNA homology, and numerical taxonomy, *A. viscosus* strains isolated from the mouths of rodents bear little relation to isolates from humans. However, rodent isolates have priority for the designation *A. viscosus* ("viscosus" because they grow as a cohesive slime) by being the first to be described under this name. They had originally been described in a new but now defunct genus *Odontomyces* ("odonto" meaning tooth; "myces" from "Actinomyces").

Identification

Appropriate classification finds its clinical significance in identification of new isolates and determination of their association with health status. Optimally, identification is the use of a minimum number of rapid tests, which allows assignment to a given species in the classification scheme. A combination of acid end-product analysis, serology, and a few biochemical tests is usually sufficient to identify these bacteria to genus level. However, at species level, fresh isolates of oral gram-positive rods frequently challenge the concept of easy identification because their response in microbiologic tests is so wide-ranging, and the classification defining species relies on a combination of "chemotaxonomic" methods. Gas chromatography of acid end products of glucose metabolism is often essential

TABLE 8–2 ✦ Filament Facts

Actinomyces bovis—Not isolated from human mouth
    —Associated with "lumpy jaw" (actinomycosis) in cattle

    A. israelii—Isolated from human plaque, calculus, tonsillar crypts
    —Associated with most cases of human actinomycosis
    —Increased proportions in plaque under nonhygienic conditions
    —Serotype II recently reclassified as *A. gereacseriae*

    A. odontolyticus—Despite name, role in caries etiology has not been established
    —Requires serum for growth; forms reddish colonies on blood agar
    —Found in dental plaque, but no specific relationship to disease established

    A. naeslundii—Preferentially colonizes tongue and other mucosal surfaces
    —Can colonize oral cavity prior to tooth eruption
    —Induces periodontal disease and root caries in animals
    —Adheres to mucosal cells and oral streptococci via type 2 fibril-borne lectin specific for β-galactosides and galactosamine
    —Associated with some cases of actinomycosis

    A. viscosus—Catalase-positive member of genus *Actinomyces;* human isolates in *A. naeslundii* genospecies 2
    —Preferentially colonizes teeth
    —Does not often colonize predentate infants
    —Induces periodontal lesions and root caries in animals
    —Numerical association with human gingivitis but not with advanced or progressive periodontitis
    —Stimulates gingival inflammatory response via several pathways
    —Prevalent in established human root caries, but also on noncarious surfaces
    —Adheres to pellicle via type 1 fibrils and to epithelial cells and oral streptococci by type 2 fibril-associated lectin

    A. meyeri—Previously classified in genus *Actinobacterium*
    —Isolated from plaque, but association with disease not established

Arachnia propionica—Produces propionic acid; cell wall has diaminopimelic acid
    —Some taxonomists have proposed moving *Arachnia* to family *Propionibacteriaceae*
    —Associated with some cases of human actinomycosis and periapical endodontic lesions

    Bifidobacterium sp.—Isolated from dental plaque and from deep dentinal carious lesions
    —Not known to be associated with etiology of any oral diseases
    —"Bifid" morphology helps to differentiate from anaerobic lactobacilli

Bacterionema matruchotii—Isolated from dental plaque
    —Not known to be associated with etiology of dental diseases
    —Long filaments with short, thick terminal bacillus yields characteristic "whip handle" morphology
    —Composes central filament of "corn-cob" formations (*S. sanguis* cells bound to *B. matruchotii*) at salivary interface of supragingival plaque
    —Has been used to study bacterial calcification and calculus formation

    Rothia dentocariosa—Despite name, role in carries etiology doubtful
    —Commonly isolated from dental plaque and root caries; associated with endocarditis
    —Aerobic
    —Highly pleomorphic; often cocci mixed with filaments
    —Has been shown to induce gingival inflammation in laboratory rodents

(see Table 8–1). For example, it is difficult to differentiate *Actinomyces israelii* from *Arachnia propionica* by typical bench microbiology tests, although they are classified in separate genera. They are best differentiated by acid end-product analysis. Both produce acetic and succinic acids, but *A. propionica* also produces propionic acid (hence its name), while *A. israelii*, like all *Actinomyces* species, produces lactic acid. Chemical analysis of cell wall sugars is also useful; diaminopimelic acid is

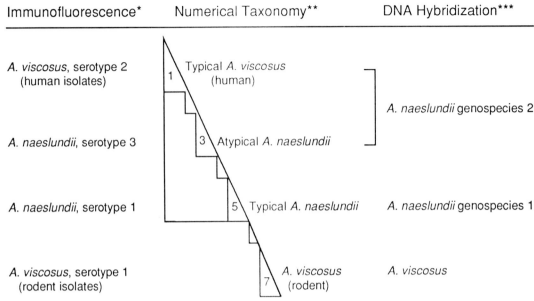

| Immunofluorescence* | Numerical Taxonomy** | DNA Hybridization*** |

A. viscosus, serotype 2 (human isolates) — 1 Typical *A. viscosus* (human) — *A. naeslundii* genospecies 2

A. naeslundii, serotype 3 — 3 Atypical *A. naeslundii*

A. naeslundii, serotype 1 — 5 Typical *A. naeslundii* — *A. naeslundii* genospecies 1

A. viscosus, serotype 1 (rodent isolates) — 7 *A. viscosus* (rodent) — *A. viscosus*

FIGURE 8–1 ✦ Comparison of three *Actinomyces viscosus* and *Actinomyces naeslundii* classification schemes based on serology,* numerical taxonomy,** and DNA hybridization.***

*Adapted from Slack, J. M. and Gerencser, M. A.: *Actinomyces,* Filamentous Bacteria. Biology and Pathogenicity. Burgess Publishing, Minneapolis, 1975.

**Adapted from Fillery, E. D., et al.: A comparison of strains of bacteria designated *Actinomyces viscosus* and *Actinomyces naeslundii*. Caries Res. 12:299, 1978, with permission of S. Karger AG, Basel.

***Adapted from Johnson, J. L., et al.: *Actinomyces georgiae* sp. nov., *Actinomyces gerencseriae* sp. nov., designation of two genospecies of *Actinomyces naeslundii,* and inclusion of *A. naeslundii* serotypes II and III and *Actinomyces viscosus* serotype II in *A. naeslundii* genospecies 2. Int. J. Syst. Bacteriol. 40:273, 1990.

found in *A. propionica* but not in *A. israelii* walls. Members of Actinomycetaceae must also be differentiated from other gram-positive bacilli, which are not members of this family, including some genera that are morphologically and metabolically rather similar *(Propionibacterium, Corynebacterium, Eubacterium).*

One of the fastest and surest identification methods for this group is the use of serology, especially by fluorescence microscopy. Immunofluorescence

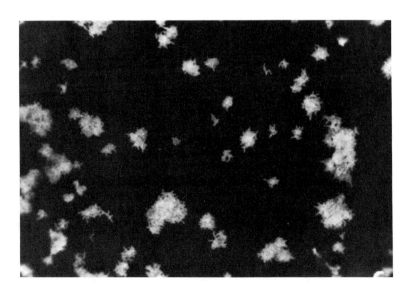

FIGURE 8–2 ✦ Example of typical *Actinomyces* morphology in a positive immunofluorescence test.

reagents can discriminate among genera and among serotypes within the genus *Actinomyces*. Figure 8–2 is an example of a positive test result, which also demonstrates typical *Actinomyces* cell morphology. The identification scheme of Slack and Gerencser, which uses specific antisera prepared by absorbing out problematic cross-reacting antibodies, has received wide acceptance. Antibody-mediated bacterial agglutination tests are also accurate for intergeneric identification and identification of major *A. viscosus* and *A. naeslundii* subgroups based on more laborious numerical taxonomy and DNA homology. It is interesting to note the degree of agreement among different approaches for grouping *A. viscosus* and *A. naeslundii* (Fig. 8–1).

PATHOGENICITY
Actinomycosis

Of the *Actinomyces* species described, all but *A. bovis, A. howellii,* and *A. hordeovulneris* are prevalent in the human oral cavity. They are often isolated in significant levels from dental plaque and calculus, as well as from the tongue, tonsils, and other soft tissues. Opportunistic infections may arise following traumatic injury and the introduction of contaminated debris into the tissues. Actinomycosis is a chronic, granulomatous, soft tissue infection with foci of abscesses and suppuration through draining sinuses. It is most common in the cervicofacial region (Fig. 8–3), draining intraorally or through the skin of the face or neck. Actinomycosis can also affect the lower respiratory tract via aspiration or inhalation of contaminated material from the mouth and may occasionally affect the abdomen following surgical or accidental trauma. Several reports have linked actinomycetes

to persistent urogenital and pelvic infections in women using intrauterine birth control devices. Actinomycosis is not a common disease, but it can be fatal.

In addition to the clinical appearance and case history, examination of draining pus from so-called sulfur granules helps to establish a tentative diagnosis of actinomycosis. The gross appearance of these granules, as seen under low-power magnification, is an irregularly shaped, yellowish mass of radiating filaments. Under high-power magnification, filaments and club-shaped extensions are clearly evident (Fig. 8–4). Infected tissues should be biopsied, sectioned, and stained for histopathologic assessment. Such preparations usually contain the granules, digested cellular debris, and mixed populations of polymorphonuclear leukocytes and lymphocytes, surrounded by fibrous connective tissue. Diagnosis of actinomycosis should be confirmed by cultivation or by immunofluorescence. For the sake of clarity, "sulfur granules," despite their yellow color, are likely devoid of significant sulfur.

Actinomycosis lesions often contain a mixed microbiota. By far, the most common species is *A. israelii,* but some lesions yield *A. naeslundii, A. viscosus,* or *Arachnia propionica. Actinomyces bovis* causes similar infections in cattle. Along with anaerobic streptococci, gram-negative bacteria have been isolated from mixed actinomycotic lesions; the most common are pigmented gram-negative anaerobic rods and *Actinobacillus actinomycetemcomitans*—this significant periodontal pathogen was named for its actinomycosis association! The relative contribution of the individual species to pathogenicity of mixed actinomycosis infections has not been clearly established, but their common colonization of teeth and periodontal

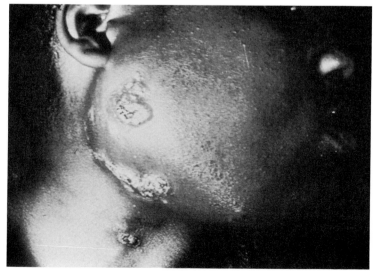

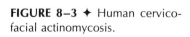

FIGURE 8–3 ✦ Human cervicofacial actinomycosis.

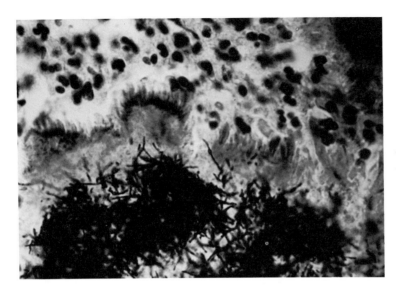

FIGURE 8-4 ✦ Microscopic appearance of a sulfur granule obtained from a human actinomycotic lesion.

pockets suggests an intraoral reservoir for infecting other tissues. It should not be surprising that trauma to the teeth or jaws and bite wounds are often the opportunistic events predisposing to actinomycosis. Treatment of actinomycosis is often difficult and protracted because the mixed flora massed in the center of the "sulfur granules" is relatively protected from host defenses. Surgical excision and drainage is usually required, as well as extended antibiotic therapy, usually with drugs in the penicillin family.

Periodontal Diseases

As a group, the gram-positive filamentous rods increase in proportion relative to other bacteria in the microbiota soon after cessation of oral hygiene practices. Thus, they have the opportunity, along with other bacteria in early plaque, to stimulate inflammatory responses in the gingiva. Yet, because their subgingival proportions decrease relative to the great increase in gram-negative species in advanced, destructive periodontal lesions in the adjacent tissues, they are not considered highly pathogenic in progressive periodontitis in humans.

A. viscosus is the only member of this group to be studied in depth for its periodontal pathogenic potential, probably because it was originally isolated from, and shown to be responsible for, naturally occurring transmissible periodontitis in laboratory rodents (Fig. 8-5). However, very few potential virulence traits that might account for direct tissue damage have been documented for this species. It produces few potent proteolytic or other hydrolytic enzymes; its acid end products are not significantly more toxic than those of other bac-

FIGURE 8-5 ✦ Periodontitis and roof surface caries induced experimentally by *A. viscosus* infection.

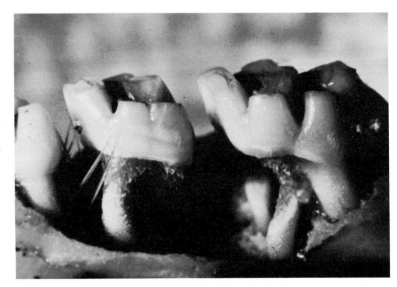

teria; and it does not produce volatile sulfur-containing compounds. In contrast, the evidence is very strong that *A. viscosus* can stimulate an inflammatory response, leading to tissue damage indirectly (Table 8–3). The fact that humans demonstrate elevated levels of *A. viscosus* and simultaneously elevated hypersensitivity reactions specific for *A. viscosus* antigens during the onset of experimental gingivitis probably means that it is involved in the etiology of gingivitis and, possibly, of mild cases of periodontitis.

Gram-positive bacteria, like *A. viscosus,* may also be involved in the sequence of events leading to more rapidly destructive periodontitis by creating an environment suitable for outgrowth of more virulent gram-negative species. It is well known that the environment in dental plaque becomes more anaerobic with time because of utilization of oxygen by bacteria. *A. viscosus* is also known to promote adhesion of the periodontal pathogen *Porphyromonas gingivalis* to dental plaque and to produce succinate, a growth-stimulating factor for *P. gingivalis*. Moreover, the increased bleeding and pocket depth occurring via the inflammatory response also encourages the emergence of fastidious, gram-negative anaerobes.

Dental Root Surface Caries

Filamentous bacteria are very numerous in supragingival root surface plaques and plaques overlying established carious lesions on roots. While these bacteria have little coronal cariogenic activity in experimental animals, *A. viscosus* and *A. naes-*

TABLE 8–3 ✦ Mechanisms by Which *Actinomyces viscosus* Affects Periodontal Health

Elaborates factors chemotactic for polymorpho-
   nuclear leukocytes
Causes release of hydrolytic enzymes from leuko-
   cytes and macrophages
Alters fibroblast function
Mitogenically stimulates lymphocytes (polyclonal
   activator)
Antigenically stimulates host hypersensitivity
Stimulates osteoclastic bone resorption

lundii strains isolated from human root decay have been shown repeatedly to induce root surface caries in laboratory rodents (see Fig. 8–6). *A. viscosus* ferments sugars, yielding acid end products, and isolates from root lesions store intracellular polysaccharides, which may contribute to prolonged acid release. However, *A. viscosus* is not as rapidly acidogenic as *Streptococcus mutans*, a known cariogenic species, when grown on a variety of dietary carbohydrates. Although *A. viscosus* might contribute to root caries activity, its similar isolation frequency and proportion of the microbiota in samples from carious and caries-free root surfaces renders it a poor choice as a microbiologic marker for assessing patients' root caries risk. There is some evidence that *A. viscosus* isolates from carious root lesions have a greater capacity for intracellular polysaccharide storage, acidogenicity, and aciduricity than isolates from caries-free roots, sug-

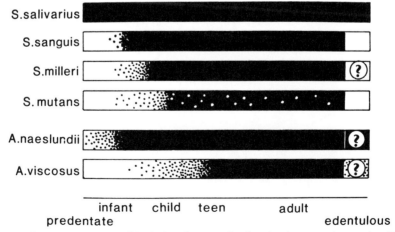

FIGURE 8–6 ✦ Comparative oral isolation frequencies for *A. viscosus, A. naeslundii,* and oral streptococci during the human lifespan. Solid black bars represent virtually 100 percent carrier state in the population. (From Ellen, R. P.: Oral colonization by gram-positive bacteria significant to periodontal disease. In Genco R. J., and Mergenhagen, S. E. (eds): Host-Parasite Interactions in Periodontal Diseases. ASM Publications, Washington, D.C. 1982, pp. 98–111, with permission.)

gesting that the root caries environment selects for biotypes with increased cariogenic potential.

ECOLOGY OF *ACTINOMYCES VISCOSUS* AND *A. NAESLUNDII*
Establishment and Distribution

In contrast to the paucity of information on the oral ecology of *A. israelii* and *A. odontolyticus,* much is known about *A. viscosus* and *A. naeslundii.* Figure 8–6 illustrates the host age at which these species establish in the human mouth, relative to some of the oral streptococci. Although almost identical in their physiologic traits and nutrient requirements, *A. viscosus* and *A. naeslundii* differ in the host age at which they appear in the mouth and in the surfaces that they preferentially colonize. *A. naeslundii* colonizes the tongue more readily and usually accounts for a greater proportion of the salivary microbiota than *A. viscosus.* Therefore, conditions favor its intraoral establishment prior to tooth eruption. In contrast, *A. viscosus* colonizes teeth more efficiently than mucosal surfaces. Thus, establishment is often delayed until after teeth erupt and even longer, depending on the effective dose transmitted by saliva of individuals with whom the child has contact. These colonization differences are relative in that, in adults, *A. naeslundii* does colonize teeth and *A. viscosus* colonizes mucosal surfaces, but not to the same extent. Differences in their colonization patterns probably reflect their relative abilities to attach to different receptors on the various surfaces of the mouth.

Surface Properties and Adherence

Both *A. viscosus* and *A. naeslundii* elaborate long surface protein appendages termed *fibrils,* or *fimbriae* (Fig. 8–7). They carry some of the antigens that differentiate the two species. The fibrils

help foster the attachment of *A. viscosus* and *A. naeslundii* to host surfaces and to other bacteria in dental plaque. Although morphologically similar, two types of distinct populations of fibrils have been described immunochemically and functionally. Type 1 is involved in adherence to salivary pellicle coating the teeth, specifically to proline-rich proteins and statherin. Type 2 functions in *Actinomyces* interactions with host epithelial and red blood cell membranes as well as with other bacteria such as various streptococci. Type 2 fibrils carry an adhesin that binds specifically to oligosaccharides terminating in beta-linked galactosides or *N*-acetyl-galactosamine. Target galactosides in membrane glycoproteins or glycolipids are often in a position penultimate to sialic acids; *A. viscosus* and *A. naeslundii* can actually promote their own adherence by cleaving the sialic acid, thereby exposing the galactosides. Relative abilities to bind to oral surfaces may reflect differences in the distribution of type 1 and type 2 fibrils on *A. viscosus* and *A. naeslundii* cell surfaces. Typical *A. naeslundii* strains are devoid of type 1 fibrils, rendering them inefficient in binding to salivary pellicle. The fibril composition on atypical *A. naeslundii* (serotype 3, see Fig. 8–1) is more closely related to *A. viscosus,* and both of these adhere efficiently to salivary pellicle. Genes encoding subunits for both types of fimbriae have been cloned. Their sequences display considerable homology, and regions of the type 1 subunit are highly conserved among *A. viscosus* and *A. naeslundii* strains from a wide range of hosts.

BIBLIOGRAPHY

Bowden, G. H., and Hardie, J. M.: Commensal and pathogenic *Actinomyces* species in man. In Sykes, G., and Skinner, F. A. (eds): *Actinomycetales:* Characteristics and Practical Importance. Academic Press, New York, 1973.

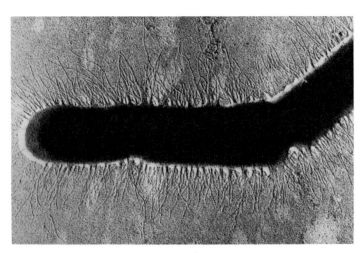

FIGURE 8–7 ✦ Electron photomicrograph of shadow cast *A. viscosus* cell. The long fibrils are clearly evident. (From Masuda, N., Ellen, R. P., and Grove, D. A.: J. Bacteriol. 147:1095, 1981.)

Cisar, J. O., Vatter, A. E., Clark, W. B., Hurst-Calderone, S., and Sandberg, A. L.: Mutants of *Actinomyces viscosus* T14 lacking type 1, type 2, or both types of fimbriae. Infect. Immunol. 56:2984, 1988.

Coykendall, A. L., and Munzenmaier, A. J.: Deoxyribonucleic acid hybridization among strains of *Actinomyces viscosus* and *Actinomyces naeslundii*. Int. J. Syst. Bacteriol. 29:234, 1979.

Ellen, R. P.: Oral colonization by Gram-positive bacteria significant to periodontal disease. In Genco, R. J., and Mergenhagen, S. E. (eds): Host-Parasite Interactions in Periodontal Diseases. American Society of Microbiologists, Washington, DC, 1982.

Fillery, E. D., Bowden, G. H., and Hardie, J. M.: A comparison of strains of bacteria designated *Actinomyces viscosus* and *Actinomyces naeslundii*. Caries Res. 12:299, 1978.

Gibbons, R. J., Hay, D. I., Cisar, J. O., and Clark, W. B.: Absorbed salivary proline-rich protein 1 and statherin: Receptors for type 1 fimbriae of *Actinomyces viscosus* T14V-J1 on apatitic surfaces. Infect. Immunol. 56:2990, 1988.

Goodfellow, M., Mordarski, M., and Williams, S. T.: The Biology of the Actinomycetes. Academic Press, London, 1984.

Holmberg, K., and Nord, C. -E.: Numerical taxonomy and laboratory identification of *Actinomyces* and *Arachnia* and some related bacteria. J. Gen. Microbiol. 91:17, 1975.

Howell, A., Jordan, H. V., George, L. K., and Pine, L.: *Odontomyces viscosus,* gen. nov., spec. nov.: A filamentous microorganism isolated from periodontal plaque in hamsters. Sabouraudia 4:65, 1965.

Johnson, J. L., Moore, L. V. H., Kaneko, B., and Moore, W. E. C.: *Actinomyces georgiae* sp. nov., *Actinomyces gerencsceriae* sp. nov., designation of two genospecies of *Actinomyces naeslundii* and inclusion of *A. naeslundii* serotypes II and III and *Actinomyces viscosus* serotype II in *A. naeslundii* genospecies 2. Int. J. Syst. Bacteriol. 40:273, 1990.

Jordan, H. V., and Keyes, P H.: Studies on the bacteriology of hamster periodontal diseases. Am. J. Pathol. 46:843, 1965.

Kolenbrander, P. E.: Intergeneric coaggregation among human oral bacteria and ecology of dental plaque. Ann. Rev. Microbiol. 42:627, 1988.

Pine, L., and George, L. K.: Classification and phylogenetic relationship of microaerophilic actinomycetes. Int. J. Syst. Bacteriol. 20:445, 1970.

Răsić, J. L., and Kurman, J. A.: Bifidobacteria and Their Role. Experientia Supplementum, Vol. 39, Birkhäuser Verlag, Basel, 1983.

Schofield, G. M., and Schaal, K. P.: A numerical taxonomy study of members of the *Actinomycetaceae* and related taxa. J. Gen. Microbiol. 127:237, 1981.

Slack, J. M., and Gerencser, M. A.: *Actinomyces,* Filamentous Bacteria. Biology and Pathogenicity. Burgess Publishing, Minneapolis, 1975.

Stackebrandt, E., and Charfreitag, O.: Partial 165r RNA primary structure of five *Actinomyces* species: Phylogenetic implications and development of an *Actinomyces israelii*–specific oligonucleotide probe. J. Gen. Microbiol. 136:37, 1990.

Yeung, M. K.: Conservation of an *Actinomyces viscosus* T14V type 1 fimbrial subunit homolog among divergent groups of *Actinomyces* sp. Infect. Immunol. 60:1047, 1992.

Yeung, M. K., and Cisar, J. O.: Sequence homology between the subunits of two immunologically and functionally distinct types of fimbriae of *Actinomyces* sp. J. Bacteriol. 172:2462, 1990.

Haemophilus *and* Pasteurella

M. Jane Gillespie

CHAPTER OUTLINE

The HAP-group of bacteria
The genus Haemophilus
The genus Pasteurella
The Rtx family of toxins
Taxonomy of the HAP-bacteria

THE HAP-GROUP OF BACTERIA

The bacterial genera *Haemophilus, Pasteurella,* and *Actinobacillus* are members of the family Pasteurellaceae. They are obligate parasites for humans and other vertebrates. Because they are causative agents of a number of devastating diseases in both humans and livestock, the Pasteurellaceae are a source of worldwide socioeconomic problems. Veterinary scientists studying these diseases have designated the three genera of the Pasteurellaceae the "HAP" bacteria. The most important human pathogen among the HAP bacteria is *Haemophilus influenzae;* other human pathogens include the etiologic agent of localized juvenile periodontitis, *Actinobacillus actinomycetemcomitans* (see Chapter 17).

THE GENUS *HAEMOPHILUS*

Sixteen species of *Haemophilus* are listed in *Bergey's Manual of Systematic Bacteriology*. The genus exhibits a pronounced host specificity with 10 species parasitic in humans. The haemophili are pleomorphic, gram-negative bacteria that are fastidious in their growth requirements. The genus name is derived from the Greek words for blood *(haemo)* and loving *(philos)* and refers to the requirement for growth factors that are found in blood. These factors have been identified as protoporphorin IX or protoheme (X factor) and nicotinamide adenine dinucleotide (V factor). The only *Haemophilus* that can grow in the absence of both X and V factor is *Haemophilus aprophilus*. The remaining members of the genus require either one or both of these growth factors. This differential requirement for X and V factors has become an important criterion for species classification (Table 9–1). Other metabolic characteristics include nitrate reduction by all haemophili, species variation in catalase, oxidase and hemolysin production, and poor or irregular fermentation of carbohydrates.

Habitat

In humans, the primary ecologic niche of *Haemophilus* sp. is the mucous membranes of the upper respiratory tract. They also are found in virtually all salivary samples and 95 percent of supragingival and subgingival plaque samples. Four species of haemophili commonly found in the human oral cavity include *H. aphrophilus, H. paraphrophilus, H. parainfluenzae,* and *H. segnis* (Table 9–1). *H. influenzae* is primarily a resident of the nasopharynx; however, it too is occasionally isolated from oral specimens.

The presence of haemophili in dental plaque is inversely related to the presence of black-pigmented bacteria and spirochetes. That is, plaque containing a high proportion of either black-pigmented bacteria or spirochetes virtually never contains a high proportion of haemophili. This may be a consequence of the differing oxygen requirements of these bacterial genera. While the black-pigmented bacteria and spirochetes are obligate anaerobes, the oral haemophili are facultative anaerobes. Therefore, differing oxygen tensions may dictate the position of the facultative haemophili

TABLE 9–1 ✦ Haemophili: Growth Requirements, Enzymatic Activity and Primary Site of Isolation

SPECIES	X FACTOR REQUIREMENT	V FACTOR REQUIREMENT	CATALASE	OXIDASE	ISOLATION SITE
H. aphrophilus	–	–	–	–	Dental plaque
H. paraphrophilus	–	+	+	+	Dental plaque
H. influenzae	+	+	+	+	Saliva and dental plaque
H. aegyptius	+	+	+	+	Nasopharynx
H. parainfluenzae	–	+	+	+	Conjunctiva
H. segnis	–	+	+	–	Saliva and dental plaque
H. ducreyi	+	–	–	–	Genitalia

and strictly anaerobic black-pigmenting bacteria and spirochetes in ecological succession as it occurs in dental plaque.

Morphology

The key word that describes the cell and colonial morphology of *Haemophilus* species is tiny. Haemophili cells are coccobacillary in shape. Encapsulated forms tend to be uniform in size ranging from 0.2 to 0.3 μm by 0.5 to 0.8 μm. Unencapsulated organisms, especially those from rough colonies, are more pleomorphic and may form long filaments.

Haemophilus species often are cultivated on chocolate agar. This medium is prepared by adding blood to agar that is equilibrated to 70°C. The blood cells lyse under these conditions and release the X and V factors that are required for growth. At 36 to 48 hours, colonies of *Haemophilus* species on chocolate agar are 0.5 to 1.5 mm in diameter. Colonial morphology is affected by encapsulation. Unencapsulated cells form small, dewlike colonies that develop a rough appearance. Encapsulated cells form colonies that are larger, glistening, and mucoid.

Ordinary blood agar will not support the growth of haemophili that require both X and V factors unless it is cross-inoculated with a V factor excreting organism such as a *Staphylococcus* species. The haemophili will grow around the *Staphylococcus* species forming colonies 3 to 4 mm in diameter. Before the use of paper strips impregnated with X and V factors, this phenomenon, known as "satellitism," was an important test for identifying the various *Haemophilus* species.

Haemophilus Species Virulence Factors and Antigens

Since *H. influenzae* is the most important human pathogen in the genus, its virulence factors and antigens are the most extensively studied. *H. influenzae* has three major classes of surface antigens, capsular polysaccharides, lipooligosaccharides (LOS) and outer membrane proteins. Among these, the most important virulence factors are the capsular polysaccharides (MW > 150,000) that divide *H. influenzae* strains into six serotypes designated a to f. The polyribosylribose phosphate capsule of *H. influenzae,* type b, (Hib) is most significant in the production of invasive disease with type b organisms causing over 95 percent of systemic infections in children. Conversely, unencapsulated *H. influenzae* are noninvasive members of the normal flora of the upper respiratory tract.

The LOS and outer membrane proteins are the major somatic antigens of the haemophili. The LOS differs from the classic lipopolysaccharide (LPS) of enteric bacteria in not possessing a long polysaccharide tail, commonly known as the O antigen, which interfaces with the bacterial environment. Instead the LOS consists of only core polysaccharide and lipid A. The lipid A of *H. influenzae* is endotoxic, producing the localized Schwartzman reaction. The lipid A is also antigenically heterogeneous among *Haemophilus* strains and species, which is evidence of diversity among the lipid A molecules of the Pasteurellaceae. Like the LPS, the LOS is an important elicitor of inflammatory mediators in host immune cells. The *H. influenzae* LOS may utilize this inflammatory response to increase the permeability of the blood–brain barrier.

Outer membrane proteins of *H. influenzae* designated P1 through P6 have been identified and characterized. With the exception of P2, which is a porin, the physiological activities of these proteins are unknown. P6 is highly conserved among both encapsulated and unencapsulated strains. Mutants lacking P2 and P6 have not been found indicating that such mutations may be lethal. Other proteins that may enhance *Haemophilus* species virulence include pili and IgA proteases. The pilus exhibits mannose resistant hemagglutination of type O human red blood cells and is likely involved in bacterial adherence to host cells. The IgA proteases hydrolyze the heavy chain of human immunoglobulin A. Because *H. influenzae* primarily infects human mucosal surfaces where host defense is mediated by secretory IgA, cleavage of IgA may contribute to the organism's virulence potential. Certain animal pathogens among the haemophili and other members of the HAP bacteria produce cytotoxins that kill host immune cells and therefore allow evasion of the host defense system. These are important to dental science because of their relationship to the leukotoxin of the oral pathogen *A. actinomycetemcomitans*. They are discussed in greater detail with the *Pasteurella* species.

Haemophilus influenzae

In the United States, encapsulated *H. influenzae* type b is responsible for 10,000 cases of meningitis per year. *H. influenzae* meningitis is age related with children under 3 months and over 6 years rarely contracting the disease. Other invasive infections caused primarily by encapsulated type b *H. influenzae* include epiglottitis, cellulitis, and pericarditis. These also occur mainly in children under the age of 2 and amount to 5000 cases per year. Noninvasive, unencapsulated *H. influenzae* that are normal inhabitants of the upper respiratory tract are associated with exacerbations of chronic bronchitis, pneumonia in elderly or immune compromised patients, otitis media in children, and lower respiratory disease in children in the developing world.

Encapsulated *H. influenzae* type b is transmitted by the respiratory route. Mortality rates in meningitis cases left untreated may reach 90 percent, and sequelae of the disease make it the leading cause of acquired deafness and mental retardation in the United States. The antibiotics ampicillin and amoxicillin are used to treat systemic *H. influenzae;* however, approximately 24 percent of all strains now isolated in the United States are resistant to ampicillin. In these cases, alternative treatment with chloramphenicol and the newer cephalosporins is used.

The Hib capsular polysaccharide was tested as a vaccine against *H. influenzae,* because antibody to the type b capsule is opsonic, bactericidal in the presence of complement, and protective against Hib. This vaccine was only partially successful in that it was 90 percent effective in protecting children 24 months or older, but it did not provide protection for younger children. In clinical trials, conjugate vaccines consisting of capsular polysaccharide coupled to toxoids such as tetanus and diphtheria were protective in younger children. As a result, the American Academy of Pediatrics has approved a number of these for vaccination of children age 2 months and older. Because antibodies to the *H. influenzae* outer membrane proteins P1, P2, and P6 are protective in the infant rat model, they may be used in future vaccine development. In particular, P6 has been recommended for protection against noninvasive *H. influenzae*.

Oral *Haemophilus* Species

The haemophili important to oral microbiology include *H. aprophilus, H. paraphrophilus, H. parainfluenzae,* and *H. segnis*. These organisms normally are found in the oral cavity; however, upon displacement from their normal habitat, they may become opportunistic pathogens. *H. aprophilus* and *H. paraphrophilus* are very closely related with greater than 70 percent homology between their DNA. The only phenotypic difference is the nutritional requirement of *H. aprophilus* for X and V factors while *H. paraphrophilus* requires only V factor. *H. aprophilus* is a frequent member of the microflora of human dental plaque particularly interproximally and in the gingival pockets. *H. paraphrophilus* is a member of the normal flora of the human oral cavity and pharynx. Plaque formation by these organisms occurs readily in vitro and is not dependent on the presence of sucrose or the production of extracellular polysaccharides. These *Haemophilus* species rarely cause infections of medical importance; however, dental treatments and predisposing conditions such as rheumatic heart disease and valvular lesions may lead to serious secondary infections with mortality rates up to 27 percent. Infections attributed to these organisms include endocarditis, brain abscess, dental abscess, and osteomyelitis of the jaw.

H. parainfluenzae is ubiquitous in the human oral cavity. It constitutes about 10 percent of the total anaerobic flora in saliva and 2 percent in mature dental plaque and predominates among the haemophili in these sites accounting for 85 percent of *Haemophilus* species isolated from saliva and 57 percent isolated from mature dental plaque (Table 9–2). The bacterium's propensity to attach to oral mucosa may reflect its ability to produce neuraminidase that binds salivary glycoproteins. It is not associated with any dental diseases; however, it is of medical importance in the etiology of infective endocarditis causing 5 percent of all cases.

H. segnis previously was confused with *H. parainfluenzae*. It has been differentiated from that species due to low DNA homology. *H. segnis* makes up about 33 percent of the haemophili found in mature dental plaque, but it is rare in saliva (Table 9–2). It is thought to be of little medical importance, but it has been isolated from an abscess of the pancreas.

TABLE 9–2 ✦ Haemophili in Saliva and Plaque

TABLE 9–2 ✦ Haemophili in Saliva and Plaque

SPECIES*	% HAEMOPHILI IN SALIVA†	% HAEMOPHILI IN MATURE PLAQUE‡
H. parainfluenzae	85	57
H. segnis	9	33
H. influenzae	2	0
H. aphrophilus	0	7
H. paraphrophilus	2	3

*Total haemophili did not include *H. actinomycetemcomitans* in this analysis.

†Haemophili comprised 10 percent of total salivary anaerobes.

‡Haemophili comprised 2 percent of total plaque anaerobes.

Other Haemophili

H. aegyptius (Koch-Weeks bacillus) is associated with communicable purulent conjunctivitis, especially in children in hot climates. It is indistinguishable from *H. influenzae* biovar III and has 78 percent DNA homology with *H. influenzae* leaving little reason to maintain it in a separate species. Presently, *H. aegyptius* is not classified in *H. influenzae* because it is more fastidious, hemagglutinates, and causes a more acute form of conjunctivitis.

H. ducreyi causes the sexually transmitted disease chancroid (soft chancre). Chancroid is characterized by a ragged ulcer on the genitalia with marked swelling and tenderness involving the regional lymph nodes. The disease is worldwide in distribution and usually associated with poor socioeconomic and unhygienic conditions. *H. ducreyi* requires blood for growth and its recovery from clinical samples is improved by the addition of fetal calf serum. These stringent growth requirements have hampered clinical and epidemiologic investigation of the disease.

THE GENUS *PASTEURELLA*

There are six species of *Pasteurella* listed in *Bergey's Manual of Systematic Bacteriology*. Only one species, *Pasteurella ureae* is found primarily in humans. The remainder are parasitic for a wide variety of mammals and birds where their natural habitat is the mucus membranes of the upper respiratory and gastrointestinal tracts. The pasteurella are gram-negative, nonmotile, facultatively anaerobic, fermentative, ovoid to rod shaped bacteria that are characterized by bipolar staining. Organisms exhibiting bipolar staining, especially in stained smears from infected tissue such as liver or spleen, are often said to be demonstrating "safety pin" morphology.

Human disease caused by pasteurella is rare; however, it may occur through one of three mechanisms: (1) infection through bites or scratches, (2) superinfection of a chronically diseased lung, and (3) focal infections that are secondary to septicemia. Complications of these infections can be severe and include osteomyelitis, meningitis, cerebellar abscess, and infectious endocarditis. The pasteurella most often associated with these diseases is *Pasteurella multocida*, which causes disease in a variety of animal species. *P. multocida* is resident in the upper respiratory tract of cats and is thus, the most frequent cause of infection resulting from cat bites. There are four serotypes of *P. multocida*, A through D, with A and D being the most frequent isolates from human infections. The serogroups are based on the organism's polysaccharide capsule, which is its most important virulence factor. Other factors contributing to virulence of *P. multocida* include neuraminidase, hyaluronidase, and a dermonecrotic toxin associated with atrophic rhinitis in swine.

THE Rtx FAMILY OF TOXINS

Numerous species of the HAP bacteria, especially those causing serious veterinary diseases, produce heat labile cytotoxins that lyse leukocytes including peripheral blood monocytes, polymorphonuclear leukocytes and macrophages (Table 9–3). These toxins are believed to inhibit host defense mechanisms at the site of infection. The designation Rtx alludes to repeating nucleotide sequences in the structural toxin genes. The relatedness of the Rtx toxin genes from the diverse bacteria listed in Table 9–3 is apparent in homologous nucleotide sequences and in cross-reactions between antisera to their structural gene products. The toxins are of similar molecular size, 100 to 115 kilodaltons, and in those examined, the genetic determinant consists of a cluster of four genes. Study of these toxins has been invaluable to periodontology, because *Actinobacillus actinomycetemcomitans*, etiologic in periodontal disease, produces an Rtx leukotoxin. The genetic homology between this oral leukotoxin and the *Escherichia coli* hemolysin and *Pasteurella haemolytica* leukotoxin, has allowed use of genetic probes and other molecular tools from these non-oral toxins in the cloning and characterization of the *A. actinomycetemcomitans* leukotoxin.

TAXONOMY OF THE HAP-BACTERIA

Like most bacteria, the original classification of the *Pasteurellaceae* was based on a limited number

TABLE 9–3 ✦ The Family of Rtx Cytotoxins

DISEASES AND HOST RANGE	BACTERIA	TOXIN TYPE
Periodontitis in humans	*Actinobacillus actinomycetemcomitans*	Leukotoxin
Respiratory infections including pneumoniae, septicemia, opportunistic infections in livestock	*Pasteurella haemolytica* *Actinobacillus pleuropneumoniae* *Actinobacillus suis* *Actinobacillus equuli*	Leukotoxin
Gastrointestinal disorders, bacteremia, urinary tract, and wound infections in humans	*Escherichia coli* *Proteus vulgaris* *Proteus mirabilis* *Morganella morganii*	Hemolysin
Whooping cough in humans	*Bordetella pertussis*	Cyclolysin
Blight, wilt, and soft rot in plants	*Erwinia chrysanthemi*	Metalloprotease

of phenotypic characteristics. Beginning in the 1980s, concerted efforts to reexamine the genotypic properties of the family were made using new DNA and RNA technologies. This resulted in an increase from 29 to 50 in the number of suggested or proposed species, as well as the suggested reclassification of a number of species. For example, *Haemophilus pleuropneumoniae* is now *Actinobacillus pleuropneumoniae*. In addition, based on serotyping, DNA hybridization, and phenotypic characteristics many have observed that the oral pathogen *A. actinomycetemcomitans* is more closely related to certain haemophili (i.e., *H. aphrophilus* and *H. paraphrophilus*) than it is to other *Actinobacillus* species. Reclassification of *A. actinomycetemcomitans* is problematic, however, because DNA from neither *A. actinomycetemcomitans* nor the two haemophili that it closely resembles shows high homology to the type species of the haemophili, *H. influenzae*. Therefore, the taxonomic organization of the family Pasteurellaceae is a subject of considerable debate, and there will likely be significant reorganization apparent in the next edition of *Bergey's Manual of Systematic Bacteriology*.

BIBLIOGRAPHY

American Academy of Pediatrics Committee on Infectious Diseases: *Haemophilus* type b conjugate vaccines: Recommendations for immunization of infants and children 2 months of age and older: Update. Pediatrics 88:169, 1991.

Barnum D. A.: Socioeconomic Significance of the HAP-group of Bacteria. Can. J. Vet. Res. 54 Suppl:S1, 1990.

Brooks, G. F., Butel, J. S., Ornston, L. N. et al.: Jawetz, Melnick & Adelberg's Medical Microbiology, ed 19. Appleton & Lange, Norwalk, Conn., 1991, p. 237 and 248.

Carter, G. R.: Genus I. Pasteurella. In Kreig, N. R. (ed.): Bergey's Manual of Systematic Bacteriology. Williams and Wilkins, Baltimore, 1984, p. 552.

Fenwick, B. W.: Virulence Attributes of the Liposaccharides of the HAP-Group Organisms. Can. J. Vet. Res. 54 Suppl:S28, 1990.

Gutman, L. T. and Willett, H. P.: Pasteurella and miscellaneous Gram-negative bacilli. In Joklik, W. K., Willett, H. P., Amos B. D., and Wilfert, C. M. (eds.): Zinsser Microbiology. Appleton & Lange, Norwalk, Conn, 1988, p. 506.

Kilian, M., and Biberstein, E. L.: Genus II. Haemophilus. In Kreig, N. R. (ed.): Bergey's Manual of Systematic Bacteriology. Williams and Wilkins, Baltimore, 1984, p. 558.

Lo, R. Y. C.: Molecular characterization of cytotoxins produced by *Haemophilus, Actinobacillus, Pasteurella*. Can. J. Vet. Res. 54 Suppl:S33, 1990.

MacInness, J. I., and Borr, J. D.: The family *Pasteurellaceae:* Modern approaches to taxonomy. Can. J. Vet. Res. 54 Suppl:S1, 1990.

Munson, R. S., Jr.: *Haemophilus influenzae:* Surface antigens and aspects of virulence. Can. J. Vet. Res. 54 Suppl:S63, 1990.

Murphy, T. F., Nelson, M. B., and Apicella, M. A.: The P6 outer membrane protein of nontypeable *Haemophilus influenzae* as a vaccine antigen. J. Infect. Dis. 165 Suppl:S203, 1992.

Nicolet, J.: Overview of the virulence attributes of the HAP-group of bacteria. Can. J. Vet. Res. 54 Suppl:S12. 1990.

Potts, T. V.: Haemophilus and Pasteurella. In Newman, M. G. and Nisengard, R. (eds.): Oral Microbiology and Immunology. W. B. Saunders Co., Harcourt, Brace, Jovanovich, Inc., Philadelphia, 1988, p. 183.

Potts, T. V., Zambon, J. J., and Genco, R. J.: Reassignment of *Actinobacillus actinomycetemcomitans* to the genus *Haemophilus* as *Haemophilus actinomycetemcomitans* comb. nov. Int. J. Syst. Bacteriol. 35:337, 1985.

Ward, J.: Prevention of invasive *Haemophilus influenzae* type b disease: Lessons from vaccine efficacy trials. Vaccine. 9 Suppl:S17, 1991.

Willett, H. P.: Haemophilus. In Joklik, W. K., Willett, H. P., Amos B. D., and Wilfert, C. M. (eds.): Zinsser Microbiology. Appleton & Lange, Norwalk, Conn., 1988, p. 393.

10 Neisseria

Anthony A. Campagnari and Michael A. Apicella

CHAPTER OUTLINE

Neisseria gonorrhoeae
Neisseria meningitidis

In the past 25 years, there has been an increase in our understanding of the genus *Neisseria,* in particular the meningococcus and the gonococcus. One of the most influential events contributing to renewed interest in *N. meningitidis* occurred in 1963 at Fort Ord, California. An epidemic of group B meningoccoci in military recruits could not be controlled by the use of sulfa prophylaxis. This emergence of the sulfonamide-resistant meningococci marked the end of a 20-year period when sulfa drugs could be used to prevent meningococcal disease in susceptible populations. The increased incidence of meningococcal disease in military recruits and the lack of effective prevention, prompted the study of the elements involved in the human immune response to the meningococcal components. These studies led to the development of an effective vaccine for serotype A and C meningococcal disease.

Similarly, an increase in the number of cases of gonococcal infection, at about the same time period, reached epidemic proportions. The lack of the available methods to contain the spread of gonorrhea stimulated a renewed interest in the immunobiology of the gonococcus.

NEISSERIA GONORRHOEAE
Morphological, Cultural, and Biochemical Characteristics

N. gonorrhoeae is a gram-negative diplococcus approximately 0.8 to 0.6 μm in size. The organism does not grow at 22°C and flourishes at 35°C in a humid atmosphere containing 2.5 to 5 percent carbon dioxide. The organism grows on chocolate media supplemented with co-carboxylase, cysteine, and glutamine, on Columbia media and on supplemented Mueller-Hinton media.

The use of selective Thayer-Martin media has improved the ability to isolate the gonococcus and the meningococcus from body sites (i,e., cervix

and nasopharynx) where it competes with other faster growing microbes. This medium contains standard chocolate agar and the antibiotics vancomycin, colistin, and nystatin. All other organisms are suppressed and this media selects for the gonococcus and meningococcus.

The gonococcus produces acid in the presence of glucose without gas formation, and will not ferment maltose or sucrose (Table 10–1). These fermentation characteristics differentiate it from the meningococcus. The gonococcus oxidizes dimethylparaphenylene diamine. This so-called oxidase test causes a conversion of a colorless dye to pink and than dark purple, which is useful in the preliminary identification of *Neisseria.*

Antigenic and Cell Surface Structures

The gonococcus contains an outer membrane similar in basic structure to that found in the Enterobacteriaceae. The outer membrane of the pathogenic *Neisseria* contains lipooligosaccharide (LOS) and a series of proteins including a principal outer membrane protein (OMP), which is a porin. This structure rests on an inner membrane linked to a single layer of peptidoglycan.

The LOS of pathogenic *Neisseria* is analogous to the lipopolysaccharide (LPS) endotoxin from other gram-negative organisms. It consists of an oligosaccharide portion that contains both common polysaccharide antigens and those that are serotypically distinct. The other portion of the LPS is the lipid A moiety, which is the principal bacterial toxin of the meningococcus and the gonococcus.

Both the meningococcus and the gonococcus express pili. These are membrane structures that allow the organisms to adhere to the mucosal cell surface of the cervix, urethra and nasopharynx. The pilus is composed of proteins called pilin, which are approximately 19,000 molecular weight in size. The pilus antigens are heterogeneous and account for numerous pilus serotypes.

TABLE 10−1 ✦ Characteristics of *Neisseria* Species

SPECIES	OXIDASE	GROWTH AT 22°C	PRODUCE IgA PROTEASE	FERMENTATIONS		
				GLUCOSE	MALTOSE	SUCROSE
N. meningitidis	+	−	+	+	+	−
N. gonorrhoeae	+	−	+	+	−	−
N. sicca	+	+	−	+	+	+
N. flavescens	+	+	−	−	−	−
N. subflava	+	+	−	+	+	V*

*V = variable.

Gonococcal Infection

Gonococcal infection is only found in humans. Epidemiological studies from the United States Navy indicate that the risk of infection after a single exposure is 20 to 30 percent. In men, the incubation period is within 3 to 10 days but occasionally intervals of up to 30 days occur before onset of symptoms.

In up to 75 percent of infected women, the disease can be asymptomatic for long periods of time. Although the presence of the asymptomatic man (1 to 2 percent of all infected) has been shown, the asymptomatic women poses the most serious problem in achieving eradication of this disease.

In men, the characteristic symptoms of acute infection is dysuria, urethritis, and a purulent discharge. In women, changes in color and odor of vaginal discharge and abdominal pain are the primary symptoms of cervical infection. Electron microscopic studies of cervical punch biopsies from patients with acute gonococcal infection have revealed gonococci ingested by stratified squamous epithelial cells on the cervical surface. The bacteria are present in the cells shed from this surface and it appears that they are rephagocytosed by leukocytes in cervical secretions. Squamous cell ingestion of the bacteria may play a role in the asymptomatic state as these intracellular organisms will not be exposed to antibiotics or host immune factors.

Pelvic inflammatory disease (PID) is a serious consequence of gonococcal infection in women. Although half the cases of PID are caused by *N. gonorrhoeae*, the mechanisms of infection are not known. It appears that gonococcal LPS alters the mucosal surface of the fallopian tubes, permitting the invasion by aerobic gram-negative and anaerobic organisms. Studies have shown that early after the onset of symptoms, the gonococcus is isolatable from the cul de sac. As the period of time increases between the onset of symptoms and the attempted culture, the ability to isolate gonococci decreases remarkably. In all of these patients, the cervical culture was positive for *N. gonorrhoeae*.

Disseminated gonococcal infection includes fever, arthralgias, arthritis, tenosynovitis, and a skin eruption. This disease occurs in approximately 1 in 300 to 1 in 600 cases of genital gonorrhea. This form of gonococcal disease occurs six times more frequently in women than in men. In over half the cases, it occurs within 1 week of menses and there also appears to be a relationship between this disease and the third trimester of pregnancy, since there is a higher disease frequency than in the general population.

Pharyngeal infection by the gonococcus can occur. It is associated with fellatio oral sex and tends to be self-limiting. Symptomatic infection can occur and should be treated with appropriate antibiotics.

Treatment of Gonococcal Infection

Because of the increasing frequency of penicillinase producing *N. gonorrhoeae*, ceftriaxone is now the principle drug used for the treatment of gonococcal infection. This treatment is given parenterally as a single dose on an outpatient basis. The treatment of extragenital and fallopian tube gonorrhea may require longer courses of therapy and may sometimes necessitate hospitalization of the patient.

Drugs to prevent gonococcal infection have been universally unsuccessful, with one exception. During passage down the birth canal, newborns can develop gonococcal conjunctivitis if the mothers' genital secretions are infected. Prophylactic treatment by the instillation of 1 percent silver nitrate into the conjunctival space immediately after birth has markedly reduced this complication of gonococcal infection.

NEISSERIA MENINGITIDIS
Morphologic, Cultural, Biochemical Characteristics

N. meningitidis is a gram-negative diplococcus (0.6 × 0.8 μ). The adjacent sides are flattened to produce the typical "biscuit" shape. Because the organism tends to readily undergo autolysis, considerable size and shape variation can be seen in older cultures. The organism is considered fastidious in its growth conditions, necessitating the use of appropriate media and growth conditions. On solid media, the meningococcus grows as a transparent, nonpigmented, nonhemolytic colony, approximately 1 to 5 mm in diameter. Optimal growth conditions are achieved in a moist environment at 35° to 37°C under an atmosphere of 5 to 10 percent carbon dioxide. The organism will grow well on a number of medium bases, including blood agar base, trypticase soy agar, supplemented chocolate agar, and Mueller-Hinton agar. Confirmation of the presence of this organism in clinical specimens is dependent on a series of carbohydrate fermentations (Table 10–1). The meningococcus will ferment glucose and maltose to acid without gas formation and fails to ferment sucrose or lactose. Indole and hydrogen sulfide are not formed.

Meningococci can be segregated by seroagglutination into nine serogroups, A, B, C, D, X, Z, (Z'), W135 and 29E. Capsular polysaccharides responsible for the serogrouping specificity of the groups A, B, C, X, and Y have been purified. Chemical analysis of these five polysaccharides has been completed (Table 10–2).

Noncapsular cell wall antigens appear to be important in understanding the immunobiology of the meningococcus. The antigen responsible for the noncapsular meningococcal serotyping system is protein in nature and resides in the outer membrane as part of a lipoprotein lipopolysaccharide complex.

The Human Immunobiology of *N. meningitidis*

At birth, due to maternal transfer of antibodies, about 50 percent of infants have bactericidal antibody titers. The prevalence of bactericidal antibody decreases after birth and reaches its nadir between 6 and 24 months of age. Thereafter, a linear incidence increase in antibody occurs until age 12. In early adulthood, the prevalence of bactericidal antibody varies with the serogroup but ranges from 67 percent for group A to 86 percent for group B. The protective nature of bactericidal antibody against homologous serogroups has been demonstrated during epidemics. It appears that bactericidal antibodies are directed against both the capsular polysaccharide and other cell wall antigens that may cross-react within the family *Neisseria* and with other bacterial genera. The meningococcal carrier state is an immunizing process and within 2 weeks of colonization production of antibodies to meningococci can be identified. Non-

TABLE 10–2 ✦ Chemical Composition of Meningococcal Capsular Polysaccharides

CAPSULAR SEROGROUP ANTIGEN	CHEMICAL COMPOSITION OF CAPSULAR POLYMER
A	*N*-acetyl mannosamine phosphate
B	*N*-acetyl neuraminic acid
C_{+1}	*O*,*N*-acetyl neuraminic acid
C_{1-}	*N*-acetyl neuraminic acid
X	2-acetamido-2 deoxy-D-glucose 4-phosphate
Y	D-glucose *N*-acetylneuraminic acid, 1:1

typable meningococcal strains, which are seen in carrier studies in children, contain cross-reacting antigens with the encapsulated strains and bactericidal antibody to these strains develops after nasopharyngeal colonization.

Meningococcal Infection
EPIDEMIOLOGY

Meningococcal disease is a major worldwide health problem. The greatest percentage of cases occurs in children. Approximately, 2500 to 3000 cases occur in the United States each year. During epidemics, the case rate rises dramatically. In an epidemic in Chile from 1940 to 1943, the case rate in the province of Valparaiso during 1942 was 188.1 per 100,000 people. In 1966, an epidemic was reported in Holland that was caused primarily by group B meningococci. There were 516 cases, with a case fatality rate of 8.5 percent. From 1974 to 1975, an epidemic in Brazil due to group A and C strains had a case fatality rate of less than 10 percent.

THE CARRIER STATE

Since 1896, it has been reported that *N. meningitidis* can exist in the nasopharynx of otherwise healthy humans. Such individuals are called meningococcal carriers. The transmission of the meningococci from carrier to carrier is probably via the respiratory route. During epidemics, the rate of new carrier acquisition can be rapid, while in nonepidemic situations, the new carrier rate can be considerably slower and the state of carriage can exist for prolonged periods of time.

The carrier state is an immunizing process. Indirect evidence for this phenomenon is the fact that while military recruits have a high frequency of meningococcal carriage disease, seasoned veterans have a much lower carriage rate and a disease incidence similar to the civilian population. In military recruits, anti-meningococci antibodies have been shown to persist for a minimum of 4 to 6 months after exposure. These antibodies are of the three major immunoglobulin classes and react with group specific and cross-reactive antigens.

MENINGOCOCCAL DISEASE

The clinical manifestations of meningococcal disease can be quite varied. This can range from transient fever and bacteremia to fulminant disease with death ensuing within hours of the onset of clinical symptoms. Four clinical situations have been described: (1) bacteremia without sepsis, (2) meningococcemia without meningitis, (3) meningitis with or without meningococcemia, and (4) the meningoencephalitic presentation.

Variations of these manifestations can occur and the patient can progress from one to the other during the course of disease. Studies have recently demonstrated the deficiency of complement components in a high percentage of patients with systemic meningococcal infection.

Meningococcal pneumonia has been a recognized clinical syndrome for over 60 years. Because of the nasopharyngeal carriage of the meningococcus, the ability to establish the diagnosis based on the sputum culture alone is hazardous.

Meningococcal upper respiratory tract infections (pharyngitis) associated with contacts of cases and as a prior symptom and sign in cases of serious meningococcal disease has been described by several authors. Suggestions that pharyngeal inflammation is the predecessor to bacteremic dissemination have been made but are unsubstantiated.

TREATMENT OF MENINGOCOCCAL INFECTIONS

Penicillin therapy for the treatment of meningococcal infections is safe and effective. The drug can be administered intravenously or intramuscularly. The intrathecal route is contraindicated because of the severe neurotoxicity of penicillin in high concentrations in the central nervous system. A dose of 200,000 U/kg/day is recommended with a maximum of 20 million U/day total dose. Chloramphenicol is an effective substitute for use in the penicillin allergic patient and should be administered intravenously in a dose of 100 mg/kg/day to a maximum of 4 g/dose. Duration of antibiotic therapy will vary somewhat with the presentation and manifestation of the disease with the response of the patient. At present, the meningococcus is quite sensitive to the agents just mentioned and 10 to 14 days of therapy is usually sufficient.

CHEMOPROPHYLAXIS

Treatment of patients carrying meningococci with rifampin or sulfonamides can eradicate carriage quickly for prolonged periods. Presently, the recommended therapy for meningococcal prophylaxis is rifampin, 600 mg every 12 hours for 2 days for adults and 10 mg/kg every 12 hours for 2 days for children.

Since the clinical onset of sulfa resistance and the problem in finding agents that are safe, and effective, more attention has been paid to the populations at greatest risk who need chemoprophylaxis. In both epidemic and endemic situations in civilian populations, household contacts have been shown to be at increased risk to infection. Similar high risk situations exist in closed populations such as college dormitories, chronic care hospitals, nursery schools and military barracks. Hospital personnel are not at increased risk and usually do not receive chemoprophylaxis, unless they experience an intimate exposure to an infected patient.

IMMUNOPROPHYLAXIS

After the emergence of sulfa resistant meningococci, intense effort was directed at developing a vaccine to prevent meningococcal infections in high risk populations. The result was two vaccine preparations derived from the capsular polysaccharide of the group A and C meningococci. The effectiveness of the group C vaccine has been demonstrated in studies of American Army recruits. Only one case of meningococcal disease occurred among 13,763 vaccinees, while 38 bacteriologically proven cases occurred in a control group of 68,072. Group A polysaccharide administered to Finnish military recruits also significantly lowered the incidence of disease due to this serogroup when compared with an unvaccinated control population. Studies from Finland during a group A epidemic showed the effectiveness of this vaccine in children 3 months to 5 years of age.

The serogroup C vaccine does not elicit protective antibodies in children under the age of 24 months. Studies of the immune response to the A and C vaccine in infants have demonstrated that detectable levels of antibody are generated but at levels significantly lower than in older children. In adults, the group C antibody titer persisted for 2 to 4 years after vaccination and in children, vaccinated with group A polysaccharide, protection wanes after 1 year.

There is no vaccine presently available for prevention of group B disease. The group B capsular polysaccharide is poorly immunogenic and fails to produce an antibody response in humans. Several solutions to this problem are being studied, including the chemical alteration of the capsular B antigen to make it more immunogenic and the search for other cell wall antigens capable of eliciting bactericidal antibodies against B meningococci with a minimum of side effects.

BIBLIOGRAPHY

Advisory Committee on Immunization Practices: Meningococcal polysaccharide vaccines. Ann. Intern. Med. 84:179, 1976.

Artenstein, M. S. and Ellis, R. E.: The risk of exposure to a patient with meningococcal meningitis. Milit. Med. 133:474, 1968.

Eisenstein, B. I. and Masi, A. T.: Disseminated gonococcal infection (DGI) and gonococcal arthritis (GCA). 1. Bacteriology, epidemiology, host factors, pathogen factors and pathology. Semin. Arthritis Rheum. 10:155, 1981.

Eschenbach, D. A.: Acute pelvic inflammatory disease: Etiology, risk factors and pathogenesis. Clin. Obstet. Gynecol. 19:147, 1976.

Feldman, H. A.: Meningococcal infections. Adv. Intern. Med. 18:177, 1972.

Griffiss, J. M.: Epidemic meningococcal disease: Synthesis of a hypothetical immunoepidemiological model. Rev. Infect. Dis. 4:159, 1982.

Hook, E. W. and Holmes, K. K.: Gonococcal infections. Ann. Intern. Med. 102:229, 1985.

Hutt, D. M. and Judson, F. N.: Epidemiology and treatment of oropharyngeal gonorrhea. Ann. Intern. Med. 104:655, 1986.

Peltola, H.: Meningococcal disease: Still with us. Rev. Infect. Dis. 5:71, 1983.

Peterson, B. H., Lee, T. J., and Synderman, R., et al.: *Neisseria meningitidis* and *Neisseria gonorrhoeae* bacteremia associated with C6, C7, or C8 deficiency. Ann. Intern. Med. 90:917, 1986.

Wiesner, P. J., Tronca, E., and Bonin, P. et al.: Clinical spectrum of pharyngeal gonorrhoeae. N. Engl. J. Med. 288:181, 1973.

11 Corynebacterium *and* Mycobacterium

Paulette J. Tempro and Joseph J. Zambon

CHAPTER OUTLINE

Corynebacterium

Mycobacterium

CORYNEBACTERIUM

The *Corynebacterium* include a group of facultatively anaerobic pathogenic and saprophytic gram-positive, nonmotile, non–spore-forming rods (Table 11–1). The name "Corynebacterium" derives from the Greek "koryne," meaning club, and "bakterion," meaning small rod. Hence, these bacteria are small straight or slightly curved rods, some having club-shaped ends, that stain irregularly. Cell division results in right angle or palisade cell groupings. The *Corynebacterium* are related

TABLE 11–1 ✦ *Corynebacterium*

Characteristics	Facultative anaerobes
	Gram-positive, nonmotile, non–spore-forming, club-shaped rods with *metachromatic granules*
	Pathogens and saprophytes
	Cell wall with meso-diamino-pimelic acid
Major species	*C. diphtheriae*
Growth	Loeffler's medium, medium containing 0.045 percent tellurite
	Colony morphologies include "gravis," "mitis," and "intermedius"
Disease	Diphtheria
Pathogenesis	Exotoxin
	β-prophage carries the structural gene for the toxin
	Clinically characterized by grayish pseudomembrane
	Schick test for circulating antibody to the toxin
Prevention	Vaccination with toxoid
Treatment	Penicillin, erythromycin, tetracycline

to the genera *Mycobacterium, Nocardia,* and *Rhodococcus* in that they possess a cell wall peptidoglycan containing mesodiaminopimelic acid; however, the latter three genera have n-glycolyl residues in their cell wall glycans, which are not found in *Corynebacterium. Corynebacterium* also possess arabinose and galactose as major cell wall sugars and have short-chain (22 to 36 carbon atoms) mycolic acids in the cell wall.

Corynebacterium diphtheriae

The most important microorganism in this genus is *Corynebacterium diphtheriae*, which causes diphtheria (croup). This disease is named after the gray pseudomembrane composed of fibrin, bacteria, and trapped leukocytes (from the Greek *diphthera*, meaning skin or membrane) that forms in the patient's throat during the course of the disease.

CHARACTERISTICS OF THE MICROORGANISM

These organisms are gram-positive, non–spore-forming, straight or slightly curved rods, with tapered ends but without flagella or capsule. The cells may have swollen or club-shaped ends and often have accumulations of polyphosphate in metachromatic granules (Babès-Ernst bodies), which stain bluish-purple with methylene or toluidine blue. The organism measures 0.3 to 0.8 μm wide by 1 to 8 μm long. *C. diphtheriae* multiplies by "snapping," resulting in accumulations of cells that are at right angles to one another and appear as Chinese or cuneiform characters. The term *diphtheroid* is used in medical microbiology to designate gram-positive rods resembling *C. diphtheriae*.

C. diphtheriae grows as an obligate aerobe at 30°C to 37°C. Complex media such as Loeffler's coagulated serum medium are required for primary isolation. Colonies appear cream-colored or grayish-white on Loeffler's medium but are characteristically dark gray or black on medium containing 0.045 percent tellurite, as a result of the organism's reduction of tellurite to tellurium. Three morphologically distinct types of colonies have been described. Each colony morphology, originally thought to relate to the patient's clinical condition, is no longer thought to have such correlation. These morphologies include (1) "gravis" strains, with short, irregular, rod-shaped bacterial cells that form large, radially striated, flat gray to black colonies on tellurite medium; (2) "mitis" strains, with long, curved, rod-shaped cells that form small, black, and convex colonies with a glossy surface; and (3) "intermedius" strains, with long, rod-shaped cells that form flat, creamy, transparent colonies.

PATHOGENESIS

Diphtheria is caused by an exotoxin produced by strains of *C. diphtheriae* that have been infected with a beta-prophage. This bacteriophage carries the structural gene (tox) for the toxin molecule. Toxigenic *C. diphtheriae* strains cured of the bacteriophage lose the ability to produce toxin and are avirulent. Furthermore, toxin production in toxigenic, lysogenic strains of *C. diphtheriae* is dependent upon environmental factors including iron. High toxin levels are produced only where iron levels are low. The toxin is a heat-labile protein of 60,000 daltons molecular weight. It originates as a larger latent precursor molecule which is converted to active toxin by cleavage of a peptide linkage 194 residues from the N-terminus. The active toxin itself is composed of two fragments— an N-terminal fragment A of 21,150 daltons, which carries the enzyme activity, and a larger fragment B of 39,000 daltons, which is responsible for binding to specific surface receptors on sensitive cells. Following this binding, fragment A is transported across the cell membrane, where it catalyzes the transfer of an ADP-ribosyl group from nicotinamide adenine dinucleotide (NAD) to elongation factor, EF2. This effectively blocks EF2 from carrying out its crucial role in cellular protein synthesis and the cell dies within a few hours.

C. diphtheriae is transmitted either by droplet infection from asymptomatic carriers and active cases or by contact with cutaneous lesions. Human disease begins as an upper respiratory tract infection in which virulent *C. diphtheriae* multiply and secrete a toxin that causes cellular necrosis in the mucosa of the oropharynx—especially of the tonsils. The microorganism rarely invades the deeper tissues; however, the toxin can be carried via the blood to other parts of the body, causing a toxemia. At the site of infection, accumulations of necrotic epithelial cells, *C. diphtheriae,* fibrin, erythro-

cytes, and leukocytes form the characteristic grayish **pseudomembrane.** Patients usually have a moderate fever, chills, malaise, sore throat, and cervical lymphadenopathy, which may become so pronounced as to give the appearance of a "bull neck." The disease may extend to adjacent areas of the larynx and trachea causing laryngeal diphtheria or extend into the nasal passages causing nasopharyngeal diphtheria. Laryngeal diphtheria is associated with respiratory tract obstructions, which may necessitate tracheotomy. Nasopharyngeal diphtheria is associated with neurologic and cardiac complications due to circulating toxin. Cardiac complications of nasopharyngeal diphtheria appear within 2 weeks and involve myocardial degeneration. Neurologic complications appear within 3 to 5 weeks and produce paralysis of cranial nerves, which can lead to both paralysis of the soft palate and polyneuritis of peripheral nerves. In tropical areas, cutaneous diphtheria may occur as a secondary infection of pre-existing skin lesions. These appear as chronic, sometimes spreading, ulcers, which do not heal and are covered by a grayish pseudomembrane.

IMMUNITY

As a result of transplacental transfer of maternal antibody to the *C. diphtheriae* toxin, newborn infants may have passive immunity for up to 2 years. However, after the first few months of life, maternal antibody levels are generally insufficient to prevent *C. diphtheriae* infection and the development of diphtheria. Children born to mothers who do not have antibody to *C. diphtheriae* likewise do not have this passive immunity. For these reasons, diphtheria toxoid is used to immunize infants as part of the DPT (diphtheria, pertussis, and tetanus) combined vaccine. The toxoid is derived from formaldehyde treatment of the *C. diphtheriae* toxin, which results in the loss of toxicity but retention of antigenicity. Active immunization with DPT vaccine produces adequate antibody levels to the *C. diphtheriae* toxin for several years. Booster immunizations, however, are necessary to maintain antibody levels during childhood.

The Schick test identifies persons with circulating antibody to the *C. diphtheriae* toxin. Following an intradermal injection of a small volume of *C. diphtheriae* toxin, persons without antibody develop a positive Schick test with red to brown pigmented areas of swelling, redness, and necrosis at the site of injection within 4 to 5 days. Persons with enough circulating antibody to neutralize the injected toxin do not develop this "positive" Schick test. Thus, a positive Schick test result identifies susceptible individuals, and a negative result identifies those with protective immunity. Often, intradermal injection with a *C. diphtheriae* toxoid preparation is used as a control to distinguish a true-positive reaction from delayed hypersensitivity reactions (allergy) to the toxin or to non-toxin antigens present in the same preparation.

DIAGNOSIS AND TREATMENT

The diagnosis of diphtheria is made by the identification of toxigenic *C. diphtheriae*. Swabs of throat lesions are cultured onto a Loeffler's slant, a blood agar plate, and a tellurite agar plate. Smears are made from colonies appearing 24 hours after incubation on any of the media. The smears are stained with methylene blue and microscopically examined for coryneform cell morphology. If colonies appear on the blood agar plate but not on the tellurite medium, the latter is reincubated for an additional 24 hours. Negative growth after the second incubation is used to rule out *Corynebacterium* infection.

After culture, *C. diphtheriae* isolates should be tested for toxin production by an in vivo assay in guinea pigs or rabbits or by in vitro gel diffusion assay. The in vivo test involves subcutaneous injections of the experimental animal with 0.2 ml of a 48-hour broth culture or 0.1 ml of a heavy bacterial suspension from the Loeffler's slant. After 4 hours, the animal is intraperitoneally injected with 500 units of diphtheria antitoxin, and after an additional 30 minutes the animal is reinjected with an additional sample of the bacterial suspension into a new site. If the *C. diphtheriae* strain is toxigenic, the site injected before administration of the antitoxin will have become necrotic within 48 to 72 hours, while the site injected after administration of the antitoxin will reveal only nonspecific inflammation.

The in vitro gel diffusion test involves pouring calf serum–peptone maltose agar into a Petri plate containing a filter paper strip impregnated with diphtheria antitoxin. The *C. diphtheriae* strain to be tested is streaked across the surface of the solidified agar at right angles to the paper strip and the plate is incubated for 24 hours. The appearance of an antigen-antibody precipitin line indicates that the *C. diphtheriae* strain produces toxin.

Since the diphtheria toxin can enter sensitive cells within a short period of time, suspected cases of diphtheria should be immediately treated with antitoxin—even before microbiologic assays are completed. Once the toxin has entered the target cells, the antitoxin is no longer effective in neutralizing it. A large single bolus of antitoxin is administered intramuscularly, 100 to 500 units per pound, to neutralize both circulating toxin and toxin that has bound to cell membranes but that has not yet entered the cell.

C. diphtheriae is susceptible to a number of antibiotics, including penicillin, erythromycin, and tetracycline. Therapy, however, should be first directed toward neutralization of the diphtheria toxin. Antibiotic therapy can then be useful in eliminating the primary *C. diphtheriae* infection.

MYCOBACTERIUM

This genus contains saprophytic microorganisms that cause non-tuberculous mycobacterial disease and parasitic microorganisms including two major human pathogens, *Mycobacterium tuberculosis* and *Mycobacterium leprae*, which cause tuberculosis and leprosy, respectively (Table 11–2). Diseases caused by mycobacteria are characterized by the development of destructive granulomas with central areas of necrosis. These organisms are classified in the order *Actinomycetales* and are closely related to the genera *Corynebacterium* and *Nocardia*. The group as a whole is sometimes referred to as *the CNM group*. The bacterial cells are slow-growing, nonmotile, non–spore-forming, acid- and alcohol-fast bacilli. They are slightly curved or straight rods, and range in size from 0.2 to 0.6 μm wide and 1 to 10 μm long. Bacilli stained with dyes during the Ziehl-Neelsen procedure or the fluorochrome technique are resistant to decolorization with acid or alcohol, owing to the high lipid content in the cell walls. Bacterial cells grow as branches, filaments, or mycelia, which can be dispersed into cocci. Microscopy is therefore a key test for identification of *Mycobacterium* in clinical specimens. *Mycobacteria* are similar to *Corynebacterium* and *Nocardium* in that they have ara-

TABLE 11–2 ✦ *Mycobacterium*

Characteristics	Acid- and alcohol-fast bacilli Ziehl-Neelsen or fluorochrome stains
Major species	*Mycobacterium tuberculosis* Obligate aerobe Grows as serpentine cords *Mycobacterium leprae*—noncultivable
Growth	Slow growth on egg yolk or oleic acid agar
Disease	Tuberculosis and leprosy
Pathogenesis	Destructive granulomas with central areas of necrosis
Prevention	Skin testing with a purified protein derivative or lepromin
Treatment	Isoniazid, rifampin, ethambutol, rifabutin, pyrazinamide, amikacin, ciprofloxacin, ofloxacin, streptomycin Dapsone (diaminodiphenylsulfone) for leprosy

binose, galactose, and mycolic acid in the cell walls. They are serologically similar, in that they have a common antigen.

Mycobacterium tuberculosis

M. tuberculosis causes tuberculosis ("consumption"), a disease affecting mankind since ancient times. Radiographic examination of Egyptian mummies, for example, revealed evidence of tuberculosis. This disease is associated with unsanitary and crowded living conditions. Until fairly recently, treatment involved isolation of tubercular patients for extended time periods in sanitariums. The discovery by Dr. Robert Koch of *M. tuberculosis* as the cause of this pulmonary disease stands as a landmark in the history of microbiology and led to the development of Koch's postulates. These have been extremely valuable in pinpointing the microbial etiology of other infectious diseases.

After nearly 30 years of decline in the incidence of tuberculosis in the United States, a dramatic increase occurred in the late 1980s. This resurgence partly resulted from an influx of immigrants from areas where tuberculosis is endemic, especially Southeast Asia and infections among patients with Acquired Immunodeficiency Syndrome (AIDS). In addition, reservoirs of tuberculosis in urban areas and in populations difficult to reach (the homeless, alcoholics, drug abusers, and the elderly poor) have persisted. Tuberculosis has once again emerged as an important infectious disease and a major public health problem.

Concomitant with this increased incidence of tuberculosis has been an increase in the prevalence of strains resistant to single and multiple antituberculosis drugs. The resistant strains are thought to have arisen from noncompliant patients taking suboptimal antituberculosis agents and to immigrants treated inadequately. Primary infections with multidrug-resistant strains in patients never treated for tuberculosis was uncommon in the United States. However, major outbreaks of nosocomial multidrug resistant (MDR) tuberculosis among hospitalized AIDS patients has occurred with increasing frequency. Smaller outbreaks of MDR-tuberculosis infections among prisoners, some with HIV and AIDS, and their contacts also have been recently documented. The movement of asymptomatic prisoners among facilities in the prison system seems to be responsible for spread in this population. Health care workers on HIV hospital wards and clinics constitute another group in which infection with MDR-tuberculosis has occurred.

CELLULAR AND COLONIAL CHARACTERISTICS

M. tuberculosis is a slow-growing, obligate aerobe. The bacterial cells are slender, slightly curved rods measuring approximately 0.3 to 0.6 μm wide by 1 to 4 μm long. The cell morphology varies from cocci to filaments, depending on the growth medium. Bacterial cells often have a beaded or banded appearance due to polymetaphosphate accumulations and glycogen granules, which stain metachromatically. The cells may grow parallel to one another in long aggregated strands known as "serpentine cords" and may form adherent moldlike clumps.

"Cord factor," responsible for serpentine growth, may also play a role in virulence. Highly virulent strains contain large amounts of cord factor, whereas cord factor–free cells are avirulent. Cord factor is toxic, and immunization against cord factor can prevent the development of tuberculosis in experimental animals.

Dispersed growth of the bacterial cells will occur with the addition of a nonionic detergent (such as Tween) to broth cultures. Cell walls contain a peptidoglycan and large amounts of glycolipid, including mycolic acids, which are unique to the CNM *(Corynebacterium-Nocardia-Mycobacterium)* group of organisms.

Bacterial colonies are slow to appear: generally 3 to 6 weeks may be required. The colonies are buff-colored, rough, and raised, with a wrinkled surface, and they produce niacin. Serpentine cord formation is seen in smears made from cultures.

ANTIGENICITY

M. tuberculosis contains species- and strain-specific antigens as well as common antigens shared with *Corynebacterium* and *Nocardia*. Patients with tuberculosis due to *M. tuberculosis* or *M. bovis,* as well as nondiseased subjects exposed to either of these microorganisms, can develop delayed hypersensitivity reactions to the organism. This can be detected by intradermal testing with a purified protein derivative (PPD) from *M. tuberculosis*. Patients with tuberculosis due to *M. bovis* also exhibit a positive reaction to this preparation.

IMMUNITY

In addition to identifying the etiologic agent in tuberculosis, Koch also demonstrated the development of partial immunity to *M. tuberculosis* in an animal model. This is known as the "Koch phenomena." The first injection of *M. tuberculosis* into an experimental animal such as a guinea pig results in a large persistent ulceration at the site of injection after approximately 2 weeks. Subsequent challenge with another dose of *M. tuberculosis* in another site results in the rapid development of an ulceration at the site of injection, but this second lesion soon heals as a result of the partial immunity developed in response to the first injection.

PATHOGENESIS

The pathogenesis of *M. tuberculosis* in tuberculosis is a classic example of the relationship between microbial virulence on the one hand and host resistance on the other. Accordingly, there is a range of host responses to infection with *M. tuberculosis*. The microorganism is generally transmitted by droplet (as from coughing) from a person with an active case of tuberculosis. The microorganism is very stable in such sputum droplets and can remain viable in even dry sputum for up to 6 weeks. *M. tuberculosis* in the droplets is then inhaled into the previously uninfected host and lodges in the highly aerobic environment of the lung, where it produces a nonspecific pneumonitis. Histologically, the initial response is exudative, followed by a granulomatous response, during which the patient develops the delayed hypersensitivity characteristic of tuberculosis. In pulmonary sites of infection, macrophages in contact with *M. tuberculosis* form complexes known as tubercles which may fuse to form giant cells. This initial infection of the lung and regional extension to the hilar lymph nodes is known as the primary complex. As the tubercular lesion progresses, there is often cheeselike necrosis in the center of the lesion, known as caseation necrosis. If host resistance is adequate at this point, these caseous lesions heal by calcification to form Ghon's complexes, which are visible on chest radiographs as radiodensities. If host resistance cannot overcome this pathogenic process, then the caseation necrosis proceeds to frank liquefaction with a liquid produced in the necrotic center. This liquefaction serves as the basis for cavity formation and rapid proliferation of *M. tuberculosis*. At this point, *M. tuberculosis* can again be spread by droplet infection. Coughing caused by the bronchial irritation of the infection brings up *M. tuberculosis*—infected sputum, which can then be transmitted to other persons. If the tubercular cavity in the lung becomes large enough, it may gain access to the vasculature and become disseminated (or miliary) tuberculosis. Within the same patient, there may, in fact, be both healing and active tubercular lesions.

Several factors relate to the pathogenesis of tuberculosis. The disease is associated with unsanitary, crowded living conditions often occurring with low socioeconomic status, stress, and malnutrition. Genetics also appear important, as evidenced by the high prevalence of tuberculosis in American Indians and Eskimos. Age and hormonal status also appear important. Prior to the first half of this century, most children were exposed to *M. tuberculosis* and became skin test–positive. The high prevalence of this infection suggested that *M. tuberculosis* represented an "endogenous" infection. However, with improvements in living conditions and sanitation, children today are rarely exposed to *M. tuberculosis*.

MDR tuberculosis is a rapid and usually fatal disease in AIDS patients. The MDR tuberculosis strains are acquired nosocomially in hospital settings. The high fatality rate is partly caused by the delay in recognizing the mycobacterial disease and in starting efficacious multidrug therapy as well as the profoundly immunosuppressed status of the patient. Following a brief period from exposure to MDR-tuberculosis until development of infection in AIDS patients, a fatality rate as high as 90 percent occurs within 4 to 16 weeks of onset of symptoms. The disease is characterized by rapid onset with fever, weight loss, cough, and commonly extrapulmonary involvement.

DIAGNOSIS

Tuberculosis can be diagnosed by several methods. First, demonstration of acid-fast bacilli in smears made from sputum samples is indicative of tuberculosis. Second, *M. tuberculosis* can be cultured from sputum or other contaminated fluids onto egg yolk containing agar or onto oleic acid—albumin agar following 2 to 4 weeks of incubation. Finally, a positive skin test is indicative of tuberculosis. Previously, an old tuberculin (OT) preparation consisting of a filtered broth from autoclaved or boiled tubercle bacilli was used in skin testing. Currently, PPD, an ammonium sulfate precipitate from tubercle bacilli cultures, is used in skin testing. In what is known as the Mantoux test, 0.1 ml of diluted PPD is injected into the skin of the forearm. If a patient has been sensitized and has developed delayed hypersensitivity to *M. tuberculosis,* then an area of induration and erythema will appear after 48 hours at the site of injection. These areas are measured with a ruler. A positive reaction, therefore, indicates sensitivity to *M. tuberculosis*. It does not distinguish between patients who currently have tuberculosis and those who have previously had tuberculosis. Delayed hypersensitivity becomes apparent 4 to 6 weeks after exposure to the organism and may remain apparent for months or years.

Diagnosis of symptomatic MDR tuberculosis in AIDS patients is often based on ruling out other etiological agents rather than isolation of *M. tuberculosis*. Roentgenographic chest findings are nonspecific with abnormalities not helpful in diagnosis. Primary isolation from clinical samples takes 2 to 3 weeks, too long for a rapidly deteriorating patient. Skin testing is not useful in this population.

TREATMENT

Before the development of appropriate antibiotics, treatment of tuberculosis involved rest, proper nutrition, and sometimes artificial collapse of one lung. When tuberculosis was epidemic, large numbers of tuberculosis sanitariums were operated for treatment and to sequester patients from the general population. Streptomycin, developed in 1945, was the first antibiotic useful for treatment of tuberculosis. This antibiotic, however, is toxic and can cause eighth nerve deafness. Also, although bactericidal, streptomycin is incapable of killing *M. tuberculosis* located intracellularly. A superior drug for treatment of tuberculosis is isoniazid (INH). INH can kill *M. tuberculosis* located in both extracellular and intracellular sites. Its low toxicity, cost, and oral route of administration have revolutionized the treatment of tuberculosis. Tuberculosis was no longer treated by long periods of confinement in sanitaria. Other drugs have been added to the treatment regimen in combination including rifampin, para-aminosalicylic acid (PAS), ethambutol (EMB), kanamycin, capreomycin, cycloserine, ethionamide, and pyrazinamide. The use of these drugs led to the practice of treating tuberculosis on an outpatient basis with decreased emphasis on prevention and control. Even so, treatment for tuberculosis requires long periods of antibiotic therapy—as long as 10 to 12 months. The laxity with which the disease had been treated in the 1970s is most likely a factor responsible for its current resurgence.

When tuberculosis was prevalent in the United States, mass screening by chest radiography and skin testing was commonplace for epidemiologic prevention. These approaches have been abandoned.

In symptomatic MDR-tuberculosis in AIDS patients, drug therapy often includes 7 or more drugs chosen on the basis of the pattern of *M. tuberculosis* drug resistance in the community. Treatment of tuberculosis in HIV-positive asymptomatic patients infected with strains not suspected of resistance begins with isoniazid, rifampin and pyrazinamide for 2 months and isoniazid and rifampin for 8 additional months as a standard regimen. When the infecting strain is suspected of being MDR, a combination regimen usually consisting of six to seven agents is selected on the basis of drug resistance surveillance data for that community. HIV-positive patients with MDR tuberculosis may be infective for long periods, and chemotherapy must continue for 6 months after three consecutive negative sputums. Healthy HIV-positive patients respond as well as non–HIV-positive patients to efficacious therapy.

In response to outbreaks of tuberculosis, renewed emphasis on once-familiar infection control procedures have been instituted: early identification and multidrug treatment of persons with active tuberculosis, isolation of hospitalized active tuberculosis patients, isolation rooms equipped with negative air pressure, six air changes per hour, air purification with ultraviolet light, and avoidance of aerosols. Personnel coming into contact with patients are required to wear proper barriers. Public health strategies under consideration are regionalization of facilities for care of tuberculosis patients as an alternative to renovation of community hospitals and supervised chemotherapy for noncompliant tuberculosis patients.

Mycobacterium leprae

Another important human pathogen in the genus *Mycobacterium* is *Mycobacterium leprae*. This microorganism, also known as Hansen's bacillus, causes leprosy, a grossly disfiguring and degenerative disease that was prevalent in biblical times and that even today affects millions worldwide.

M. leprae is morphologically indistinguishable from *M. tuberculosis;* however, this microorganism has never been cultured. It can be found in high numbers of lepromatous lesions and propagated in mice foot pads and in the nine-banded armadillo. Even though *M. leprae* has not been cultured, an extract known as lepromin can be obtained by boiling *M. leprae*–rich human tissue for use as a skin test reagent.

PATHOGENESIS

M. leprae apparently is transmitted from infected cutaneous lesions through skin abrasions where it may lie dormant for months to decades. It then forms chronic granulomatous lesions similar to those of tuberculosis, with epithelioid and giant cells but without caseation necrosis. *M. leprae* affects mainly skin and nerve tissue. The cutaneous form of leprosy results in the production of numerous firm nodules. The neural form results in peripheral nerve paresthesia and anesthesia. Subjects with this form of leprosy are liable to injure their extremities, with the development of secondary infection and severe cosmetic defects.

Lepromin is useful in determining the prognosis and progression of the disease, similar to tuberculin skin testing. The development of a hypersensitive granuloma following injection of lepromin into a sensitized patient is known as a Mitsuda reaction.

Leprosy presents with a spectrum of diverse clinical manifestations. At one pole of the spectrum, tuberculoid leprosy, there are few acid-fast bacilli in the tissues and patients develop high levels of cell-mediated immunity. Ultimately, the bacilli are killed and cleared from the tissues, often with concomitant immunologic damage to the nerves. At the lepromatous pole, patients exhibit selective unresponsiveness to antigens of *M. leprae* and the organisms multiply in the skin, often to numbers as high as 10^{10}/g tissue. Lepromatous patients have few lymphocytes in their lesions, are negative to skin testing with antigens of *M. leprae,* and show little or no lymphocyte transformation to *M. leprae* antigens in vitro. Lepromatous disease presents clinically as erythematous nodules in the skin, presumed to be caused by immune complexes in the tissue and concomitant immunologic nerve damage. The disease for the majority of patients exists in categories between the two poles, and if untreated, progresses towards one or the other pole of the clinical and immunological spectrum over the course of infection. Patients do not die of leprosy per se, but rather of secondary infections by other microorganisms and of a systemic disease known as amyloidosis, which results in the deposition of waxy substances in internal organs.

DIAGNOSIS AND TREATMENT

Leprosy can be diagnosed by the demonstration of acid-fast bacilli in skin lesions. Often there is a false-positive reaction to the serologic test for syphilis. Leprosy is treated with the drug dapsone (diaminodiphenylsulfone). Immunotherapy of leprosy with intradermal injection of killed *M. vaccae,* a nonpathogenic, environmental mycobacterium, and protein antigens of *M. tuberculosis* along with chemotherapy has led to skin test responsiveness in lepromatous leprosy patients and clearance of bacilli from tissues. This preparation also has been used in immunoprophylaxis in areas where leprosy is endemic. It is not yet known whether induction of a positive lepromin skin test confers protection.

Nontuberculous *Mycobacterium*

Mycobacterium other than *M. tuberculosis* were identified soon after Koch's discovery of the tubercle bacillus. It was not until the 1950s that they were recognized as human pathogens. Patients with pulmonary diseases similar to tuberculosis due to nontubercular mycobacteria (NTM) made up 1–2 percent of the population in tuberculosis sanitariums. The patients with NTM differed from those with tuberculosis in that they were older and had underlying chronic lung disease. Reaction to PPD was also less common than in tuberculosis patients and close contacts were generally PPD negative.

NTM, commonly isolated from soil and water, were classified as environmental bacteria and opportunistic parasites. Table 11–3 shows a partial

TABLE 11–3 ✦ Some Common *Mycobacterium* and Associated Diseases

MYCOBACTERIUM	ASSOCIATED DISEASES
Obligate Pathogens	
M. tuberculosis	Tuberculosis
M. bovis	Tuberculosis in humans and animals
M. leprae	Leprosy
Opportunistic Pathogens	
M. avium-intercellulare complex	Disseminated infection in AIDS and inflammatory bowel disease
M. marinum	Deep tissue infection associated with aquatic activity
M. scrofulaceum	Disseminated infection in AIDS
M. kansasii	Pulmonary disease
M. fortuitum complex	Nosocomial wound infection
M. ulcerans	Superficial skin infection
Nonpathogens	
M. gastri	Rare pulmonary disease
M. gordonae	Rare disseminated infection in AIDS
M. terrae complex	Rare pulmonary disease

list of the more common environmental mycobacteria and associated infections. Recently, NTM have been implicated in fatal disseminated disease in an increasing number of AIDS patients and in colon biopsies of patients with Crohn's disease (inflammatory bowel disease).

NTM infection is the most common systemic opportunistic bacterial infection in AIDS patients. The predominant isolate in HIV-infected patients is *M. avium* complex (*M. avium* and *M. intracellulare*). In AIDS patients, NTM disease most frequently presents as a non-pulmonary, disseminated infection. The infection is rarely the AIDS-defining illness but occurs in the later stages of disease when immunosuppression is most profound. *M. kansasii* and *M. fortuitum* are two environmental mycobacteria causing a smaller proportion of opportunistic NTM infections in AIDS patients.

M. avium complex organisms are ubiquitous in the environment and are acquired by AIDS patients through food, water, soil, and dust leading to colonization of the gastrointestinal (GI) tract or lungs followed by hematogenous dissemination. The relationship between GI and pulmonary colonization and subsequent dissemination is not clear. *M. avium* are phagocytized by macrophages and carried to the organs of the reticuloendothelial system. Examination of biopsy material at this stage reveals large numbers of organisms as high as 10^9 to 10^{10} organisms per gram of tissue. The organisms are present within macrophages, with little evidence of granuloma formation or inflammation. *M. avium* infection is common in AIDS patients who are symptomatic and have absolute CD4 (see Chapter 2) counts of less than $100/\mu l$. The most prevalent symptoms are fever, sweating, anorexia, weakness, and sometimes diarrhea. Any febrile illness in AIDS patients with a CD4 count below $100/\mu l$, once infections with *Pneumocystis carinii,* cytomegalovirus, and diarrheal pathogens have been ruled out, is likely to be disseminated NTM infection.

DIAGNOSIS AND TREATMENT

Diagnosis of *M. avium* infection is made by peripheral blood and tissue culture. The organism also can be observed histologically in lymph node, bone marrow, and liver biopsy material.

Resistance of the *M. avium* complex to multiple antimycobacterial agents has made therapy challenging. Therapeutic regimens are still evolving for this newly recognized infectious disease but combination therapy with several bactericidal agents appears to yield a favorable response. Based on in vitro sensitivity testing and clinical data, the optimal regimen should include clofazimine (a macrolide), ethambutol, rifamycin, ciprofloxacin (a quinolone), and amikacin. Four-drug therapy should continue even after symptoms improve until blood cultures are clear of organisms (about 4 to 6 weeks) followed by an indefinite perioid of maintenance with fewer drugs to suppress infection.

Crohn's disease is a chronic low grade granulomatous inflammation of the terminal ileum or colon. The disease was first described by Crohn, Ginzberg, and Oppenheimer in 1932. At that time, a mycobacterial etiology was suspected because the inflammatory disease resembled intestinal tuberculosis clinically and pathologically although no caseating granulomas or acid fast bacilli could be demonstrated in the tissues. After nearly 60 years of efforts to find the infectious agent, recent preliminary data has implicated NTM, particularly *M. avium,* in the disease. Despite the preliminary nature of the data, the similarities of Crohn's disease to other mycobacterial intestinal diseases, the familial occurrences, the ectopic sites of disease often occurring concurrently with intestinal infection, and recurrence of the disease at the resection margins points to the disease having a mycobacterial etiology.

BIBLIOGRAPHY

Bailey, W. C., Albert, R. K., Davidson, P. T., Farer, L. S., Glassroth, J., Kendig, E., Loridan, R. G., and Inselman, L. S.: Treatment of tuberculosis and other mycobacterial diseases. Am. Rev. Respir. Dis. 127:790, 1983.

Busillo, P. C., Lessnau, K., Sajana, V., Soumakis, S., Davidson, M., Mullen, M. P., Talavera, W.: Multidrug resistant *Mycobacterium* tuberculosis in patients with human immunodeficiency virus infection. Chest 102:797, 1992.

Dutt, A. K., and Snead, W. W.: Present chemotherapy for tuberculosis. J. Infect. Dis. 146:698, 1982.

Kim, T. C., Blackman, R. S., Heatwole, K. M., Kim, T., and Rochester, D. F.: Acid-fast bacilli in sputum smears of patients with pulmonary tuberculosis. Am. Rev. Respir. Dis. 129:264, 1984.

Bloom, B. L., and Mehra, V.: Immunologic unresponsiveness in leprosy. Immunol. Rev. 80:5, 1984.

Collins, F. M.: Mycobacterial disease, immunosuppression and acquired immunodeficiency syndrome. Clin. Micro. Rev. 2:360, 1987.

Leysen, D. C., Haemers, A., and Pattyn, S. R.: Mycobacteria and the new quinolones. Antimicrob. Agents Chemother. 33:1, 1989.

MacDonnell, K. B., and Glassroth, J.: *Mycobacterium avium* complex and other nontuberculous mycobacteria in patients with HIV infection. Semin. Respir. Infect. 4:123, 1989.

Stanford, J. L., Rook, G. A., Bahr, G. M., Dowleti, Y., Ganapati, R., Ghazi Saidi, K., Lucas, S., Ramu, G., Torres, P., Minh, Ly, H., et al.: *Mycobacterium vaccae* in immunoprophylaxis and immunotherapy of leprosy and tuberculosis. Vaccine 8:525, 1990.

12 Enterobacteriaceae and Vibrionaceae

Eugene A. Gorzynski

CHAPTER OUTLINE

Enterobacteriaceae

Vibrionaceae

Laboratory diagnosis of gram-negative infections

ENTEROBACTERIACEAE

During the past 35 years, there has been a gradual decline in the frequency of infectious diseases caused by certain pathogenic bacteria. Whereas serious, life-threatening infections caused by these bacteria still exist, diagnosis, treatment, and management have benefited from new techniques in laboratory medicine, from the marketing of new and effective antimicrobial agents, and from the introduction of devices that monitor the patient's progress during treatment and recovery. Although rapid diagnosis and specific treatment are welcome benefits that reduce hospital stay and prolong life, these same benefits frequently play a major role in altering the patient's capacity to accept and survive new challenges to well-being. Many invasive devices and heroic measures designed to prolong or improve the quality of life, may reduce innate or acquired competency to resist infection. Until competency is restored, the compromised patient remains inordinately susceptible to microbial agents, including saprophytic commensals, and even to

the host's normal or indigenous microbial flora. This chapter addresses the microorganisms associated with the intestinal tract and their role in disease.

NORMAL FLORA, LARGE INTESTINE

Microorganisms encountered in the colon (Table 12–1) of the healthy human being are responsible for many infections that ensue in the compromised individual. Significantly, by the second to third year of life, an individual has more bacteria per gram of feces (about 10^{11}) than found in any other site; 95 to 98 percent of these are anaerobes and outnumber by 1000:1 to 10,000:1 the facultative anaerobes (e.g., *Escherichia coli*) present. Of the microorganisms listed in Table 12–1, only members of the family Enterobacteriaceae will be considered in this chapter.

TAXONOMY

Fifteen years ago, there were 11 genera and 26 species in the family Enterobacteriaceae. At present, 26 genera and 100 species are assigned to this family of enteric bacteria. More than 99 percent of clinical isolates belong to only 23 species. Of the latter, *E. coli, Klebsiella pneumoniae*, and *Proteus mirabilis* are responsible for most infections caused by Enterobacteriaceae.

GENERAL CHARACTERISTICS

The family Enterobacteriaceae is composed of gram-negative, aerobic and facultatively anaerobic, rod-shaped bacteria that do not produce spores. Many species have flagella; nonmotile variants of motile species may be encountered. Nitrates are reduced to nitrites and glucose is used fermentatively. The percentages of positive reactions to identifying or differentiating biochemical substrates are shown in Table 12–2.

TABLE 12–1 ✦ Normal Flora: Large Intestine

Staphylococcus epidermidis	*Pseudomonas aeruginosa*
Staphylococcus aureus	*Alcaligenes faecalis*
Viridans streptococci	*Bacteroides* sp.
Enterococcus sp.	*Fusobacterium* sp.
Streptococcus pyogenes*	*Actinomyces* sp.
Peptostreptococcus sp.	*Candida* sp.
Lactobacillus sp.†	Protozoans
Corynebacterium sp.	Viruses
Enterobacteriaceae	Bacteriophages
Mycobacterium sp.	*Mycoplasma* sp.

*Occasionally.
†Especially in infants.

179

TABLE 12–2 ✦ Biochemical Reactions of Enterobacteriaceae Causing Human Infections Most Frequently (% Positive)

ENTEROBACTERIACEAE	INDOLE PRODUCTION	METHYL RED	VOGES PROSKAUER	CITRATE (SIMMONS)	H₂S PRODUCTION	UREA HYDROLYSIS	LYSINE DECARBOXYLASE	ARGININE DIHYDROLASE	ORNITHINE DECARBOXYLASE	MOTILITY AT 36°C	D-GLUCOSE, GAS	LACTOSE FERMENTATION	SUCROSE FERMENTATION	D-MANNITOL FERMENTATION
Citrobacter freundii	5	100	0	95	80	70	0	65	20	95	95	50	30	99
Citrobacter diversus	99	100	0	99	0	75	0	65	99	95	98	35	45	100
Enterobacter aerogenes	0	5	98	95	0	2	98	0	98	97	100	95	100	100
Enterobacter cloacae	0	5	100	100	0	65	0	97	96	95	100	93	97	100
Escherichia coli	98	99	0	1	1	1	90	17	65	95	95	95	50	98
Hafnia alvei	0	40	85	10	0	4	100	6	98	85	98	5	10	99
Klebsiella pneumonia	0	10	98	98	0	95	98	0	0	0	97	98	99	99
Klebsiella oxytoca	99	20	95	95	0	90	99	0	0	0	97	100	100	99
Morganella morganii	98	97	0	0	5	98	0	0	98	95	90	1	0	0
Proteus mirabilis	2	97	50	65	98	98	0	0	99	95	96	2	15	0
Proteus vulgaris	98	95	0	15	95	95	0	0	0	95	85	2	97	0
Providencia rettgeri	99	93	0	95	0	98	0	0	0	94	10	5	15	100
Providencia stuartii	98	100	0	93	0	30	0	0	0	85	0	2	30	0
Providencia alcalifaciens	99	99	0	98	0	0	0	0	1	96	85	0	15	2
Salmonella typhi	0	100	0	0	97	0	98	3	0	97	0	1	0	100
Salmonella paratyphi A	0	100	0	0	10	0	0	15	95	95	99	0	0	100
Salmonella, most serotypes	1	100	0	95	95	1	98	70	97	95	96	1	1	100
Shigella sonnei	0	100	0	0	0	0	0	2	98	0	0	2	1	99
Shigella serogroups A, B, C	50	100	0	0	0	0	0	5	1	0	2	0	0	93
Yersinia enterocolitica	50	97	2	0	0	75	0	0	95	2	5	5	95	98
Yersinia pestis	0	80	0	0	0	5	0	0	0	0	0	0	0	97
Yersinia pseudotuberculosis	0	100	0	0	0	95	0	0	0	0	0	0	0	100

Data from Farmer et al: J. Clin. Microbiol. 21:46, 1985.

Requirements for Pathogenicity

Bacteria vary significantly in their capacity to cause disease (i.e., in their pathogenicity). The degree of pathogenicity or virulence reflects not only the particular microbial species or strain per se, but also the number of these required to produce infection. To avoid confusion, the adjectives "pathogenic" and "virulent" may be used as synonyms. That is, one may characterize a microorganism as being either more or less pathogenic or more or less virulent under certain conditions. The major requirements for pathogenicity (virulence) can be addressed according to the microorganism's ability to (1) colonize the host, (2) penetrate mucous surfaces, (3) invade and multiply in tissue, (4) circumvent or inhibit local or systemic defense mechanisms, and (5) directly or indirectly cause damage. The requirements are summarized in Table 12–3.

Determinants of Pathogenicity
ADHESINS

These macromolecules are on the surface or appendages of many bacteria and promote attachment to specific receptors on some eukaryotic cells. Adhesins may reside on fimbriae (nonflagellar, proteinaceous, filamentous appendages), pili (filamen-

tous appendages involved in the conjugative transfer of DNA), or glycocalyx (a loose network of fibrils extending outward from the cell). The microbial flora identified as normal in certain body sites (skin, oral cavity, intestinal tract) reflects selective colonization by microorganisms bearing adhesins; a portion of the bacterium is adsorbed to the animal-cell surface while the remaining portion divides and releases its progeny. Studies in oral microbiology have contributed significantly to our knowledge of colonization and the persistence of microorganisms despite the flushing action of oral (saliva) and lumen (e.g., intestinal) contents. Desquamation of surface epithelial cells, releasing both cells and adherent bacteria, contributes to host defense against pathogens. Also, intercepting bacterial adsorption by blocking or neutralizing specific-receptor loci with antibodies, mannose-binding plant protein (concanavalin A), secreted glycoproteins, or antimicrobial agents has clinical applicability.

ENDOTOXINS

The cell walls of gram-negative bacteria contain the following three components outside of the peptidoglycan layer: lipoprotein, outer membrane, and lipopolysaccharide. The lipoprotein stabilizes the outer membrane by anchoring it to the peptidogly-

TABLE 12–3 ✦ Requirements for Pathogenicity

PROGRESSION	COMMENTS
Colonization	The establishment and growth of an exogenous microbial strain on or in a host; clinical manifestations or immune responses may or may not ensue.
Penetration	Whereas any microorganism can invade tissue damaged by burn or trauma, most gain access after initial colonization of mucosal surfaces of the respiratory, alimentary, and urogenital tract. Normally, mucosal surfaces are protected from invasion by the (1) normal microbial flora, (2) bactericidal or bacteriostatic influences present in mucous secretions, (3) mechanical flushing of lumen contents, including mucus. However, some bacteria produce substances that enhance adsorption to mucosal surfaces or promote phagocytosis by surface cells, which protects against the flushing action of lumen contents.
Multiplication in vivo	To produce infection, bacteria must multiply on mucosal surfaces or within the host's tissue. However, multiplication is initiated and continues only when the nutritional conditions are favorable and the microorganism either circumvents or fails to stimulate host defense mechanisms.
Inhibition of host defenses	Aggressins are products of bacterial growth that inhibit host defense mechanisms, e.g., bactericidal factors present in body fluids, action of phagocytes (mobilization, contact, ingestion, intracellular killing). In addition, cytoplasmic factors or endotoxins of gram-negative bacteria may interfere with humoral or cell-mediated immunity. The clinical outcome depends on the results of interplay between the microorganism and its host's or tissue environment.
Damage to the host	Species of *Enterobacteriaceae* can harm the host by one or several of the following: (1) production of exotoxin, (2) liberation of endotoxin, (3) elicitation of hypersensitivity responses to continued or subsequent infection by the identical pathogen.

can layer; the outer membrane protects enteric bacteria from bile salts and hydrolytic enzymes of the host environment; the lipopolysaccharide (LPS) is composed of a polysaccharide attached to a potent nonprotein toxin, a complex lipid called lipid A. The polysaccharide of LPS represents the major surface (O) antigen of the bacterial cell; specificity of antigen is conferred by terminal repeat units (linear trisaccharides or branched tetra- or pentasaccharides) that branch from a core polysaccharide constant in all species of Enterobacteriaceae. The endotoxin moiety is stable at 100°C; it can be extracted with phenol water from intact cells and further separated into lipid A and polysaccharide components by mild acid hydrolysis. Significantly, both in vitro and in situ, LPS is liberated when bacteria lyse. The pathophysiologic effects are similar, independent of enterobacterial origin, and range from self-limited fever, at one extreme, to refractory endotoxic shock. Major biologic effects are presented in Table 12–4.

ENTEROTOXINS

These are extracellular toxins (exotoxins), protein in character, and intrinsically different from cell-wall endotoxins. In contradistinction to the latter, enterotoxins

1. Do not cause fever in the host
2. Are unstable at temperatures above 60°C
3. Stimulate the formation of enterotoxin-neutralizing antibodies (antitoxins)
4. Are excreted by living cells
5. Are toxic to laboratory animals in nanogram amounts
6. Activate adenyl cyclase present in the intestinal epithelial membrane causing a rise in intracellular cyclic adenosine monophosphate (cAMP) levels and, accordingly, affect electrolyte transport

Exotoxin production has been demonstrated by many strains of enteric bacteria *(Vibrio cholerae, V. parahaemolyticus, Yersinia enterocolitica, Escherichia coli, Shigella dysenteriae, Klebsiella*

TABLE 12–4 ✦ Biologic Effects of Enterobacterial Lipopolysaccharide

EFFECT	COMMENT
Fever	Caused by release of endogenous pyrogen from polymorphonuclear leukocytes
Leukopenia	Within minutes after the administration of LPS, the number of leukocytes per mm³ may be reduced more than 70%, leukopenia is transient
Leukocytosis	Occurs after initial (transient) leukopenia
Phagocytosis	Enhanced by small doses; depressed by large doses
Complement activation	In vitro, via the alternative pathway; however, lysis of endotoxin coated erythrocytes likely does require the classical pathway
Macrophage activation	Results in markedly augmented, nonspecific microbicidal activity
Elicitation of Shwartzman phenomenon	Subcutaneous injection into a rabbit of a few micrograms of LPS causes slight inflammation at the site of administration. If, 24 hours later, the same amount of any LPS is injected intravenously, a hemorrhagic or necrotic lesion appears within a few hours at the skin site injected initially.
Activation of intravascular coagulation	A very serious consequence of endotoxin intoxication. Fibrin deposition in the microcirculation of vital organs contributes significantly to ensuing death. Heparin, administered prophylactically during sepsis, may ameliorate an untoward intravascular reaction.
Adjuvant activity	Similar to other adjuvants (Freund's, alum, aluminum hydroxide, dextran sulfate), LPS enhances the immunogenicity of adsorbed soluble proteins. Macrophage and T (helper) cell activities are increased by most adjuvants. LPS is a polyclonal B cell activator and, likely, promotes proliferation of B cells.
Altered resistance to infection	Endotoxin affects resistance to bacterial infection nonspecifically. Whereas large doses depress phagocytosis and resistance, small doses enhance both phagocytosis and synthesis of antibody. To an appropriate dose, the response is biphasic (i.e., depression followed by enhancement as the concentration in situ decreases).
Endotoxemia	Toxemia that follows the administration or acquisition of a large amount of LPS presents hypoglycemia, high blood lactate/pyruvate ratios, and decreased tissue oxygen utilization. As noted previously, other events occur simultaneously or progressively. Irreversible shock and death are predictable sequelae.

pneumoniae, species of *Citrobacter* and *Enterobacter*) and even *Pseudomonas aeruginosa.* The exotoxins of *E. coli* and *V. cholerae* have characteristics in common and will be addressed later.

CAPSULAR POLYSACCHARIDES

Certain species of Enterobacteriaceae have capsules composed of polysaccharide antigens that are external to the O antigens of LPS. The extracellular layer of capsule provides a good means of circumventing host defense and, as a result, contributes to the pathogenic asset of the microorganism per se, by shielding against the bactericidal action of complement and phagocytes. In *E. coli,* the capsular antigen is called K. Specific K determinants are numbered; K-12 antigen is often encountered in *E. coli* causing urinary tract infection; *E. coli* containing K-1 is a significant cause of neonatal meningitis. Certain K antigens of *E. coli* cross-react; e.g., K-12 with K-14. Also, other K antigens of *E. coli* bear strong similarities to polysaccharide antigens present in species of other genera; e.g., *E. coli* K-27 with *Klebsiella* K antigen; *E. coli* K-14 with the capsular polysaccharide of *Neisseria meningitidis* group 29-E. It is of interest that the capsular polysaccharide of *N. meningitidis* Group B (see Chapter 10) and K-1 of *E. coli* have an identical structure and are etiologic agents of the same disease, neonatal meningitis. The latter is an excellent example of intergeneric identity (or structural relatedness) and pathogenicity.

PLASMIDS

Extrachromosomal genetic elements composed of circular, double-stranded DNA molecules, distinct from the chromosomes of the bacterial host, are called plasmids. The following are characteristics or markers attributable to plasmids:

1. Production of enterotoxin
2. Production of beta hemolysin
3. Production of bacteriocins
4. Resistance to antimicrobial agents
5. Unique or altered metabolic activity
6. Physiologic mechanisms that mediate bacterial mating (conjugation)

A plasmid may replicate autonomously, in synchrony with its bacterial-host chromosome, or integrate with the latter chromosome and replicate as a single unit (replicon) and, by conjugation, transfer donor characteristics or markers to recipients of the same or heterogeneric species.

BACTERIOCINS

These are proteins produced by many gram-negative microorganisms that have antimicrobial properties active against other strains of the same bacterial species. Bacteriocins are named according to respective bacterial hosts; for example, marcescins *(Serratia marcescens),* colicins *(Escherichia coli),* and pyocins *(Pseudomonas aeruginosa,* formerly *P. pyocyaneus).* Bacteriocins are encoded by plasmid genes and are nonconjugative. After release from host cells, bacteriocins attach to specific receptors on susceptible cells and induce a specific metabolic block, that is, cessation of nucleic acid or protein synthesis, or of oxidative phosphorylation; the recipient cell dies. Bacteria can be identified or "typed" according to their susceptibility to a specific bacteriocin.

SUMMARY

Enterobacteriaceae vary in their capacity to cause infection; this variation occurs not only among species of the same genus but also among strains of the same species. Pathogenicity is highly polygenic. That is, it requires the action of several different genes and can be affected by mutation or changes in a microorganism's nutrition, growth rate, or environment. The degree of pathogenicity is determined by virulence factors, that is, by inheritable or transmissible toxins and by surface molecules that are antiphagocytic or promote adsorption to susceptible eukaryotic cells. Virulence can be measured under appropriately controlled laboratory conditions. As a result, by manipulating the physiologic requirements or determinants of a microbial strain and by addressing routes of administration to a suitable animal host, specific factors can be characterized, modes of action can be predicted, and modulation by chemotherapeutic intervention can be studied.

Antigenic Structure

The etiologic agent of an enterobacterial disease can be identified with a measurable degree of certainty by biochemical tests (see Table 12–2). Usually, appropriate treatment and management of an infected patient will be started after identification is made by biochemical profile. To confirm the identification of an isolate for therapeutic, epidemiologic, or academic reasons, an analysis of the bacterium's antigenic structure or composition may be required. This is accomplished by serologic typing; that is, by employing antisera containing antibodies directed against antigenic determinants on a microorganism, its fraction, or substrate. The antigens of Enterobacteriaceae are classified under three main groups: somatic (O antigens), flagellar (H antigens), capsular (K antigens).

SOMATIC (O) ANTIGENS

These are complexes located on the most external part of the cell wall lipopolysaccharide.

Specificity is determined by the nature of the terminal groups and the order in which these groups occur in the repeating units of the polysaccharide chain. Eighteen different monosaccharides have been identified in certain genera; some species have as many as nine.

Somatic antigens of Enterobacteriaceae are stable at 100°C and are resistant to ethanol and dilute acid. Whereas each genus of the family Enterobacteriaceae is characterized by the presence of certain O antigens, species may carry one or several additional O antigens. Moreover, species of different genera may share O (heterogeneric) antigens. For example, most Enterobacteriaceae share the O14 antigen with *E. coli*. Therefore, on the basis of determining the presence of both generic and species antigens, a microorganism can be identified serologically to species level if one uses care to preclude or account for cross-reactions.

FLAGELLAR (H) ANTIGENS

These proteins, called flagellins, are found in flagella. Specificity is determined by amino acid content and by the order in which these acids occur in the flagellins. Flagellins are heat-labile, inactivated by ethanol, and form loosely knit floccular aggregates in the presence of anti-H antibodies. Unless removed chemically or destroyed by heat, H antigens may interfere with the serologic detection of the microorganism's O antigen. Uniquely, in the genus *Salmonella,* a reversible variation (phase variation) of H antigen(s) may occur. In phase variation, the antigenic identity of flagellin may shift during culture of a flagellated species from a specific (homologous) to a nonspecific (heterologous) serotype. The shift designations are called phase 1 (specific) and phase 2 (nonspecific). On further subculturing the phases may shift back and forth. Not all salmonellae are diphasic; some are irreversibly monophasic, others are multiphasic.

CAPSULAR (K) ANTIGENS

Capsules, if present, are topographically external to the somatic antigens of Enterobacteriaceae. Most capsules are composed of polysaccharide that protect the bacterial cell against the bactericidal action of phagocytes and complement. Like flagellin, capsular antigen is heat-labile and may interfere with O agglutination by anti-O antibodies. Many antigenically different K antigens have been identified; they are labeled numerically. As noted earlier, certain K antigens are associated with virulence (e.g., *E. coli* with K1 antigen is a frequent cause of neonatal meningitis). Also, some species of *Salmonella* possess a capsular antigen, called Vi, that may be associated with invasiveness. Of note, a Vi-related antigen has been reported for certain serotypes of *Citrobacter,* a genus with species less frequently associated with invasive disease.

ENTEROBACTERIAL COMMON ANTIGEN (ECA)

This heat-stable, ethanol-soluble antigen exists in one or both of two forms in species of Enterobacteriaceae; one form is immunogenic in laboratory animals and the other is "nonimmunogenic," although both forms contain the identical antigenic determinant. The immunogenic form is present in only few bacterial species, probably covalently linked to LPS; *E. coli* O14 is the prototype. The "nonimmunogenic" form is present in most other species of Enterobacteriaceae. Significantly, after separation from LPS by ethanol extraction, the "nonimmunogenic" form elicits anti-ECA antibodies that may protect against infection induced against heterologous enteric species containing ECA. Taxonomically, a determination that a microorganism produces ECA may be a significant aid to assigning a new species to the family Enterobacteriaceae.

Clinical Infection

Whereas a few enterobacterial species have always been characterized as causes of overt intestinal infection, it is likely that all species of Enterobacteriaceae have the capability of causing infection outside of the intestinal tract. It is important to emphasize, however, that the mere presence of enteric microorganisms in urine, sputum, wounds, burns, or specimens obtained from normally sterile body fluid (e.g., blood, peritoneal, cerebrospinal) does not indicate the unequivocal cause of disease. These microorganisms may be contaminants or may represent a transient population of commensal or saprophytic microbial strains. Definition of the (potential) role these microorganisms play requires clinical judgment supported by the careful and timely acquisition of appropriate specimens, and laboratory data obtained from tests that are sensitive and provide specific and quality-controlled information. In the subsequent sections, the Enterobacteriaceae most frequently encountered in human disease will be addressed. General morphologic and physiologic attributes were presented in the previous section on general characteristics in Table 12–2.

ESCHERICHIA COLI

This is the most prominent aerobic species in the large bowel. Whereas more than 150 serotypes have been identified, only a few serotypes or strains have been shown to cause intestinal disease or to produce enterotoxin. The presence of *E. coli,* regardless of serotype, outside its host (e.g., food, water, soil, solutions, instruments, and devices) always indicates fecal contamination. The presence in clinical specimens may indicate contamination, colonization, or infection.

Intestinal Disease

Infantile Diarrhea. At least 12 antigenic types (e.g., O111, O55, O26, and O127) have been identified as causes of severe, life-threatening diarrhea in infants. Responsible strains are designated by the acronym EPEC (enteropathogenic *E. coli*). EPEC strains do not cause intestinal disease in older children or adults; therefore, except in outbreaks of infantile diarrhea, serotyping is not indicated.

Traveler's Diarrhea. Enterotoxin-producing strains of *E. coli*, designated ETEC, are responsible for a diarrhea, milder than infantile diarrhea and usually self-limited, that may affect people traveling abroad or relocating to a different geographic area. ETEC strains produce one or each of two kinds of enterotoxins; a heat-labile toxin (LT), which resembles the toxin of *Vibrio cholerae,* and a heat-stable toxin (ST). LT activates adenyl cyclase; ST activates guanyl cyclase. The toxins are active in the small bowel and, likely, in the colon. Enterotoxin production is mediated by plasmids.

Hemorrhagic Colitis. *E. coli* serotype 0157:H7 produces a unique toxin called verotoxin, which is associated with diarrhea, hemorrhagic colitis, and hemolytic-uremic syndrome. Verotoxin has characteristics of structure and mode of action in common with Shigella toxin, which will be discussed later.

Extraintestinal Infection. Of the more than 150 serotypes, about 10 percent are encountered most frequently in urinary tract, meningeal, wound, postsurgical, and peritoneal infections caused by *E. coli*. The presence of a particular capsular polysaccharide antigen (K-1) is associated with pyelonephritis and neonatal meningitis. Of interest are reports of immunochemical similarity between certain *E. coli* K antigens and capsular antigens of other invasive microorganisms, e.g., *Haemophilus influenzae* (serotype b), *Neisseria*

meningitidis (serogroups B and C), and several serotypes of *Streptococcus pneumoniae*.

SHIGELLA

This genus contains four species. Significant characteristics are presented in Table 12–5. It is noteworthy that, in contrast to most other enterobacterial causes of intestinal infections, shigellae are not motile. All species are pathogens and cause bacillary dysentery (shigellosis) in humans. The infective dose is low, less than 10^3 microorganisms. Shigellosis is transmitted by the fecal-oral route, primarily by hand to mouth contact. Outdoor latrines and the density of flies can be related to the occurrence of bacillary dysentery. Usually, infections are limited to the terminal ileum and the colon, where mucosal ulcerations, covered by a pseudomembrane, evolve after initial invasion of intestinal epithelial cells. Endotoxic lipopolysaccharide, released upon autolysis of shigellae, likely contributes to the death of epithelial cells. Rarely do *Shigella* species invade the blood stream or cause infection at sites other than the intestinal tract. *S. dysenteriae* produces a heat-labile exotoxin that is both neurotoxic and enterotoxic.

Bacillary dysentery has a brief incubation period (less than 4 days) and is characterized by a sudden onset of abdominal pain, diarrhea, and fever. The loss of water and salts may cause dehydration and electrolyte imbalance. Mucus and blood in feces are common findings.

During convalescence, most persons develop fecal (copro) and humoral antibodies; these do not protect against reinfection.

ENTEROBACTER

Species of this genus are found normally in 40 to 80 percent of fecal specimens obtained from human subjects. In examining food and water supplies for evidence of fecal contamination, it is important to distinguish *E. coli,* the index microorganism, from species of *Enterobacter*. The latter are found commonly on plants and can be differentiated from *E. coli* by biochemical tests (Table 12–6).

Enterobacter species may cause extraintestinal

TABLE 12–5 ✦ Species and Characteristics of *Shigella* Species

SPECIES	MOTILITY	GROUPS	TYPES	MANNITOL*	ORNITHINE DECARBOXYLASE*
S. dysenteriae	−	A	1 to 10	−	−
S. flexneri	−	B	1 to 6	+	−
S. boydii	−	C	1 to 15	+	−
S. sonnei	−	D	1	+	+

*− = 95% or more negative in 24 to 48 hours; + = 95% or more positive in 24 to 48 hours.

TABLE 12–6 ✦ **Percentages Positive Metabolic Reactions of *Escherichia coli* and Species of *Enterobacter***

	REACTIONS			
	I	**MR**	**VP**	**C**
Escherichia coli	96.3	99.1	0	0.2
Enterobacter				
aerogenes	0.8	1.6	100	92.6
cloacae	0	3.3	100	98.9

I = Indole formation in media containing tryptophan, MR = Methyl red as indicator of mixed acid fermentation, VP = Voges-Proskauer reaction, a color test for acetoin, a product of butylene glycol fermentation, C = Citrate as the only source of carbon

Reprinted by permission of the publisher from W. H. Ewing, Edwards and Ewing's Identification of Enterobacteriaceae, ed. 4. Appleton & Lange, Norwalk, Conn, 1986, Ch. 6, 9, and 14.

infections. Often they are isolated as secondary invaders or as opportunists from patients compromised by malignancy, instrumentation, or therapy. They have characteristics in common with species of *Klebsiella* (see next section), causes of respiratory and urinary tract infections, with major differences in susceptibility to antimicrobial agents.

KLEBSIELLA

This genus has seven species; *K. pneumoniae* (Friendlander's bacillus) and *K. oxytoca*, biochemically similar to *K. pneumoniae*, are the most frequent clinical isolates. *K. pneumoniae* is a major cause of community and hospital acquired infections. It is encapsulated and the most virulent *Klebsiella* species; varients (rough strains) are not virulent. Whereas *K. pneumoniae* may be found in the respiratory tract and feces of healthy individuals, it is a significant cause of acute bacterial pneumonia and, next to *E. coli*, the most common cause of urinary tract infection. Because of its capsule

(K antigen), *K. pneumoniae* produces large, moist, mucoid colonies on nutrient media. In situ, these capsules preclude phagocytosis and interfere with antimicrobial therapy.

Unlike *K. pneumoniae*, *K. oxytoca* produces indole in media containing tryptophan. Although not a frequent pathogen, *K. oxytoca* has been recovered from blood, urine, wounds, and sputum; it may be found in feces of healthy hosts. Administration of an aminoglycoside or a cephalosporin or, in severe cases, a combination of both antimicrobic agents, remains the most effective therapy of klebsiellae infections. As a rule, antimicrobials should be used only after susceptibility tests have been performed and only when indicated.

SALMONELLA

This genus has three species: *typhi* (one serotype), *choleraesuis* (one serotype), and *enteritidis* (more than 1800 serotypes). Serotypes reflect the presence of one to several major and none to several minor O antigens. Serotypes with the same major O antigens are placed in the same lettered O serogroup. Representative antigenic formulas of salmonellae are shown in Table 12–7. Whereas *Salmonella* serotypes are not species, reporting these microorganisms as species is a convenient way to avoid long names; for example, *S. enteritidis* serotype *typhimurium* may be reported simply as *S. typhimurium*. Approximately 95 percent of the *Salmonella* serotypes causing human infection belong to the five serogroups shown in Table 12–8. The 10 serotypes isolated most frequently are presented in Table 12–8 according to median age of infected persons. For diagnostic, management, and epidemiologic reasons, identifying *Salmonella* species by serotyping is important. The application of molecular and biologic methods to epidemiologic studies assists in identifying the antigenic serotypes in salmonellae outbreaks.

In humans, species of *Salmonella* cause the clinical diseases summarized in Table 12–9. Independent of source or mode of transmission, the mean

TABLE 12–7 ✦ **Representative Antigenic Formulae of *Salmonella* Species**

SEROGROUP	SEROTYPE ("SPECIES")	0	H1	H2
A	*S. paratyphi* A	1,2,12	a	—
B	*S. typhimurium*	1,4,5,12	i	1,2
C	*S. choleraesuis*	6,7	c	1,5
D	*S. typhi*	9,12,Vi*	d	—
E	*S. anatum*	3,10	e,h	1,6

H1 = Phase 1 flagellar antigen(s), H2 = Phase 2 flagellar antigen(s).

*Vi may not be present.

Reprinted by permission of the publisher from W. H. Ewing, Edwards and Ewing's Identification of Enterobacteriaceae, ed. 4. Appleton & Lange, Norwalk, Conn, 1986, Ch. 6, 9, and 14.

TABLE 12–8 ✦ Serotypes of *Salmonella* Isolated Most Frequently from Humans

SEROTYPE	NO. OF ISOLATES	PERCENTAGE OF TOTAL	MEDIAN AGE OF PERSONS FROM WHOM ISOLATES WERE OBTAINED
S. typhimurium	12,176	34.2	8.0
S. enteritidis	2,554	7.2	19.0
S. newport	2,134	6.0	15.0
S. heidelberg	2,049	5.8	4.0
S. infantis	1,497	4.2	5.0
S. agona	1,205	3.4	2.0
S. saint-paul	861	2.4	17.5
S. montevideo	739	2.1	18.5
S. muenchen	644	1.8	15.5
S. typhi	604*	1.7	26.0
Subtotal†	24,463	68.8	
Total *Salmonella*	35,625		12.0

*38 (6.3%) of the 604 isolates of *S. typhi* were from carriers, 195 (32.3%) from overt infections, and the remaining 371 (61.4%) undesignated.

†Most frequent isolates.

Reprinted by permission of the New England Journal of Medicine, from Morbidity and Mortality Weekly Report 31/No. 45; November 1982.

infecting dose usually is high, 10^6 to 10^8 microorganisms. As expected in individuals compromised by age, diet, underlying disease, or environment, the infectious dose may be lower—for example, 10^3 or less. Additional salient features of salmonellosis are as follows.

Enterocolitis. This is the most common manifestation of infection by salmonellae (see Table 12–8). Although any serotype of *S. enteritidis* may cause this condition, *S. typhimurium* is responsible most frequently (about 34 percent).

Nausea, vomiting, profuse diarrhea, and low-grade fever are the most common symptoms. Most infections are self-limited; moreover, antimicrobial treatment may prolong excretion of the etiologic agent.

Enteric Fever (Typhoid). After ingestion, microorganisms infect the small intestine and invade the blood stream through lymphatics. After infecting many organs and multiplying in lymphatic tissue, these microorganisms reach the intestine in large numbers and are expelled in the feces.

Usual symptoms include fever, constipation, prostration, abdominal tenderness and, frequently,

TABLE 12–9 ✦ Clinical Diseases Caused by *Salmonella* Species

OBSERVATION	ENTEROCOLITIS	ENTERIC FEVER	SEPTICEMIA
Etiology	*S. typhimurium*	*S. typhi*†	*S. choleraesuis*
Source	Animals*	Humans‡	Animals (swine)
Modes of transmission	Contaminated food, drink, direct contact, and insects (flies) as couriers		
Incubation period	1–2 days	7–14 days	Variable
Duration	2–5 days	18–32 days	Variable
Blood cultures	Negative	Positive during the initial 12–14 days	Positive
Stool cultures	Usually positive	Negative early in disease; positive after blood cultures become negative	Usually negative

*Turtles, poultry, pigs, rodents, and so on.

†*S. paratyphi* A causes less grave enteric fever with a briefer incubation period.

‡Most laboratory animals are resistant, unless the infectious dose is suspended in mucin.

distention; an enlarged spleen and leukopenia are also common. Rarely, intestinal hemorrhage and perforation of the bowel with subsequent peritonitis may occur with fatal sequelae.

Septicemia. This feature is characterized by an abrupt onset with high, remittent fever and bacteremia. Gastrointestinal involvement is not apparent. Focal suppurative lesions may develop in kidneys, heart, meninges, spleen, lungs and joints. The septicemia may be prolonged and is difficult to control by treating with antimicrobial agents active in vitro.

PROTEUS

Species of this genus are found commonly in sewage, manure, soil, and normal human feces. Owing to peritrichous flagella, *Proteus* species are actively motile; unless inhibited by chemicals (such as phenylethyl alcohol) incorporated in a medium, "swarming" on the medium's surface will occur, masking or covering colonies of other bacterial species that may be present.

Proteus species are frequent causes of urinary tract infection; the urine becomes alkaline, promoting stone formation and making acidification very difficult. The high pH results from the liberation of ammonia that occurs after the hydrolysis of urea by urease-producing species. Outside of the intestinal tract, species of *Proteus* may cause wound infections, pneumonia, and focal infections in debilitated patients. Although not an established cause of diarrhea, the number of *Proteus* species increases in patients receiving antimicrobial therapy or during diarrheal diseases caused by other microorganisms. *P. vulgaris,* which usually produces indole, is more resistant to antimicrobial agents than is *P. mirabilis.* The latter may be inhibited readily by a cephalosporin or an aminoglycoside; even a penicillin-like agent may be effective.

MORGANELLA

The single species of this genus, *morganii,* has been implicated as a cause of diarrhea. More significantly, it causes urinary tract infections and is recovered as a potential pathogen from many other body sites. Tests for indole, H_2S production, and ornithine decarboxylase activity are useful for separating *M. morganii* from species of *Proteus.*

PROVIDENCIA

Hospital-borne infections of the urinary tract occasionally are caused by a species of *Providencia,* either *stuartii* or *alcalifaciens.* The latter is present in the feces of healthy individuals. Whereas *P. alcalifaciens* is frequently isolated from feces of children with diarrheal gastroenteritis, its etiologic role has not been established. In contrast, *P. stuartii,* rarely found in feces, is a cause of infection in patients compromised by instrumentation, intensive antimicrobial treatment, or burns. In burn patients, septicemia and pneumonia are frequent complications.

YERSINIA

This genus has at least 10 species that have animals as their natural hosts. *Y. pestis, Y. enterocolitica,* and *Y. pseudotuberculosis* infect animals and, through insect vectors, humans.

Y. pestis. This is the etiologic agent of plague (black death), a disease that killed millions of people during pandemics of the 6th century A.D., of the 14th century, and at the close of the 19th century. Although plague declined worldwide during the first half of the 20th century, there has been a recent, gradual increase on various continents. In the United States, sylvatic (wild) plague is epizootic among pack rats, prairie dogs, squirrels, and rabbits. As a result, rare and sporadic cases in humans do occur, especially in western states (e.g., New Mexico, Arizona, and California) where certain sylvatic plague is epizootic.

Plague is transmitted among rodents and from rodents to humans through the bite of fleas infected by blood sucked from their infected hosts. From the bite, *Y. pestis* extends to regional lymph nodes via lymphatic channels. There is rapid and progressive hemorrhagic inflammation at the bite site, along the lymphatic channels, and in the infected lymph nodes. The nodes, most frequently located in the axilla or groin, become very large "bubos." This phase of infection is called bubonic plague. Often, infection progresses via efferent lymphatics and the thoracic duct to the blood and, as a consequence, to all organs of the host. Rapid proliferation in the blood is the septicemic form of plague. The parenchymatous lesions produced in infected organs are hemorrhagic; disseminated intravascular coagulation may ensue. If metastatic pneumonia (pneumonic plague) develops, the infection may be transmitted readily by droplets from the respiratory tract. Pneumonic plague is extraordinarily malignant and resistant to therapy, and prognosis is poor.

Strains of *Y. pestis* produce the following factors, which significantly influence virulence:

1. Fraction 1 (F1), an envelope (heat-labile protein) antigen
2. VW antigen, comprising a protein (V) and a lipoprotein (W)
3. Lipopolysaccharide (endotoxin)
4. Murine toxin, lethal to mice and rats but not to rabbits or monkeys
5. Enterobacterial common antigen (ECA)

It is important to note that both F1 and VW are antiphagocytic antigens; effective vaccines must contain both complexes.

Y. enterocolitica. This enterotoxigenic microorganism causes in humans a diffuse and severe enterocolitis with mucosal ulcers and mesenteric lymphadenitis. Symptoms simulate appendicitis and include fever, severe abdominal pain, and diarrhea. An outbreak affecting 218 children in Oneida County, New York, was traced to the consumption of contaminated chocolate milk (*Morbidity and Mortality Weekly Report,* a publication of United States Public Health Service, 18 February 1977).

Y. pseudotuberculosis. This microorganism, which has an extensive animal reservoir, may cause mesenteric lymphadenitis in children and young adults. Food and water contaminated by animal excreta appear to be the main modes of transmission. However, institutional outbreaks suggest transmission also through direct contact with infected patients.

HAFNIA ALVEI

Compared with other Enterobacteriaceae, this microorganism is less frequently encountered as a cause of extraintestinal infection. Until recently, the species *alvei* was classified under the genus *Enterobacter.*

CITROBACTER

The two species, *freundii* and *diversus,* are well-recognized human pathogens found to be primary or secondary causes of a variety of diseases in humans compromised by age or invasive procedures. Certain strains of *C. freundii* produce H_2S and therefore may be confused with species of *Salmonella.* Differentiation is made by biochemical tests.

SERRATIA MARCESCENS

This microorganism, long considered a harmless saprophyte, has emerged as a significant cause of opportunistic, nosocomial, and iatrogenic infections, with bacteriuria, wound infections, pneumonia, and septicemia as serious sequelae, especially in patients compromised by age, malignancy, or therapy. Its relative frequency as a cause of sepsis is 5 to 7 percent. *S. marcescens* may produce an intense red pigment in culture; more frequently, nonpigmented variants are isolated as etiologic agents.

Highlights of the Enterobacteriaceae associated with diarrhea are presented in Table 12–10.

VIBRIONACEAE

This family is composed of gram-negative, facultative, oxidase-positive, motile bacilli with predominantly polar flagellation when grown in a liquid medium and, frequently, peritrichous flagella when grown on a solid medium. Water sources are the normal habitats of representatives of this family. Several species of *Vibrio* and *Aeromonas* have clinical significance.

VIBRIO

Species are curved rods on initial culture and become straight, resembling Enterobacteriaceae,

TABLE 12–10 ✦ Bacterial Causes of Diarrhea: Highlights

ETIOLOGIC AGENT	SITE	SALIENT CHARACTERISTICS
Invasive		
Escherichia coli	Small bowel? colon?	EPEC; >12 antigenic types
Salmonella sp.	Small bowel, colon	*S. typhimurium* causes self-limiting gastroenteritis
Proteus sp.	?	May be responsible for diarrhea in patients receiving antibiotics
Noninvasive		
Shigella sp.	Ileum, colon	Infecting dose, <10^3; ulcers covered by pseudomembrane
Vibrio cholerae	Large bowel	Massive loss of fluid and electrolytes
Vibro parahaemolyticus	Large bowel	Self-limiting enteritis requiring restoration of fluid and electrolytes
Enterotoxin producers		
Escherichia coli	Small bowel, colon?	ETEC strains producing LT and/or ST; cause of traveler's diarrhea
Shigella dysenteriae	Small bowel, colon	Infecting dose, <10^3; neurotoxic
Yersinia enterocoliticia	Intestinal lymph nodes	Cause mucosal ulcers and mesenteric lymphadenitis; symptoms simulate appendicitis
Campylobacter jejuni	Proximal small intestine	Causes acute diarrhea; stools may contain blood and inflammatory cells

after prolonged or repeated cultivation. The microscopic recognition of curved gram-negative bacilli in a fresh, appropriately collected diarrheal sample may guide a preliminary report and subsequent speciation and treatment. *Vibrio* species are uncommon isolates in most inland laboratories in the United States; strains are encountered more frequently in laboratories serving coastal areas. Whereas 28 species of *Vibrio* have been characterized, 10 are considered human pathogens. Two, *V. cholerae* and *V. parahaemolyticus,* are encountered most frequently.

V. cholerae. This is the etiologic agent of cholera, endemic in India for centuries with periodic epidemics in Southeast Asia and China. Seven pandemics have been recorded since 1817; the most recent, in the 1960s, spread from Indonesia to the Far East, India, the Middle East, and Africa. Later, sporadic outbreaks were reported in several European nations bordering the Mediterranean Sea. In the United States, during recent years, sporadic cases and minor outbreaks have been reported from Louisiana, Florida, and Texas. Likely, *V. cholerae* now is endemic in the coastal waters of the Gulf of Mexico. Whereas the diagnosis of cholera during an epidemic presents no problem on the basis of clinical findings alone, sporadic or mild cases are not readily differentiated from other diarrheal infections. The high infecting dose (more than 10^8) required for infection likely contributes to its low prevalence in industrialized areas where water contaminated with feces, the primary mode of transmission, is monitored and controlled.

Cholera is not an invasive infection. Enterotoxigenic strains of *V. cholerae,* present in contaminated water supplies and marine food, multiply and remain localized in the intestinal tract; they do not invade the bloodstream. In the intestines, enterotoxin, endotoxin, and, likely, mucinases are released by the rapidly multiplying *V. cholerae.* The enterotoxin is adsorbed onto epithelial cell gangliosides; absorption of sodium is inhibited. Because of a hypersecretion of water and chloride, and the elution of fluid and electrolytes into the small intestine, massive diarrhea results 2 to 5 days after consuming a toxigenic dose of *V. cholerae.* The loss of luminal fluid, rice waterlike in appearance, may reach 10 to 15 liters per day; without intervention, dehydration, acidosis, shock, and death ensue. The prompt and adequate replacement of fluid and electrolytes is life-saving. Whereas the administration of antimicrobial agents may eliminate intestinal *V. cholerae,* only heroic rehydration and infusion of electrolytes will preclude shock and death.

V. parahaemolyticus. This is a halophilic microorganism (requiring 3 to 7 percent sodium chloride for growth) found in marine water and fauna throughout the world. It has been recovered from seafood (e.g., plankton, shellfish, and crustaceans); in Japan it is responsible for at least 70 percent of all cases of bacterial food poisoning. In the United States, *V. parahaemolyticus* is isolated from feces with increasing frequency as a cause of vomiting and diarrhea. The incubation period is brief: 12 to 24 hours after ingestion of contaminated seafood. The enteritis is self-limiting, usually requiring only the restoration of fluids and electrolytes.

AEROMONAS HYDROPHILIA

This microorganism, classified in the family *Vibrionaceae* because of its characteristic morphology, biochemical reactions, and ecology, may cause serious human infection. Although *A. hydrophilia* has been isolated from many body fluids without evidence of pathogenicity, it has been reported as a cause of septicemia, pneumonia, and gastroenteritis. Patients with severely impaired host defenses are most vulnerable.

Campylobacter

Formerly, on the basis of gram-negative, slightly curved, monotrichous morphology, species of this genus were considered vibrios that infected various animals, including sheep, cattle, poultry, and wild birds. During the past decade, classification at the species level has been undergoing changes. These changes reflect, in part, the fact that certain *Vibrio* species have different nucleotide-based compositions and are not able to use sugars either oxidatively or fermentatively. Accordingly, these species were placed in a new genus, *Campylobacter* instead of the family Vibrionaceae. At present, at least seven species of *Campylobacter* have been identified on the basis of DNA hybridization studies. At least two, *C. jejuni* and *C. fetus* subspecies *fetus* (formerly called subspecies *intestinalis*), are unequivocal human pathogens acquired by direct contact with infected animals or by consuming contaminated water or food. Human campylobacteriosis is manifested most frequently as a self-limiting gastroenteritis, usually due to *C. jejuni,* and infrequently as a systemic disease (bacteremia, endocarditis, pericarditis, arthritis), usually caused by *C. fetus* subspecies *fetus.* Recent reports implicate additional species of *Campylobacter* as causes of disease in humans.

Species of *Campylobacter* will not grow on simple nutrient media; they are fastidious and require enriched media supplemented with hemin, vitamin K, and 5 percent defibrinated sheep blood. A microaerophilic atmosphere (5 percent O_2, 5 percent CO_2, and 90 percent N_2) is required for growth. Duplicate sets of media should be inoculated for incubation in parallel at 25°C and 42°C; *C. fetus* subspecies *fetus* grows at 25°C and not 42°C, *C. jejuni* thrives better at 42°C than at 25°C. All *Campylobacter* species grow at 35°C to 37°C.

The highlights of the bacterial causes of diarrhea addressed in this chapter are presented in Table 12–10.

LABORATORY DIAGNOSIS OF GRAM-NEGATIVE INFECTIONS

Diagnosis of an infectious disease starts in the clinic or at the patient's bedside where a history is recorded, physical examination is undertaken, tentative diagnosis is made, and orders for specimen acquisition are written. Laboratory diagnosis ends when the primary care physician or dentist receives and assesses data or results from specimen analysis. It is obvious that the length of time between history-taking and the receipt of laboratory results depends on factors directly controlled by the clinician, healthcare personnel (including couriers of specimens), laboratorians, and the communication system. With certain exceptions, the laboratorian is unable to measure the integrity of a specimen; that is, whether or not the specimen was obtained from the proper site and under conditions that exclude or minimize contamination. The specimen will be examined and results reported according to routine protocol of the testing laboratory.

The most convincing way of identifying the etiologic agent of an infection is initiated by separating the (potential) pathogen from other microorganisms that may be present as contaminants or representatives of a normal flora. Usually, this is accomplished by spreading a minute sample of specimen over the surface of a nutrient agar medium. Frequently, on the basis of the morphology, color, and texture of bacterial colonies that form after the required period of incubation, and stained, microscopic characteristics of the microbial population, an experienced technologist can provide a presumptive identification to genus level. In many cases, knowledge of genus alone is sufficient for clinical decision making. Speciation, if required, is accomplished by interpreting the isolated microorganism's phenotypic characteristics, including biochemical and antigenic profiles.

The Enterobacteriaceae grow readily on simple nutrient media; isolation of species from normally sterile body sites presents no problem. However, media for specimens likely to contain mixtures of

TABLE 12–11 ✦ Media for Primary Isolation of Gram-Negative Enteric Bacilli

MICOORGANISM	MEDIA	INCUBATION		REMARKS
		°C	DAYS	
Escherichia, Enterobacter,	BA	35	1	
Klebsiella, Serratia	MC	35		On MC, colonies of lactose fermenting bacteria are pink to red.
Proteus	PEA	35	1	Gram-negative microorganisms other than *Proteus* are markedly or completely inhibited.
Salmonella, Shigella	BA	35	2	
	MC	35	2	Colorless colonies on MC.
	XLD	35	2	Red colonies on XLD; may have black center.
	HEK	35	2	Blue or blue-green colonies on HEK; may have black center.
Vibrio	TCBS	35	2	Yellow or blue colonies.
Yersinia enterocolitica	YSAB*	25	2	Red colonies.
	S	4	21	Transfer from S to YSAB once each week.
Campylobacter				
jejuni	CBA(B)	42	2	Requires atmosphere of 5% O_2,
fetus subsp. *fetus*	CBA(B)	35	2	5% CO_2, and 90% N_2; only *C. jejuni* will grow at both 25°C and 42°C

BA = blood agar, MC = MacConkey, PEA = phenylethyl alcohol agar, XLD = xylose-lysine-deoxycholate agar, HEK = hektoenteric agar, TCBS = thiosulfate-citrate-bile-sucrose agar, YSAB = yersinia selective agar base, S = saline, CBA(B) = campy blood agar (Blaser).
*Preferably supplemented with cefsulodin and novobiocin to improve inhibition of normal enteric bacteria

microorganisms (feces, saliva, sputum, urine, wound) should be selected on the basis of their ability to enhance growth when small numbers of Enterobacteriaceae are present, eliminate or reduce growth of normal flora or saprophytes, or provide distinguishing characteristics to bacterial colonies that form during incubation at an appropriate temperature. Media that may be employed to grow microorganisms addressed in this chapter are presented in Table 12–11.

Less sensitive and more costly, albeit more rapid, methods are available for detecting the presence of certain bacteria in selected specimens. Dedicated antisera or monospecific antibodies are used; detection is on the basis of recognizable antigen-antibody reactions. Whereas positive data may have clinical significance, if quality controlled reagents and protocols are employed, negative data do not rule out the presence, in small numbers, of a specified microorganism.

A retrospective diagnosis of a specific cause of infection, in the absence of successful culture, may be feasible by using serologic techniques; i.e., testing serum samples for the presence and concentration (titer) of antibodies against known antigens. However, resulting data may be difficult to interpret because of unaccountable or uncontrollable variables. For example, in the serodiagnosis of typhoid fever (Widal test) the following must be considered: (1) *Salmonella typhi* shares antigens with other Enterobacteriaceae; (2) anti-O and anti-H antibody titers to typhoid and other antigens may rise during unrelated febrile illness or in recently immunized individuals; (3) the predictive values of both elevated and low or unchanged titers depend upon the prevalence of similar titers in a given population or geographic area; (4) *S. typhi* antibodies may be absent or in low titer owing to the stage of infection, poor antigenic stimulus, immunoincompetence of the host, or nutritional hypoproteinemia; (5) the patient may have a history of typhoid infection or may have been specifically immunized; and (6) in endemic areas, significantly elevated titers are encountered during early stages of typhoid.

After the microbiologic cause of an infection is established, multiple antibiotics with specific or broad-spectrum designations are available for judicious use. However, the empirical or arbitrary use of a chemotherapeutic agent is never justified without knowledge of its potential efficacy and without considering its pharmacokinetics, effect on normal microbial flora, and cost.

BIBLIOGRAPHY

Balows A, Hausler W. J., Jr., Herrmann K. L., Isenberg H. D., and Shadomy H. J.: Manual of Clinical Microbiology. Am. Society of Microbiology, Washington, D.C., 1991, pp. 360–395.

Brenner, D.J., Farmer, J. J. III, Hickman, F. W., Asbury, M. A., and Steigewalt, A. G.: Taxonomic and Nomenclature Changes in Enterobacteriaceae. Centers for Disease Control, Atlanta, 1977, pp. 1–15.

Edwards, P. R., and Ewing, W. H.: Identification of Enterobacteriaceae. Ed 4. Elsevier Science Publishing Co., New York, 1986.

Farmer, J. J. III, Davis, B. R., Hickman-Brenner, F. W., McWhorter, A., Huntley-Carter, G. P., Asbury M. W., Riddle, C., Wathen-Grady, H. G., Ellis, C., Fanning, G. R., Steigerwalt, A. G., O'Hara, C. M., Morris, G. K., Smith, P. B., and Brenner, D. J.: Biochemical identification of new species and biotypes of *Enterobacteriaceae* isolated from clinical specimens. J. Clin. Microbiol. 21:46, 1985.

Urbaschek, B., Urbaschek, R., and Neter, E.: Gram-Negative Bacterial Infections. Springer-Verlag, New York, 1975, p. 8–15.

13 *Pseudomonadaceae*

Joseph J. Zambon and Russell J. Nisengard

CHAPTER OUTLINE

Characteristics

Habitat

Clinical significance

Transmission

The slime layer

Leukocidin

Control

The family of the Pseudomonadaceae is one of the most diverse in the microbial world and has very simple growth requirements.

The family consists of four genera of bacteria: *Pseudomonas, Xanthomonas, Frateuria,* and *Zoogloea* (Table 13–1). *Pseudomonas* species are pathogenic to humans, animals, and plants. *Xanthomonas,* while not pathogenic to humans, is an important plant pathogen. *Zoogloea* is found in polluted water and *Frateuria* species are associated with plants.

The organisms of the Pseudomonadaceae family are straight or curved gram-negative rods, motile via polar flagella, strictly aerobic chemo-organotrophs with a respiratory metabolism. They grow at temperatures ranging from 2°C to 45°C and are capable of utilizing diverse organic compounds as carbon and energy sources. They are catalase-positive and usually oxidase-positive. Since the most important genus is *Pseudomonas,* this chapter will concentrate on *P. aeruginosa.*

CHARACTERISTICS

Pseudomonas aeruginosa is a gram-negative rod, 0.5 to 1.0 μm wide by 3 to 4 μm long, motile by means of one to three polar flagella. The cell wall structure is similar to *Escherichia coli* except the lipid A moiety lacks β-hydroxymyristic acid and the carbohydrate side chain consists of amino rather than neutral sugars. The organism is a strict aerobe but can grow anaerobically if provided with an alternate electron acceptor (such as nitrate or arginine). Like other members of the family, it is catalase-positive and usually oxidase-positive and produces a variety of water-soluble pigments. It is, however, the only pseudomonad that produces a chloroform-soluble pigment (pyocyanin).

Clinical identification is based on cell and colony morphology, gram-stain reaction, odor (often described as a sweet, fruity odor), pigmentation, absence of spores, motility, mode of glucose utilization, production of certain enzymes, hydrogen sulfide production, carbohydrate utilization patterns, and growth temperature.

HABITAT

Pseudomonas can be routinely isolated from a wide range of sources including soil, ground water, a variety of foods, house plants, animals, humans, jet fuel, and various medical instruments (Table 13–2). Any moist environment can harbor *P. aeruginosa.* The organism's simple metabolic requirements enable it to grow in aquatic environments

TABLE 13–1 ✦ Family Pseudomonadaceae

GENUS	IMPORTANCE
Pseudomonas	Human pathogens, plant pathogens
Xanthomonas	
Frateuria	Plant organisms
Zoogloea	Polluted water

TABLE 13–2 ✦ Sources from Which
Pseudomonas aeruginosa **Has Been Isolated**

HOSPITALS	OTHER
Sink traps and drains	Faucet aerators
Ice machines	Water filters
Water pitchers	Soap dishes
Mops	Hand creams
Soiled linen	Medications
Respiratory equipment	Heated whirlpools
Turbo jets	Swimming pools
Nebulizers	Water filters
Medications	Water deionizers
	Disinfectants
	Hexachlorophene soaps
	Milk

where substrates are often very dilute. In fact, the organism can even grow in distilled water. The organism produces many extracellular enzymes, which enable it to take advantage of a diversity of soil components. The pigments of *P. aeruginosa* are potent antimicrobials. One pigment, pyocyanin, also decreases oxygen consumption by tissues and leukocytes. This organism is notorious for its antibiotic resistance, not surprising in view of the fact that the vast majority of the known antibiotics have been isolated from soil organisms. The slime layer of *P. aeruginosa* is protective against amebic predators and hydraulic forces and is antiphagocytic.

CLINICAL SIGNIFICANCE

Recently, there has been a significant increase in the number of infections involving *P. aeruginosa,* especially nosocomial infections. In fact, *P. aeruginosa* has now replaced *Staphylococcus aureus* as the primary cause of nosocomial infection. This change is caused by several factors including the inappropriate use of antibiotics. *P. aeruginosa* is resistant to many antibiotics and also acquires antibiotic resistance genes easily.

P. aeruginosa also is very resistant to many disinfectants, particularly phenolic-based disinfectants. The extensive use of disinfectants in the hospital where antibiotic use is also high, favors colonization by resistant organisms. Because of improved medical care, there are greater numbers of immunocompromised patients susceptible to *Pseudomonas* infection. The increased use of "hot tubs" and extended-wear contact lenses result in *Pseudomonas folliculitis* and ocular infection, respectively.

Pseudomonas infections have been associated with open root canals, removal of impacted molars, and oral surgery in the soft tissue and bones. They also have been associated with osteomyelitis of the mandible and maxilla. Virtually every tissue of the body is susceptible to infection by this organism.

Other species of *Pseudomonas* are known pathogens, including *P. cepacia, P. maltophilia, P. mallei, P. pseudomallei,* and *P. fluorescens. P. mallei* causes glanders in horses and donkeys and can be transmitted to humans through abrasions or cuts. *P. pseudomallei* causes a glanderslike disease in humans; however, it has rarely been observed in the Western hemisphere.

TRANSMISSION

P. aeruginosa colonization of the upper and lower respiratory tract has been studied extensively because of its importance in cystic fibrosis. The first step in colonization is attachment to epithelial cells in the respiratory tract. Attachment of *P. aeruginosa* is prevented by fibronectin coating these cells. If this coating is absent or lost, the pili of *P. aeruginosa* can mediate attachment. Increased colonization has been associated with salivary proteolytic activity degrading fibronectin. *P. aeruginosa* also has lectinlike molecules on its surface that can specifically bind galactose, mannose, and sialic acid residues. These sugars are important moieties in cell surface glycoproteins and are found in very high concentration in mucins.

After colonization, *P. aeruginosa* proteases play a role in pathogenesis. The two most studied proteases are elastinase (neutral protease) and alkaline protease. The elastinase is a heat-stable zinc containing metalloprotease that causes the hemorrhagic lesions observed in *Pseudomonas* infection by attacking the elastic lamina of the blood vessels. The elastinase cleaves and inactivates IgG antibodies and certain complement components. The alkaline protease causes tissue necrosis.

P. aeruginosa (also *P. fluorescens* and *P. aureofaciens*) produces an extracellular phospholipase C (PLC) that hydrolyzes phospholipids and is similar to enzymes in *Clostridium perfringens* and *Staphylococcus aureus*. The PLC of *P. aeruginosa* has a rather large range of lipid species that can act as substrate, allowing it to play a role in the damage of many different tissues. In vivo it probably functions combined with the proteases causing considerable necrosis. The PLC contributes to pneumonia by attacking the pulmonary surfactant leading to atelectasis (incomplete expansion of the lungs) and necrosis.

P. aeruginosa also produces two hemolysins and three potent exotoxins (A, B, and C). The latter are lethal when injected into mice and dogs and cause hypotensive shock in monkeys. Exotoxin A is the most potent toxin and is produced by 90 percent of the clinical isolates under iron-limited conditions. The toxic activity appears to be identical to that of the diphtheria toxin in inhibiting protein synthesis. It causes local tissue necrosis and inhibits granulocytic and macrophage progenitor cells in the bone marrow.

Lipopolysaccharides (LPS), or endotoxins, in *P. aeruginosa,* as in all gram-negative organisms, are responsible for many of the toxic effects observed in gram-negative sepsis: adult respiratory distress syndrome, fever, oliguria, hypotension, leukopenia/leukocytosis, and disseminated intravascular coagulation. The LPS activates the complement, fibrinolytic and clotting systems, as well as stimulating release of vasoactive peptides.

THE SLIME LAYER

Many clinical isolates of *P. aeruginosa* possess an external polysaccharide layer referred to as "the slime layer," "mucoid substance," or "glycocalyx" composed of repeating sugar chains. This layer is not considered a capsule because it is amorphous and is easily dispersed or removed from cells. It may be involved with bacterial attachment or protection from deleterious agents. The slime layer is antiphagocytic, a permeability barrier to certain antibiotics, and reduces susceptibility to opsonizing antibody.

Isolates from cystic fibrosis patients have an overproduction of the slime layer, which is easily recognized by the mucoid appearance on culture.

LEUKOCIDIN

P. aeruginosa produces a leukocidin that destroys PMNs without lysis. Since PMNs are the body's main defense against *Pseudomonas,* the importance of this toxin is obvious. Unfortunately, little is known about this substance. It is cell-associated and is activated and released via the action of proteases (elastinase).

CONTROL

In patients with advanced periodontitis *P. aeruginosa* has been isolated from 11.2 percent of pockets, particularly where previous therapy included antibiotics. Ciproflaxin was most effective on the periodontitis isolates. Beta-lactam and tetracycline antibiotics were largely ineffective. Chlorhexidine (0.12 percent), a mouthwash for reduction of gingival inflammation, may be of limited value for *Pseudomonas* infections of the mouth, since the organisms are relatively resistant to this antimicrobial agent.

BIBLIOGRAPHY

Bock, S. S.: Disinfection, sterilization, and preservation. Lea and Febiger, Philadelphia, 1977.

Doggert, R. G.: *Pseudomonas aeruginosa* clinical manifestations of infection and current therapy. Academic Press, San Francisco, 1979.

Lory, S., and Tai, P. C.: Biochemical and genetic aspects of *Pseudomonas aeruginosa* virulence. In Goebel, W. (ed.): Current Topics in Microbiology and Immunology.

Palleroni, N. J., Family 1. *Pseudomonadaceae.* Winslow, Broadhurst, Buchanan, Krumwiede, Rogers and Smith, 1917. In Krieg, N. R., and Holt, J. G. (eds.): Bergey's Manual of Systematic Bacteriology. Williams and Wilkins, Baltimore, 1984.

Reviews of Infectious Diseases 6 (Suppl. 3), 1984. (Special issue on *Pseudomonas* infection.)

Slots, J., Felk, D., and Rams, T. E.: In vitro antimicrobial sensitivity of enteric rods and pseudomonads from advanced adult periodontitis. Oral Microbiol. Immunol. 5:298, 1990.

Slots, J., Felk, D., and Rams, T. E.: Prevalence and antimicrobial susceptibility of *Enterobacteriaceae, Pseudomonadaceae,* and *Acinetobacter* in human periodontitis. Oral Microbiol. Immunol. 5:149, 1990.

Slots, J., Rams, T. E., and Schonfeld, S. E.: In vitro activity of chlorhexidine against enteric rods, and pseudomonads and acinetobacter from human periodontitis. Oral Microbiol. Immunol. 6:62, 1991.

Young, V. M.: *Pseudomonas aeruginosa:* Ecological aspects and patient colonization. Raven Press, New York, 1977.

14 Brucella, Yersinia, *and* Francisella

Joseph J. Zambon and Paulette J. Tempro

CHAPTER OUTLINE

Brucella

Yersinia

Francisella

BRUCELLA

The bacterial genus *Brucella* is a group of gram-negative bacterial species that exist as obligate parasites in a variety of animal hosts (Table 14–1). The genus is named after Sir David Bruce, who isolated *Brucella* from the spleens of British soldiers who had died of undulant fever on the island of Malta (Malta fever) after drinking contaminated goat's milk. Three species of *Brucella* are human pathogens that cause acute or chronic brucellosis characterized by an acute or relapsing (undulant) fever. They are classified by their animal reservoirs: *B. melitensis*, derived from goats and sheep; *B. abortus*, derived from cattle; and *B. suis*, derived from swine (also hares and reindeer). Three other species—*B. ovis*, found in sheep; *B. neotomae*, found in desert wood rats; and *B. canis*, found in dogs—are not usually associated with disease in humans.

Characteristics of Bacterial Cells and Colonies

Brucella are nonmotile, short, slender bacilli, sometimes appearing as cocci, coccobacilli, or short rods that are 0.5 to 0.7 μm in diameter. The cells generally have slightly convex sides and rounded ends, and usually are found singly but sometimes may occur in pairs, short chains, or small clusters. The bacterial cells sometimes exhibit bipolar staining. Bacterial colonies are small, moist-appearing, translucent, convex, and raised, with an entire edge and a smooth, shiny surface.

The *Brucella* are generally aerobic but can utilize nitrate anaerobically. Optimum growth is at 36°C to 38°C but can occur between 20°C to 40°C. Primary cultures are slow growing and fastidious, with colonies rarely visible before 48 hours, at

TABLE 14–1 ✦ *Brucella*

Characteristics	Nonmotile, short, slender bacilli, cocci, or coccobacilli; or short rods Bipolar staining Aerobic but *B. abortus* requires 5 to 10 percent CO_2 for primary isolation
Major species	*B. melitensis* from goats and sheep—relapsing fever *B. abortus*—abortions in cattle *B. suis* from swine *B. ovis* in sheep *B. neotomae* in rats *B. canis* in dogs
Growth	Media containing special dyes, thionine, and basic fuchsin
Disease	Brucellosis
Pathogenesis	Contaminated milk, cheese, or animal tissues Viscerotropism based on erythritol Intracellular parasites Granuloma formation
Prevention	Vaccination of cattle
Treatment	Doxycycline plus rifampin IMP-SMZ plus rifampin Doxycycline alone

which time they are 0.5 to 1.0 mm in diameter. Of all the *Brucella* species, only *B. abortus* requires 5 to 10 percent CO_2 for primary isolation. These microorganisms grow on media containing special dyes, thionine, and basic fuchsin. They produce catalase and decompose urea but, with the exception of *B. neotomae*, do not ferment sugars. Initial isolates of *Brucella* exhibit a smooth colony morphology, which is indicative of a highly virulent form. The organism undergoes change in colony morphology from the original smooth (S) form through an intermediate (I) form to a mucoid (M) or a rough (R) colony that is less virulent than the original and that also exhibits less agglutination. For example, the smooth form, unlike the rough form, is able to multiply in nonimmune monocytes. Transformations in colony morphology are thought to result from production and accumulation of D-alanine, as well as reduction in the pO_2 by the smooth form. Both factors favor the emergence of the rough form.

There are two major antigens shared among the *Brucella* species, A and M, which are part of the protein-lipopolysaccharide complex. The A antigen is a major antigen in *B. abortus* and *B. suis* but only a minor antigen in *B. militensis*. The M antigen is a major antigen in *B. militensis* but is minor in the other two species. *Brucella* species also have antigens that cross-react with *Escherichia coli*, *Francisella tularensis*, *Vibrio cholerae*, and *Yersinia enterocolitica*. *Brucella* species do not exhibit antiphagocytic factors or exotoxins. In fact, the pathogenesis of the organism is partly dependent on its ability to undergo phagocytosis as a means of gaining access to the host lymphatic tissues.

The Pathogenesis of *Brucella* Infections

Brucella often produces a generalized infection and bacteremia in animal hosts before localizing in the reproductive and reticuloendothelial systems. This is an example of *viscerotropism*—a specific infection of certain tissues by a bacterial pathogen. *Brucella* viscerotropism is dependent on the presence of erythritol, a four-carbon polyhydric alcohol, found in high concentrations in bovine allantoic and amniotic fluids as well as in the chorion, cotyledons, and fetal fluids of other animals. *Brucella* infection in pregnant animals often results in abortion; hence, the name *B. abortus* for the organism responsible for abortions in cattle. Animal infection can also localize in the mammary glands, resulting in contaminated milk. Humans become infected by ingesting contaminated milk and animal tissues or by handling contaminated animal tissue. The organism enters the host through

breaks in the skin or mucosa of the gastrointestinal tract, through the conjunctiva, and possibly by inhalation of contaminated aerosol sprays. Once the organism gains entrance, the bacterial cells are phagocytosed by polymorphonuclear leukocytes and monocytes, which provide the setting for intracellular growth by the organism. As intracellular parasites, they can be transported to regional lymph nodes, liver, spleen, bone marrow, and kidneys, where they form granulomas.

Following infection, clinical symptoms of human brucellosis appear after a long incubation period of weeks or months. This is followed by an insidious onset. Symptoms include malaise, chills, fever, sweats, weakness, myalgia, and headache, as well as vague gastrointestinal and nervous complaints. Clinical examination of these patients reveals enlarged lymph nodes, spleen, and liver, with approximately 20 percent of the subjects demonstrating bacteremia. Liver involvement is common and characterized by small noncaseating granulomas, which become larger, sometimes calcify, and develop suppurative abscesses. This is especially true in chronic brucellosis due to *B. suis*. *B. melitensis* causes a form of brucellosis characterized by relapsing fever, diffuse hepatitis with focal areas of necrosis in the liver, and occasionally epididyorchitis. Brucellosis also can result in acute meningoencephalitis, osteomyelitis, endocarditis, and interstitial nephritis with focal glomerular lesions.

Humoral immunity in brucellosis is detected by agglutination, precipitin, opsonization, and bactericidal tests. However, these antibodies do not confer protection. On the other hand, exposure to contaminated animal tissues appears to produce relative immunity in slaughterhouse workers. Cellular immunity appears to be important in resistance to *Brucella* infection as demonstrated by the fact that brucellae in macrophages taken from actively immunized animals survive for shorter periods of time in culture than in macrophages taken from nonimmunized animals.

Diagnosis and Treatment

Diagnosis of brucellosis is based on history, clinical findings, and laboratory examinations. The patient typically has a history of unexplained fever. The organism can be identified from blood or biopsy specimens cultured on *Brucella* agar, on trypticase soy broth in 10 percent CO_2, or by serologic tests for antibodies to *Brucella*. Since there is a long incubation period before symptoms become apparent, serum antibodies to the organism are generally present at the time of initial examination. As with other humoral immune responses, there is an initial elevation in IgM antibody titers to *Brucella* followed by an elevation in IgG titers.

Tube agglutination assays for serum antibodies utilize phenol-killed suspensions of *B. abortus.* The presence of IgG titers between 1:640 and 1:2560, as well as the presence of IgG agglutinins resistant to degradation with 2-mercaptoethanol suggest an active *Brucella* infection. Chronic active brucellosis is similarly associated with elevated IgG titers. There can be cross-reaction between serum antibodies to *F. tularensis, V. cholerae, V. fetus,* or *Y. enterocolitica* and *Brucella* in serologic assays.

Chemotherapy for human brucellosis is directed toward prompt control of symptoms and prevention of complications and relapse. Most *Brucella* species are sensitive to ampicillin, chloramphenicol, erythromycin, kanamycin, novobiocin, tetracycline, and streptomycin. Most of these organisms are resistant to penicillin, cephalosporins, clindamycin, lincomycin, polymyxin, nalidixic acid, and nystatin. As a result of randomized controlled drug trials, combination chemotherapy has emerged as most effective in eliminating *Brucella* organisms from tissues and preventing relapse. The recommended therapy for acute and subacute brucellosis in adult men and nonpregnant adult women is doxycycline plus rifampin orally. This combination is nontoxic and effective, and relapses are infrequent. Doxycycline alone is an acceptable alternative in pregnant women. Sulfamethoxazole-trimethoprim plus rifampin is a safe and effective combination in children. Since these microorganisms can exist intracellularly, it is important that antibiotic therapy be continued for 3 to 6 weeks, or relapse is likely to occur.

The incidence of brucellosis in cattle and subsequent transmission to humans can be reduced by vaccination with live attenuated *B. abortus* strain 19. Such vaccination produces partial immunity and limits *Brucella* infection.

Similar to diagnosis of brucellosis in humans, detection of infected cattle can be determined by agglutination assays on serum or milk. Alternatively, the organism can be directly detected in animal tissues such as abortion material by immunofluorescence. If detected, infected animals are destroyed. *Brucella* infection also is limited by vaccination of calves and pasteurization of milk. At present, human brucellosis is seen primarily in persons who work with animals or animal tissues, including veterinarians and workers in meat-packing plants, although 10 percent of cases are associated with ingestion of raw milk or imported cheese.

YERSINIA

Yersinia species cause a group of infections in which the microorganism normally resides in a lower vertebrate host and is transmitted to humans (Table 14–2). These types of infections (like brucellosis) are known as *zoonoses.* Bubonic plague is the best known of the *Yersinia* infections and is caused by *Y. pestis* (formerly classified as *Pasteurella pestis*). This disease is the "Black Death" of the Middle Ages, which was responsible for the death of approximately one quarter of the inhabitants of Europe. Even today, there are significant numbers of cases of bubonic plague.

Yersinia pestis

Y. pestis is a gram-negative, nonmotile, short, ovoid bacillus named after Alexandre Yersin (1863–1943), who is credited with the discovery of this microorganism as the causative agent of plague during the 1884 epidemic in Hong Kong.

Y. pestis infects the gastrointestinal tract of the fleas such as *Xenopsylla cheopis* and *Xenopsylla brasiliensis,* which reside on urban and domestic rats and on sylvatic rodents such as squirrels and prairie dogs. The fleas are, in turn, transmitted to humans.

Initially, the fleas become infected with *Y. pestis* by feasting on blood from infected rats. The microorganism multiples and finally blocks a part of the insect's gastrointestinal tract, the proventriculus. When the infected flea next bites the rodent vector, it cannot eat because of the blockage. It does, however, regurgitate *Y. pestis* cells into the wound. The microorganism can also be transmitted through contamination of abraded skin with flea

TABLE 14–2 ✦ *Yersinia*

Characteristics	Gram-negative, nonmotile, short, ovoid bacillus
Major species	*Yersinia pestis*—bubonic and other forms of plague
	Yersinia pseudotuberculosis—acute mesenteric lymphadenitis
	Yersinia enterocolitica—enterocolitis
Pathogenesis	Plague—transmitted from rats and rat fleas, invades vasculature, proliferates in lymph nodes to form buboes
	Other yersinioses—ingestion of contaminated food or water, invasion of the gastrointestinal tract
Prevention	Plague—control of rat and invertebrate populations
	Other yersinioses—proper cooking of animal products and sanitation
Treatment	Streptomycin, tetracycline, chloramphenicol

feces. Epidemics of plague are thus associated with increases in the rodent population and reflect the intimacy with which people live with these infested animals.

Y. pestis exhibits a capsule on initial isolation. The microorganism also exhibits bipolar staining using Wayson's stain, which consists of methylene blue and carbol-fuchsin, as well as with Giemsa's stain. After 2 days' growth at 28°C on blood agar, the colonies appear brown and without hemolysis. The organism ferments glucose and mannitol with gas production but does not ferment lactose, sucrose, rhamnose, or adonitol.

ANTIGENS

Yersinia species possess three plasmids, 10, 70, and 100 kilobase (kb) chromosomally independent hereditary elements, that encord factors essential for virulence expression. The 100 kb Tox plasmid is also *Y. pestis*–specific and encodes the plague exotoxin and the capsular antigens. The capsular or envelope antigen (also known as fraction 1, or F1) is a glycoprotein that enables *Y. pestis* to resist complement-mediated phagocytosis. Even in the absence of a bacterial capsule, this microorganism can resist phagocytosis by means of virulence determinants encoded on the 70 kb Lcr plasmid which is also possessed by *Y. pseudotuberculosis* and *Y. enterocolitica*. This plasmid mediates nutritional stepdown of *Yersinia* at 37°C and in low calcium environments. In this restricted state, the synthesis of virulence factors called *Yops (Yersinia* outer membrane peptides) and soluble V antigens ensues. Reduction of the temperature to 26°C or the addition of calcium results in repression of the Lcr plasmid. The function of Yops is not fully known; however, *Yersinia* with the Lcr plasmid can resist phagocytosis and attach and grow in tissues.

The 10 kb Pst plasmid is unique to *Y. pestis* and codes for a monometric 63 kilodalton protein, pesticin, which is responsible for the singular ability of the organism to invade deep tissues. This factor is an *N*-acetylglucosaminidase, which hydrolyzes bacterial cell wall lipoproteins and acts as a bacteriocin against other species in this genus, including *Y. pseudotuberculosis* and *Y. enterocolitica*.

There are several other *Y. pestis* toxins involved in the pathogenesis of plague, including a murine toxin and a lipopolysaccharide endotoxin. The murine toxin is a protein composed of a 240 kilodalton toxin A and 120 kilodalton toxin B. As the name indicates, the murine toxin is highly lethal for mice and rats but less toxic for other species. Less than 1 μg can cause death in mice and rats. The murine toxin acts as an antagonist of adenosine $3':5'$-cyclic monophosphate and causes beta-adrenergic blockade. The lipopolysaccharide endotoxin is similar to that produced by other enteric bacilli.

PATHOGENESIS

As previously described, the primary reservoir of *Y. pestis* is the gastrointestinal tract of wild and domestic rats. It can cause the death of these animals through an acute bacteremia, or remain as a chronic infection. In the rat flea, *Y. pestis* is found in the gut and has neither a capsule nor the VW antigens. The microorganism is apparently nonvirulent in the flea, owing to its normally low body temperature (25°C), but the organisms can proliferate at this temperature and cause blockage of the proventriculus. *Y. pestis* multiples in the flea, which then transmits the organism to other rats or to human beings through bites. *Y. pestis* can also be transmitted to humans through infected meat, through contact with other infected humans via droplet infection, or by means of a bite from the human flea, *Pulex irritans*.

Once transmitted to humans, the organism makes its way to the lymphatic system and to the regional lymph nodes, where it proliferates and after 2 to 8 days forms a large oval swelling known as a bubo—hence the name *bubonic plague*. Although buboes may develop in the axilla or neck, they most frequently are found in the groin and are accompanied by intense pain. If the bacilli are not confined to the lymph nodes, they extend through the efferent lymphatics to the vasculature, resulting in septicemic plague, which may occur without formation of buboes. The microorganism can then seed to internal organs such as the lungs and spleen. Septicemia can develop into disseminated intravascular coagulation, which may be characterized by skin lesions (purpura), high fever, tachycardia, pain in the limbs and back, and gangrenous necrosis of distal extremities—the *black* in the *black death*. Plague septicemia can also result in infection of the meninges (meningeal plague) and of the pharynx (plague pharyngitis), the latter clinically resembling acute tonsillitis. After 3 to 5 days, the patient may die.

Secondary involvement of the lungs can result in pneumonic plague, which carries a very high mortality rate. This is the most fulminant form of the disease. Patients with pneumonic plague produce large amounts of bloody, frothy sputum. This form is so virulent that patients can die of pneumonic plague on the very same day that they develop symptoms. Pneumonic plague produces infected sputum and other bronchial secretions, which may be transmitted to uninfected persons by droplet infection.

Exposure to *Y. pestis* may produce immunity to the antiphagocytic F1 and VW antigens; however, antisera to the toxins is not protective.

DIAGNOSIS

Bubonic plague can be diagnosed by culture of *Y. pestis* from aspirates taken of the buboes as well as from sputum, throat swabs, and autopsy material plated onto blood agar or into infusion broth. The resulting colonies can be identified by colony and biochemical characteristics. Inoculation of the suspected microorganism into animals such as mice or guinea pigs can also differentiate *Y. pestis* from other *Yersinia* species. Serologic tests including identification of the microorganism by means of fluorescent antibody staining, agglutination by specific antiserum, or lysis with a specific bacteriophage can also be useful.

Antibody assays of human or animal sera can be useful for retrospective diagnostic confirmation, seroepidemiology, and for monitoring *Y. pestis* in animals. Serum antibodies to the F1 antigen can, for example, be detected by passive hemagglutination.

TREATMENT

There is an extremely high mortality rate associated with plague. More than 50 percent of patients with untreated bubonic plague, and almost 100 percent of those with pneumonic plague, will die. With antibiotic treatment, however, the mortality rate drops to 5 to 15 percent. Streptomycin is the drug of choice, and the dosage is 30 mg per kg of body weight administered intramuscularly for 10 days. Tetracycline is useful in patients who are allergic to streptomycin or when an orally administered drug must be used. Tetracycline is administered at a dosage of 2 to 4 gm per day for 10 days. Intravenous chloramphenicol is used in patients with meningeal plague.

PREVENTION

It is impossible to eliminate the animal reservoir or the vector for bubonic plague. However, the incidence can be controlled first by the use of insecticides to kill the rat flea and the human flea; second, by the isolation of patients with pneumonic plague; and third, by immunization with killed or attenuated microorganisms to provide short-term immunity.

Other *Yersinia* Species

Other *Yersinia* species—*Y. pseudotuberculosis* and *Y. enterocolitica*—can cause disease in humans known as yersinioses. Both microorganisms are gram-negative coccobacilli that are found in domestic and wild mammal and bird reservoirs.

Y. pseudotuberculosis is found in rabbits, deer, racoons, turkeys, ducks, geese, pigeons, pheasants, and canaries and only rarely infects humans. The microorganism is transmitted by ingestion of improperly cooked and contaminated food or by direct contact with infected animals. This microorganism causes a yersiniosis characterized by acute mesenteric lymphadenitis. *Y. pseudotuberculosis* is highly invasive; it enters humans usually through the gastrointestinal tract and spreads to the mesenteric lymph nodes and bloodstream. It has a lipopolysaccharide endotoxin and VW antigens as does *Y. pestis* but, in contrast to *Y. pestis,* it lacks fibrinolysin and coagulase. Expression of the V and W antigens is plasmid-mediated. There are six serotypes of *Y. pseudotuberculosis* (I through VI) and eight subtypes based on combination of 15 heat-stable somatic O antigens and heat-labile H antigens. Serotype I *Y. pseudotuberculosis* is the most prevalent serotype and is found in about 90 percent of human yersiniosis due to *Y. pseudotuberculosis*. Several of these antigens cross-react with antigens present on salmonella. *Y. pseudotuberculosis* infection is effectively treated by several antibiotics including kanamycin, tetracycline, and chloramphenicol.

The other organism responsible for the non-plague yersinioses is *Y. enterocolitica*. Humans and pigs are the main reservoirs for this microorganism. The organism is transmitted mainly in rural areas through food, especially improperly cooked meat; through feces-contaminated water; and through person-to-person contact. There is no known invertebrate vector. Once the organism is ingested, it proliferates in the bowel lumen and in the associated lymphoid tissue. It is highly invasive and can invade cells in culture. The organism's pathogenicity is also temperature dependent. Strains of *Y. enterocolitica* grown at 37°C are much less pathogenic than strains cultured at 25°C. A key feature in this disease is the enterotoxin produced by *Y. enterocolitica*. This enterotoxin is a 9000 dalton, heat-stable protein consisting of two toxic components, ST-1 and ST-2.

An acute gastroenteritis or enterocolitis is produced. This occurs predominantly in young children and may be clinically indistinguishable from gastroenteritis due to salmonella, shigella, or toxigenic *Escherichia coli*. The patients experience considerable pain, which resembles acute appendicitis, as well as acute nonsuppurative polyarthritis, erythema nodosum, and Reiter's syndrome (arthritis with urethritis and conjunctivitis) in adults.

There are 34 serotypes of *Yersinia enterocolitica* based on somatic O antigens. The predominant human isolate in the United States is serotype 8. Serotypes 3 and 9 are predominant in Europe, Africa, Japan, and Canada. Antibodies to these O antigens are usually absent at the onset of the disease but may be demonstrated by hemagglutination at the peak of the disease and during convalescence. There is cross-reaction between *Y. enterocolitica* serotype 9 and *Brucella abortus,* which can be shown in coagglutination assays. There are also a number of biotypes of *Y. enterocolitica* based on reactions with indole, xylose, and trehalose and on the presence of lipase and DNAse. The prevalent human biotype is biotype 4.

Yersinial enterocolitis due to *Y. enterocolitica* can be diagnosed by identification and culture of the organism. *Y. enterocolitica* is distinguished by biochemical tests and agglutination with specific antisera. The organism is also identified by susceptibility to specific bacteriophages. *Y. enterocolitica* can be distinguished from *Y. pestis* and other Enterobacteriaceae on the basis of cellular motility, which is apparent at from 22°C to 28°C but not at 37°C.

Other *Yersinia* species include *Y. intermedia*, *Y. frederiksenii*, and *Y. ruckeri*, which is the cause of red mouth disease in salmon and trout.

FRANCISELLA

Francisella contains three species: *F. tularensis* and *F. novicida*, both responsible for tularemia in humans and animals, and a species formally classified in the genus *Yersinia*, *F. philomiragia*, which causes infection in near-drowning victims and immunocompromised humans especially those with chronic granulomatous diseases. *F. tularensis* can be divided into two main types: *F. tularensis* subsp. *tularensis* found in North America and *F. tularensis* subsp. *palaearctica* which occurs in Asia and Europe and to a minor extent in North America. The genus is named after the American microbiologist Edward Francis, who extensively studied tularemia.

Characteristics of Bacterial Cells and Colonies

These microorganisms are gram-negative, short, nonmotile, nonspore-forming, obligately aerobic rods that occur singly and stain poorly. *F. tularensis* measures 0.2 μm by 0.2 to 0.7 μm. Older cultures exhibit significant pleomorphism with coccoid, bacillary, and filamentous forms. Virulent *F. tularensis* possesses a thick capsule; loss of virulence is associated with loss of the capsule. Culture of *F. tularensis* requires special media such as cysteine-glucose-blood agar, coagulated egg yolk medium, or thioglycolate broth, all of which contain sulfhydryl compounds. Primary isolates are visible after 2 to 10 days of culture at 37°C as smooth (S), gray, minute, transparent, easily emulsified colonies. They are catalase-positive, oxidase-negative, and slowly ferment carbohydrates, producing acid. Smooth forms are transformed to rough (R) forms, which are less virulent. Highly virulent strains of *F. tularensis* ferment glycerol and are generally isolated from tick-borne

tularemia in rabbits, whereas less virulent strains do not ferment glycerol and are associated with water-borne disease of rodents.

Pathogenesis

F. tularensis was first isolated from squirrels in Tulare County, California, in 1912. Francis cultured this microorganism from jack rabbits and showed them to be an important source of human tularemia. The organism can be transmitted from deer flies, ticks, infected muskrats, and polluted water. *F. tularensis* subsp. *tularensis* has been found so far only in North America associated with ticks and rabbits and is highly virulent to humans. *F. tularensis* subsp. *palaearctica* occurs in Asia, Europe, and to a small extent in North America associated with mosquitoes and rodents and is less virulent to humans. While *F. tularensis* can be found everywhere except Antarctica and Australia, tularemia is generally considered a disease of the Northern hemisphere. *F. tularensis* biotype *nearctica* causes most tularemia in the United States. There are several types of human tularemia, each of which is related to the primary route of infection:

1. An ulceroglandular form, in which an ulcerating papule develps at the site of the primary skin lesion. This form occurs by transmission through abraded skin or through bites from infected animals.
2. An oculoglandular form, in which the initial infection occurs through the conjunctivae.
3. A pneumonic form, resulting from inhalation of infected droplets during processing of animal products or by hematogenous dissemination from the site of local infection.
4. An abdominal (typhoidal) form, caused by ingestion of contaminated meat. Patients with the typhoidal form exhibit gastrointestinal symptoms, toxemia, and fever similar to typhoid fever.

Symptoms usually appear 3 to 4 days after infection, but the incubation period can range from 2 to 10 days. Tularemia is an acute disease with symptoms including headache, fever, and general malaise. As the disease progresses, the patient may experience delirium and coma, and may die. The mortality rate in untreated ulceroglandular tularemia is 5 percent, and in typhoidal and pneumonic tularemia 30 percent.

Once the organism infects the host, it is phagocytized by monocytes and remains alive as an intracellular parasite for extended periods of time, which explains why patients have occasional relapses and a persistent immune response. The organism is transported within monocytes throughout the lymphatics to regional lymph nodes. From there, the organism can cause transitory bacteremia and spread to the lungs, liver, and spleen, where it can form abscesses and granulomatous, caseating nodules.

F. philomiragia–associated diseases contrast markedly with the clinical features of disease caused by *F. tularensis*. A febrile illness and bacteremia usually occurs 4 to 5 days after exposure, and pneumonitis is common. Several cases of infection with *F. philomiragia* have been described in near-drowning in salt water, suggesting saltwater exposure as a risk factor for infection. The major routes of transmission for *F. tularensis* are contact with the tissues or fluids of wild animals and tick bites. The population at risk for *F. philomiragia* infection also differs from that at risk for development of tularemia. The majority (86%) of reports of infection with *F. philomiragia* involved hosts with either impaired physical barrier to infection as in near-drowning or impaired immunologic defenses as in chronic granulomatosis disease or myeloproliferative disease. Most tularemia infections occur in immunocompetent individuals, suggesting that *F. tularensis* is the more virulent species.

Diagnosis and Treatment

F. tularensis has cell wall antigens including an endotoxin, a polysaccharide antigen, and a protein antigen that cross-reacts with *Brucella* species. Skin tests with the polysaccharide antigen in convalescent patients elicit characteristic delayed hypersensitivity reactions transferable with spleen cells. Agglutinating serum antibodies are also demonstrable in convalescent sera by the second week of the infection and may persist for years. Since *F. tularensis* is an intracellular parasite, however, exacerbations of the disease can occur even in the presence of high serum antibody titers.

Laboratory diagnosis of tularemia and other *Francisella*-associated infections is based on the identification of the organism either by culture of clinical specimens such as gastric washings, sputum, and tissue specimens or by fluorescent antibody tests on smears. The microorganisms cultured on special sulfhydryl-containing media are often confirmed by fluorescent antibody tests or biochemical characteristics (Table 14–3). The presence of serum antibodies to *F. tularensis* also is useful in the diagnosis and treatment of tularemia. A rise in antibody titer indicates a recent infection, while a positive skin test reaction to polysaccharide antigen suggests either a present or a past infection.

Streptomycin is the drug of choice for treatment of tularemia, but bacteriostatic drugs such as tetracycline and chloramphenicol are also effective in mild cases. Antibiotic treatment reduces the mortality of tularemia to approximately 1 percent. Pa-

TABLE 14–3 ✦ *Francisella*

Characteristics	Gram-negative, short, nonmotile, nonspore-forming, obligately aerobic rods
Major species	*Francisella tularensis* subsp. *tularensis*
	Francisella tularensis subsp. *palearctica*
Growth	Sulfhydryl compound—containing medium, such as glucose-blood agar, coagulated egg yolk medium, or thioglycolate broth
Disease	Tularemia in humans and animals
	Infections in near-drowning victims and immunocompromised humans
	Forms
	Ulceroglandular
	Oculoglandular
	Pneumonic
	Typhoidal
Pathogenesis	Infected rabbits, deer flies, ticks, infected muskrats; saltwater exposure
	Headache, fever, and general malaise
	Intracellular parasite spread through lymphatics
	Transitory bacteremia, spread to lungs, liver, and spleen
	Abscesses, granulomatous, caseating nodules
Prevention	Attenuated live vaccine
	Mechanical barriers
Treatment	Streptomycin, tetracycline and chloramphenicol

tients may relapse if antibiotic therapy is not continued for a sufficient period of time or if the antibiotic is not able to eliminate the intracellular infection.

An attenuated live vaccine is available for laboratory workers and other persons likely to come into contact with infected material. Mechanical barriers such as gloves and face masks are also recommended for persons who skin and dress rabbits.

BIBLIOGRAPHY
Brucella

Hall, W. H.: Modern Chemotherapy for *Brucella* in humans. Rev. Infect. Dis. 12:1060, 1990.

McAllister, T. A.: Laboratory diagnosis of human brucellosis. Scot. Med. J. 21:129, 1976.

Smith, L. D. and Ficht, T. A.: Pathogenesis of *Brucella*. Crit. Rev. Microbiol. 17:209, 1990.

Young, E. J. Human brucellosis. Rev. Infect. Dis. 5:821, 1983.

Yersinia

Brubaker, R. R.: Factors promoting acute and chronic diseases caused by Yersiniae. Clin. Microbiol. Rev. 4:309, 1991.

Pollitzer, R.: Plague. W. H. O. Monograph Series No. 22, World Health Organization, Geneva, 1954.

Yersin, A.: Ann. Pasteur Inst. (Paris) 8:662, 1894.

Francisella

Hollis, D. G., Weaver, R. E., Steigerwalt, A. G., Wenger, J. D., Moss, C. W., and Brenner, D. J.: *Francisella philomiragia* comb nov (formerly *Yersinia philomiragia*) and *Francisella tularensis* biogroup *novicida* (formerly *Francisella novicida*) associated with human disease. J. Clin. Microbiol. 27:1601, 1989.

Owen, C. R.: Francisella infections. In Bodily, H. L., Updyke, E. L., and Mason, J. O. (eds.): Diagnostic Procedures for Bacterial, Mycotic and Parasitic Infection, ed. 5. American Public Health Association, New York, 1970.

Wenger, J. D., Hollis, D. G., Weaver, R. E., Baker C. N., Brown, G. R., Brenner, D. J., Broome, C. V.: Infection caused by *Francisella philomiragia* (formerly *Yersinia philomiragia*): A newly recognized human pathogen. Ann. Intern. Med. 1:888, 1989.

15 Bacillus *and* Clostridium

Sydney M. Finegold

CHAPTER OUTLINE
Bacillus
Clostridium

BACILLUS

The ninth edition of *Bergey's Manual of Systematic Bacteriology* lists 34 species of *Bacillus;* several of these are found in infectious processes in humans on occasion. *Bacillus* species are widely distributed in nature and are relatively common contaminants in laboratory cultures. Contamination of alcohol swabs and of radiometric blood culture apparatus has led to false-positive blood cultures. Most true infections involving this genus are in immunocompromised hosts, including patients with implanted devices of one type or another.

Description and General Characteristics

Most organisms in the genus *Bacillus* are gram-positive, obligately aerobic bacilli that produce endospores. Occasional species or strains are gram-negative or facultatively anaerobic. They closely resemble *Clostridium*, but the latter is characteristically obligately anaerobic. *Bacillus* species may be differentiated from each other on the basis of morphologic and biochemical characteristics, but speciation is not important for routine clinical purposes except for *B. anthracis*, the causative agent of anthrax. Most strains of *Bacillus* produce characteristic large, flat colonies with beta hemolysis.

Pathogenesis of *Bacillus* Infections

Capsules and exotoxins are the primary features in *Bacillus* strains that account for pathogenicity. The capsule permits strains to resist phagocytosis and the exotoxins are responsible for the pathology produced. The exotoxin (enterotoxin) produced by *B. cereus* is involved in food poisoning caused by this organism. *B. cereus* also is involved in true infection.

Host Defense Mechanisms

Certain species, such as rats, chickens, and dogs, are relatively resistant to anthrax, compared with many other warm-blooded animals; this is at least partly due to a high degree of phagocytic activity against *B. anthracis*. Antibodies to the exotoxin provide specific immunity. Vaccines have been developed.

Clinical Features

The most serious *Bacillus* infection is **anthrax,** which is seen in three forms in humans. **Cutaneous anthrax** (malignant pustule) is the most common type in the United States. The organisms gain entrance via an abrasion of the skin, usually on the hands or forearms. There is a serosanguinous discharge in which the organisms may be readily recognized. A second form of the disease is **pulmonary anthrax** or woolsorter's disease; the infection is acquired by inhalation of spores during shearing or handling of animal hair. Bacilli are found in large numbers in the sputum. The most severe and rarest form of anthrax is gastrointestinal anthrax. Infection is initiated by swallowing of the organisms or its spores.

B. cereus is the cause of a variety of infections, often serious (Table 15–1). This organism is an important cause of food poisoning. A short-incubation-period type of food poisoning is most often associated with fried rice that has been held warm for extended periods; this is due to preformed toxin

TABLE 15–1 ✦ Types of Infection Caused by *Bacillus cereus*

Septicemia	Destructive ophthalmitis
Endocarditis	Peritonitis
Pericarditis	Wound infection
Necrotizing pneumonia	Myonecrosis
Empyema	Osteomyelitis
Meningitis	Food-poisoning

and is characterized primarily by vomiting. The long-incubation variety of food poisoning due to this organism often is associated with meat or vegetable dishes; toxin is formed in vivo, and the disease is characterized chiefly by diarrhea. Factors predisposing to infection with *B. cereus* are listed in Table 15–2.

Other species of *Bacillus* may cause infection in immunocompromised hosts or in relation to trauma and foreign bodies.

Identification

The clinical picture of anthrax is often distinctive enough to suggest the diagnosis. *B. anthracis* is a facultative, large, square-ended, gram-positive rod with a centrally located spore that does not cause the cell to bulge. Frequently, the bacterial cells occur in long chains with a bamboolike appearance. Capsules may be evident. Colonies are 4 to 5 mm in diameter, opaque, raised, and irregular with a curled margin. The organism is nonhemolytic on sheep blood agar. In broth, growth occurs in the form of a heavy surface pellicle. The organism is dangerous to work with; all work should take place in a bacteriologic safety hood. All areas should be decontaminated with a sporicidal germicide. Specific identification can be made by public health laboratories using a gamma bacteriophage.

The clinical picture of *B. cereus* infection is usually not distinctive. Colonies of this organism vary from small, shiny, and compact to large, spreading, and feathery; on sheep blood agar, one

TABLE 15–2 ✦ Factors Predisposing to *B. cereus* Infection

Disease or therapy leading to immunocompromise
Surgery
Trauma
Burns
Intravenous drug abuse
Implanted prosthetic devices
Indwelling catheters
Hemodialysis
Peritoneal dialysis

sees a lavender colony with beta hemolysis. In contrast to *B. anthracis*, *B. cereus* is resistant to gamma phage, is usually resistant to penicillins and cephalosporins (because of β-lactamase production) and does not form capsules on bicarbonate agar.

Therapy

Penicillin G is the drug of choice for the treatment of anthrax, although rare strains of *B. anthracis* are resistant. In systemic forms of the disease, the mortality may be significant if treatment is delayed. Alternative drugs for the penicillin-allergic patient include tetracycline, erythromycin, and chloramphenicol.

B. cereus food poisoning is of short duration and requires no specific therapy. *B. cereus* infections cannot reliably be treated with penicillin G or other beta lactam drugs. Clindamycin and vancomycin should generally be effective and ciprofloxacin was effective in one patient. In certain situations, surgical drainage or debridement may be important considerations.

CLOSTRIDIUM

There are 85 species of *Clostridium* recognized in the ninth edition of *Bergey's Manual of Systematic Bacteriology*. Of these, 20 are important human pathogens. Clostridia are widely distributed in nature, but most disease in humans is of endogenous origin except for intoxications such as *C. perfringens*–induced food poisoning, tetanus, and botulism, many cases of *C. difficile* colitis, and a small percentage of cases of gas gangrene. The endogenous infections derive primarily from the intestinal flora and, to a lesser extent, the indigenous flora of the female genital tract or other mucosal surfaces.

Description and General Characteristics

Clostridia are chiefly spore-forming, anaerobic, gram-positive rods. However, some species become aerotolerant on subculture, and some (*C. carnis*, *C. histolyticum*, and *C. tertium*) grow aerobically. *Clostridium* species sporulate anaerobically only, grow much better anaerobically, and are usually catalase-negative, whereas *Bacillus* species sporulate aerobically only, usually grow better aerobically, and are usually catalase-positive. A few species of clostridia are gram-negative, and older cultures may appear gram-negative. Sporulation may be difficult to demonstrate in some species. Differentiation between species of clostridia is based on the shape and location of spores and bio-

TABLE 15–3 ✦ Characteristics of Clostridial Species[1]

	GELATIN HYDROLYSIS	GLUCOSE FERMENTATION	LECITHINASE	LIPASE	INDOLE	BUTYRIC ACID PRODUCED IN PYG	ISOACIDS PRODUCED IN PYG	AEROBIC GROWTH	UREASE	MILK REACTION
Saccharolytic— proteolytic										
C. bifermentans	+	+	+	−	+	(+)	(+)	−	−	d
C. sordellii	+	+	+	−	+	(+)	(+)	−	+⁻	d
C. perfringens	+	+	+	−	−	+	−	−	−	dᶜ
C. novyi type A	+	+	+	+	−	+	−	−	−	c
						+	+	−		d
C. cadaveris	+	+	−	−	+	+	−	−	−	dᶜ
C. septicum	+	+	−	−	−	+	−	−	−	cdᶜ
C. difficile	+	+	−	−	−	+	+	−	−	−
C. putrificum	+	+	−	−	−	+	+	−	−	d
Saccharolytic— nonproteolytic										
C. baratii	−	+	+	−	−	+	−	−	−	c
C. tertium	−	+	−	−	−	+	−	+	−	c
C. butyricum	−	+	−	−	−	+	−	−	−	c
C. innocuum	−	+	−	−	−	+	−	−	−	−
C. ramosum	−	+	−	−	−⁺	−	−	−	−	c
C. clostridioforme	−	+	−	−	−	−	−	−	−	c
Asaccharolytic— proteolytic										
C. tetani	+	−	−	−	+⁻	+	−	−	−	d⁻
C. hastiforme	+	−	−	−	−	+	+	−	−	dᶜ
C. subterminale	+	−	−	−	−	+	+	−	−	dᶜ
C. histolyticum	+	−	−	−	−	−	−	+⁻	−	d
C. limosum	+	−	+	−	−	−	−	−	−	d

Note: [1]*C. botulinum* types vary in proteolytic, saccharolytic, and lipase reactions. Send suspected isolates or suspected *C. botulinum*—containing material to the appropriate local or state agency.

[2]Spores rarely observed.

Reactions:
  − = Negative reaction
  + = Positive reaction for majority of strains; includes weak as well as strong acid production from carbohydrates in saccharolytic organisms
  V = Variable reaction
  (+) = Delayed reaction
  c = Clot formed in milk
  d = Milk digested

PRAS carbohydrate fermentation:
  + = pH <5.5
  W = pH 5.5–5.7
  − = pH >5.7
  V = variable

LACTOSE	MALTOSE	FRUCTOSE	CELLOBIOSE	ARABINOSE	MANNOSE	XYLOSE	NITRATE REDUCTION	SPORE LOCATION	END PRODUCTS FROM PYG
			FERMENTATION OF						
$-$	W$^-$	V	$-$	$-$	$-$^{w}	$-$	$-$	OS	A (p ib b iv ic l s)
$-$	W$^+$	V	$-$	$-$	$-$^{w}	$-$	$-$	OS	A (p ib b iv ic l)
$+$	$+$	$+$	$-$$^+$	$-$	$+$	$-$	V	OS^2	A B L (p s)
$-$	V	$-$^{w}	$-$	$-$	$-$	$-$	$-$	OS	A P B
$-$	$-$^{w}	$-$^{w}	$-$	$-$	$-$	$-$	$-$	OS	A B ib iv (p v ic l s)
$-$	$-$	V	$-$	$-$	$-$^{w}	$-$	$-$	OT	A B (l s)
$+$	$+$	$+$	$+$^{w}	$-$	$+$	$-$	V	OS	A B (p l)
$-$	$-$	$+$	$-$^{w}	$-$	W$^-$	$-$^{w}	$-$	OS	A ib B iv IC (v l)
$-$	$-$^{w}	$-$^{w}	$-$	$-$	$-$	$-$	$-$	OT	A ib B iv (p v ic l s)
$+$^{w}	$+$^{w}	$+$	$+$	$-$	$+$	$-$	$+$$^-$	RS	A B L (p s)
$+$	$+$	$+$	$+$	$-$	$+$	V	$+$$^-$	OT	A B L (s)
$+$	$+$	$+$	$+$	$+$$^-$	$+$	$+$	$-$	OS	A B (l s)
$-$	$-$	$+$	$+$	$-$	$+$	$-$^{w}	$-$	OT	A B L (s)
$+$	$+$	$+$	$+$	$-$	$+$	$-$^{w}	$-$	OT^2	A l (s)
$+$^{w}	$+$	$+$	V	V	$+$^{w}	$+$	$+$$^-$	OS^2	A (l s)
$-$	$-$	$-$	$-$	$-$	$-$	$-$	$-$	RT	A p B (l s)
$-$	$-$	$-$	$-$	$-$	$-$	$-$	$-$$^+$	S	A B ib iv (p ic)
$-$	$-$	$-$	$-$	$-$	$-$	$-$	$-$	OS	A B ib IV (p ic l s)
$-$	$-$	$-$	$-$	$-$	$-$	$-$	$-$	OS	A (l s)
$-$	$-$	$-$	$-$	$-$	$-$	$-$	$-$	OS	A (l s)

Fatty acid end products from PYG
    A = Acetic
    P = Propionic
    IB = Isobutyric
    B = Butyric
    IV = Isovaleric
    V = Valeric
    IC = Isocaproic
    L = Lactic
    S = Succinic
Note: (1) Capital letters indicate major metabolic products; (2) Lower case letters indicate minor products; (3) Parentheses indicate a variable reaction; (4) Superscripts indicate less common reaction; (5) Isoacids are primarily from carbohydrate-free media (such as PY) in the case of saccharolytic organisms.
From Summanen, Baron, Citron, Strong, Wexler, and Finegold: Wadsworth Anaerobic Bacteriology Manual, ed 5, 1993. Reprinted with permission of Star Publishing Company, Belmont, CA.

chemical tests; Table 15–3 lists the characteristics of the clostridia most often encountered in the clinical setting.

Pathogenesis of Clostridial Infections

Clostridial infection of wounds or soft tissue, like other anaerobic infections, occurs primarily in an anaerobic tissue environment due to impaired arterial or venous circulation, trauma, surgery, and malignant or other disease. The various factors listed previously may also account for the breach in the mucosal surface of the intestinal or female genital tract that permits the endogenous clostridial flora to enter the tissues that ultimately become infected. The vast majority of clostridial infections are mixed, involving other anaerobes, aerobic and/ or facultative bacteria.

Capsules may be important in protecting clostridia from the body's host defenses, particularly with *C. perfringens*. The major virulence factors, however, are **exotoxins.** The toxins produced by *C. tetani* and *C. botulinum* are among the most potent poisons known to mankind (one million times more potent than rattlesnake poison). **Tetanus toxin** (tetanospasmin) binds to gangliosides in the central nervous system and suppresses the central inhibitory balancing influences on motor neuron activity; this leads to spasticity and convulsions and intensified reflex responses to various stimuli. This toxin also acts on the sympathetic nervous system and on the neurocirculatory and neuroendocrine systems. **Botulinal toxin** attaches to individual motor nerve terminals to prevent acetylcholine release at the nerve endings. Other species of clostridia produce numerous toxins. For example, *C. perfringens* produces an alpha toxin (a lecithinase, phospholipase C); this toxin is a hemolysin and also is active against white blood cells and platelets and has necrotizing activity. The nu

toxin is an RNAse. The theta toxin is a hemolysin. The kappa toxin is a collagenase, the mu toxin a hyaluronidase, and the epsilon and iota toxins lead to increased capillary permeability. This organism also produces a neuraminidase and an enterotoxin. *C. difficile* produces at least three toxins—a cytotoxin, an enterotoxin, and a motility-altering toxin.

Host Defense Mechanisms

The normal intestinal flora clearly is an important defense mechanism against infant (and perhaps some cases of adult) botulism and against pseudomembranous colitis due to *C. difficile* and certain other enteric infections or intoxications involving clostridia. Infant botulism is not seen after the age of eight months, by which time the normal intestinal flora is well established. Antitoxic immunity is clearly important in preventing tetanus, botulism, and necrotizing enterocolitis due to type C *C. perfringens* and may operate in other situations as well. Active immunization is useful in these settings.

Clinical Features

The classic infections involving *C. perfringens* are clostridial myonecrosis (gas gangrene), gangrenous cholecystitis (with or without visceral gas gangrene), and postabortal sepsis with intravascular hemolysis. Clostridial myonecrosis is a rapidly advancing infection, which may prove rapidly fatal. Onset is characterized by sudden pain in the region of a wound that steadily increases in severity and remains localized to the area of the spreading infection. Soon there is local swelling and edema, and a thin hemorrhagic exudate may be apparent. There is relatively little fever but a disproportionately rapid pulse rate. Early, the skin is tense,

TABLE 15–4 ✦ In Vitro Susceptibility of Clostridia to Antimicrobial Agents

BACTERIA	CHLORAMPHENICOL	CLINDAMYCIN	ERYTHROMYCIN‡	METRONIDAZOLE
C. perfringens	+ + +	+ + +†	+ + +	+ + +
Other				
Clostridium sp.	+ + +	+ +	+ + to + + +	+ + +

Key: + = Poor or inconsistent activity; + + = moderate activity; + + + = good activity.
*Piperacillin, mezlocillin, azlocillin, carbenicillin, ticarcillin.
†Rare strains are resistant.
‡Not approved by FDA for anaerobic infections.
§Other penicillins and cephalosporins are frequently less active. Ampicillin and amoxicillin are roughly comparable to penicillin G in activity. Addition of beta-lactamase inhibitors, such as clavulanic acid and sulbactam, remarkably increase the activity against beta-lactamase producers.

white, and colder than normal. Bronzed discoloration appears and increases with time. Eventually, the discharge becomes more profuse; the skin becomes dusky; and hemorrhagic bullae appear. Gas is usually present, but only in limited amounts early. Involvement of the underlying muscle is the major pathology and the hallmark of the disease. Early changes in the muscle include pallor and edema, but there is progression to marked change in color, loss of contractility, and then frank gangrene to liquefaction. *C. perfringens* is involved in 80 to 95 percent of cases, with *C. novyi* and *C. septicum* other important causes in civilian cases of clostridial myonecrosis.

Clostridia account for only a small percentage of postabortal infections, but often produce the most dramatic and severe illnesses of this type. With severe clostridial sepsis due to *C. perfringens*, there is a very dramatic clinical picture consisting of hemolytic anemia, hemoglobinemia, hemoglobinuria, disseminated intravascular coagulation, hyperbilirubinemia, shock, and anuria.

The clinical pictures just described are very dramatic and the illnesses are life-threatening. However, *C. perfringens* and a number of other clostridia are more commonly involved in diverse infections throughout the body similar to the type caused by non–spore-forming anaerobes and other bacteria. Included are brain abscesses, subdural empyema, aspiration pneumonia, thoracic empyema, intra-abdominal infection, infection related to gynecologic disease or surgery, wound infections following other types of surgery, and soft tissue infections. Bacteremia may be seen as a complication of some of these types of infection. There is a distinct association between infection involving *C. septicum* and *C. tertium* and malignancy and other diseases of the cecum.

Clostridia are infrequently involved in dental or oral infections. *C. perfringens* has been isolated in mixed culture from a case of pyogenic granuloma and two cases of periostitis with subperiosteal abscess. Clostridia also have been found in mixed culture from a gingival abscess and *C. sporogenes*, along with other organisms, from a case of cervical actinomycosis of buccodental origin.

Tetanus and **botulism** are classic clostridial intoxications. Adult botulism also may be secondary to wound infection with *C. botulinum*.

It is important to note that tetanus may result from infected gingiva or teeth or from surgery for such problems. Dental sources accounted for 1.2 percent of cases of tetanus in the United States in 1970–1971. It also is important to note that trismus related to dental problems may be confused with tetanus, and vice versa.

Early findings in tetanus include tension or cramps and twitching in muscles about a wound and stiffness of the jaw muscles with mild pain in facial muscles. In full-blown tetanus, the most typical complaint is lockjaw or trismus—inability to open the mouth because of spasm of the masseter muscles. Spasm of facial muscles leads to risus sardonicus, the characteristic grotesque, grinning facial expression. Spasms or contractions of the muscles of the trunk and extremities may be widespread and result in boardlike rigidity, in painful intermittent tonic convulsions and opisthotonos, a condition in which the back is bowed backward so that the back of the head and heels approach each other. External stimuli of even minor degree may precipitate extended painful tonic convulsions. Spasm of pharyngeal and laryngeal muscles may lead to difficulty in swallowing, cyanosis, and even respiratory arrest and death.

Botulism also has a distinctive clinical picture. As with tetanus, fever is absent and the patient's mentation is clear. There is a descending symmetrical motor paralysis first affecting muscles supplied by the cranial nerves. Common symptoms include

CEFOXITIN	UREIDO- AND CARBOXY- PENICILLINS*	PENICILLIN G§	TETRACYCLINE	VANCOMYCIN‡
+ + +	+ + +	+ + +	+ +	+ + +
+ to + +	+ + +	+ + +	+ +	+ + to + + +

diplopia, dysarthria, and dysphagia. Pupils are often dilated and fixed. Mucous membranes of the mouth, tongue, and pharynx may be extremely dry and even painful. Gastrointestinal symptoms are variable and are seen in about one third of patients.

Food poisoning due to certain serotypes of type A *C. perfringens* is common. It is a benign, self-limited process typically lasting only 24 hours. Symptoms include abdominal pain, nausea, and acute watery diarrhea without fever. Outbreaks are common and follow ingestion of contaminated foods, notably meat, poultry, or gravy.

C. difficile is the primary cause of pseudomembranous colitis related to antimicrobial therapy and certain antineoplastic agents. Rare cases of this problem are caused by type C *C. perfringens* and other clostridia as well as by *Staphylococcus aureus*. Nonspecific colitis also appears commonly due to *C. difficile*. Diarrhea without colitis that follows antimicrobial therapy may also involve *C. difficile* on occasion, and there is evidence to implicate type A *C. perfringens* in some of these cases as well. The hallmark of pseudomembranous colitis is a characteristic yellowish elevated plaque that may be seen by endoscopic examination of the colon.

On the basis of the disease syndromes they produce or are involved in, clostridia may be placed in five groups:

> Group 1—the **gas gangrene group.** This includes type A *C. perfringens, C. novyi, C. septicum, C. bifermentans, C. histolyticum, C. sordellii, C. sporogenes,* and others.
>
> Group 2—*C. tetani,* the etiologic agent of **tetanus.**
>
> Group 3—the **botulism group.** This includes various types of *C. botulinum,* as well as strains of *C. baratii* and *C. butyricum* that produce an identical toxin.
>
> Group 4—the **enteric group.** This includes *C. difficile,* responsible for most cases of antimicrobial-associated pseudomembranous colitis as well as other clostridia that may be involved in this process, including type C *C. perfringens, C. sordellii,* and others. In addition, type A *C. perfringens* is included as a cause of antibiotic-associated diarrhea without colitis and as a cause of food poisoning. Type C *C. perfringens* is the cause of enteritis necroticans.
>
> Group 5—the miscellaneous infection group (wound infection, abscesses, bacteremia, and so forth). This group includes *C. perfringens, C. ramosum, C. bifermentans, C. sphenoides, C. sporogenes,* and a number of others.

Identification

The clinical picture of certain entities such as gas gangrene, tetanus, botulism, and postabortal *C. perfringens* sepsis is usually distinctive enough

to permit definitive diagnosis. The diagnosis is made by nonbacteriologic means in other cases— for example, by detection of the pathognomonic plaques in the colon of patients having pseudomembranous colitis.

The colonial and microscopic morphology of clostridia vary widely. As noted earlier, it may be difficult to determine that they are anaerobes, that they are gram-positive, and that they are spore-formers. In some cases, however, the morphology is distinctive enough to suggest that a *Clostridium* is involved and even to indicate a particular species. Examples of such unique morphology include medusa-head colonies, the double zone of hemolysis around colonies of *C. perfringens* on sheep blood agar, lipase- and lecithinase-positive colonies on egg yolk agar, the large colonies that fluoresce chartreuse on cycloserine cefoxitin fructose agar (a highly selective medium for *C. difficile*), the box carlike shape of *C. perfringens* (particularly in a clinical Gram stain in which the white blood cells have been severely damaged or destroyed by the organism's toxin), and gram-positive rods whose cells clearly contain spores. There are tests available for detection of toxins or other products of *C. difficile,* such as the cytotoxicity test in tissue culture and immunoassays for toxins. There is a mouse lethality test and also an ELISA procedure for detection and confirmation of botulinal toxin in gastrointestinal contents and in implicated food specimens. Culture and biochemical reactions, as indicated in Table 15–3, are useful for diagnosis and identification in the vast majority of commonly encountered clostridial infections. It should be noted that collection of specimens so as to avoid indigenous flora and transport of such specimens in a manner designed to avoid exposure to air are very important for success in recovery of clostridia, as with all anaerobes.

Therapy

Antitoxin therapy is important in intoxications such as tetanus and botulism, and toxoids may be used to induce immunity prophylactically. Surgical debridement and drainage are of particular importance in the management of clostridial infections, especially the more serious ones such as clostridial myonecrosis.

Antimicrobial therapy is also important in the proper management of most clostridial infections. Penicillin G is an excellent drug against clostridia but some strains, including some of *C. perfringens,* are resistant and others, such as some strains of *C. ramosum,* are relatively resistant (minimal inhibitory concentrations as high as 8 units per ml). *C. ramosum,* often overlooked or misidentified, is commonly encountered in infection and is relatively resistant to antimicrobial agents. About 15 percent of strains of this species are highly resistant to clindamycin, and many strains are resistant to tetracycline and erythromycin. About 20 to 30 percent of strains of a number of clostridial species other than *C. perfringens* are resistant to clindamycin. One-third of clostridia other than *C. perfringens* are resistant to cefoxitin. Metronidazole and chloramphenicol are essentially always active against clostridia. Table 15–4 summarizes the in vitro susceptibility of clostridia to some of the agents commonly employed in anaerobic infections or in infections of uncertain cause. For pseudomembranous colitis due to *C. difficile,* oral metronidazole, vancomycin, or bacitracin is the preferred antimicrobial agent.

BIBLIOGRAPHY

Baron, E. J. and Finegold, S. M.: Bailey and Scott's Diagnostic Microbiology, ed 8. C. V. Mosby, St. Louis, 1990.

Finegold, S. M.: Anaerobic Bacteria in Human Disease. Academic Press, New York, 1977.

Finegold, S. M. and George, W. L.: Anaerobic Infections in Humans. San Diego, Academic Press, Inc., 1989.

Sneath, P. H. A., Mair, N. S., Sharpe, M. E., and Holt, J. G.: Bergey's Manual of Systematic Bacteriology, Vol. 2 ed 9, Williams and Wilkins, Baltimore, 1986.

Summanen P., Baron, E. J., Citron, D. M., Strong, C., Wexler, H. M. and Finegold, S. M.: Wadsworth Anaerobic Bacteriology Manual, ed 5. Star Publishing, Belmont, CA, 1993.

Willis, A. T.: Clostridia of Wound Infection. Butterworths, London, 1969.

16 Black-Pigmenting Bacteria

Joseph J. Zambon and Russell J. Nisengard

CHAPTER OUTLINE

Taxonomy of the black-pigmenting bacteria

Organisms in this group include gram-negative, obligately anaerobic, nonmotile, nonspore-forming rods. These species are of prime importance in oral infections and are thought to play major roles in the pathogenesis of both periodontal disease and endodontic infections. Members of this group of organisms are also associated with significant, sometimes life-threatening soft tissue infections of the head and neck region. In addition, they comprise a major component of the microflora not only in the human oral cavity, but throughout the human gastrointestinal tract and are associated with diseases of the colon, upper respiratory tract and urogenital tract.

TAXONOMY OF THE BLACK-PIGMENTING BACTERIA

Major changes have occurred in the taxonomy of this group of organisms. Formerly, many of these organisms were referred to as the "black-pigmented *Bacteroides*" or the "BPB" group of organisms since the bacterial colonies often produce a black or beige pigment especially when these species are cultured on media containing rabbit blood. In recent years, however, many species have been reclassified from the genus *Bacteroides* into other genera, particularly the newly defined genera *Porphyromonas* and *Prevotella*. For that reason, the term black-pigmented *Bacteroides* is no longer appropriate although it is still commonly used.

Oliver and Wherry in 1921 first isolated these organisms from the oral cavity and noted that the colonies produced a black or beige pigment that they mistakenly referred to as melanin, and, which recently has been shown to be protoheme. They consequently named these organisms *Bacterium melaninogenicum* ("melanin producing"). This single species has been subdivided over the ensuing years into a number of subspecies and has led to the present classification. (Refer to Fig. 14–1

which describes the evolution of the taxonomy of oral *Bacteroides* species).

In extra-oral sites, the *Bacteroides* species best known are those in the *B. fragilis* group, which includes the species *B. fragilis*, *B. distasonis*, *B. eggerthii*, *B. vulgatus*, *B. thetaiotaomicron*, *B. ovatus*, and *B. uniformis*. Species in the *B. fragilis* group cause infections in the abdomen and colon and may be associated with infections elsewhere in the body. These infections may be especially difficult to treat since these species frequently exhibit resistance to various antibiotics. Two members of the *B. fragilis* group, *B. bivius* and *B. disiens* are found mainly in the female genital tract.

The *B. fragilis* group often cause infections in combination with other anaerobes, particularly anaerobic cocci such as members of the *Peptostreptococcus*. The pathogenesis of the *B. fragilis* group of organisms is related to the production of lipopolysaccha.ide endotoxins and capsular polysaccharides which can elicit abscesses upon injection into animal models. This group also produces beta lactamase, which can inhibit antibiotic therapy with antimicrobials such as penicillin G.

Bacteroides species can be divided into those species that produce pigment (i.e., the black-pigmenting *Bacteroides* species) and those species that do not. It should be noted, however, that the oral *Bacteroides* are not the only oral bacteria that can produce black or dark pigmented colonies. For example, *Actinomyces odontolyticus* also can produce darkly pigmented colonies. Among the black-pigmenting group, Holdeman and Moore in 1970 were able to distinguish subgroups based on the ability of some strains to ferment sugar. Categorization based on this phenotypic trait resulted in three subspecies—*Bacteroides melaninogenicus* subspecies *asaccharolyticus* for those organisms which did not ferment sugar, *B. melaninogenicus* subspecies *melaninogenicus* for those organisms that showed the ability to strongly ferment sugar, and *B. melaninogenicus* subspecies *intermedius* for those organisms that were intermediate in their ability to ferment sugars. Subsequently these subspecies were all elevated to species level as *B. melaninogenicus*, *B. intermedius*, and *B. asaccharolyticus*. Further work demonstrated that oral strains of *B. asaccharolyticus* were genetically distinct from nonoral strains and the oral species were renamed *B. gingivalis* in reference to their frequent colonization of gingiva. Additional work by a number of investigators on this group of oral black-pigmenting species has resulted in the current classification (see Table 16–1). The black-pigmenting species can be differentiated by a series of biochemical characteristics as summarized in Table 16–2. These include sugar fermentations and enzymatic activity.

These species are not unique to the human oral cavity. Similar species have been isolated from the oral cavity of a variety of different animals including dog and nonhuman primates. These latter species have facilitated the study of virulence factors in black-pigmenting *Bacteroides* species infecting humans. Studies by Holt et al. have shown that monoinfection with *Porphyromonas gingivalis* in the monkey ligature model can result in alveolar bone loss similar to that seen in human periodontitis.

Aside from being relatively strict anaerobes, the BPB species also require certain levels of hemin and vitamin K_1 for growth. Hemin serves as an iron and protoporphyrin source for the growth of these organisms, however, excess levels of hemin can inhibit growth. Estradiol, progesterone, and other steroid-based hormones have chemical structures similar to vitamin K_1 and can serve as substitutes for vitamin K_1. The presence of high levels of these hormones in adolescents at the time of puberty, in people under psychological stress, and in pregnant women is associated with particular forms of periodontal disease characterized by infections with *Bacteroides* species. The high levels of these hormones are thought to favor the growth of these species and to facilitate periodontal infections.

The black-pigmenting species are found in the following genera:

Bacteroides

Most oral species once categorized in this genera have recently been recategorized into the *Porphyromonas* and *Prevotella* listed below. One notable exception is *Bacteroides forsythus*, first isolated by Dr. Anne Tanner of Forsyth Dental Center. This was originally described as "fusiform" *Bacteroides* based on the microscopic appearance of the cells that have tapered (fusiform) ends and may have central swellings. *B. forsythus* is a slow growing, strict anaerobe that has unique growth requirements. The colonies often appear on primary culture as satellites of *Fusobacterium nucleatum* and isolates will grow only in the presence of "feeder" colonies of *F. nucleatum* or *Porphyromonas gingivalis* or upon addition of *N*-acetyl-muramic acid to agar or broth media. This species is often found in subgingival dental plaque in association with sites of peridontal attachment loss.

Porphyromonas

Porphyromonas is a new genera that includes species previously classified among the asaccharolytic black-pigmenting *Bacteroides*. *B. gingivalis*, *B. endodontalis*, and *B. asaccharolyticus* have been reclassified as *Porphyromonas gingivalis*, *P. endodontalis*, and *P. asaccharolytica*, respectively. These species differ from other members of the *Bacteroides* based on the G + C content that ranges from 46 to 54 percent for the porphyromonads compared with 40 to 48 percent for the *Bacteroides*.

PORPHYROMONAS GINGIVALIS

P. gingivalis (formerly *Bacteroides gingivalis*) is an anaerobic, non-fermenting, gram-negative short rod that also may appear as cocci, that is, pleomorphic. *P. gingivalis* is frequently isolated from subgingival plaque samples in patients with adult and other forms of periodontitis. The major oral ecologic niche for this species appears to be subgingival plaque although Van Winkelhoff and

TABLE 16–1 ✦ Human Black-Pigmenting Bacteria

CURRENT NOMENCLATURE	PREVIOUS NOMENCLATURE(S)
Bacteroides Species	
Bacteroides forsythus	
Bacteroides salivosus	
Porphyromonas Species	
Porphyromonas asaccharolytica	Bacteroides asaccharolyticus
Porphyromonas endodontalis	Bacteroides endodontalis
Porphyromonas gingivalis	Bacteroides gingivalis
Prevotella Species	
Prevotella denticola	Bacteroides denticola
Prevotella disiens	Bacteroides disiens
Prevotella intermedia	Bacteroides intermedius
Prevotella loescheii	Bacteroides loescheii
Prevotella melaninogenica	Bacteroides melaninogenicus

TABLE 16–2 . Differential Characteristics of Important Black-Pigmenting Bacteria

	BACTEROIDES FORSYTHUS	PORPHYROMONAS ASACCHAROLYTICA	PORPHYROMONAS ENDODONTALIS
Indole	+	+	+
Lipase	−	−	−
Esculin hydrolysis	+	−	−
Fermentation of			
Cellobiose	−	−	−
Glucose	−	−	−
Lactose	−	−	−
Maltose	−	−	−
Sucrose	−	−	−
Enzymes:			
α-glucosidase	−	−	−
α-fucosidase	+	+	−
N-acetyl-β-glucosaminidase	+	−	−
Phenylacetic acid production	−	−	−
Trypsin	+	−	−

*most strains are positive but a few are negative.
†V = variable
‡most strains are negative but a few are positive.

others found this species in other sites within the human oral cavity including the tonsil, lateral border of the tongue, and buccal mucosa. The role of *P. gingivalis* in the pathogenesis of human periodontitis is based partially on the fact that it rarely occurs in the gingival sulci associated with healthy periodontal tissues while it is found in high prevalence as an increased proportion of the total microflora in subgingival sites associated with periodontitis. There are at least three serogroups or antigenically distinct groups within the species *P. gingivalis*, serotypes A, B, and C. *P. gingivalis* produces a number of factors that can be associated with virulence including fimbria, collagenase, lipopolysaccharide, and endotoxin (Table 16–3).

Electron microscopic studies of *P. gingivalis* show the presence of a capsule and fimbria. *P. gingivalis* fimbria, like fimbria from other species, are filamentous surface structures. They may be important in mediating bacterial adherence to tooth structure, to other bacteria, or to human epithelial cells such as those lining the gingival sulcus. The fimbria are composed of 43,000 molecular weight repeating subunits. Other components associated with *P. gingivalis* fimbria may mediate the ability to bind red blood cells, that is, a hemagglutinating activity.

In addition to the monkey ligature model, a mouse abscess model also has been used to study the virulence of *P. gingivalis*. These studies show significant differences among various *P. gingivalis*

strains in their ability to produce abscesses. Certain strains produced localized lesions while other usually highly proteolytic strains produce spreading lesions.

Among the virulence factors produced by *P. gingivalis* are collagenase, a trypsinlike enzyme, keratinases, hemolysins, fibrinolysins, hyaluronidases, phospholipase, alkaline phosphatase, acid phosphatase, and other toxic proteases (see Table 16–3). The trypsinlike activity is capable of degrading various synthetic substrates among them is *N*-benzoyl-DL-arginine-2-naphthylamide (BANA). This trypsinlike activity is shared by other oral bacterial species including spirochetes and has been used in the formulation of a rapid, in-office diagnostic test for the presence of this group of organisms in patient plaque samples.

Capsular polysaccharide also is a significant virulence factor for *P. gingivalis*. Capsular polysaccharides, in general, engender a number of advantages to bacteria, primarily the ability to inhibit phagocytosis by host immune cells. Ultrastructural studies of *P. gingivalis* show that avirulent variants tend to demonstrate lesser amounts of extracellular capsular material than virulent variants. Further, the *P. gingivalis* polysaccharide capsule also may be important in cell adherence. Recent studies by Schifferle, et al. show that a crude vaccine composed of a capsular polysaccharide/protein conjugate from *P. gingivalis* was protective in the experimental mouse abscess model.

PORPHYROMONAS GINGIVALIS	*PREVOTELLA INTERMEDIA*	*PREVOTELLA LOESCHEII*	*PREVOTELLA MELANINOGENICA*
+	+	−	−
−	+*	V†	−‡
−	−	V	−
−	−	+	−
−	+	+	+
−	+	+	+
−	+	+	+
−	+	+	+
−	+	+	+
−	+	−	+
+	−	+	−
+	−	−	−
+	−	−	−

PORPHYROMONAS ENDODONTALIS

This organism originally was isolated from severe odontogenic abscesses associated with endodontic infections and is a strict anaerobe as opposed to *P. gingivalis*, which can survive short periods of exposure to air. In view of this, *P. endodontalis* may actually be more frequently associated with endodontic infections than demonstrated by culture. Studies by Pantera et al., for example, shows that this organism can be frequently detected from endodontic lesions by immunofluorescence microscopy. *P. endodontalis* may contribute to the pathogenesis of endodontic infections by its ability to degrade type IV collagen and proteolytic activity to gelatin.

PORPHYROMONAS ASACCHAROLYTICA

This name is one of the original classifications of the black-pigmented *Bacteroides* and represents those nonfermenting species not included within *P. endodontalis* or *P. gingivalis*. This organism can be differentiated from *P. gingivalis* on the basis of DNA-DNA hybridization and by the absence of both the trypsinlike activity and the hemagglutinating activity that is present in *P. gingivalis* but not in *P. asaccharolyticus*. This organism is infrequently found in oral sites and is mainly restricted to other areas of the gastrointestinal tract.

Prevotella

The newly described genus *Prevotella* (named after the French anaerobic microbiologist, Prevot) includes those organisms formerly classified mainly with the *Bacteroides intermedius* and *B. melaninogenicus* group. These are anaerobic, gram-negative rods which ferment sugar and includes both pigmenting and non-pigmenting species.

PREVOTELLA INTERMEDIA

Formerly known as *Bacteroides intermedius*, this species contained three DNA homology groups, one of which was separated into a species named *Bacteroides* (now *Prevotella*) *corporis*. *P. intermedia* ferment sugars as do *P. melaninogenica*, but less strongly. The colonies of *P. intermedia* are unique in that they give off a brick red fluorescence when exposed to ultraviolet light. This feature has been used in the laboratory to differentiate the black colonies of *P. intermedia* from other black colonies that may appear on a primary culture plate. The ability of *P. intermedia* to produce β-galactosidase also differentiates this species from other black-pigmenting colonies (Table 16–2).

P. intermedia is associated with moderate-to-severe gingival inflammation, acute necrotizing ulcerative gingivitis, and chronic adult periodontitis. Recent evidence suggests that there may be differences within *P. intermedia* with certain subgroups related to gingivitis and others related to periodontitis. Some factors associated with its virulence are summarized in Table 16–3.

PREVOTELLA MELANINOGENICA

Formerly known as *Bacteroides melaninogenicus*, *Prevotella melaninogenica* and two

TABLE 16–3 ✦ Bacterial Virulence Factors

	PORPHYROMONAS GINGIVALIS	*PREVOTELLA INTERMEDIA*
Colonization Factors		
Capsules	+	+
Pili	+	+
Tissue Destructive Factors		
Abscess former	Strong	Moderate
Enzymes:		
Acid phosphatase	+	+
Alkaline phosphatase	+	+
Aminopeptidases	±	−
Collagenase type I	+	−
type IV	+	−
Elastase	+	−
Gelatinase	Strong	Moderate
Trypsinlike	+	+
Toxic factors:		
Ammonia	+	+
Butyric and proprionic acids	+	−
Endotoxin	Weak	Weak
Epitheliotoxin	+	+
Fibroblast growth inhibitors	+	+
Fibronectin degradation	+	
Indole	+	+
LPS bone resorption	+	+
Host Defense Factors		
C3 degradation	+	
Fibrinolysin	Strong	Weak
IgA proteases	+	+
IgG proteases	+	+
Polymorphonuclear leukocytes:		
Leukotoxin	−	−
Decreased phagocytosis and intracellular killing	+	+
Superoxide dismutase	+	+

other closely related species, *P. denticola* and *P. loescheii* (named after Dr. Walter Loesche) strongly ferment sugars. The role of *P. melaninogenica, P. denticola,* and *P. loescheii* in oral disease is not well established although they do not appear to be prominent pathogens.

BIBLIOGRAPHY

Jousimies-Somer, H. R. and Finegold, S. M.: Anaerobic gram-negative bacilli and cocci. In Ballows, A., Hausler Jr., W. J., Herrmann, K. L., Isenberg, H. D., and Shadomy, H. J. (eds): Manual of Clinical Microbiology, ed. 5. American Society of Microbiology, Washington, D.C.

Lantz, M. S., Allen, R. D., Duck, L. W., Switolski, L. M., Hook, M.: *Porphyromonas gingivalis* surface components bind and degrade connective tissue proteins. J. Periodont. Res. 26:283, 1991.

Shah, H. N. and Collins, M. D.: Proposal for reclassification of *Bacteroides asacchararolyticus, Bacteroides gingivalis,* and *Bacteroides endodontalis* in a new genus, *Porphyromonas.* Int. J. Syst. Bacteriol. 38:128, 1988.

Shah, H. N. and Collins, M. D.: Proposal to restrict the genus *Bacteroides* (Castellani and Chalmers) to *Bacteroides fragilis* and closely related species. Int. J. Syst. Bacteriol. 39:85, 1989.

Shah, H. N. and Collins, M. D.: *Prevotella,* a new genus to include *Bacteroides melaninogenicus* and related species formerly classified in the genus *Bacteroides.* Int. J. Syst. Bacteriol. 40:205, 1990.

Slots, J. and Genco, R. J.: Microbial Pathogenicity. Black-pigmented *Bacteroides* species, *Capnocytophaga* species, and *Actinobacillus actinomycetem-*

comitans in human peridontal disease: Virulence factors in colonization, survival, and tissue destruction. J. Dent. Res. 63:412, 1984.

Tanner, A. C. R., Listgarten, M. A., Ebersole, J. L., and Strzempko, M. N.: *Bacteroides forsythus* sp. from the human oral cavity. Int. J. Syst. Bacteriol. 36:213, 1986.

Uitto, V-J., Haapasalo, M., Laakso, T., and Salo, T.: Degradation of basement membrane (type IV) collagen by proteases from some anaerobic oral microorganisms. Oral Microbiol. Immunol. 3:97, 1988.

Van Winkelhoff, A. J., van Steenbergen, T. J. M., and de Graaf, J.: The role of black-pigmented *Bacteroides* in human oral disease. J. Clin. Periodontol. 15:145, 1988.

17 Actinobacillus actinomycetemcomitans

Jørgen Slots

CHAPTER OUTLINE

Morphology

Cultivation and other detection methods

Antigenic composition

Oral colonization

Plasmids and bacteriophages

Potential virulence mechanisms

Actinobacillus actinomycetemcomitans is a gram-negative, small, nonspore-forming, nonmotile, facultatively anaerobic rod. It was isolated originally from human cases of actinomycosis, first by Klinger in Germany in 1912, then by Comstock in England in 1920, and by Bayne-Jones in the United States in 1925. The organism's early name *Bacterium actinomycetem-comitans* (*comitans*, from accompanying the bacterium *Actinomyces*) reflected its association with actinomycosis. *A. actinomycetemcomitans* is now isolated mainly from periodontitis and occasionally from endocarditis lesions, and it can be detected in various focal infections. Of the five recognized *Actinobacillus* species, *A. actinomycetemcomitans* is the only one indigenous to man. *A. actinomycetemcomitans* also may colonize the oral cavity of apes, monkeys, dogs, cats, and other animals. The four other *Actinobacillus* species are pathogenic in cattle, horses, and pigs.

The *Actinobacillus* genus is closely related to the *Haemophilus* and *Pasteurella* genera. In particular, *A. actinomycetemcomitans* and *Haemophilus aphrophilus* share many nucleotide base sequences, surface antigens, and biochemical features. *A. actinomycetemcomitans* is more closely related genetically to *H. aphrophilus* than to *Actinobacillus lignieresii*, the type species of the *Actinobacillus* genus. Therefore, this taxon was recently proposed to be transferred to the *Haemophilus* genus. However, the proposed transfer was rejected because the taxonomic status of *H. aphrophilus* remains unresolved as well.

MORPHOLOGY

Fresh clinical isolates of *A. actinomycetemcomitans* appear as circular convex colonies about 1.0 mm in diameter with slightly irregular edges (Fig. 17–1). Primary colonies are translucent, glistening, and exhibit a starlike inner structure. They adhere to the agar surface and are difficult to break up. Growth in broth is granular with clumps of cell strongly adherent to the side of a test tube. The ability of the colonies to adhere to agar medium, the inner structure of the colonies, and the granular growth in broth disappear on repeated subculture.

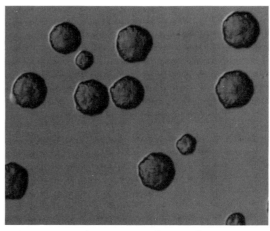

FIGURE 17–1 ✦ Primary isolation of *A. actinomycetemcomitans* on TSBV selective medium showing the characteristic star-shaped inner structure.

A. actinomycetemcomitans cells are about 1.0 to 1.5 × 0.4 to 0.5 μm in size, and occur singly, in pairs, or in small clumps. In old cultures or after several transfers some strains show longer cell forms.

CULTIVATION AND OTHER DETECTION METHODS

A. actinomycetemcomitans grows best on serum or blood agar in an anaerobic atmosphere or in 10 percent CO_2. Cultures may be stimulated by 1 percent $NaHCO_3$. Steroid hormones including estrogen, progesterone, and testosterone are capable of enhancing the growth of *A. actinomycetemcomitans* and may influence the population of the organism during puberty. Growth is optimal at 37°C. Hemin (X-factor) and nicotinamide adenine dinucleotide (V-factor), which are important growth factors for the *Haemophilus* genus (*H. aphrophilus* exhibits no requirement for X and V factors), are not required by *A. actinomycetemcomitans*.

Recovery of *A. actinomycetemcomitans* from oral specimens often requires the use of a selective medium to detect small levels of the organism, which may have clinical significance, and to avoid in vitro inhibition by sampled streptococci. Tryptic soy agar-serum-bacitracin-vancomycin (TSBV) is a commonly used selective medium for *A. actinomycetemcomitans* recovery. Detection of *A. actinomycetemcomitans* in oral specimens also can take place using immunological and DNA probe technologies.

A. actinomycetemcomitans can be divided into 10 biotypes on the basis of dextrin, maltose, mannitol, and xylose fermentation reaction patterns, five serotypes on the basis of cell surface antigens, and a large number of genotypes using chromosomal restriction endonuclease digestion pattern (REDS), restriction fragment length polymorphism (RFLP), and arbitrarily primed polymerase chain reaction (AP-PCR). Fingerprinting the genome of *A. actinomycetemcomitans* by means of the AP-PCR technique represents a particularly powerful tool in understanding the molecular epidemiology of the organism.

ANTIGENIC COMPOSITION

The *A. actinomycetemcomitans* species contains five serotypes (a through e). The serotype-determining antigens are heat-stable surface polysaccharides that appear to be unique for the species. *A. actinomycetemcomitans* serotype b is the most common serotype in localized juvenile periodontitis. Serotypes d and e occur with lowest prevalence. The serotype determining antigens comprise up to 95 percent carbohydrate, including rhamnose, fucose, and deoxy-talose-polymers.

Shared antigens occur among the *A. actinomycetemcomitans* serotypes and among *A. actinomycetemcomitans* and various *Haemophilus* species.

ORAL COLONIZATION

A. actinomycetemcomitans occurs more frequently in the oral cavity of African-Americans than of Caucasians. The organism is transmitted from family member to family member in localized juvenile periodontitis and some forms of adult periodontitis.

A. actinomycetemcomitans is one of the few oral bacteria capable of colonizing buccal mucosa as well as dental plaque. The establishment of *A. actinomycetemcomitans* in the human oral cavity is dependent on appropriate attachment sites for initial colonization and is influenced by the interacting microflora and various host factors (Table 17–1).

Fimbriae (pili) are thin surface appendages that serve as adhesion determinants for many medical pathogens and also seem to be a major determinant of the initial attachment of *A. actinomycetemcomitans* to oral surfaces. Freshly isolated *A. actinomycetemcomitans* strains are strongly adherent to agar, glass, and other surfaces. This adherent capability is lost on repeated subculture. The adherent colony type demonstrates an abundance of fimbriae on the cell surface whereas established, nonadherent laboratory strains rarely show fimbriae. It is not known if the change in attachment potential and fimbriation is caused by mutation or phenotypic regulation due to environmental changes.

A. actinomycetemcomitans elaborates numerous vesicles, or "blebs," on the cell surfaces. Their role in initial colonization, if any, remains to be determined.

Bacterial interactions seem to be another determinant of oral colonization of *A. actinomycetemcomitans*. *Streptococcus sanguis*, *Actinomyces viscosus*, and *Streptococcus uberis* inhibit the in vitro growth of *A. actinomycetemcomitans*. The ability of *S. sanguis* to inhibit the growth of *A. actinomycetemcomitans* is due to production of hydrogen peroxide at levels inhibitory to *A. actinomycetemcomitans*. On the other hand, *A. actinomycetem-*

TABLE 17–1 ✦ *A. actinomycetemcomitans* Colonization Factors

Pili or fimbriae
Capsule
Interactions with other bacteria
Vesicles?

comitans also displays bacteriocin properties capable of inhibiting in vitro growth of *S. sanguis, A. viscosus,* and other common dental plaque microorganisms. Possibly, whether *A. actinomycetemcomitans* or certain gram-positive plaque bacteria are the first organisms to colonize an oral site will determine the potential for later colonization of various streptococci or *A. actinomycetemcomitans,* respectively.

PLASMIDS AND BACTERIOPHAGES

Plasmids and bacteriophages are genetic elements that may alter the physiological properties of a microorganism, contribute to virulence, modify taxonomic status, and spread biological properties among different strains, species, and genera.

About 5 percent of clinical isolates of *A. actinomycetemcomitans* show small or larger cryptic (i.e., with unknown function) plasmids. Many *A. actinomycetemcomitans* strains harbor bacteriophages and at least three morphologically distinct types of phages can infect the organism. It is not known whether the phage's gene products can affect the pathogenic potential of *A. actinomycetemcomitans.* Some studies have related high levels of free *A. actinomycetemcomitans* bacteriophages to actively progressing periodontal disease.

POTENTIAL VIRULENCE MECHANISMS

A. actinomycetemcomitans and most other members of the *Actinobacillus* genus appear both as commensal and pathogenic organisms. The translation of several actinobacilli species from the commensal to the pathogenic status usually involves factors that aid the organism in entering and colonizing eucaryotic cells and tissues. Invasiveness may be an important virulence determinant for *A. actinomycetemcomitans* as well. If so, microbial factors that enable the organism to overcome various host defenses are critical for virulence.

A. actinomycetemcomitans produces several biologically active substances that individually or collectively could be involved in the production of disease (Table 17–2). Of particular interest are those factors of *A. actinomycetemcomitans* that are not shared by other putative periodontopathic bacteria. The *A. actinomycetemcomitans* leukotoxin and *A. actinomycetemcomitans* immunosuppressive factor have not, for example, been identified in a large number of other plaque organisms. The capacity of *A. actinomycetemcomitans* to mediate bone resorption, depress fibroblast proliferation, or produce polyclonal B-cell activators is seen in many groups of bacteria. Differences in the biologic potentials of *A. actinomycetemcomitans* versus other bacteria may help to explain the peculiar features of periodontal lesions infected by *A. actinomycetemcomitans.*

TABLE 17–2 ✦ *A. actinomycetemcomitans*—Host Interactions

Leukotoxin
Inhibition of neutrophil functions
Immunosuppression via T-suppressor cell activation
Resistant to complement-mediated killing
Polyclonal cell activation
Endotoxin-mediated complement activation

Leukotoxin

Neutrophils are key cells in the periodontal defense against microbial pathogens. Neutrophils can kill *A. actinomycetemcomitans* under aerobic and anaerobic conditions in vitro. On the other hand, *A. actinomycetemcomitans* also can kill human neutrophils and monocytes-macrophages in vitro. The killing of neutrophils is due to a proteinaceous, heat-labile leukotoxin. Although neutrophils and monocytes from several nonhuman primates are also destroyed by the leukotoxin, human leukocytes seem to be especially sensitive. Some human T and B cell lines are also sensitive to the leukotoxin. Interestingly, other human cells (such as platelets, erythrocytes, fibroblasts, and endothelial and epithelial cells) as well as leukocytes from other species (such as dogs, rabbits, rats, and mice) are not affected by the leukotoxin. The leukotoxin-mediated killing is extremely rapid (a matter of minutes) and is caused by formation of pores in the cell membrane of the target cells. If the leukotoxin acts in vivo as it does in vitro, it could have profound effects on the course of *A. actinomycetemcomitans* infection by depleting neutrophils as they migrate into the area, thereby crippling innate resistance to bacterial attack. Furthermore, leukotoxin-damaged cells release lysosomal products into the extracellular milieu, which also may contribute to tissue injury. Finally, killing of monocytes in the gingival tissues may perturb adaptative resistance (the immune response) and delay antibody synthesis against the leukotoxin or other bacterial antigens.

The *A. actinomycetemcomitans* leukotoxin gene has been cloned and expressed in *Escherichia coli.* Analysis of nucleoside sequence data shows a similarity with the *Pasteurella haemolytica* leukotoxin gene and the *E. coli* hemolysin gene. Although these leukotoxin molecules seem to form a family of related cytotoxins, *A. actinomycetemcomitans* is the only organism that can produce cell lysis by intact whole cells. Cell specificity of the leukotoxins vary as well. These differences may be due, in part, to the close association of the *A. actinomycetemcomitans* leukotoxin with the bacterial cell envelope or the membrane vesicles on the outer bacterial cell surface. The *P. haemolytica* and *E. coli* toxins are secreted into the cell media.

Immunosuppressive Factor

Patients with localized juvenile periodontitis show a high incidence of infection by *A. actinomycetemcomitans,* and the vast majority also demonstrate antibodies to *A. actinomycetemcomitans*–derived antigens (including the leukotoxin) in serum and gingival exudates. Thus, there is a vigorous immune response to *A. actinomycetemcomitans* and this may be critical in limiting the extent of *A. actinomycetemcomitans* attack on the host. However, during the early phases of a periodontal infection, it is conceivable that *A. actinomycetemcomitans* may impede the local and/or systemic humoral immune response and hence secure sufficient time to become "firmly" established in the area. As discussed above, the *A. actinomycetemcomitans* leukotoxin could contribute to immunosuppression by killing monocytes. Also, the leukotoxin may kill some T cell clones by damaging the plasma membrane ("necrosis") or activating a nuclease able to cleave chromosomal DNA ("programmed cell death"). In addition, *A. actinomycetemcomitans* possesses a unique heat-labile immunosuppressive factor that inhibits various critical functions of lymphoid cells such as blastogenesis, antibody production, and lymphokine synthesis. The immunosuppressive factor does not kill cells but selectively activates T-suppressor cells. While several other plaque bacteria inhibit lymphoid responsiveness to antigens or mitogens, none appears to operate in this manner. The immunosuppressive factor, unlike the leukotoxin, can affect lymphoid cells from primates as well as other species and also is found in non-leukotoxic *A. actinomycetemcomitans* strains (see further on). This substance, together with the leukotoxin, may represent a potent mechanism for overwhelming local host defense systems.

Perturbation of Neutrophil Functions Unrelated to Leukotoxin Activity

A. actinomycetemcomitans can affect neutrophil behavior without killing these cells. For example, strains of *A. actinomycetemcomitans* that lack the toxin (or have very low levels of leukotoxin) are not phagocytosed by neutrophils unless opsonized by antibodies or other serum components. Further, leukotoxic as well as nonleukotoxic strains contain unidentified substances that inhibit neutrophil che-

motaxis. They also produce catalase and superoxide dismutase and seem to be relatively insensitive to hydrogen peroxide and superoxide anion. These data suggest that neutrophils may have difficulty dealing with *A. actinomycetemcomitans* even in the absence of leukotoxin. This might be relevant in situations when the host has formed neutralizing antibodies to the leukotoxin or in patients infected with nonleukotoxic *A. actinomycetemcomitans* strains. In this context, cross-sectional studies in patients with localized juvenile periodontitis suggest that there may be a shift from leukotoxic to nonleukotoxic *A. actinomycetemcomitans* during the course of infection. The basis for this change in biologic activity is not presently understood.

Inhibition of Fibroblasts, Endothelial Cells, and Epithelial Cell Activities

A. actinomycetemcomitans can modulate the behavior of fibroblasts, endothelial cells, and epithelial cells without actually killing these resident tissue cells (Table 17–3). The relevant factors have not been adequately defined but they are heat-sensitive and inactivated by proteolytic enzymes. For example, extracts of either leukotoxic or nonleukotoxic *A. actinomycetemcomitans* can inhibit DNA, RNA, and protein synthesis in cultures of fibroblasts or endothelial cells. Likewise, epithelial cell proliferation and attachment to plastic tissue culture growth surfaces are depressed by *A. actinomycetemcomitans* extracts. Obviously, if the functions of resident tissue cells are compromised in vivo there are likely to be profound changes in the ability of infected tissues to resist or respond to injury.

Lipopolysaccharide Activity

Bacterial endotoxic lipopolysaccharides have been advocated as important virulence factors in the pathogenesis of many forms of periodontal disease, and *A. actinomycetemcomitans* contains very potent lipopolysaccharides. These substances, for example, act as B-cell mitogens (see further on), and activate the alternative complement pathway.

TABLE 17–3 ✦ *A. actinomycetemcomitans* Effects on Tissue

Inhibition of fibroblasts, endothelial cells, and epithelial cells
Endotoxin-mediated bone resorption
Endotoxin-mediated tissue toxicity
Collagenase
Invasion

In addition, endotoxin can stimulate bone resorption in vitro. In this context, *A. actinomycetemcomitans* also contains nonendotoxic factors that cause bone destruction in tissue cultures. Patients often show high serum antibody levels to the polysaccharide moiety of the *A. actinomycetemcomitans* endotoxin.

Polyclonal Cell Activation

A. actinomycetemcomitans stimulates polyclonal antibody production as well as mitogenic responses in human blood lymphocytes. Stimulatory effects of *A. actinomycetemcomitans* on B cells may be mediated by both endotoxic as well as nonendotoxic components. Polyclonal cell activation could result in overproduction in immunologic effector molecules (e.g., antibodies, lymphokines) that may have potential beneficial and/or harmful effects on the host (e.g., hypersecretion of bone-destroying factor might lead to bone resorption; formation of "inappropriate" immune complexes could nonspecifically activate the complement system, stimulate neutrophil degranulation, and so forth).

Invasion of Host Tissues

A. actinomycetemcomitans often is localized at the "apical front" of subgingival deposits and is thus in a very strategic position to penetrate underlying soft tissues. Indeed, gram-negative organisms, including those resembling *A. actinomycetemcomitans*, has been identified in gingival specimens from patients with severe localized juvenile periodontitis. *A. actinomycetemcomitans* is able to invade epithelial cells in laboratory experiments and the invasion phase seems to correspond to a rough-to-smooth colonial phenotype phase variation. The rough, fimbriated form of *A. actinomycetemcomitans*, which is the natural inhabitant of the oral cavity, may serve as a reservoir from which the smooth, nonfimbriated, and invasive forms may derive. If so, the factors that modulate the rough-to-smooth phenotypic variation

may play important roles in pathogenicity. Observation on whether *A. actinomycetemcomitans* also colonizes soft tissue during initial or early phases of disease may help to settle whether *A. actinomycetemcomitans* invasiveness is a factor in the etiology of juvenile periodontitis.

From the foregoing it is apparent that *A. actinomycetemcomitans* possesses biologic properties that could allow it to attack the host. The capacity of *A. actinomycetemcomitans* to overwhelm or evade antibacterial defense systems in the gingival region may be particularly relevant in explaining how this organism causes disease.

BIBLIOGRAPHY

McArthur, W. P., Tsai, C. C., and Taichman, N. S.: Non-cytolytic effects of *Actinobacillus actinomycetemcomitans* on leukocyte functions. In Genco, R. J., and Mergenhagen, S. E. (eds.): Host-Parasite Interactions in Periodontal Diseases. American Society for Microbiology, Washington, D.C., 1982, p. 179.

Saglie, F. R.: Bacterial invasion and its role in the pathogenesis of periodontal disease. In Hamada, S., Holt, S. C., and McGhee, J. R. (eds.): Periodontal Disease: Pathogens & Host Immune Responses. Quintessence Publishing Co., Tokyo, 1991, p. 27.

Shenker, B. J., Tsai, C. C., and Taichman, N. S.: Suppression of lymphocyte responses by *Actinobacillus actinomycetemcomitans*. J. Periodont. Res. 17:462, 1982.

Slots, J.: Selective medium for isolation of *Actinobacillus actinomycetemcomitans*. J. Clin. Microbiol. 15:606, 1982.

Slots, J. and Schonfeld, S. E.: *Actinobacillus actinomycetemcomitans* in localized juvenile periodontitis. In Hamada, S., Holt, S. C., and McGhee, J. R. (eds.): Periodontal Disease: Pathogens & Host Immune Responses. Quintessence Publishing Co., Tokyo, 1991, p. 53.

Slots, J., Liu, Y. B., Di Rienzo, J. M., and Chen, C.: Evaluating two methods for fingerprinting genomes of *Actinobacillus actinomycetemcomitans*. Oral Microbiol. Immunol. 8, 1993.

Zambon, J. J.: *Actinobacillus actinomycetemcomitans* in human periodontal diseases. J. Clin. Periodontol. 12:1, 1985.

18 Veillonella, Wolinella, *and* Campylobacter

Paulette J. Tempro and Joseph J. Zambon

CHAPTER OUTLINE

Veillonella *species*

Wolinella *species*

Campylobacter *species*

VEILLONELLA SPECIES

The *Veillonella* are gram-negative, anaerobic cocci found in the human intestinal and respiratory tracts as well as in some animals (Table 18–1). This genus is classified together with the genera *Acidaminococcus* and *Megasphaera* in the family Veillonellaceae. The bacteria, 0.3 to 0.5 μm in diameter, occur as diplococci and in short chains are nonmotile and grow best at 30°C to 37°C. They are oxidase- and catalase-negative. On agar they may form lens-, diamond-, or heart-shaped colonies that are opaque, grayish white. One distinguishing feature is the ability of the bacterial colonies to exhibit a pink to red fluorescence when illuminated with a long-wave ultraviolet light. This fluorescence characteristic is shared with black pigmented species such as *Prevotella intermedia*. The *Veillonella* can ferment pyruvate, lactate, malate, fumarate, and oxaloacetate but do not ferment carbohydrates. They exhibit between 36 and 43 mol% G + C.

Seven species of *Veillonella* have been identified—*V. parvula, V. rodentium, V. atypica, V. ratti, V. criceti, V. dispar,* and *V. caviae*—of which three species, *parvula, atypica,* and *dispar,* have been isolated from humans, especially from the oral cavity. These species, which are phenotypically similar can be distinguished from one another only by DNA/DNA hybridization. *V. parvula* and *V. dispar* have been isolated from human dental plaque in patients with periodontal disease. There is, however, no evidence to indicate that these species are important in the etiology of human periodontal disease.

TABLE 18–1 ✦ *Veillonella*

Characteristics	Gram-negative, anaerobic cocci
	Found in the human GI and respiratory tract
	Found in alimentary canal of animals
Major species	*V. parvula* ⎫ species
	V. atypica ⎬ found
	V. dispar ⎭ in humans
Growth	Anaerobic at 30°C–37°C
Disease	Possible association with human periodontal disease
Pathogenesis	Unknown

WOLINELLA SPECIES

The *Wolinella* are gram-negative, motile anaerobes found as helical, curved, or straight bacterial cells 0.5 to 1.0 μm by 2 to 6 μm with tapered or round ends (Table 18–2). A rapid, darting type of bacterial motility by means of flagella located at one pole of the bacterial cell is exhibited. This motility can be observed by phase contrast microscopy. The bacteria form three types of colonies on agar: (1) a pale, translucent, nonspreading yellow colony, (2) a gray translucent colony, which may be mistaken for a water droplet on the agar, and (3) depending on the growth medium, a pit on the agar surface. The microorganism grows best at 37°C in an anaerobic environment of 85 percent N_2, 10 percent H_2, and 5 percent CO_2. The G + C content of the DNA ranges from 42 to 48 mol%.

Recently, an extensive phylogenetic study was undertaken of *Campylobacter* and *Wolinella* spe-

TABLE 18–2 ✦ *Wolinella*

Characteristics	Gram-negative anaerobe
	Motile by means of polar flagella
	Three colony types
	Hexagonal subunits on the outer cell membrane
Major species	*Campylobacter rectus* (*W. recta*)
	W. succinogenes
	Campylobacter curvus (*W. curva*)
Growth	Anaerobic at 37°C
Disease	*C. rectus* is associated with adult periodontitis
Pathogenesis	Unknown

cies, using DNA-rRNA hybridization and immunotyping. On the basis of numerous genotypic and phenotypic similarities, a proposal was tendered to include *W. curva, W. recta* and the unnamed *Wolinella* sp. strain CCUG 11641 in the genus *Campylobacter* as *Campylobacter curvus, Campylobacter rectus* and *Campylobacter* sp. *incertae sedis,* respectively. The description of these bacteria is the same as that given above. *W. succinogenes,* previously referred to as *Vibrio succinogenes,* remains in the genus *Wolinella* because it resides in a separate rRNA homology group than *C. curvus* and *C. rectus.*

These microorganisms occur in large numbers in the subgingival dental plaque of adult periodontitis patients and may be involved in the pathogenesis of this form of periodontal disease. They also are found in infected root canals and in the gastrointestinal tract of cows. The genus *Wolinella* is part of the family Bacteroidaceae, which includes other gram-negative microorganisms that can be found in subgingival dental plaque, such as the black-pigmenting bacteria.

C. curva appears as spiral or curved cells and thus can be distinguished from *C. rectus,* which appears mainly as straight cells. Electron microscopy demonstrates an unusual feature of *C. rectus.* The outer cell membrane is covered by hexagonal subunits. *W. succinogenes,* as the name implies, has a growth requirement for succinate or for compounds such as pyruvate and bicarbonate, which can be converted to succinate during bacterial metabolism. *C. rectus* can also be differentiated from *C. curvus* and *W. succinogenes* on the basis of sensitivity to various dyes and antibiotics.

As previously mentioned, *C. rectus* can be found in high numbers in subgingival dental plaque in adult periodontitis patients. In fact, this microorganism is, along with black-pigmenting bacterial species, one of the predominant bacterial isolates from certain patients. For example, this is a predominant bacterial species in subgingival plaque

from periodontitis patients with AIDS (Table 18–3).

CAMPYLOBACTER SPECIES

The *Campylobacter* (curved rod) are gram-negative, motile, S- or spiral-shaped bacilli ranging from 0.2 to 0.5 μm wide by 0.5 to 5 μm long. These organisms cause abortion in cattle and sheep and diarrheal disease in humans, including "traveler's diarrhea." The first studies of *Campylobacter* involved their role in causing veterinary disease in domestic animals, particularly abortion in cattle.

The sizable body of literature that has accumulated on the genus *Campylobacter* in the last 20 years has placed the genus in a state of flux. New species are being described at a rapid pace, and others are being reclassified to new genera. An extensive phylogenetic study was undertaken of *Campylobacter* sp. and related taxa using DNA-rRNA hybridization and immunotyping. Within the phylogenetic tree of gram-negative bacteria, it is possible to distinguish at least five major rRNA superfamilies. The DNA-rRNA hybridization between *Campylobacter* strains and gram-negative reference strains belonging to superfamilies I to V indicate that the genus *Campylobacter* constitutes a sixth rRNA superfamily and a separate eubacterial phylum. Within superfamily VI, three rRNA clusters are identified. Ribosomal RNA cluster I contain 11 species considered true *Campylobacter,* several of which are pathogenic for humans and animals (Table 18–4). All other *Campylobacter* species are now considered generically misnamed.

Campylobacter species range in oxygen sensitivity from microaerophilic to strict anaerobes. The genus *Campylobacter* together with the genus *Spirillum* compose the bacterial family Spirillaceae. The *Campylobacter* species can be distinguished from the *Spirillum* by their inability to accumulate intracellular granules of polyhydroxybutyric acid (PHB), by a mol% G + C content of 30 to 46 percent, and by the presence of a single flagellum on one or both ends. This flagellum enables the *Campylobacter* species to move with a characteristic darting and corkscrew motion similar to the movement of *Wolinella.* The *Spirillum,* by contrast, can accumulate intracellular PHB, have a mol% G + C of 38 to 65 percent, and have tufts of flagella at the poles. The *Campylobacter* species are oxidase-positive but neither ferment nor oxidize carbohydrates.

The catalase test is useful for differentiating some species, and in the past, *Campylobacter* were grouped on the basis of catalase activity. The test

TABLE 18–3 ✦ **Predominant Bacterial Species in Subgingival Plaques from Periodontitis Patients with AIDS**

BACTERIAL SPECIES	BACTERIAL ISOLATES NUMBER (%)*	POSITIVE SITES NUMBER (%)†	POSITIVE PATIENTS NUMBER (%)‡	RANGE % VIABLE COUNT
Actinomyces israelli	1 (0.2)	1 (4.7)	1 (9.0)	0.0– 3.1
Actinomyces meyeri	1 (0.2)	1 (4.7)	1 (9.0)	0.0– 3.6
Actinomyces naeslundii	50 (7.5)	17 (80.9)	9 (81.8)	0.0–23.3
Actinomyces odontolyticus	2 (0.3)	1 (4.7)	1 (9.0)	0.0– 6.7
Actinomyces viscosus	31 (4.7)	14 (66.6)	9 (81.8)	0.0–16.7
Arachnia propionica	1 (0.2)	1 (4.7)	1 (9.0)	0.0– 3.3
Bacteroides gracilis	3 (0.5)	2 (9.5)	2 (18.1)	0.0– 6.7
Bacteroides melaninogenicus	1 (0.2)	1 (4.7)	1 (9.0)	0.0– 3.3
Campylobacter concisus	12 (1.8)	5 (23.8)	5 (36.3)	0.0–12.5
Campylobacter sputorum	4 (0.6)	4 (19.0)	4 (36.3)	0.0– 3.3
Campylobacter rectus	20 (3.0)	3 (14.2)	3 (27.2)	0.0–10.0
Capnocytophaga sp.	6 (0.9)	4 (19.0)	2 (18.1)	0.0– 9.4
Clostridium clostridiiforme	2 (0.3)	2 (9.5)	1 (9.0)	0.0–13.9
Clostridium difficile	5 (0.8)	1 (4.7)	1 (9.0)	0.0–13.9
Clostridium sp.	1 (0.2)	1 (4.7)	1 (9.0)	0.0– 6.3
Corynebacterium matruchotii	2 (0.3)	1 (4.7)	1 (9.0)	0.0– 6.3
Eikenella corrodens	2 (0.3)	2 (9.5)	2 (18.1)	0.0– 3.3
Enterococcus avium	1 (0.2)	1 (4.7)	1 (9.0)	0.0– 4.3
Enterococcus faecalis	3 (0.5)	1 (4.7)	1 (9.0)	0.0– 8.6
Enterococcus faecalis 3	1 (0.2)	1 (4.7)	1 (9.0)	0.0– 3.3
Eubacterium sp.	4 (0.6)	3 (14.2)	1 (9.0)	0.0– 6.3
Fusobacterium nucleatum	76 (11.4)	16 (76.1)	10 (90.9)	0.0–44.4
Fusobacterium sp.	5 (0.8)	2 (9.5)	2 (18.1)	0.0–13.3
Gemella haemolysans	2 (0.3)	2 (9.5)	2 (18.1)	0.0– 4.3
Klebsiella pneumoniae	1 (0.2)	1 (4.7)	1 (9.0)	0.0– 3.3
Lactobacillus acidophilus	81 (12.2)	13 (61.9)	6 (54.5)	0.0–54.2
Leptotrichia buccalis	1 (0.2)	1 (4.7)	1 (9.0)	0.0– 3.3
Peptostreptococcus micros	33 (5.0)	11 (52.3)	7 (63.6)	0.0–20.0
Peptostreptococcus prevotii	1 (0.2)	1 (4.7)	1 (9.0)	0.0– 3.3
Porphyromonas gingivalis	80 (12.0)	11 (52.3)	5 (45.4)	0.0–55.6
Prevotella intermedia	5 (0.8)	5 (23.8)	5 (45.4)	0.0–13.9
Propionibacterium acnes	1 (0.2)	1 (4.7)	1 (9.0)	0.0– 3.3
Rothia denticariosa	2 (0.3)	1 (4.7)	1 (9.0)	0.0– 5.7
Staphylococcus epidermidis	58 (8.7)	6 (28.5)	6 (54.5)	0.0–86.7
Streptococcus bovis	1 (0.2)	1 (4.7)	1 (9.0)	0.0– 4.2
Streptococcus milleri	2 (0.3)	2 (9.5)	2 (18.1)	0.0– 4.3
Streptococcus mitis	3 (0.5)	3 (14.2)	3 (27.2)	0.0– 3.1
Streptococcus mutans	2 (0.3)	1 (4.7)	1 (9.0)	0.0– 6.7
Streptococcus salivarius	4 (0.6)	2 (9.5)	2 (18.1)	0.0–12.5
Streptococcus sanguis I	3 (0.5)	2 (9.5)	2 (18.1)	0.0– 6.7
Streptococcus sanguis II	123 (18.5)	16 (76.1)	8 (72.7)	0.0–60.9
Veillonella dispar	11 (1.7)	3 (14.2)	3 (27.2)	0.0–20.0
Wolinella sp.	4 (0.6)	4 (19.0)	1 (9.0)	0.0–21.9
Lost through transfer	14 (2.1)			

From Zambon, J. J., Reynolds, H. S., and Genco, R. J.: Studies of the subgingival microflora in patients with acquired immunodeficiency syndrome. J. Periodontol 61:699, 1990.

permitted differentiation of catalase positive *C. fetus*, a bovine pathogen, from catalase negative commensal campylobacteria. This grouping has become less relevant in the last decade because of the increased number of pathogenic *Campylobacter* species described and the need to develop additional tests to differentiate these.

A limited number of properties and biochemical reactions are presently used to distinguish species (Table 18–5). There is a wide range in temperature for culturing campylobacteria, extending from 15°C to 42°C. *C. jejuni* and *C. coli* are considered thermotolerant campylobacteria because they grow at 42°C, although growth is more abundant at 37°C.

TABLE 18–4 ✦ *Campylobacter*

Characteristics	Gram-negative, motile, S- or spiral-shaped bacilli Microaerophilic to anaerobic Catalase-positive and -negative species
Major species and diseases	*C. fetus*—sporadic abortion in cattle and sheep and enzootic sterility *C. jejuni*—human gastroenteritis, sporadic abortion in sheep *C. sputorum*—commensal in humans and animals *C. concisus*—human oral commensal *C. curvus*—human oral commensal *C. coli*—human gastroenteritis
Prevention	Thorough cooking of meat products
Treatment	Self-limiting, antibiotics of limited use

The hippurate test is important for distinguishing between positive *C. jejuni* and negative *C. coli*. The H$_2$S test is notable for causing variable reactions in undefined medium because of variation in cysteine content of peptones used in media preparation. Triple sugar iron (TSI) medium has been used most consistently in microbiology labs, and with this medium, H$_2$S production is not detected in *C. jejuni*, *C. coli*, and *C. lari*. Positive urease activity and resistance to nalidixic acid distinguishes *C. lari* from *C. jejuni* and *C. coli*. Growth of *C. rectus* and *C. curvus* is stimulated by the presence of formate and fumarate.

Among the catalase-positive *Campylobacter* species is *C. fetus*, which causes enzootic sterility and abortion in cattle. Enzootic sterility, also known as venereal bovine campylobacteriosis, is the result of transmission of the microorganism from the prepuce of an infected bull to the vagina of a cow following sexual intercourse. In the cow, the organism multiplies and causes abortion. *C. fetus* subsp. *venerealis* serotype A and *C. fetus* subsp. *fetus* serotype B cause enzootic sterility. *C. fetus* subsp. *fetus* serotype A causes sporadic abortion. Here, the organism may be present as a commensal in the gallbladder or gut of the cow and may spread to the developing placenta where it can cause anoxia and spontaneous abortion late in the course of the pregnancy.

The important human pathogens among the *Campylobacter* include *C. coli*, *C. fetus* subsp. *fetus*, and *C. jejuni*, all of which can cause diarrheal

disease. *C. fetus* subsp. *fetus* can also cause septicemia, cardiac disease, meningitis, arthritis, and localized suppuration. It usually affects patients who are already debilitated as a result of another underlying disease. *C. fetus* subsp. *fetus* is susceptible to several antibiotics including tetracycline, aminoglycosides, and erythromycin. The organism is found in domestic animals—especially pigs—and is found as a commensal in the gastrointestinal tract of sheep, in which it can cause abortion.

C. jejuni infection in humans, including "traveler's diarrhea," usually starts with a prodromal period of 24 to 48 hours characterized by a high fever, sometimes with delirium. Over the next 2 to 3 days, the patient experiences periumbilical pain, abdominal cramps, and produces profuse, watery, slimy stools, sometimes with blood. Microscopic examination of feces can demonstrate *Campylobacter* and polymorphonuclear leukocytes. Antibiotic therapy is usually not indicated, since the disease rarely lasts longer than 1 week.

Other catalase-positive *Campylobacter* species include the nalidixic acid-resistant thermophilic *C. lari*, which has been isolated from seagulls and children with diarrheal disease, and *C. sputorum* subsp. *fecalis*, which has been isolated from birds and cattle. The pathogenicity of these two species is still under investigation.

Among the catalase-negative *Campylobacter* species is *C. sputorum* subspecies *sputorum*, which is found as a commensal in the human oral cavity. The pathogenic potential of this species is unknown. *C. concisus* and *C. curvas*, formerly *Wolinella curva*, are also catalase-negative *Campylo-*

TABLE 18–5 ✦ *Campylobacter* Species

SPECIES	DISEASE
Catalase Positive	
C. fetus subsp. *fetus*	Sporadic abortion in cattle and sheep
C. fetus subsp. *venerealis*	Enzootic sterility and abortion in cattle
C. jejuni	Human gastroenteritis, sporadic abortion in sheep
C. coli	Human gastroenteritis
C. sputorum subsp. *fecalis*	Isolated from seagulls Isolated from birds and cattle
Catalase Negative	
C. sputorum subsp. *sputorum*	Human oral isolate
C. sputorum subsp. *bubulus*	Genital tract of cattle and sheep
C. concisus	Human oral isolate

bacter found in the human oral cavity. *C. rectus*, formerly *W. recta*, is found in high numbers in subgingival dental plaque in adult periodontitis and is thought to play a role in its etiology. *C. sputorum* subspecies *mucosalis* is found in pigs and is associated with porcine gastrointestinal diseases, including ileitis and hemorrhagic enteropathy. *C. sputorum* subspecies *bubulus* can be isolated from the genital tract of cattle or sheep.

In 1984, bacteria resembling campylobacteria were recovered from biopsy specimens of human gastric mucosa taken from patients with gastritis and peptic ulceration. This was the first indication that campylobacteria species were etiologic factors in these diseases. This species was named *C. pyloridis* and later corrected to *C. pylori*. However, mounting analytic biochemical and genetic studies showed that the organism was very different from other species of campylobacteria. Therefore, *C. pylori* was transferred to the newly created genus *Helicobacter*.

HELICOBACTER SPECIES

The new genus *Helicobacter* was proposed by Goodwin et al. in 1989 with emendation of the generic description by Vandamme et al. in 1991. The genus name refers to the in vivo helical morphology of the organisms. The phylogenetic position of the four species included in this genus, *Helicobacter pylori* (*Campylobacter pylori*), *Helicobacter mustelae* (formerly *Campylobacter mustelae*), *Helicobacter cinaedi* (formerly *Campylobacter cinaedi*), and *Helicobacter fennelliae* (formerly *Campylobacter fennelliae*), is based upon 16S ribosomal RNA sequencing, immunotyping, DNA-rRNA hybridization, and DNA-DNA hybridization.

Helicobacter are helical, curved, or short unbranched gram-negative cells that are 0.3–1.0 μm wide and 1.5–5 μm long with rounded ends and spiral periodicity. Darting mobility is accomplished by means of a single polar flagella (*H. cinaedi* and *H. fennelliae*) or triple unipolar or bipolar and lateral flagella (*H. pylori* and *H. mustelae*). *Helicobacter* are microaerophilic with a respiratory type of metabolism. Carbohydrates are not oxidized or fermented, and energy is obtained from amino acids or tricarboxylic acid cycle intermediates. Growth is optimum at 37°C and hydrogen stimulates growth. Catalase and oxidase are produced, but no pigment or H_2S is produced.

Two other recently described human pathogens are *H. cinaedi* (*cinaedi*, of a homosexual) and *H. fennelliae* (*fennelliae*, feminine form of the name of the technologist C. L. Fennell who first isolated the organism). These organisms cause enteritis in homosexual men.

H. pylori (as in *pyloris*, the lower half of the stomach) is strongly associated with chronic type B gastritis and peptic ulcer disease in humans. It produces several virulence factors, including a urease that neutralizes gastric secretions and enables the microorganism to colonize the gastric mucosa. It also produces a vacuolating toxin that is thought to injure gastric epithelial cells.

The presence of *H. pylori*–associated gastritis and peptic ulcer disease is positively correlated with the presence of *H. pylori* DNA in dental plaque. Dental plaque is likely to be a reservoir of the organism because no other source for the organism has yet been demonstrated.

BIBLIOGRAPHY

Butzler, J. P. (ed.): Campylobacter infection in man and animals. CRC Press, Orlando, FL, 1982.

Bloser, M. J., Berkowitz, I. D., LaForce, F. M., Cravens, J., Reller, L. B., and Wang, W.-L. L.: Campylobacter enteritis: Clinical and epidemiologic features. Ann. Intern. Med. 91:179, 1979.

Desai, H. G., Gill, H. H., Shan Karan, K., Mehta, P. R., Prabhu, S. R.: Dental plaque: A permanent reservoir of *Helicobacter pylori*? Scand. J. Gastroenterol. 26:1205, 1991.

Lai, C.-H., Listgarten, M. A., Tanner, A. C. R., and Socransky, S. S.: Ultrastructures of *Bacteroides gracilis, Campylobacter concisus, Wolinella recta,* and *Eikenella corrodens,* all from humans with periodontal disease. Int. J. Syst. Bacteriol. 31:465, 1981.

Tanner, A. C. R., Badger, S., Lai, C.-H., Listgarten, M. A., Visconti, R. A., and Socransky, S. S.: *Wolinella* gen. nov. *Wolinella succinogenes (Vibrio succinogenes)* Wolin et al. comb. nov., and description of *Bacteroides gracilis* sp. nov., *Wolinella recta* sp. nov., *Campylobacter concisus* sp. nov., and *Eikenella corrodens,* all from humans with periodontal disease. Int. J. Syst. Bacteriol. 31:432, 1981.

Vandamme, P., Folsen, E., Rossau, R., Hoste, B., Segers, P., Tytgat, R., and De Lay, J.: Revision of *Campylobacter, Helicobacter,* and *Wolinella* taxonomy: Emendation of generic descriptions and proposal of *Arcobacter* gen. nov. Int. J. Syst. Bacteriol. 41:88, 1991.

19 *The Spirochetes*

Walter J. Loesche

CHAPTER OUTLINE

ORAL SPIROCHETES

While many bacterial species live in the dental plaque, the most recognizable of these organisms are the **spirochetes.** The spirochetes are long, thin, corkscrewlike gram-negative anaerobic bacteria whose characteristic motility and morphology can readily be discerned by darkfield and/or phase contrast microscopic examination of subgingival plaque. Spirochetes are observed mainly in plaques removed from diseased periodontal sites, which has led some investigators to consider these organisms as periodontopathogens. Others have suggested that the pre-eminent spirochetes are secondary, opportunistic organisms thriving on the nutrients that are relatively abundant in a periodontally inflamed site. In either case, the increase of spirochetes in plaque is not a favorable sign, and efforts should be made to reduce and/or eliminate them from the subgingival plaques.

MORPHOLOGY AND TAXONOMY

Spirochetes are unique bacteria in that they have internal flagellalike structures called *axial fila-ments,* which are located between an outer osmotically labile envelope and an inner rigid protoplasmic cylinder (Fig. 19–1). A variable number of axial fibers insert at each end of the cylinder and flow back along the cylinder for about two-thirds of its length. The number of fibrils can be used to classify the spirochetes. In Figure 19–1, a 1-2-1 spirochete is shown, a designation based upon the insertion of one axial filament at each end of the spirochete and the overlap of these two filaments in the middle section. A classification scheme based upon ultrastructure is shown in Table 19–1. Small spirochetes have 1-2-1 or 2-4-2 fibril patterns, and their protoplasmic cylinder has a diameter of 100 to 250 nm. Some of these spirochetes have been cultivated and, on the basis of biochemical and physiologic criteria, can be divided into three species: *Treponema denticola, T. pectinovorum,* and *T. socranskii.*

The intermediate-sized spirochetes have a protoplasmic cylinder that is 200 to 500 nm in diameter and from 3 to 20 axial fibrils inserted at each end. These spirochetes have rarely been cultured and may contain several species, including the cultiv-

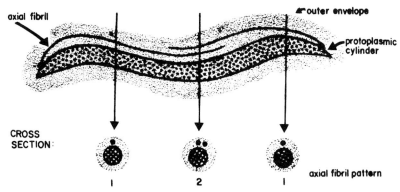

FIGURE 19–1 ✦ Schematic diagram of a 1-2-1 small oral spirochete. Note that one axial fibril inserts at each end of the protoplasmic cylinder and that they overlap in the center. The axial fibrils are inside the outer envelope, so they are not true flagella. (From Loesche, W. J.: Dental Caries: A Treatable Infection. University of Michigan School of Dentistry, 1987. Used by permission.)

able organism known as *T. vincentii*. Microscopic evidence implicates these spirochetes in acute necrotizing ulcerative gingivitis (ANUG). Undoubtedly, they include the *Treponema* that Vincent originally described in ANUG, which was subsequently referred to as *Borrelia vincentii*. The large spirochetes have a protoplasmic cylinder with diameters in excess of 50 nm and at least 12 axial fibers. They have also never been cultured. Hence, when the term "oral spirochetes" is used it should be understood that this is a general morphologic description and that, within this grouping, morphologically and biochemically distinct species exist.

ACQUISITION OF SPIROCHETES

Definitive information on the acquisition of the oral spirochetes is lacking. Human oral spirochetes appear to be distinct from human genital and intestinal spirochetes, from animal species, from overtly pathogenic species, and from free-living forms. This implies that the oral spirochetes are acquired from other humans via oral contact. Spirochetes have been detected by darkfield microscopy in the dental plaque of about 50 percent of the 3- to 5-year-old and 6- to 12-year-old children whom we have examined. However, their numbers were less than 0.5 percent of the flora and they were uncultivable. Almost all 6- to 12-year-old Dutch and Tanzanian children examined had detectable spirochetes in their plaques, and their numbers and proportions were greater when the plaques were removed from sites of gingival bleeding.

This suggests that most, if not all, individuals acquire some type of spirochete in their early life. As the oral spirochetes comprise at least four species (Table 19–1) and undoubtedly more, one as-

sumes from the above frequency data that the acquisition of any one of these spirochetes is a likely event once the teeth erupt. Once acquired, the spirochetes show a predilection for the subgingival plaque presumably because in this ecosystem, these motile organisms are not at as great a risk of being swept away by the saliva and masticatory forces. Also, the lower oxygen tension present in these plaques, combined with the availability of preformed nutrients derived from the host and cohabitating plaque bacteria, enable them to grow and persist.

With good oral hygiene, the spirochetes remain in low proportions and are often undetectable in plaque smears. However, if oral hygiene is suspended, as in the experimental gingivitis model, spirochetes invariably become detectable after 15 to 21 days. The universality of this emergence of the spirochetes reflects the growth of the indigenous spirochetes in response to increased nutrient availability, secondarily to gingival inflammation, rather than to de novo colonization from the outside.

These data from children and from the experimental gingivitis model form the basis for the assumption that spirochetes are ubiquitous to the subgingival plaque and are normally members of our supplemental flora. They contribute to gingival pathology only when their numbers increase beyond a certain threshold, and in this sense, periodontal disease can be considered an endogenous infection.

ISOLATION AND CHARACTERIZATION

The spirochetes are notoriously difficult to isolate and most oral species—especially the inter-

TABLE 19–1 ✦ Taxonomic Characteristics of Oral Spirochetes

SPECIES	SIZE	NO. OF AXIAL FIBRILS	CARBOHYDRATE FERMENTATION	% G + C
Treponema denticola	Small	2-4-2, 5-10-5	No	37–38
T. vincentii	Intermediate	5-10-5	No	44
T. socranskii	Small	1-2-1	Yes	51
T. pectinovorum	Small	2-4-2	Pectin	39
T. oralis	Small	1-2-1	No	?
T. macrodentium	Small	1-2-1	Yes	?

mediate and large size spirochetes—have probably never been cultivated. In many instances, this can be attributed to the failure of the isolating medium to contain specific nutrients that these organisms require. A case in point is the requirement for pectin or its constituents galacturonic and glucuronic acids by the recently described species *Treponema pectinovorum*. If these unusual substrates were not present in the isolation medium, then this species would not have been isolated. Most investigators use complex media that are supplemented with biologic fluids such as serum, rumen fluid, or ascitic fluid. This approach has led to the isolation of *T. denticola* and *T. vincentii,* which grow well on most commercially available media supplemented with rabbit serum, whereas *T. pectinovorum*'s and *T. socranskii*'s requirement for rumen fluid can be replaced by volatile short chain fatty acids.

Spirochetes are delicate organisms relative to the other bacterial types found in dental plaque. This affects their isolation, as procedures used to disrupt the plaque in order to facilitate the cultivation of the maximum colonies usually lyse the spirochetes. This was demonstrated by experiments in which subgingival plaques were gently disrupted by mechanical mixing to obtain a microscopic count, and then were subjected to vigorous disruption by either sonication or by homogenization (Table 19–2). Spirochetes averaged 55 percent of the microscopic count but only accounted for about 0.5 percent of the viable count. Since *T. denticola* was the most common spirochetal isolate, and readily grows by the cultural conditions employed, these data indicate that its failure to be cultured reflected its destruction by the dispersal procedures normally used in cultural studies.

Thus, harsh dispersal procedures and exacting nutrient requirements, and **not** anaerobiosis, are the main obstacles toward the isolation and subsequent characterization of the oral spirochetes. Until investigators can reliably identify and quantitate which spirochetes are indeed present in the plaque, it will be difficult to implicate any specific spirochetal species, or for that matter any other bacterial

species, as periodontopathic. This uncertainty is lessened in regard to the cultivable species such as *T. denticola* and *T. vincentii,* as highly specific antibodies and DNA probes have now been used to quantify these organisms in plaque samples.

ASSOCIATION STUDIES

Spirochetes either are not detectable or, when detectable, are present in low proportions in plaques from healthy tooth sites. However, they most likely are always present in these nondiseased plaques, given the universality of their detection in the 3- to 4-week-old plaques formed when periodontally healthy individuals refrain from oral hygiene procedures while participating in the experimental gingivitis model.

Studies in 6- to 12-year-old children show a relationship between bleeding and increased proportions of spirochetes (Table 19–3). When the gingivitis is long-standing, the proportions of spirochetes increase still further to account for 8 to 20 percent of the plaque organisms. If the gingivitis is acute, as in ANUG, or of a severe generalized nature, the spirochetes can account for over 30 percent of the plaque flora.

Numerous investigators have noted elevated levels and proportions of spirochetes in adult periodontitis (AP) and early onset periodontitis (EOP). Table 19–4 lists several studies that showed spirochetes to average 37 percent of the flora in AP (range 21 to 56 percent). An uncultivable spirochete that reacts with an antibody specific for *Treponema palladium,* has been demonstrated in tissue specimens taken from ANUG and from periodontitis. This spirochete known as pathogen-related oral spirochete (PROS), could be important in periodontal disease as it is the dominant spirochete in some plaque samples. Only in localized juvenile periodontitis are spirochetes not conspicuously associated with periodontal morbidity. These findings in toto would seem to make the spirochetes pathognomonic of periodontal disease.

TABLE 19–2 ✦ Effect of Dispersal Procedures on Recovery of Spirochetes from Subgingival Plaque Samples (n = 15)

DISPERSAL PROCEDURE	MORPHOTYPE			
	SMALL	INTERMEDIATE	LARGE	TOTAL
	Spirochetes as % of microscopic count			
Gentle mechanical	31%	15%	8%	54%
	Spirochetes as % of viable count			
Harsh mechanical	0.8%*	No growth	No growth	0.8
Homogenization	0.9%	No growth	No growth	0.9
Sonification	0.1%	No growth	No growth	0.1

*91% of isolates were *Treponema denticola,* 5% were *T. socranskii,* and 4% were unspeciated.

LONGITUDINAL STUDIES

The development of periodontal disease from gingivitis to periodontitis has not been documented. However, in recent years, two clinical situations or models have been described that monitor the further loss of attachment around periodontally involved teeth. In one study, 20 patients previously treated for moderate to advanced periodontitis were not given any further treatment during recall visits. During a 1-year-period, 7 patients had 2 or more teeth which lost 3 mm or more of attachment, whereas 6 patients exhibited no teeth with 3 mm attachment loss. The patients with the attachment loss had significantly higher proportions of spirochetes in pooled plaques than did patients with no attachment loss. This attachment loss was also correlated with baseline proportions of spirochetes but could not be correlated with plaque or gingivitis scores, probing depth or gingival recession. This suggested that plaque proportions of spirochetes were predictors of subsequent tissue loss.

RESPONSE TO TREATMENT

If spirochetes are of etiologic significance in periodontal disease, then their demise in the subgingival plaque should coincide with the restoration of periodontal health. Many studies show that mechanical debridement with and without antimicrobial agents such as metronidazole, chlorhexidine, or tetracycline result in a decrease in spirochetes and a concurrent improvement in periodontal health as measured by reduced probing depth or increased apparent attachment, or both.

The proportions of spirochetes remaining after these treatments may be a sensitive indicator of the efficacy of treatment. In a study in which monoclonal antibodies to *T. denticola* and to *Porphyromonas (Bacteroides) gingivalis* were used as probes, improved health as measured by a decrease in probing depth was significantly associated with a decrease in *T. denticola,* but not with *P. gingivalis.* In double-blind studies involving systemic metronidazole or placebo treatment (250 mg tablets taken 3 times a day for 1 week) superimposed upon rigorous mechanical debridement, the levels and proportions of spirochetes were reduced in both groups but significantly more so in the metronidazole groups (Table 19–5). This bacteriologic difference was associated with a reduced need for surgery in the metronidazole group. Thus, the clinician who examined the patients, without knowing

TABLE 19–3 ✦ Prevalence of Spirochetes in the Subgingival Plaque of 6- to 12-Year-Old Dutch and Tanzanian Children

	% SPIROCHETES				ISOLATION FREQUENCY
	SMALL	MEDIUM	LARGE	TOTAL	
Dutch					
Bleeding (77)*	1.5	1.20	0.006	2.6	66%
Nonbleeding (67)	0.1	0.06	0.000	0.2	19
Tanzanian					
Bleeding (69)	6.5 ↕	3.1 ↕	0.06	9.7 ↕	100%
Nonbleeding (71)	2.5	1.4	0.07	3.8	93

*Number of sites.

↕ Values connected by arrows are significantly different.

Adapted from Mikx, F. H., Matee, M. I., Schaeken, M. J.: J. Clin. Periodontol. 13:289, 1986. © 1986 Munksgaard International, Publishers Ltd., Copenhagen.

TABLE 19–4 ✦ Reported Studies That Associate Spirochetes with Periodontal Disease

% SPIROCHETES IN PLAQUE		
HEALTHY GINGIVA	GINGIVITIS	PERIODONTITIS
0.2%*	2%*	21%	38%*
0.6	3	23	38
0.8	8	30	44
1.8	10	32	45
2.0	18	34	49
4.0	30	34	50
	36	35	52
	36	38	56
n = 6	n = 8	n = 16	
ave. 1.6%	ave. 17.8%	ave. 37%	

*Each percentage value is taken from a published study.

which group they were in, initially estimated that the metronidazole patients had an average of 19 teeth and the placebo group 17 teeth that would require either periodontal or oral surgery. When he re-examined the patients, those patients in the metronidazole group had eight fewer teeth that required periodontal surgery, whereas those in the placebo group had three fewer teeth. This difference between groups was significant and was reflected only by the spirochetal parameters of the more than 30 bacteriologic parameters that were monitored.

These data indicate that the spirochetal levels and/or proportions are sensitive indicators of treatment efficacy.

VIRULENCE MECHANISMS

If spirochetal overgrowth is synonymous with the presence of clinical inflammation, then it is likely that these organisms are active contributors to this inflammation. Spirochetes contain endotoxin and therefore would contribute to those toxic and pharmacologic effects attributed to the total endotoxin load found in the subgingival plaque. More importantly, however, the small size of the spirochetes and their motility enable some of them to invade the periodontal tissue and release their endotoxin and other toxic components directly adjacent to fibroblasts, epithelial cells, and other tissue components.

The availability of cultivable species has permitted in vitro studies of virulence mechanisms. A surprising finding was that *T. denticola, T. socranskii,* and possibly *T. vincentii* are not immunologically reactive in the periodontal patient. Thus, there was no correlation between the number of spirochetes in the plaque sample (despite the fact that high numbers of spirochetes came from patients and low numbers came from healthy subjects), and either the titers of antibodies or the lymphocyte blastogenic response of the sera to *T. denticola* or *T. vincentii.* In another study, the serologic response to *T. denticola* and *T. socranskii* was reduced in individuals with severe periodontal involvement compared with healthy controls and to individuals with less periodontal morbidity.

These studies raise the possibility that high antigen loads of these spirochetes may lead to some type of immune suppression, which would enable the spirochetes to escape the normal host defense mechanisms and thereby remain in high numbers in the plaque. This suppression concept was verified in vitro in regard to lymphocyte response to various antigens and mitogens. Thus, sonicates of some strains of *T. denticola,* when preincubated with human lymphocytes, caused a dose-dependent inhibition of responsiveness to mitogens, ConA, PHA, PWM, and SKSD. This inhibitory effect, seen only with *T. denticola* and not with *T. vin-*

TABLE 19–5 ✦ Effect of Debridement of Root Surfaces with and without Systemic Metronidazole for One Week on Proportions of Spirochetes and Periodontal Surgical Needs

	METRONIDAZOLE PLUS MECHANICAL (17)*		PLACEBO PLUS MECHANICAL (20)*	
	BEFORE	AFTER	BEFORE	AFTER
% Spirochetes	52%	‡ ⟷ 22%§	57%	42§
No. of teeth needing surgery†	19	‡ ⟷ 11	17	14

*Number of patients in each group.
†Surgery includes both periodontal surgery and tooth extraction because of periodontal disease.
‡Values connected by arrow are significantly different.
§Difference between metronidazole and placebo groups is significant.

centii, was dependent on the presence of monocytes and was reversed by the addition of both
indomethacin and catalase to the mixture.

T. denticola and *T. vincentii* also inhibit polymorphonuclear leukocyte (PMN) function in vitro.
Thus, the PMNs can readily phagocytize these spirochetes but were unable to degrade them. This
was associated with a failure of the lysosomal granules to degranulate and suggested that the spirochetes may limit the fusion of the lysosomes to the
phagosomes. If this is the case, then these spirochetes could evade the host protective effects of
the PMNs and persist in the plaques. These studies
indicate that the cultivable spirochetes can evade
the normal host immunologic and phagocytic surveillance. These mechanisms could account then
for their high levels and proportions in subgingival
plaques removed from diseased sites.

DIAGNOSTIC IMPLICATIONS OF SPIROCHETES

The association and response to treatment studies indicate that subgingival plaque levels and/or
proportions of spirochetes could be used clinically
to identify those sites and/or individuals requiring
periodontal treatment. This information can be routinely obtained by the use of phase or darkfield
microscopy. However, if other periodontopathic organisms are also involved, these other organisms
would not be detected microscopically. Thus, a
more broad-base diagnostic procedure would be
preferred.

The screening of periodontopathic organisms
with various enzyme assays have shown that *Treponema denticola, Porphyromonas gingivalis,
Bacteroides forsythus*, and an unspeciated *Capnocytophaga* possess a trypsinlike enzyme that can
be detected by the hydrolysis of benzoyl-DL-ar-
ginine-2-naphthylamide (BANA). This BANA hydrolytic enzyme could also be detected in subgingival plaque samples and was statistically related
to the plaque levels and proportions of spirochetes
and with probing depth. Thus, a BANA-positive
plaque was indicative of subgingival plaques containing more than 30 percent spirochetes that were
removed from sites with probing depths of 7 mm
or more. Subsequent studies using DNA probes
and highly specific antibodies indicated that *T. denticola* was making more of a contribution to the
BANA reaction than was *P. gingivalis* or *B. forsythus*.

Seventy-one percent of the plaques removed
from untreated periodontal patients were BANA
positive. These sites averaged 40 percent spirochetes, and came from sites that had average probing depths of 7 mm. The BANA-negative plaques
in these patients averaged 12 percent spirochetes

and came from sites that had average probing
depths of 5.4 mm. In contrast, only 8 percent of
the plaques removed from treated patients at recall
visits were BANA positive, and these plaques had
significantly higher proportions of spirochetes and
came from deeper pockets than the BANA-negative
plaques.

These data indicate that the ability of subgingival plaque to hydrolyze BANA is a reliable
marker for the presence of high proportions of spirochetes, *T. denticola, P. gingivalis* and *B. forsythus* and as such could be used to diagnose an
anaerobic periodontal infection. If so, BANA hydrolysis has the potential to be an objective indicator of periodontal disease activity and could be
used in combination with clinical criteria both to
initiate therapy and as a means to monitor the efficacy of treatment.

OTHER SPIROCHETES
Other Infections

Spirochetes are also found on the intestinal and,
to a lesser extent, the genital-urinary surfaces of
humans. Most of these spirochetes are presumed
to be nonpathogenic, but notable exceptions occur,
such as *T. pallidum* being the etiologic agent of
syphilis, *T. pertenue* being the etiologic agent of
the childhood infection known as yaws, and *T.
carateum* being the etiologic agent of pinta.

There are other types of spirochetes, such as the
very thin aerobic species classified in the genus
Leptospira, and the larger anaerobic species classified in the genus *Borrelia*. Pathogenic leptospira
reside in domestic and wild animals, where they
can cause life-threatening infections that are a major concern to the meat and dairy industry. Humans
can become accidentally infected with leptospira
when they come into contact with soil or water that
has been contaminated with urine from the infected
animal. Rarely does the individual develop a fatal
infection, but on occasion a severe icteric infection
(jaundice), known as *Weil's disease,* occurs.

Human infections due to *Borrelia* species are
more common than those due to leptospira and
invariably involve transmission by infected lice or
ticks. Many of these infections manifest as febrile
diseases characterized by a remittent fever and are
known as *relapsing fevers*. The louse-borne infection occurs under conditions of poor personal hygiene and sanitation, and for this reason it can reach
epidemic proportions in communities devastated by
wars or natural disaster. The tick-borne infection
occurs only in individuals exposed to infected
ticks, and these infections are called *endemic relapsing fever*. Recently, a new type of tick-borne
infection was described in residents of Lyme, Connecticut, who exhibited skin and joint lesions and

involvement of the heart and nervous system. This complex of symptoms has been called *Lyme disease,* and the high number of reported cases since its initial description has made Lyme disease an important public health problem.

The salient features of these other spirochetal infections are given in Table 19–6. Syphilis, the most important of these nonoral spirochetal infections, will be briefly described subsequently.

Syphilis

Syphilis invoked as much dread and censure in the 19th and early 20th century as AIDS does in the late 20th century. The advent of effective chemotherapeutic agents and an apparent decreased virulence of *Treponema pallidum* have made syphilis a considerably less fearsome disease today. Syphilis was the target disease for Paul Ehrlich's magic bullet, and the conceptual and therapeutic breakthrough of his arsenic compound, arsphenamine, ushered in the modern age of antimicrobial chemotherapy. Penicillin has long since replaced arsphenamine as the drug of choice, and the remarkable effectiveness of this agent against *T. pallidum* has led to the general easing of concern over syphilis as a major health concern. Yet syphilitic infections still occur with a greater frequency than is necessary, given today's knowledge of venereal disease control. Also, the possibility that *T. pallidum* will develop clinical resistance to penicillin cannot be ignored.

Syphilis is transmitted from person to person usually by sexual intercourse, but the lesions of secondary syphilis, which would include oral lesions, are also infectious. Spirochetes can be transferred across the placenta to the fetus, but congenital syphilis can be prevented by aggressive treatment of the mother with penicillin in the early stages of pregnancy, and still later by treating the newborn. Such treatments have made a diagnostic rarity of Hutchinson's triad observed in congenital

syphilis, which included tooth deformities (notched incisors, moon molars), interstitial keratitis, and nerve deafness.

Syphilis was known as "the great imitator," because the diverse array of lesions that it caused in many organ systems often resembled the symptoms of other diseases. The clinical course of untreated syphilis has a primary, secondary, and often fatal tertiary phase. The **primary phase** reflected the erythema and induration that followed the multiplication of the spirochetes at the entry site. The hard chancre that forms is highly contagious and should cause the individual to seek prompt medical care. If untreated, the lesion heals leaving remnants of scar tissue. After an asymptomatic period of 2 to 24 weeks the **secondary stage** begins with a high fever and culminates with a mucocutaneous rash that spreads from the palms and soles to include almost all surface areas of the body and many internal organs. White mucoid patches of moist papules or condylomata occur on the mucous membranes of the mouth, vagina, and anus. These lesions are also highly contagious and care should be exercised when examining them.

Within several weeks the host mounts an effective immune response and the lesions heal, although in about 25 percent of patients there may be several recurrences of the rash. After clinical resolution *T. pallidum* seems to disappear from the skin and mucous membranes but can still be detected in the spleen and lymph nodes. Tertiary syphilis occurs from 5 to 30 years later, when potentially fatal cardiovascular (80 percent of cases) and neurologic (20 percent of cases) symptoms occur.

Most syphilitic infections do not progress through the three stages. The natural history of the infection was followed for 30 to 50 years in 1000 untreated Norwegian patients in the early part of this century. Twenty-five percent of the subjects progressed to secondary syphilis, and only 13 percent developed tertiary syphilis. This indicates that

TABLE 19–6 ✦ Aspects of Various Human Spirochetal Infections

	LEPTOSPIRA	*BORRELIA*		*TREPONEMA*		
Disease	Weil's disease	Relapsing fever	Lyme disease	Syphilis	Yaws	Pinta
Agent	*L. interrogans* serotype icterohaemorrhagiae	*B. recurrentis*	*B. burgdorferi*	*T. pallidum*	*T. pertenue*	*T. carateum*
Age group	All	All	All	Adults	Children	Children
Spread	Contact with contaminated animal urine	Louse or tick bite	Tick bite	Venereal	Skin	Skin
Cultivable	Yes	Yes	Yes	No	No	No
Treatment	Penicillin Tetracycline	Tetracycline	Tetracycline	Penicillin	Penicillin	Penicillin

the host mounts a protective immune response that can thwart the progression of the infection in the majority of infected individuals who are untreated. This protection also prevents new instances of primary syphilis. Thus, individuals who have once been infected appear to be resistant to subsequent new infections. However, in the modern era, this protective immunity rarely develops, as most individuals with primary syphilis are promptly treated prior to the mounting of a protective immune response.

Children with yaws and pinta infections rarely develop syphilis as adults. This was dramatically demonstrated by a public health program, which was successful in treating yaws in children, but led eventually to an outbreak of syphilis in these children when they became older and sexually active. Apparently the immune response to *T. pertenue* included antibodies that recognized *T. pallidum*, and thus the yaws infection served as a vaccine against syphilis.

These findings indicate that a vaccine against *T. pallidum* would be protective. Indeed, prior to the demonstration of the efficacy of penicillin in syphilis, the pursuit of a vaccine against *T. pallidum* was of the highest medical priority. The main problem in vaccine development was and remains to this day the inability to identify, isolate, and purify those antigens that conferred immunity. As noted earlier, the discovery of penicillin reduced the importance of a vaccine, and medical science has since moved on to other matters. Syphilis, however, remains endemic in the United States, with approximately 10 cases per 100,000 individuals reported annually, for a total of about 23,000 cases per year.

SUMMARY

The spirochetal accumulation in subgingival plaques appears to be a function of the clinical severity of periodontal disease. It is not known how many different spirochetal species colonize the plaque, but based on size alone, there are small, intermediate, and large spirochetes. Four species of small spirochetes are cultivable, and of these *T. denticola* has been shown to possess factors or mechanisms that suppress lymphocyte blastogenesis and inhibit fibroblast and PMN function. This species also contains a BANA hydrolytic enzyme, which can be detected directly in plaque samples, and such detection may be useful for the diagnosis of periodontal disease activity.

BIBLIOGRAPHY

Boehringer, H., Berthold, P. H., and Taichman, N. S.: Studies on the interaction of human neutrophils with plaque spirochetes. J. Periodont. Res. 21:195, 1986.

Keyes, P. H., and Rams, R. E.: A rationale for the management of periodontal diseases: rapid identification of microbial "therapeutic targets" with phase-control microscopy. J. Am. Dent. Assoc. 106:803, 1983.

Listgarten, M. A.: Subgingival microbiological differences between periodontally healthy sites and diseased sites prior to and after treatment. Int. J. Periodont. Restor. Dent. 4:27, 1984.

Listgarten, M. A. and Socransky, S. S.: Electron microscopy as an aid in the taxonomic differentiation of oral spirochetes. Arch. Oral Biol. 10:127, 1965.

Loesche, W. J.: The identification of bacteria associated with periodontal disease and dental caries in vitro and in vivo by enzymatic methods. Oral Microbiol. Oral Immunol. 1:19, 1986.

Loesche, W. J., Syed, S. A., Laughon, B., and Stoll, J.: The bacteriology of acute necrotizing ulcerative gingivitis. J. Periodontol. 53:223, 1982.

Loesche, W. J., Syed, S. A., Schmidt, E., and Morrison, E. C.: Bacterial profiles of subgingival plaques in periodontitis. J. Periodontol. 56:447, 1985.

Loesche, W. J.: The role of spirochetes in periodontal disease. Adv. Dent. Res. 2:275, 1988.

Loesche, W. J., Lopatin, D. E., Giordano, J., Alcoforado, G., Hujoel, P. P.: Comparison of the benzoyl-DL-arginine-naphthylamide (BANA) test, DNA probes, and immunological reagents for ability to detect anaerobic periodontal infections due to *Porphyromonas gingivalis*, *Treponema denticola* and *Bacteroides forsythus*. J. Clin. Microbiol. 30:427, 1992.

Loesche, W. J., Schmidt, E., Smith, B. A., Morrison, E. C., Caffesse, R., and Hujoel, P. P.: Effects of metronidazole on periodontal treatment needs. J. Periodontol. 62:247, 1991.

Mangan, D. F., Laughon, B. E., Bower, B., and Lopatin, D. E.: In vitro lymphocyte blastogenic responses and titers of humoral antibodies from periodontitis patients to oral spirochete isolates. Infect. Immunol. 37:445, 1982.

Mikx, F. H., Matee, M. I., and Schaeken, M. J.: The prevalence of spirochetes in the subgingival microbiota of Tanzanian and Dutch children. J. Clin. Periodontol. 13:289, 1986.

Riviere, G. R., Elliot, K. S., Adam, D. F., Simonson, L. G., Forgas, L. B., Nilius, A. M., and Lukehart, S. A.: Relative proportions of pathogen-related oral spirochetes (PROS) and *Treponema denticola* in supragingival and subgingival plaque from patients with periodontitis. J. Periodontol. 63:131, 1992.

Saglie, F., Carranze, F., Newman, M., Ching, L., and Lewin, K.: Identification tissue-invading bacteria in human periodontal disease. J. Periodont. Res. 17:452, 1982.

Shenker, B. J., Listgarten, M. A., and Taichman, N. S.: Suppression of human lymphocyte responses by oral spirochetes: A monocyte-dependent phenomenon. J. Immunol. 132:2039, 1984.

Simonson, L. G., Robinson, P. J., Pranger, R. J., Cohen, M. E., and Morton, H. E. *Treponema den-*

ticola and *Porphyromonas gingivalis* as prognostic markers following periodontal treatment. J. Periodontol. 63:270, 1992.

Smibert, R. M., and Burmeister, J. A.: Treponema pectinovorum sp. nov. isolated from humans with periodontitis. Int. J. Syst. Bacteriol. 33:852, 1983.

Tew, J. G., Smibert, R. M., Scott, E. A., Burmeister, J. A., and Ranney, R. R.: Serum antibodies in young adult humans reactive with periodontitis associated treponemes. J. Periodont. Res. 20:580, 1985.

20 *Mycoplasmas, Chlamydiae, and Rickettsiae*

Joseph J. Zambon and Violet Haraszthy

CHAPTER OUTLINE

Mycoplasmas

Chlamydiae

Rickettsiae

MYCOPLASMAS

The mycoplasmas are a group of more than 80 species including approximately 11 of which are human pathogens (Table 20–1). They are very small, generally microaerophilic or anaerobic microorganisms, although one species, *Mycoplasma pneumoniae,* is an aerobe (Table 20–2). The mycoplasmas are, in fact, the smallest free-living organisms known to exist. The mycoplasmas are pleomorphic exhibiting coccoid, star-shaped, or filamentous forms. Mycoplasma cells lack a peptidoglycan cell wall and any internal membrane structures. They are composed of a cell membrane, ribosomes, and nucleoid. This lack of structural rigidity may explain why the mycoplasmas have a highly pleomorphic cell morphology. The cells are very small, and coccoid, ranging from 0.2 to 0.3 μm. The mycoplasmas, like viruses chlamydiae and rickettsiae, are able to pass through a 450-nm pore size filter. However, unlike these other microorganisms, the mycoplasmas can be cultured on artificial media. The mycoplasmas do not react to Gram stain; they do stain with Giemsa, although

poorly. The cells possess a *terminal structure,* which permits the mycoplasma to attach to host eukaryotic cells and that may be responsible for the gliding motility these organisms exhibit. Reproduction is by binary fission, although budding is evident in some species. The mycoplasma are distinguished from bacteria not only by their small size but also by their slow growth rate. The mean generation time is as long as 1 to 2 weeks. They also can be distinguished from bacteria in that they have 43 to 48 percent guanine plus cytosine in ribosomal RNA as compared with 50 to 54 percent seen in bacteria. These data suggest that mycoplasmas have a different evolutionary path than bacteria. Mycoplasmas have unique nutritional requirements, especially in their need for lipids and cholesterol, which are used in the mycoplasma cell membrane. One group, the *Acholeplasma,* does not, as the name implies, require cholesterol in its growth medium. Since the mycoplasmas do not possess a cell wall, antibiotics that inhibit cell wall synthesis do not affect the growth of these microorganisms as they do that of bacteria.

TABLE 20–1 ✦ Taxonomy of the Mycoplasmas

CLASS	ORDER	FAMILY	GENUS	CHARACTERISTICS
Mollicutes	Mycoplasmatales	Mycoplasmataceae	*Mycoplasma* *Ureaplasma*	Requires urea for growth
	Acholeplasmatales	Acholeplasmataceae	*Acholeplasma*	Does not require exogenous cholesterol *A. laidlawii* unusual in its rapid growth—18–24 hours
		Spiroplasmataceae	*Spiroplasma* *Anaeroplasma*	

TABLE 20–2 ✦ Mycoplasmas

Features	Small coccoid cells (0.2–0.3 μm), nonmotile, non–Gram-staining
	Generally microaerophilic or anaerobic
Species	*M. pneumoniae*—aerobic, causes primary atypical pneumonia
	M. hominis—cervix
	M. salivarium—in gingival crevice
	M. orale ⎫
	M. buccale ⎬ oral species
	M. faucium ⎭
	M. genitalium—urogenital tract
	Ureaplasma urealyticum (T-strain mycoplasma)—nongonococcal urethritis
	Acholeplasma laidlawii—found in burns
Diseases	Primary atypical pneumonia
	Nongonococcal urethritis
Diagnosis	Culture on specific media
	Immunofluorescence microscopy
	Increase in serum antibody titer
Treatment	Tetracycline and erythromycin

The colony morphology of the mycoplasmas also is unusual. The colonies exhibit a "fried egg" appearance as a result of the colony center growing down into the agar. These microorganisms produce tiny colonies from 10 to 600 μm in diameter, which can be seen only with a magnifying glass or under low power on a microscope. The mycoplasma grow only on complex media containing peptones, yeast extract, and serum. In broth, mycoplasmas grow as a faint haze and are best detected by pH color change. Penicillin is often added to the isolation medium to inhibit bacterial growth and amphotericin is added to inhibit yeasts. *Mycoplasma* species may be identified by inhibition of growth in proximity to a disk containing specific antisera—similar to an antibiotic susceptibility test.

Mycoplasma pneumoniae

In the first half of this century, it became apparent that significant numbers of cases of pneumonia, mainly in children and young adults, were culture-negative; that is, a specific bacterium could not be identified. These cases of culture-negative pneumonia also could be distinguished on clinical criteria. The patients developed cough, fever, and headache but the disease usually was self-limited. This type of pneumonia came to be known as primary atypical pneumonia. Studies by Eaton, however, suggested that there was a microbial origin

to primary atypical pneumonia. He was able to take patient material, inoculate it into eggs, blindly passage the infectious agent, and then use it to produce pneumonia in rats and hamsters. In 1962, Chanock, Hayflick, and Barile developed a medium and were able to culture the agent responsible for primary atypical pneumonia, which was a mycoplasma, *M. pneumoniae*. This microorganism cannot penetrate epithelial cells but is able to adhere to these cells in the respiratory tract by means of neuraminic acid receptors on the epithelial cell surface. Following attachment, the cilia on the epithelial cell cease movement (ciliostasis), are lost, and the cells die. This is thought to occur as a result of hydrogen peroxide production by *M. pneumoniae*.

Mycoplasma may also damage host tissues by means of hypersensitivity reactions. The major mycoplasmic antigens are cell membrane proteins and glycolipids, which may induce cross-reacting antibodies. In *M. pneumoniae*, for example, the major antigen is a glucose- and galactose-containing glycolipid, which induces antibodies that can cross-react with certain host tissues such as human brain. Patients with an initial mycoplasma infection can develop these cross-reactive antibodies. During a second mycoplasma infection, the antibody response may then damage host tissues as well as the microorganism.

M. pneumoniae generally causes only a mild upper respiratory infection but may cause primary atypical pneumonia. The peak incidence for this disease is in children 5 to 15 years of age, and the microorganism is responsible for up to half of all cases of pneumonia in children and young adults.

Other Mycoplasmas

Other mycoplasmas such as *M. hominis* and *M. orale* may exist as commensals on human mucous membranes. Certain mycoplasmas such as *Ureaplasma urealyticum* and *M. genitalium* exist on the mucous membranes of the urogenital tract. *U. urealyticum* has been implicated in the etiology of nongonococcal urethritis and pelvic inflammatory disease. Mycoplasmas are also frequently found as contaminants in animal cell cultures.

Diagnosis and Treatment

Mycoplasma infection can be diagnosed by culture of the microorganism on one of several special media, by the immunofluorescent detection of the organism from culture of patient specimens, by the polymerase chain reaction (for *M. pneumoniae*), and by increased serum antibody titers to mycoplasma antigens. Once cultured, the mycoplasma also can be speciated by immunofluorescence using species-specific antisera. Speciation also can be performed by growth inhibition and by metabolic inhibition. In these latter assays, the mycoplasma is grown on media on which a disk that contains species-specific antisera has been placed. If the unknown mycoplasma is the same species as the species-specific antisera, then growth will be inhibited much like in an antibiotic sensitivity test. Metabolic inhibition makes use of changes in, for example, sugar fermentation as a means of assessing the effect of the species-specific antisera.

CHLAMYDIAE

The chlamydiae are an unusual group of human and animal microbial pathogens that are a leading cause of human blindness and venereal disease (Table 20–3). They are nonmotile, gram-negative microorganisms similar to the rickettsiae in being obligate intracellar parasites. The chlamydiae can be differentiated from viruses in having both DNA and RNA and in being susceptible to broad-spectrum antibiotics such as tetracycline. They have a limited metabolic capacity however and use ATP produced by the host cell. They are smaller than other bacteria (less than 1 μm) and have an unusual two-stage life cycle. One stage, the elementary body (0.3 nm), is adapted for extracellular survival and the other stage, the reticular body, is adapted for intracellular growth and multiplication by means of cytoplasmic vesicles known as *inclusions*. The elementary body is taken up into susceptable cells by receptor-mediated endocytosis and forms an endosome. Subsequent fusion with cellular lysosomes and formation of a phagolysosome is prevented. The elementary body reforms into a reticular body. After about 8 hours, they

TABLE 20–3 ✦ Chlamydiae

Features	Small (<1 μm), nonmotile, gram-negative, obligate intracellular parasite
	Two stage life cycle:
	elementary body—infectious stage
	reticular body—intracellular stage
	Forms intracellular inclusions visible by light microscopy
Species	*C. trachomatis* causes
	1. Trachoma—leading cause of human blindness
	2. Inclusion conjunctivitis
	a. "Swimming pool" conjunctivitis in adults
	b. Inclusion blenorrhea in infants
	3. Sexually transmitted disease—infertility
	4. Lymphogranuloma venereum—Frei test
	C. psittaci causes psittacosis
	C. pneumoniae causes respiratory disease

divide by binary fission and are re-formed into elementary bodies. After an additional 18 to 24 hours, these elementary bodies are released during lysis of the infected host cell and can go on to infect other host cells. There are three main species, *Chlamydia trachomatis*, *C. pneumoniae* (causing respiratory disease) and *C. psittaci*. Each microorganism exhibits heat-labile cell surface protein antigens that are species-specific, as well as heat-stable lipopolysaccharide antigens that are group-specific.

Chlamydia trachomatis

C. trachomatis causes disease primarily in humans, including both trachoma, the leading cause of human blindness, and inclusion conjunctivitis. Trachoma is caused by *C. trachomatis* serotypes A, B, Ba and C. *C. trachomatis* also causes sexually transmitted diseases such as lymphogranuloma venereum (LGV), which is due to serotypes L1, L2, and L3, and nongonococcal urethritis and epididymitis, from serotypes D through K. Humans are the only known reservoir of *C. trachomatis*.

The elementary body is that stage of the chlamydial life cycle in which the microorganism is transmissible between hosts. The elementary body has a rigid, impermeable cell envelope that contains a hemagglutinin. It is transmitted by person-to-person contact and is a problem especially in Third World countries where sanitation and personal hygiene may be poor. The elementary body can attach to human epithelial cells as in the conjunctiva and is taken up by the cell. The reticular body is a noninfectious form that multiplies intracellularly 1 to 2 days after infection. It prevents DNA and protein synthesis by the host and destroys the host cell.

Clinically, the pathogenesis of *C. trachomatis* in trachoma is characterized by inflammation of the conjunctiva with follicle formation. The cornea becomes vascularized, injected, and, as a result, partial or complete blindness develops. Scarring may cause inversion of the eyelids and scarring of the cornea by the eyelashes. Alterations in the lacrimal glands can lead the way to secondary bacterial infections by other microorganisms. *C. trachomatis* infection results in a short-lived humoral immunity. IgG and secretory IgA are found in the eye secretions. Most *C. trachomatis* infections resolve spontaneously without severe complications such as blindness. However, approximately 10 percent of infected persons will become partially or completely blind.

The diagnosis of trachoma is based on clinical signs including conjunctival follicles, scars and corneal infiltration, and vascularization. The microorganism can be recovered from the conjunctiva and isolated by culture in a eukaryotic cell line. Cytoplasmic inclusion bodies can be seen by fluorescent antibody tests. Chlamydial antigens can be detected by ELISA and with DNA probes. Antibodies in serum or eye secretions can also be detected by serologic tests. Antibiotic therapy by means of orally administered tetracycline and ophthalmic ointment is effective in eliminating the infection.

A variant of trachoma is known as inclusion conjunctivitis or "swimming pool conjunctivitis." This disease occurs in adults and is similar to another variant of trachoma that occurs in infants known as inclusion blenorrhea. Clinically, both of these diseases exhibit conjunctival inflammation, but the diseases are self-limiting and do not generally cause blindness. Inclusion conjunctivitis is caused by ocular infection with genitourinary strains of *C. trachomatis* transmitted either by genital-to-hand-to-eye contact, sometimes through towels, or through genitourinary chlamydial contamination of improperly chlorinated swimming pools.

C. trachomatis, particularly serotypes D and K, can cause sexually transmitted genitourinary tract infections including nongonococcal urethritis and epididymitis in men and pelvic inflammatory disease in women. *C. trachomatis* is therefore a major cause of sexually transmitted disease and resulting infertility. Another form of *C. trachomatis*–related sexually transmitted disease is lymphogranuloma venereum. This is clinically apparent as herpetiform vesicles on the genitals with the development of enlarged and even suppurative regional lymph nodes referred to as *venereal buboes*. This disease can be detected by means of the Frei test in which heat-killed *C. trachomatis* is injected as a skin test and produces a delayed hypersensitivity reaction in infected individuals.

Chlamydia psittaci

C. psittaci affects mainly domestic fowl and birds, causing a disease known as psittacosis. This disease can kill large numbers of infected birds. In humans, this microorganism causes only slight respiratory disease although severe cases of human pneumonia due to *C. psittaci* have been reported. Human disease is almost always related to contact with infected birds.

In birds, *C. psittaci* produces a widely disseminated infection throughout the animal, and the microorganism is eventually shed through secretions and feces. In certain species, *C. psittaci* can be transmitted through eggs to infect the next generation. Dust contaminated with bird feces can be inhaled to cause human disease. The diagnosis of ornithosis is made by culture of *C. psittaci* or by immunofluorescence.

Diagnosis

Chlamydial infection can be detected by culture of appropriate clinical specimens or by serologic techniques. Chlamydiae can be cultured in egg yolk sacs or in the brain, liver, or spleen of mice; however, the most widely used method is by culture in eukaryotic cells such as the McCoy cell line. The clinical specimen to be tested is inoculated into cycloheximide-treated McCoy cells, incubated for 48 to 72 hours, stained with iodine or Giemsa, and examined by light microscopy for the development of the glycogen-rich inclusion bodies. Staining with fluorescent antibody enables detection after only 24 hours.

RICKETTSIAE

The rickettsiae are a group of gram-negative, obligate intracellular parasites that are transmitted to humans through the bites of arthropod vectors including insects such as lice or arachnids such as ticks (Table 20–4). Once these microorganisms gain access to the vasculature, they infect endothelial cells, resulting in hyperplasia and focal obstruction. The resulting clinical diseases are characterized by a typical clinical course including fever, headache, and skin rash. The type and distribution of skin rash is, itself, clinically useful in diagnosing rickettsial disease as well as in distinguishing different types of rickettsial disease. One type of rickettsial disease, Q fever, results from inhalation of contaminated aerosols.

TABLE 20–4 ✦ Rickettsiae

Rickettsia	Obligate intracellular parasites
	Requires an extracellular energy source
Species	*Rick. prowazekii*
	Causes
	Primary louse-borne typhus
	Recrudescent typhus (Brill-Zinsser disease)
	Features
	Rash develops from trunk to arms and legs
	Rick. rickettsii
	Causes
	Spotted fever, tick-borne
	Features
	Intracytoplasmic and intranuclear parasite
	Rash from arms and legs to trunk

The rickettsiae are distinguished from bacteria by a number of important criteria:

1. The rickettsiae are obligate intracellular parasites which parasitize phagocytic and nonphagocytic cells. Bacteria, by contrast, can sometimes exist as intracellular parasites but they also can survive extracellularly.
2. The rickettsiae require an outside energy source. ATP, NAD, and CoA can diffuse from the cytoplasm of the host cell into the rickettsiae to serve as an energy source.
3. They are smaller than bacterial cells, generally 0.3 to 0.5 nm in diameter, and they approximate the size of eukaryotic intracellular organelles such as mitochondria.

Classification of Rickettsial Disease
TYPHUS GROUP

This group of rickettsial diseases includes: (1) primary louse-borne typhus, (2) recrudescent typhus, and (3) murine typhus.

Primary louse-borne typhus is caused by *Rickettsia prowazekii,* which lives only in humans and in the human louse, *Pediculus humanus.* The transmission cycle is, therefore, louse-to-human-to-louse-to-human. Humans, however, are the reservoir for this organism since *Rick. prowazekii* infection is fatal to lice. Lice become infected by feeding on contaminated human blood. The organism multiplies in the insect's gastrointestinal tract and contaminates the feces. When the insect subsequently bites a human, it defecates on the skin and the contaminated feces are inoculated into the underlying tissues by scratching.

About 2 weeks after being bitten, the person will experience headache, rash, fever, and chills. The organism then multiplies in the endothelial cells lining the small blood vessels and causes hyperplasia and focal obstruction of these vessels. This vascular obstruction is responsible for the signs and symptoms of the disease. Thrombosis and obstruction of small vessels in the skin result in a rash, while thrombosis and obstruction of small vessels in the meninges cause headache and stupor.

The rash is clinically characteristic. It develops about 1 week after the first symptoms and it starts on the thorax and spreads to the arms and legs but does not involve the palms of the hands or the soles of the feet. The rash also changes from a maculopapular lesion to petechial hemorrhages.

Recrudescent typhus (Brill-Zinsser disease) represents a second subsequent episode of typhus in persons who previously have had primary louse-borne typhus. After the primary course of typhus, the patient recovers but the microorganism enters a latent stage. The patient may then undergo repeated bouts of typhus if, in response to stress and/or decreased host immunity, *Rick. prowazekii* leaves the latent stage and multiplies in host cells. Similar to repeated episodes of other infectious diseases, recrudescent typhus is of shorter duration and is milder, and it produces an immediate secondary IgG immune response. No vector is involved in recrudescent typhus, since the original infection may have occurred years or decades before. The patients may or may not develop a rash.

Murine typhus is, as the name suggests, spread by rats and rat fleas. The rat flea is infected with *Rick. typhi* (syn. *mooseri*) by feeding on an infected rat. The flea can then spread the microorganism from rat-to-rat or from rat-to-human through contaminated feces, the same as in primary louse-borne typhus. It also produces a similar but less virulent human disease in areas where rats are found in high numbers, such as coastal areas. This human disease is called Toulon fever in France, Moscow typhus in Russia, and red fever in the Congo.

The spotted fevers, the best known of which is Rocky Mountain spotted fever, are caused by *Rick. rickettsia.* This microorganism is spread by ticks—primarily the wood tick in the Western United States and the dog tick in the Eastern United States. Other rickettsiae that are antigenically similar to *Rick. rickettsia* produce Marseilles fever, Siberian tick typhus, and Queensland tick typhus. *Rick. rickettsia* differs from other rickettsiae in that it can be found in the nucleus of host eukaryotic cells as well as in the cytoplasm. The resulting disease is also different from that caused by the typhus group in that the rash starts on the arms and legs, including the palms of the hands and the soles of the feet, and proceeds to include the thorax. Like typhus, the primary lesion is intravascular thrombosis, which can be so severe as to cause disseminated intravascular coagulation. There is a 5 percent mortality from this disease, even with antibiotic treatment.

Ticks become infected with *Rick. rickettsia* but do not die of the infection as in primary louse-borne typhus. The organism can be passed on to the next generation of tick through transovarial infection. Eggs harboring *Rick. rickettsia* transform from larva to nymphs to adults. Ticks may also have *Rick. rickettsia* in saliva. When they bite humans, infected saliva is injected into the skin.

Scrub typhus (tsutsugamushi disease) is a disease seen in Japan, Southeast Asia, and the South Pacific islands and is spread by trombiculid mites infected with *Rick. tsutsugamushi.* The mites spread the microorganism by biting both rodents and humans. The organism is then spread to a subsequent generation of mites through infected eggs.

The site of the bite in humans develops into a black, ulcerated scar and produces regional and later generalized lymphadenopathy, which is distinct from other rickettsial diseases. Like the other rickettsial diseases, the patient develops fever, headache, and rash 1 to 2 weeks after the bite.

Q FEVER

Q fever occurs not only by means of an insect or arachnid bite, but is also spread by inhalation of infected aerosols. The primary site of human infection is the lung as opposed to the vasculature. The infectious agent is *Coxiella burnetii,* named after its discoverers, Cox in the United States and Burnett in Australia. It is differentiated from the other rickettsiae in being stable outside the eukaryotic host cells and also is antigenically distinct. *C. burnetii* can infect a variety of ticks worldwide. The ticks, in turn, bite domestic animals, which then harbor *C. burnetii* in a latent stage (similar to that of recrudescent typhus). When a period of stress occurs such as during parturition the organism multiples. It then increases to high numbers in chorionic fluid, placental tissues, feces, and urine. Q fever occurs in people, therefore, who come in contact with infected animals or animal tissues such as livestock tenders, slaughterhouse workers, textile workers (from contaminated wool), and laboratorians. The microorganism also can be spread through infected dust or aerosols that are inhaled. Clinical symptoms include headache, fever, and pneumonia.

Laboratory Diagnosis of Rickettsial Disease

Serologic tests provide the primary means for the laboratory diagnosis of rickettsial disease; however, often patients develop severe symptoms prior to an antibody response. Therefore, clinicians often rely on patient history and clinical signs and symptoms, especially the characteristic skin rash, in order to diagnose the rickettsial diseases. Serologic tests generally detect patient antibodies to one of two types of rickettsial antigens—the soluble group antigens, which are shared by most of the rickettsia, and the insoluble, type-specific antigens, which are unique to each species. The serologic assays used to detect patient antibodies include complement fixation to measure common antigens, immunofluorescence, and the Weil-Felix reaction. This latter test is based on the presence of cross-reactive polysaccharide antigens shared by the rickettsia and certain species of *Proteus.* The test is performed by mixing a drop of the patient's blood with each of three *Proteus* strains. The presence of antibody to the rickettsiae can be detected by bacterial cell agglutination, which appears after approximately 5 minutes.

Certain rickettsial diseases produce other laboratory results, which can be useful in diagnosis. Patients with Rocky Mountain spotted fever, for example, will often exhibit leukopenia and thrombocytopenia.

Treatment and Prevention

The rickettsial diseases generally respond to systemic antibiotics, particularly those antibiotics that can eliminate intracellular parasites. These include chloramphenicol and the tetracyclines.

There are two main approaches to the prevention of rickettsial disease. These are immunization with appropriate vaccines and elimination of the rickettsial vector. Vaccines have been used to prevent primary louse-borne typhus but have only ameliorated the course of the disease rather than providing complete protection. Rickettsial diseases have been better prevented by elimination of the vector. Primary louse-borne typhus and subsequent recrudescent typhus have been controlled through the use of DDT to eliminate the human lice. Murine typhus is controlled by killing rat fleas and by the elimination of rodent populations.

BIBLIOGRAPHY
Mycoplasmas

Chanock, R. M., Hayflick, L., and Barile, M. F.: Growth in artificial media of an agent associated with atypical pneumonia and its identification as a PPLO. Proc. Nat. Acad. Sci. (USA) 48:41, 1962.

Razin, S.: The mycoplasma. Microbial Reviews 42:414, 1978.

Tully, J. G., and Whitcomb, R. F. (eds.): The Mycoplasma. Academic Press, New York, 1979.

Chlamydiae

Schachter, J.: Chlamydial infections. N. Engl. J. Med. 298:428; 490; 540, 1978.

Schachter, J., and Caldwell, H. D.: Chlamydiae. Ann. Rev. Microbial. 34:285, 1980.

Rickettsiae

Weiss, E.: The biology of the rickettsiae. Ann. Rev. Microbial. 36:345, 1982.

21 Legionella

Joan Otomo-Corgel

CHAPTER OUTLINE

Clinical-epidemiologic patterns
Epidemiology
Laboratory diagnosis
Microbiology
Pathogenesis
Immunology
Treatment

In July 1976, the Pennsylvania American Legion was having its 50th Annual Convention. A mysterious illness that took 29 lives shrouded the event. Approximately 6 months later, a gram-negative bacterium was isolated by techniques used for the isolation of rickettsial agents. Survivors demonstrated antibodies against the isolate. The first description of the legionnaires' disease bacterium had just been introduced.

Earlier outbreaks were later retrospectively linked to the same etiologic organism: 81 patients became ill and 14 died in 1965 at St. Elizabeth Hospital, Washington, D.C.; 144 cases related to air conditioning in a health department building occurred in Pontiac, Michigan, and two deaths from pneumonia were associated with an Oddfellows Convention in Philadelphia in 1974. Recognition of legionnaires' disease bacterium (LDB, or *Legionella pneumophila*) brought to light a sporadic epidemic that is increasing in frequency. While it is broadly referred to as legionnaires' disease or legionellosis, a number of species within the genus *Legionella* (i.e., *L. wadsworthii, L. gormanii,* or *L. micdadei*) are linked to disease.

CLINICAL-EPIDEMIOLOGIC PATTERNS

There are three distinct clinical-epidemiologic patterns.

1. **Pontiac fever** or **nonpneumonic legionnaires' disease** is devoid of mortality and pneumonia. After a 5- to 66-hour incubation period, flulike symptoms of abrupt-onset fever, chills, headache, and myalgia develop. Neurologic and gastrointestinal symptoms are similar to those of other legionnaires' outbreaks. In the Pontiac outbreak, the suspected source of *Legionella* was the air-conditioning system since once the evaporator condenser was cleansed and relocated, the outbreak was suppressed.

2. **Pneumonic legionnaires' disease**, exemplified by the 1976 Philadelphia outbreak, has an incubation period of 2 to 10 days and a low attack rate. The clinical course begins with malaise, myalgia, headache with ensuing fever, pneumonia, and sometimes death. Central nervous system symptoms of slurred speech, clumsiness, ataxia, and confusion occur early. Lower respiratory symptoms (dyspnea and nonproductive cough) are present in 4 to 7 days without previous upper respiratory symptoms. In half of the cases, coughs became productive. Once respiratory symptoms predominate, progression to pneumonia occurs. Diarrhea, vomiting, abdominal pain, abnormalities in serum electrolytes, leukocytosis, and renal abnormalities also have been noted.

3. The third form of legionnaires' disease has been described as **nosocomial.** Attack rates are low, but fatality rates are high. An outbreak occurred in 1978 at the Veterans Ad-

ministration Medical Center, West Los Angeles, Wadsworth Division, where 75 people contracted the disease and 25 percent died. The clinical course was similar to the pneumonic form, but renal disease was absent and pneumonia progression was different. *Legionella pneumophila* was isolated from the water supply and treated primarily by hyperchlorination.

EPIDEMIOLOGY

The sex distribution in legionnaires' disease is 2 to 3:1 males to females. The average age of a patient is 60 years; however, there is a broad age range. It is also apparently more benign in children. A majority of patients have one or more predisposing underlying conditions including immunosuppression, malignancy, heart disease, and chronic renal failure.

LABORATORY DIAGNOSIS

Laboratory diagnosis is based on cultural isolation, identification in clinical specimens by direct immunofluorescence, elevated antibody titers in convalescent sera, and identification of bacterial antigens in body fluids. Newer tests for antibody determination include an indirect enzyme-linked immunosorbent assay (ELISA) using six serogroups of whole *L. pneumophila* and a microagglutination assay, which are both rapid and sensitive. *Legionella* antigens also can be detected by ELISA. At present, DNA probes are being investigated for identifying species of *Legionella*.

TABLE 21–1 ✦ Members of Legionellaceae Implicated in Pneumonia

Legionella pneumophila
Pittsburgh pneumonia agent
  Tatlockia micdadei
  Legionella micdadei
L. bozemanii
L. dumoffi
L. longbeachae
L. jordania
L. gormanii
L. feeleii
L. hackeliae
L. maceachernii
L. wadsworthii
L. birminghamensis
L. cincinnatiensis
L. oakridgensis
L. anisa
L. cherrii
L. sainthelensi

MICROBIOLOGY

The initial classification of *Legionella* was family Legionellaceae, genus *Legionella,* and single species *pneumophila*. There are now over 25 species classified in the Legionellaceae family, 18 of which are implicated in human pneumonias (Table 21–1). The genus identification is based on ability to grow on buffered charcoal yeast agar or other media containing cysteine and iron salts. This genus fails to grow on blood agar. Species identification is done serologically and, more recently, by DNA relatedness. Species designation then may be supported by antigen analysis and cell wall fatty acid profiles supported by gas-liquid chromatography. The bacterial cell wall is composed of diaminopimelic acid, typical of gram-negative bacilli, but with an unusually high cross-linkage of 80 to 90 percent.

PATHOGENESIS

L. pneumophila is an opportunistic facultative organism with a number of serotypes. Infection is thought to be via inhalation or ingestion. Small particles (less than 5 μm) are necessary to ensure respiratory bronchiole penetration. Potable water ingestion with entry into the lymphatics and lung dissemination may also occur. Mortality ranges from 10 to 20 percent of untreated cases. *Legionellosis* is an acute fibropurulent pneumonia affecting the sinus with leakage of the edema and fibrin from damaged capillaries affecting gaseous exchange leading to hypoxia. The bacterium causes cellular damage besides lung infiltration and consolidation. Histologically, there are intra-alveolar macrophages and monocytes. There is either direct tissue invasion or systemic-toxic effects of the bacterium (pyrexia or gram-negative septicemia) on extrapulmonary organs: renal, hepatic, gastrointestinal, and neurologic. Inflammation and tissue injury can occur in the absence of organisms, suggesting production of an "endotoxin-like polysaccharide substance."

IMMUNOLOGY

There is no agreement on the chemical structure of serogroup-specific and species-specific antigens, but antigenic activity of serogroup-specific antigens of *L. pneumophila* resides in the polysaccharide portion of the antigen. The antigen has a molecular weight of approximately 4×10^4 and consists of less than 10 percent carbohydrate, 15 percent protein, 1.1 percent phosphate, and a lipid. There is a similarity between serogroup antigens of *L. pneumophila* (cell-like surface location, high molecular weight, and chemical composition) and the lipopolysaccharide endotoxin classically associated with other gram-negative bacteria. *L. pneumophila* produces compounds similar to classic endotoxin in biologic activity and chemical structure, but further study is required to implicate serotype-specific antigens to endotoxin activity. Skin testing for antigens specific to legionellosis is also being developed.

L. pneumophila may multiply intracellularly in human mononuclear phagosomes (facultative, intracellular parasite), thus belonging to a special group of pathogens that can evade host defenses by parasitizing mononuclear phagocytes. Humans are probably incidental hosts for legionnaires' disease bacteria, which developed a capacity for intracellular survival in amoebae and mononuclear phagocytes. In vitro antibody studies suggest that humoral immunity may not be effective against *L. pneumophila* and that a vaccine that elicits only antibody protection also may be ineffective. The organism inhibits phagosome-lysosome fusion, which is important to its survival in mononuclear phagocytes (comparable to *Mycobacterium tuberculosis* and *Toxoplasma gondii*). In contrast to humoral defense, cell-mediated immunity seems to play a major role. Patients with legionnaires' disease develop a mononuclear response to *L. pneumophila* antigens with proliferation and generation of monocyte-activating cytokinins. Mononuclear phagocytes activated by the cytokinins inhibit intracellular multiplication of *L. pneumophila*. Monocytes and PMNs phagocytose a limited portion of an inoculum of antibody and complement-coated bacteria.

TREATMENT

Owing to the ubiquity of the organism, eradication is not feasible and control in water is difficult. Hyperchlorination is effective in nosocomial legionellosis from potable water. Low hot water temperatures, water stagnation, and faucet obstructions (rubber washers) act as reservoirs for bacterial growth. Cooling towers provide an environment for amplification of *L. pneumophila* due to thermal enhancement. Legionnaires' disease bacteria are not active at 45°C and are relatively inactive at 75°C. Therefore, current recommendations for hospitals are chlorination at or raising temperatures of hot water systems to above 63°C.

In clinical treatment, erythromycin and tetracycline decrease mortality and provide clinical improvement. Differences exist, however, between clinical response to antibiotic therapy and in vitro susceptibility studies. Based on data from epidemics, antibiotics are indicated for suspected or diagnosed legionellosis (Table 21–2). Erythromycin and rifampin inhibit *L. pneumophila* intracellular multiplication but do not kill intracellular bacteria even at high concentrations. Once the antibiotic is stopped, multiplication in monocytes resumes. Therefore, antibiotics provide an opportunity for the host to mount an immune defense against the unique bacterium. A combination of erythromycin and rifampin may be best because erythromycin does not prevent widespread lung lesions, but rifampin penetrates well into the macrophage to reach the legionnaires' disease bacteria and confines the lung lesions.

TABLE 21–2 ✦ Antimicrobial Therapy for *Legionella* Disease

ANTIMICROBIAL	DOSE	ROUTE	DURATION	MISCELLANEOUS
Erythromycin gluceptate or erythromycin lactobionate	25–50 mg/kg not to exceed 4 g/day	IV	3 wk	Dilute 0.5–1 g in 250 ml 5% dextrose or 0.9% sodium chloride solution for continuous 6 hr infusion
Tetracycline	250–500 mg q6h not to exceed 2 g/day	IV	2 wk	In children >8 yrs 15 mg/kg q12h When clinical improvement is noted, 500 mg qid oral.
Doxycycline	100 mg q12h	IV	2 wk	For patients with renal insufficiency
Rifampin	10–20 mg/kg not to exceed 600 mg/day	Oral dose + erythromycin or tetracycline on empty stomach		For critically ill Increases hepatic enzymes
Imipenem Imipenem + cilastatin	500 mg each tid	Oral dose	Minimum 5 days	New carbapenem β-lactam antibiotic Studied by Farrell et al. and Beasley et al. in 1985

Supportive care for the patients with legionnaires' disease must be maintained. Because of the pyrexia, lung infiltration, fibrosis, and septicemia associated with this disease, attention should be placed on prevention of hypotension, renal failure, and respiratory failure. Maintenance of fluid-electrolyte and acid-base balance also is important. Secondary infection also is a potential complicating factor.

Dental Treatment Considerations

Recent studies indicate prevalence of antibodies to *L. pneumophila* among dental personnel, especially dentists constantly exposed to high-speed handpiece generated aerosols. There are no clinical guidelines for treating patients with a history of or active legionnaires' disease in the dental environment. There is a paucity of information relating to transmission of legionnaires' disease bacteria infections. Dental personnel should be aware of clinical signs and symptoms and suspect patients with pneumonia of unknown etiology. Elective dental treatment should not be performed on a legionnaires' disease patient. For an emergency, the physician should be consulted and infection control procedures should be followed closely:

Barrier technique
Minimal use of air or water syringes
Strict septic technique
Slow-speed handpiece only
In-hospital treatment only (isolation)

The patient should not be placed in a fully reclining position, if this is uncomfortable. Stress reduction protocols should be employed.

In patients who have recovered from legionellosis, there are no contraindications to routine dental therapy. The dentist should be aware of patients with possible lung fibrosis, permanent cerebellum dysfunction, cranial nerve palsies, seizures, renal dysfunction, peripheral neuropathy, and even endocarditis. The disease is not spread from person to person but from water sources to immunosusceptible hosts. Relapse of the infection is infrequent.

The incidence of legionnaires' disease is increasing. It is epidemic and sporadic, but bacterial identification is rapid. Identification of reservoirs and mechanisms of aerosolization, transmission, and bacterial virulence are better understood but need greater focus. Prophylaxis is of paramount importance, especially in hospitals, where the immunocompromised patient is a prime target. Extrathoracic manifestation of legionellosis is poorly understood, and protective immunity from prior infection with bacteria of a different serogroup is unknown. Great strides have been made since 1976, but further knowledge is necessary before a solution to the problem will be found. Along with improvements in diagnosis and treatment, the management of dental patients will become clearer.

BIBLIOGRAPHY

Agrawal, L., Dhunjibhoy, K. R., and Nair, K. G.: Isolation of *Legionella pneumophila* from patients of respiratory tract disease and environmental samples. Indian J. Med. Res. 93:364–365, 1991.

Barka, N., et al.: ELISA using whole *Legionella pneumophila* as an antigen. Comparison between monovalent and polyvalent antigens for the serodiagnosis of human legionellosis. J. Immunol. Methods 93:77, 1986.

Beasley, C. R.: Treatment of pneumonia with imipenem/cilastatin. N. Z. Med. J. 98:494, 1985.

Beaty, H. N.: Clinical features of legionellosis. Legionella Proceedings of the International Symposium, American Society for Microbiology, Washington, D.C., pp. 6–10, 1984.

Blackmon, J. A., et al.: Legionellosis. Am. J. Pathol. 103:429, 1981.

Brenner, D. J., et al.: Classification of Legionnaires' disease bacterium: *Legionella pneumophila*, genus novum, species nova of the family *Legionellaceae*, familia nova. Ann. Intern. Med. 90:656, 1979.

Broome, C. V. and Fraser, D. W.: Epidemiologic aspects of legionellosis. Epidemiol. Rev. 1:1, 1979.

Cameron, S., Roder, D., Walker, C., and Feldheim, J.: Epidemiological characteristics of Legionella infection in South Australia: Implications for disease control, Australia and N. Z. Med. J. 21:65–70, 1991.

Centers for Disease Control: Respiratory infection—Pennsylvania. MMWR 25:244, 1976.

Fang, G. D., Yu, V. L., and Vickers, R. M.: Disease due to the Legionellaceae (other than Legionella pneumophila). Historical, microbiological, clinical, and epidemiological review. Medicine 68:116–132, 1989.

Farrell, I. D., et al.: The activity of imipenem on *Legionella pneumophila*, with a note on the treatment of two cases. J. Antimicrob. Chemother. 16:61, 1985.

Flesher, A. R.: Isolation of a serogroup 1-specific antigen from *Legionella pneumophila*. J. Infect. Dis. 145:224, 1982.

Fliermans C. B.: Measure of *Legionella pneumophila* activity *in situ*. Curr. Microbiol. 6:89–94, 1981.

Fraser, D. W., et al.: Legionnaires' disease: Description of an epidemic of pneumonia. N. Engl. J. Med. 297:1189, 1977.

Glavin, F. L.: Ultrastructure of lung in Legionnaires' disease. Observation of three biopsies done during the Vermont epidemic. Ann. Intern. Med. 90:555, 1979.

Glick, T. H., et al.: Pontiac Fever. An epidemic of unknown etiology in a health department. I. Clinical and epidemiological aspects. Am. J. Epidemiol. 107:149, 1978.

Haley, C. E.: Nosocomial Legionnaires' disease. A continuing common-source epidemic at Wadsworth Medical Center. Ann. Intern. Med. 90:583, 1979.

Hart, C. A. and Makin, T.: Legionella in hospitals: A review. J. Hosp. Infect., 18 Suppl. A:481–489, 1991.

Horwitz, M. A.: Interactions between *Legionella pneumophila* and human mononuclear phagocytes. Legionella, American Society for Microbiology, Washington, D.C., 159–166, 1984.

Horwitz, M. A. and Silverstein, S. C.: The Legionnaires' disease bacterium multiplies intracellularly in human monocytes. J. Clin. Invest. 66:441, 1980.

Johnson, W., et al.: Serospecificity and opsonic activity of antisera to *Legionella pneumophila*. Infect. Immunol. 26:698, 1979.

Kirby, B. D., et al.: Legionnaires' disease: Report of sixty-five nosocomial acquired cases and review of the literature. Medicine 59:188, 1980.

Lattimer, G. L., and Ormsbee, R. A.: Legionnaires' Disease. Marcel Dekker, New York, 1981.

McDade J. E., et al.: Legionnaires' disease. Isolation of a bacterium and demonstration of its role in other respiratory diseases. N. Engl. J. Med. 297:1197, 1977.

Meyer R. D.: Legionella infections: A review of five years of research. Rev. Infect. Dis. 5:258, 1983.

Muder, R. R., et al.: Pneumonia due to the Pittsburgh pneumonia agent: New clinical perspective with a review of the literature. Medicine 62:120, 1983.

Pfaller, M., Hollis, R., Johnson, W., Massanari, R. M., Helms, C., Wenzel, R., Hall, N., Moyer, N., and Joly, J.: The application of molecular and immunologic techniques to study the epidemiology of *Legionella pneumophili* serogroup 1. Diag. Microbiol. & Infect. Dis. 12:295–302, 1989.

Reinthaler, F. F., Mascher, F., and Stunzner, D.: Serological examinations from antibodies against *Legionella* species in dental personnel. J. Dent. Res. 57:942–943, 1988.

Ruf, B., Schrumann, D., Horback, I., Fehrenback, F. J., and Pohle, H. D.: Prevalence and diagnosis of Legionella pneumonia: A 3-year prospective study with emphasis on application of urinary antigen detection. J. Infect. Dis. 162:1341–1348, 1990.

Shands, K. N., et al.: Potable water as a source of Legionnaires' disease. JAMA 253:1412, 1985.

Tang, P. W. and Toma, S.: Broad-spectrum enzyme-linked immuno-absorbent assay for detection of Legionella-soluble antigens. J. Clin. Microbiol. 24:556, 1986.

Thacker, S. B., et al.: An outbreak in 1965 of severe respiratory illness caused by the Legionnaires' disease bacterium. J. Infect. Dis. 138:512, 1978.

Tsai, T. F., et al.: Legionnaires' Disease: Clinical features of the epidemic in Philadelphia. Ann. Intern. Med. 90:509, 1979.

U.S. Dept. of Health, Education and Welfare, Centers for Disease Control: Epidemiology of Legionnaires' Disease. Baine, W.B. 1980.

Wong, K. H.: Endotoxicity of the Legionnaires' disease bacterium. Ann. Intern. Med. 90:624, 1979.

22 *Virology*

No-Hee Park

CHAPTER OUTLINE

General structure of viruses
Classification of animal viruses
Virus replication
Diagnosis of viral diseases
Effect of viruses on host cell
Host response to viral infections
Respiratory viruses
Herpesviruses
Hepatitis viruses
Oncogenic viruses
AIDS and human immunodeficiency virus
Antiviral therapy
Vaccines

GENERAL STRUCTURE OF VIRUSES

Over the past two decades, significant advances have occurred in understanding the nature of viruses as well as the pathogenesis and treatment of human viral infections. Viruses are a major cause of disease in humans, being responsible for illnesses ranging in severity from the common cold to fatal encephalitis and AIDs. To establish the etiologic diagnosis, effective prophylaxis, and therapeutic measures, it is essential to understand the mechanism and pattern of that virus' dissemination within the population, its mode of entry into and spread within the hosts, the nature of its interaction with host cells, and its mode of replication within individual host cells. All of these parameters are closely related to virus structure and composition. The main structural components of a virion are nucleic acid, capsid, and viral envelope (Figs. 22–1 and 22–2).

Nucleic Acids

Viruses contain DNA or RNA, the genetic information that directs the cell to construct a series of proteins. The size of nucleic acid differs among viruses and determines the complexity of virions. The nucleic acid genome can be double-stranded (ds) circular or linear DNA, single-stranded (ss) linear DNA, ds or ss broken linear RNA, ss intact linear RNA, or ss broken circular RNA.

Capsid

Proteins are indispensable components of all virions together with nucleic acids. The protein coat that surrounds the nucleic acid genome of all viruses is called the capsid. Nucleocapsid is the complex of the capsid and the nucleic acid. In a virion lacking an envelope, the capsid provides the only protection for the nucleic acid. The capsid also determines the host range and is responsible for the initiation of infection. Most viral capsids exhibit one of two types of symmetry: icosahedral (cubic) or helical (certain complex viruses, such as the poxviruses and T-even bacteriophages exhibit bilateral symmetry). The capsids are composed of subunits called capsomeres, which may be composed of more than one polypeptide mol-

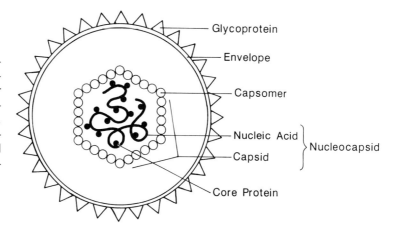

FIGURE 22–1 ✦ A schematic representation of an enveloped virion. The viral nucleic acid, either RNA or DNA, is enclosed by protein molecules forming the capsid. The capsid is enclosed in an envelope to whose outer surface viral specific glycoproteins are attached.

ecule. In addition to capsid proteins, some viruses contain a variety of virion enzymes. Some enzymes may be of host cell origin, serving no apparent useful function for the virus. Some virus-coded enzymes, however, are essential for viral infectivity. One of the most important enzymes found in some virions is **transcriptase** (or polymerase). Four different transcriptases have been found in the virion: DNA-dependent RNA polymerase in poxvirus, RNA-dependent RNA polymerase in all negative-stranded RNA viruses, RNA transcriptase in viruses with ds RNA genomes, and RNA-dependent DNA polymerase (or reverse transcriptase).

Envelope

Many viruses have a lipid envelope surrounding their nucleocapsid. Envelopes are derived from host cell nuclear membranes, endoplasmic reticulum, Golgi apparatus, plasma membranes, or vacuolar membranes. Therefore, the viral envelopes are structurally similar to cellular membranes—a lipid bilayer with protein molecules embedded in it and, frequently, with glycoprotein spikes protruding on the outer surface. The envelope represents the outer-most barrier of the virion. It contributes to the virus' resistance to various physical and chemical agents, and also determines the host range of the virus.

CLASSIFICATION OF ANIMAL VIRUSES

Animal viruses are classified by various criteria: host tissue and cell trophism, pathology and symptomatology, epidemiology, virion morphology, nu-

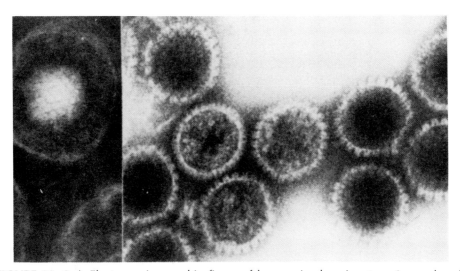

FIGURE 22–2 ✦ Electron micrographic figure of herpes simplex virus type 1, enveloped *(left)* and naked capsids *(right)*. Magnification × 189,000. (From Fields, B. N. and Knipe D. M.: In Fields, B. N., et al. (eds): Fields' Virology. Raven Press, New York, 1985, p. 12, with permission.)

cleic acids, and immunologic properties. In general, viruses are classified according to the characteristics of the virion itself, using a combination of criteria. In practice, however, weight is given to certain properties, depending upon the needs and the point of view of the classifier.

The nomenclature used for animal viruses consisted of giving the name of the disease produced in the major host followed by the word "virus." However, one faces the problem of the choice of criteria: the nature of the major hosts, the type of disease, properties of virions, or reproductive cycle. Therefore, the International Committee on Nomenclature of Viruses has proposed a dual system of nomenclature consisting of generic names ending in "-virus" for individual virus groups and eight-digit cryptograms to describe each virus according to a conventional key.

In general, animal viruses are divided into RNA viruses and DNA viruses. RNA viruses that cause diseases in humans include picornavirus, togavirus, paramyxovirus, orthomyxovirus, rhabdovirus, reovirus, and retrovirus. DNA viruses are parvovirus, papovavirus, adenovirus, herpesvirus, and poxvirus (Table 22–1).

RNA Viruses

Human RNA viruses are classified as follows (Table 22-2).

1. **Picornaviruses:** Picornavirus is small (27 nm in diameter) and naked, contains single-stranded RNA of 2.7×10^6 daltons, and exhibits icosa-hedral symmetry. This group includes poliovirus, coxsackievirus, rhinovirus, and the foot and mouth disease virus of cattle (Table 22–1). Coxsackievirus causes a variety of symptoms, especially myositis. There are three serotypes of poliovirus that can cause paralysis. Rhinoviruses, consisting of more than 100 serotypes, are the most important agents of the "common cold" in humans.

2. **Togaviruses:** Togavirus is an enveloped virus with an icosahedral capsid and is 50 to 70 nm in diameter. It has a single-stranded infectious RNA of 4×10^6 daltons. Togavirus, formerly known as "arbovirus," infects animals, birds, insects, and humans. Two subgroups of togavirus are known. Type A (alphaviruses) is mosquito-borne and includes 20 viruses that exhibit serologic cross-reactivity. Alphaviruses can cause fatal encephalitis in humans and other mammals. Type B (flaviviruses) is either mosquito-borne or tick-borne and includes several dozen cross-reacting species. Flaviviruses also cause encephalitis and other serious systemic illnesses.

3. **Paramyxoviruses:** Members of the paramyxovirus family are enveloped and pleomorphic with a diameter of approximately 150 nm. These viruses contain single-stranded "negative-strand" RNA of 7×10^6 daltons. Of the paramyxoviruses, mumps virus and the Newcastle disease virus of chickens contain neuraminidase and hemagglutinin in a single protein and are infectious for many tissues. Measles virus and respiratory syncytial virus of humans do not contain neuraminidase, but have hemagglutinin.

TABLE 22–1 ✦ Classification of Animal Viruses and Their Characteristics

CLASS	NUCLEIC ACID	CAPSID	ENVELOPE	POLARITY	INFECTIVITY OF NAKED NUCLEIC ACID
Poxvirus	ds DNA	Complex	+		
Herpesvirus	ds DNA	Icosahedron	+		+
Adenovirus	ds DNA	Icosahedron	0		+
Papovavirus	ds DNA	Icosahedron	0		+
Parvovirus	ss DNA	Icosahedron	0	+, −	+
Reovirus	ds RNA	Icosahedron	0		−
Orthomyxovirus	ss RNA	Helix	+	−	−
Paramyxovirus	ss RNA	Helix	+	−	−
Rhabdovirus	ss RNA	Helix	+	−	−
Coronavirus	ss RNA	Helix	+	+	+
Oncornavirus	ss RNA	Helix	+	+	−
Retrovirus	ss RNA		+		
Picornavirus	ss RNA	Icosahedron	0	+	+
Togavirus	ss RNA	Icosahedron	+	+	+
Hepatitis B	ds DNA	Icosahedron	+		−
Hepatitis A	ds RNA	Icosahedron	+		

ss DNA = single-strand DNA; ds DNA = double-strand DNA; ss RNA = single-strand RNA; ds RNA = double-strand RNA.

TABLE 22–2 ✦ Examples of Human RNA Viruses

CLASS	NAME OF VIRUS	MAJOR CLINICAL DISEASES
I. Picronaviruses	Poliovirus	Poliomyelitis
	Coxsackievirus A	Herpangina, aseptic meningitis, paralysis, common cold syndrome
	Coxsackievirus B	Pleurodynia, aseptic meningitis
	ECHO viruses	Paralysis, diarrhea, aseptic meningitis
	Human enterovirus 72 (hepatitis A virus)	Infectious hepatitis, jaundice
	Rhinoviruses	Common cold, bronchitis
II. Togaviruses	Rubella virus	Rubella
	Yellow fever virus	Yellow fever
III. Orthomyxoviruses	Influenza virus A, B, C	Influenza
IV. Paramyxoviruses	Measles virus	Measles
	SSPE (subacute sclerosing panencephalitis)	Chronic degeneration of CNS
	Mumps virus	Mumps
	Parainfluenza viruses	Respiratory tract infection
	Sendai virus	Croup, common cold syndrome
V. Rhabdoviruses	Rabies virus	Encephalitis, almost invariably fatal
	Vesicular stomatitis virus	Mostly occurs in cattle
VI. Reoviruses	Reovirus types 1, 2, 3	Not known
	Rotavirus	Diarrhea in infants
VII. Retroviruses	HIV-1, HIV-2	AIDS (acquired immunodeficiency virus)

4. **Orthomyxoviruses:** Members of the orthomyxovirus family are enveloped, have pleomorphic shapes, and are 80 to 120 nm in diameter. They contain a helical nucleocapsid with a diameter 6 to 9 nm. The RNA is segmented and single stranded, with a molecular weight of 2.4×10^6 daltons. Examples of orthomyxoviruses are influenza viruses A, B, and C. These viruses contain neuraminidase and hemagglutinin in separate proteins. The A strain is the most important for human disease and undergoes constant antigenic variation.

5. **Rhabdoviruses:** Rhabdoviruses are enveloped, bullet-shaped virions 70×175 nm in size, and contain helical nucleocapsids with single-stranded negative-strand RNA of 4×10^6 daltons and virion mRNA polymerase. Vesicular stomatitis virus and rabies virus belong to the rhabdovirus family.

6. **Reoviruses:** Viruses within the family of reoviruses are naked, icosahedral, and double-shelled virions. The virion contains 10 or more double-stranded RNA molecules ranging from 0.4 to 2.8×10^6 daltons and virion transcriptase. Reovirus types 1, 2, and 3, human rotavirus types 1 and 2, and Colorado tick fever virus belong to the reoviruses. Reovirus type 1 may cause diarrhea in children, and rotaviruses cause acute diarrhea in infants of many species.

7. **Retroviruses:** Members of the retrovirus family are enveloped and roundish particles about 100 nm in diameter with a helical nucleocapsid containing 6×10^6 daltons of RNA consisting of two identical molecules 3×10^6 each. They also contain reverse transcriptase and multiply by integration into DNA of the host and may cause leukemia, sarcoma, and other various malignancies.

DNA Viruses

Human DNA viruses are classified as follows (Table 22–3).

1. **Parvoviruses:** Parvoviruses are naked virions with a diameter of 18 to 26 nm and include an icosahedral nucleocapsid with 32 capsomeres. Virions contain single-stranded DNA of 1.2 to 1.8×10^6 daltons. Both defective and infectious types of parvoviruses exist: minute virus of mice (nondefective) and adeno-associated virus (AAV; defective).

2. **Papovaviruses:** Members of the papovavirus family are naked virions with icosahedral capsids, 45 to 55 nm in diameter. They contain closed, circular, double-stranded DNA from 3 to 5×10^6 daltons. Members include polyoma virus of mice, simian virus 40 (SV 40), Shope papilloma virus, and human wart virus. These viruses can cause cell transformation and tumors in animals.

3. **Adenoviruses:** The members of the adenovirus family are naked DNA viruses 80 to 90 nm in size. They are 20 to 30×10^6 daltons in molecular weight and can transform cells. Human adenovirus types 1 and 2 belong to this family. Some adenovirus types can cause respiratory illness and conjunctivitis in humans.

TABLE 22–3 ✦ Examples of Human DNA Viruses

CLASS	NAME OF VIRUS	MAJOR CLINICAL DISEASES
I. Parvoviruses	Adeno-associated virus	No known symptoms
II. Papovaviruses	Human papilloma viruses	Plantar warts
	Human polyoma virus	Isolated from brains of patients with progressive multifocal leukoencephalopathy
III. Adenoviruses	Adenovirus A	No known pathogenicity
	Adenovirus B and E	Acute respiratory disease
	Adenovirus C	Mild infections of respiratory tract, latent infection in lymphoid tissue
	Adenovirus D	Epidemic keratoconjunctivitis
IV. Herpesviruses	Herpes simplex virus type 1	Primary herpes stomatitis, recurrent herpes labialis, upper respiratory infections, herpes keratitis and genitalis, fetal encephalitis
	Herpes simplex virus type 2	Mainly herpes genitalis, rarely keratitis and stomatitis, recurrent herpes labialis, fatal encephalitis and meningitis
	Varicella zoster virus	Chickenpox in children, shingles, fatal encephalitis, keratitis
	Cytomegalovirus	Jaundice, hepatosplenomegaly, brain damage, birth defect, mononucleosis, death
	Epstein-Barr virus	Burkitt's lymphoma, nasopharyngeal carcinoma, infectious mononucleosis
V. Poxviruses	Variola virus (major)	Smallpox
	Variola virus (minor)	Alastrim
	Monkeypox virus	Smallpox-like disease
	Vaccinia virus	Vesicular eruption of the skin
VI. Hepatitis B virus	Hepatitis B virus	Hepatitis B (serum hepatitis)

4. **Herpesviruses:** The herpesviruses are enveloped and contain icosahedral 100 nm nucleocapsids with double-stranded linear DNA of 100×10^6 daltons. They grow in the nucleus, bud through the nuclear membrane, and cause latent infections. Herpes simplex virus types 1 and 2, Epstein-Barr virus, varicella zoster virus, and cytomegalovirus cause diseases in humans. Pseudorabies virus causes "mad itch" in swine and cattle, and Lucke virus causes frog adenocarcinoma.

5. **Poxviruses:** Poxviruses are enveloped, complex brick-shaped virions ($300 \times 200 \times 100$ nm) with double-stranded, linear DNA of 160×10^6 daltons in molecular weight. The virions contain many enzymes and at least 30 proteins including virion RNA polymerase. Poxviruses include human variola virus, human vaccinia virus, mammalian poxviruses for many species, and myxoma-fibroma virus. Human variola virus causes smallpox and human vaccinia virus can provide immunity to smallpox.

VIRUS REPLICATION

Viruses have a unique mode of reproduction that differentiates them from the more complex cellular microorganisms. The mechanism by which virions replicate within the cells can be divided into a number of distinct steps. The steps in the replication of a typical animal virus are as follows (Figs. 22–3 and 22–4):

1. Attachment (adsorption)
2. Penetration
3. Uncoating of the viral nucleic acid
4. Transport of virion, core, or virion nucleic acid to site of replication
5. Synthesis of viral messenger RNA (mRNA)
6. Synthesis of viral proteins
7. Replication of the virion nucleic acid
8. Assembly (maturation) of virions
9. Egress of virions from the cell

It is, however, important to recognize that in the case of animal viruses, the susceptible cells are always part of a complex multicellular organism. The virus infects a susceptible host, replicates (or at least persists) within it, exits at some time prior to the host's demise, and then infects another susceptible host. Viral multiplication in cells accompanies general cellular cytopathic changes including rounding and the appearance of large intranuclear eosinophilic inclusion bodies (Fig. 22–5).

Attachment (Adsorption)

Physical contact of the infecting virion with the host cell is the first requirement of replication.

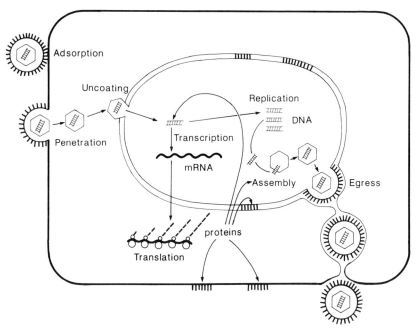

FIGURE 22–3 ✦ Replicative cycle of adenovirus (DNA virus).

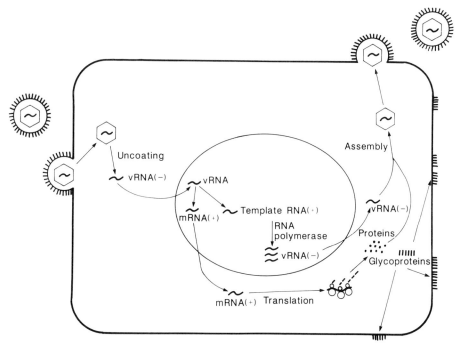

FIGURE 22–4 ✦ Replicative cycle of influenza virus (RNA virus).

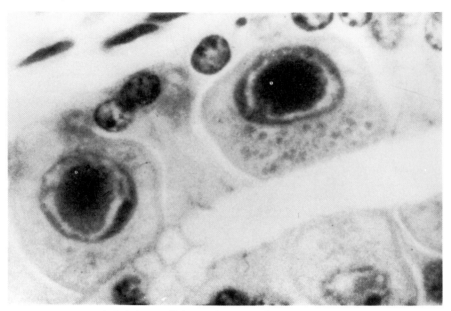

FIGURE 22–5 ✦ Epithelial duct cell from a human submaxillary gland infected with human cytomegalovirus, showing typical eosinophilic nuclear and basophilic cytoplasmic inclusions. Magnification × 1500. (From Nelson, J. S. N. and Wyatt, J. P. W.: Medicine 38:223, 1959, with permission.)

Brownian movement of virions may allow them to randomly collide with cell surfaces, where they bind electrostatically. Infections are primarily determined by the ability of viruses to bind to cells of a particular animal species. Tropism results from localization of viruses to different cells as determined by the presence of receptors. Receptors are virus-specific; even closely related viruses do not share the same receptors. However, rarely, unrelated viruses may share common receptors. The viral receptors have not been characterized, but may be glycoprotein.

Penetration

The virion attached to the surface of a cell enters into the cell by penetration. Penetration and internalization of adsorbed virions can occur by three mechanisms.

1. **Pinocytosis or viropexis:** Pinocytosis, which is akin to phagocytosis, is the most common mode of penetration by animal viruses. Both naked and enveloped virions enter the cell by this mechanism.

2. **Direct entry:** In some instances the virion appears to cross the cell membrane by direct entry without gradual engulfment. The actual mechanism is unknown. Only naked virions are taken up by this mode of entry.

3. **Fusion of viral envelope with cellular plasma membrane:** After the viral membrane fuses with the host cell plasma membrane, the nu-

cleocapsid is introduced into the cellular cytoplasm. Most enveloped virions appear to enter the cells by this mechanism.

Uncoating

Uncoating is the release of nucleic acid from the nucleocapsid after it has entered the host cell. Although there is no evidence that the uncoating process results from cellular enzymatic removal of viral capsid proteins, conformation of capsid proteins may change following the viral attachment to cell receptors. These changes in capsid protein conformation may then trigger the release of the nucleic acid. The cytoplasmic locations where the uncoating takes place differ among viruses. In simple plus-stranded RNA viruses (i.e., picornavirus and togavirus), uncoating occurs immediately after engulfment near the cellular plasma membrane. The uncoating of adenoviruses and herpesviruses takes place mainly in the vicinity of nuclear pores, the viral DNA thus gaining access into the nucleus.

Transport to Site of Replication

After penetration and uncoating, the virion must be transported to a site where the subsequent steps in the replication can take place. For example, adenovirus virions which are taken up by either endocytosis or direct transport across the cell membrane, are rapidly moved to the vicinity of nuclear pores. This transport takes place in the cytoplasmic matrix, probably along the network of microtubules. Adenovirus DNA then enters the nucleus through the nuclear pore, while the empty capsid stays outside the nucleus.

Synthesis of Viral mRNA

At the site of replication, the viral genome transcribes viral mRNA. Animal viruses are divided into six classes according to the mode of duplication of genetic material and a characteristic pattern of genetic information.

Class I: double-stranded DNA viruses (poxvirus, herpesvirus, adenovirus, and papovavirus)
Class II: single-stranded DNA viruses (parvovirus)
Class III: double-stranded RNA viruses (reovirus)
Class IV: plus-stranded RNA viruses (picorna and togavirus)
Class V: minus-stranded RNA viruses (orthomyxovirus, paramyxovirus, and rhabdovirus)
Class VI: RNA viruses with DNA intermediate (retrovirus)

Only the RNA genome of class IV viruses can act as mRNA. In other viruses, mRNA must be synthesized from the viral genome. For synthesis of mRNA, viral encoded enzymes are required if the host cell cannot provide the appropriate enzyme. Pox-, orthomyxo-, paramyxo-, rhabdo-, reo-, and retroviruses contain the virion-associated polymerases for transcription.

The synthesized mRNA is spliced after its synthesis. Spliced RNA is covalently continuous RNA composed of sequences that are encoded in separate regions of a DNA genome. The RNA sequence that is colinear with a DNA sequence is referred to as a colinear transcript. Thus, the spliced RNA is composed of two or more colinear transcripts. The splicing of mRNA has been shown to occur in SV40 and adenovirus.

Synthesis of Viral Proteins

The major function of viral mRNA is as a template for the synthesis of viral proteins. Viral proteins are referred to as structural and nonstructural proteins. Structural proteins are found on purified virions, and nonstructural proteins are found in infected cells but not as virion proteins or precursors to virion proteins. Some DNA viral genes are expressed during the early phase of replication while other genes are expressed during the late phase. In general, enzymes for nucleic acid replication and proteins that inhibit the host cell's macromolecular synthesis are termed early proteins. The capsid pro-

teins and envelope proteins are synthesized during the late phase of replication. Viral proteins are synthesized in the cytoplasm, utilizing cellular protein-synthesizing machinery.

Replication of Virion Nucleic Acid

Viral nucleic acids are synthesized in either the nucleus or the cytoplasm. In general, DNA replication takes place in the nucleus (except for poxvirus) and RNA replication in the cytoplasm. Viral infected cells show inclusion bodies, structures observed microscopically in the nucleus or cytoplasm of virus-infected cells. The location or staining characteristics of inclusion bodies may differ among viruses. For instance, poxvirus inclusion bodies occur in the cytoplasm, while herpesvirus inclusion bodies are found in the nucleus. The rabies inclusion bodies called Negri bodies are found in the cytoplasm and the measle inclusion bodies occur in both cytoplasm and nucleus. Both herpesvirus and adenovirus inclusion bodies occur in the nucleus, but the former is eosinophilic while the latter is basophilic.

Assembly and Maturation

Assembly is the formation of capsid around the viral genome or encapsidation of the viral nucleic acid. Maturation refers to the genesis of progeny virions. Assembly and maturation are one in the same event for naked virions, but the nucleocapsid of an enveloped virion must obtain an envelope for maturation. After the synthesis of individual components of the virion, they are transported to the site of nucleocapsid assembly. The nucleocapsid assembly of most DNA viruses takes place in the nucleus, whereas the final assembly of RNA-containing nucleocapsids occurs in the cytoplasm. Little is known about the regulation of intracellular transport of newly synthesized viral proteins. In general, assembly of viral components is an autocatalytic process that does not require mediation of enzymes.

Release and Envelopment

After assembly and maturation, nucleocapsids of naked viruses accumulate in the cells, and then are usually released simultaneously in a relatively short period of time. In contrast, enveloped viruses are released individually as they mature. During the late phase of replication, the enveloped viral nucleic acids express glycoproteins, which are inserted into the cell membrane. The assembled nucleocapsid moves toward the area of the cell membrane containing viral glycoproteins. These regions loop out (reverse phagocytosis) and by doing so include the nucleocapsids. The loop is eventually pinched off from the membrane and an enveloped virion is released from the cell. Replication of enveloped viruses often is not cytocidal, so the host cell may survive and continuously produce progeny virus.

DIAGNOSIS OF VIRAL DISEASES

Viruses are detected, identified, and quantitated by various methods. Specific diagnosis of a virus infection is important to delineate an etiologic agent for an observed illness.

Determination of Viral Antibodies

Although a certain virus may be isolated, it does not always prove an etiologic relationship to the illness. Therefore, the patient's sera must be examined for antibodies during the acute and convalescent periods of an illness. An acute-phase serum is obtained when the patient is first seen, hopefully within 7 days after the onset of disease, and the convalescent specimen is drawn 2 to 3 weeks later. When specimens are received by the laboratory, the viral antibody levels are measured by neutralization, hemagglutination inhibition (HI), or complement fixation (CF) tests. In viral infections, antibody titers rise fourfold or greater.

1. **Neutralization test:** Since neutralizing antibodies are highly specific, this test is extremely accurate and sensitive for determination of specific viral antibodies. Neutralizing antibodies appear early in the course of illness and persist for a long period of time. After incubating patient serum with the suspected virus, it is then placed into the appropriate cell culture system. The presence of neutralizing antibodies in the serum to the virus prevents the cytopathic effects of the virus.

2. **Hemagglutination inhibition (HI) test:** This test is only for the determination of viruses possessing hemagglutinin, including influenza, mumps, measles, the parainfluenzae, rubella, variola, arboviruses, reoviruses, some adenoviruses, and some echoviruses. These viruses cause certain types of red cells to clump together, or hemagglutinate. If antibody specific for the virus is added to the virus, hemagglutination is inhibited. In the HI test, each dilution is mixed with virus, and the mixtures are added to red blood cells to ascertain the highest dilution that prevents hemagglutination. This test is very sensitive and type-specific.

3. **Complement fixation (CF) test:** This test is a rapid and efficient method of screening a number of viral antibodies. In general, antibodies detected are group-specific, but not type-specific. For example, herpes simplex virus antibodies are distinguished from the adenovirus antibodies, but antibodies to herpes simplex virus type 1 cannot be distinguished from antibodies to herpes simplex virus type 2. Complement fixation antibodies disappear earlier than neutralizing antibodies.

Determination of Viral Antigen

Recently, new methods such as ELISA (enzyme-linked immunoabsorbent assays), RIA (radioimmunoassays), immunoprecipitation, and immunoelectrophoresis have been applied for the determination of viral antigen in clinical specimens (Chapter 34). The introduction of monoclonal antibodies tremendously increases the sensitivity and specificity of viral antigen determination.

1. **ELISA:** By this extremely sensitive technique, viral antigen is immobilized on a surface, such as the wells of plastic microtiter plate or metal beads, and test serum is added to allow the formation of antigen-antibody complex. Then antiglobulin coupled with a label of alkaline phosphatase or peroxidase attaches to the bound antigen-antibody complex. Following extensive washing, substrate (e.g., p-nitrophenyl phosphate) is added to induce visible color change, which can be determined with spectrophotometry. This technique is more than 100 times more sensitive than the complement fixation test.

2. **Immunofluorescence:** This technique has been used for the rapid determination of viral infections such as respiratory tract infections and vesicular exanthem. The cells obtained from the viral lesions are examined by indirect immunofluorescence for the presence of viruses.

3. **Determination of viral nucleic acids and proteins:** After immobilizing viral DNA, RNA, or proteins in nitrocellulose paper, the nucleic acids or proteins can be detected with enzyme or radiolabeled probe. This method is extremely sensitive and is the backbone of molecular biology research.

Cell Cultures and Quantitation of Virus

Specimens can be cultured in monolayers of cells to isolate viruses. Most viruses replicate, damage, and eventually kill the infected cells, which is called the cytopathic effect (CPE) of virus and can be readily examined under light microscope (Fig. 22–6). Numerous types of CPE can occur including rounding of cells, cell swelling, and fusion of several cells into a syncytium. Adenovirus CPE are grapelike clusters of rounded, refractile cells that have intranuclear inclusions when stained with hematoxylin and eosin. The amount of infectious virus is determined in many different ways, such as by a plaque formation as-

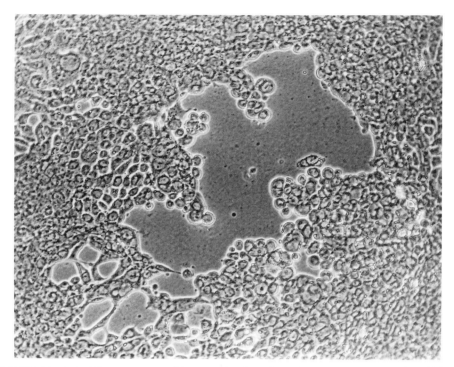

FIGURE 22–6 ✦ Microanatomy of herpes simplex virus plaque on green monkey kidney cells.

say, pock formation assay, focus formation assay, and the serial dilution end-point methods.

PLAQUE FORMATION ASSAY

This is the fundamental assay technique for determination of viral infectivity, and it is also important in viral diagnosis. It is highly reproducible, accurate, and extremely simple. When virions infect a cell monolayer, progeny viruses are produced, released, and then infect adjoining cells. This eventually allows one to see the infected area with the naked eye. These infected areas are called "plaques." To ensure that progeny virus particles liberated into the medium do not diffuse away and initiate separate plaques, agar or specific antiserum is incorporated into the culture medium. This assay technique is widely used for the titration of viruses and the units are expressed as plaque forming units per milliliter (PFU/ml) (Fig. 22–7).

POCK FORMATION ASSAY

When transparent epithelium of the chorioallantoic membrane of a chick embryo is infected by certain viruses, macroscopically recognizable foci (pocks) appear within 36 to 72 hours. These white opaque or red areas are caused by cell disintegration, migration, and proliferation. This assay is readily available, and numerous viruses such as herpes simplex virus and poxvirus produce the pocks.

FOCUS FORMATION ASSAY

Instead of producing plaques, many tumor viruses alter the morphology of infected cells and increase their rate of growth. The transformed cells develop into foci that gradually become large enough to be observable by the naked eye.

SERIAL DILUTION END-POINT METHOD

Serial dilutions of virus are inoculated onto monolayers of cells and incubated until the CPE of virus is observable. The highest viral dilution inducing CPE is the titer of the virus. This method of viral titration is extremely accurate and is also useful in titrating virus in laboratory animals.

EFFECT OF VIRUSES ON HOST CELLS

The effect of viruses on cells is diverse causing lytic infections, persistent infections (chronic, slow, and latent infections), transformations, and induction of interferon.

Lytic Infection

Lytic cytopathic effects are easily observed during the course of productive viral infections in tissue culture. Microscopically, the shape of cells is changed (e.g., cell rounding or cell fusion). The

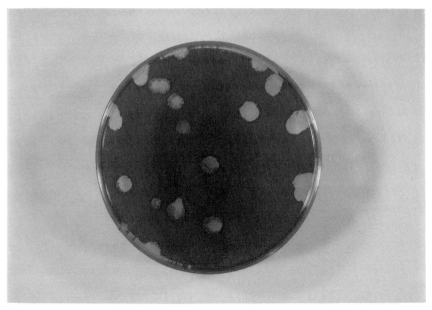

FIGURE 22–7 ✦ Plaques of herpes simplex virus type 1 on monolayers of green monkey kidney cells, 3 days after inoculation. The monolayers were stained with crystal violet.

mechanism of viral-induced morphologic cellular alterations is not completely understood. Many events may contribute to the cytopathic changes and cell death.

1. An inhibition of host cell DNA, RNA, and protein synthesis may occur during the lytic infection.
2. Some virion proteins may exert toxic effects on the host cell.
3. Activation of lysosomal enzymes may occur in cells infected with some viruses.
4. The normal ionic environment inside cells may be altered with increased intracellular Na concentration because of the inhibition of Na^+-K^+ pump by the lytic viral infection.

Persistent Infections

Following infection, some viruses persist intracellularly for extended periods or for life. There are three forms of persistent infections: chronic infections, latent infections, and slow viral infections. In **chronic infections,** viral infections are easily detectable. The individual is a carrier of the viral disease. In **latent infections,** the virus goes into hiding after primary infection and later is activated leading to recurrent viral diseases. For example, herpes simplex virus induces primary herpes stomatitis or nonsymptomatic primary infectious diseases followed by the establishment of latent infection in autonomic or sensory neuronal ganglia. This latent herpes simplex virus is later reactivated, leading to recurrent herpes labialis.

One of the best examples of **slow viral infections** is systemic sclerosing panencephalitis (SSPE). SSPE, a disease of children and adolescents, occurs years after recovery from measles.

Transformation

Some viral infections may convert normal cells into transformed or tumorigenic cells. These cells are characterized by a hereditary phenotype change to the transformed phenotype. Both DNA (papovaviruses, adenoviruses, and herpesviruses) and RNA (retroviruses) viruses cause malignant cell transformation in culture and tumors in some animals. Transformation by most DNA viruses occurs in the absence of virus multiplication.

Induction of Interferon

Viral infections induce the biosynthesis of interferon, a glycoprotein. Interferon, synthesized by viral infected cells, produces antiviral activity in secondary cells by inducing synthesis of new proteins, which make these cells resistant to viral infection. A detailed mechanism of action of interferon in its antiviral activity will be discussed later.

HOST RESPONSE TO VIRAL INFECTIONS

Upon viral infection, the host responds immunologically with antibody and cell-mediated immune responses and nonimmunologically.

Antibodies

Antibodies are classic markers of immunity to viruses and play an important role in the control of viral infections. IgA antibodies at the portals of entry (i.e., respiratory, alimentary, and urogenital mucosal surfaces) are important in resistance to reinfection, but also play a role in resistance and recovery from primary infections. Both IgM and IgG antibodies are responsible for virus neutralization in serum, while IgA antibodies neutralize viruses on mucosal surfaces. IgM antibodies, as larger molecules, do not enter extravascular tissue spaces to any great extent and are not transmitted to the fetus. IgM antibodies appear earlier than IgG antibodies during primary infections by 1 or 2 days, and thus could be of critical importance in initial resistance to viral infection. Little is known regarding the response of IgE to viral infections.

Cell-Mediated Immunity

Cell-mediated effector mechanisms against viruses are natural killer (NK) cells, antibody-dependent cell-mediated cytotoxicity, delayed-hypersensitivity, and virus-specific cytotoxic T lymphocytes. Human peripheral blood lymphocytes (NK cells) produce a spontaneous lysis of virus-infected cells. This lysis does not show specificity but is a natural cytotoxicity. The cytotoxic activity of NK cells is enhanced by interferon and interleukin-2 (IL-2). Among the peripheral blood lymphocytes, K (killer) cells lyse the cells bearing IgG antibody on the surface. This phenomenon is called antibody-dependent cell-mediated cytotoxicity (ADCC). Delayed hypersensitivity is an inflammatory reaction in tissues characterized by infiltration with activated macrophages at the site of antigen. The sensitized T cells produce numerous mediators responsible for the activation of macrophages. Delayed hypersensitivity plays an important role in host resistance to viral infections. In many viral infections, virus-specific T cells appear to be critical in the recovery from infection. For instance, patients with thymic aplasia are unable to limit poxvirus infections and develop measles giant cell pneumonia without a rash. Virus-specific cytotoxic T cells have been demonstrated in both acute and persistent infections in humans.

Nonimmunologic Factors

Fever, interferon, and genetic factors are nonimmunologic factors that provide resistance to viral infections. The role of interferon will be discussed in the section on antiviral therapy. Fever may play an important role in resistance because (1) elevated body temperature can decrease viral replication in target tissue, (2) elevated body temperature can prevent otherwise fatal herpes simplex viral infection in puppies, and (3) certain viral strains grow slowly and poorly in tissue cultures at high temperature.

RESPIRATORY VIRUSES

Respiratory viruses are the most common infectious viruses causing a variety of respiratory infectious diseases in man. Most infections are of minor consequence such as the common cold, sore throat, and low grade fever. However, some infections are more severe such as croup, bronchiolitis, or pneumonia, and lead to secondary bacterial infections resulting in serious complications, that is, sinusitis, otitis media, and bacterial pneumonia. Though all respiratory viruses can induce syndromes such as the common cold, pharyngitis, influenza, bronchitis, and pneumonia, these viruses cause more specific syndromes than others. For example, influenza viruses tend to cause influenza, while parainfluenza type 1, respiratory syncytial virus (RSV), mumps virus, and rhinoviruses tend to produce croup, bronchiolitis, mumps, and common cold, respectively. These viruses enter the host through the respiratory mucosa. After 2 to 5 days of incubation, they induce symptoms on the mucosal surfaces with infrequent systemic viremia. Though the host develops immunity against the viral infections through IgA (G and M) antibody and local T cell responses, the immunity tends not to be lifelong. Repeat infections can occur.

Influenza Viruses

Influenza viruses belong to orthomyxovirus family, and, so far, three serotypes of influenza viruses, types A, B, and C, have been discovered. The viruses cause influenza that has been recognized since the mid-19th century, when it led to a large epidemic. In fact, influenza swept the world, killing about 20 million people in 1918 and 1919. Influenza A virus was first isolated in England in 1933 by Smith, Andrews, and Laidlaw. The second influenza virus found was named influenza B virus, and the third antigenic type was isolated and named influenza C virus in 1949. Type A infects many animal species and exhibits wide antigenic diversity in their antigenicity. Type B is a human virus, and produces illness similar to type A. However, type B changes its antigenicity less frequently than type A, and therefore is of less public health concern except for Reye's syndrome. The influenza C virus has not been responsible for epidemics.

The size of influenza virus is heterogenous, 80 to 120 nm in diameter with round or ovoid shape. The virus is an enveloped virus with a nucleocapsid. The nucleocapsid (the internal component) is enveloped in a lipid-protein membrane into which are inserted evenly spaced, short (14 nm), narrow (4 nm) glycoprotein spikes. The nucleocapsid consists of eight pieces of single-stranded, negative sense RNA combined with nucleoprotein (NP) and RNA polymerase. The nucleoprotein determines the type specificity of a strain, that is, influenza A, B, and C. The envelope of virus consists of lipids, glycoprotein spikes (hemagglutinin [HA] and neuraminidase [NA]) and one glycoprotein (matrix antigen [M1]). The HA is the major determinant of immunity to antibody or T cells, while NA plays some role in protection and recovery. The function of M1 is not clearly known. The replication of influenza virus is well known. The virus attaches to cellular receptors through HA, which induces fusion of viral envelope and cellular membrane and release of the nucleocapsid into cell cytoplasm. In the cell nucleus, the negative-sense viral RNA is transcribed using RNA dependent RNA polymerase, and viral proteins such as NP, HA, and NA are synthesized. Then viral RNA is replicated: negative strand to positive strand to negative strand. The viral proteins and RNA are assembled in cytoplasm, and the virus buds with incorporation of cell membrane lipids and viral antigens.

The influenza virus selectively infects and injures the ciliated epithelial lining of the respiratory tract. In the acute stage, the ciliated epithelial linings of the nasal respiratory tract, trachea, and bronchioles are destroyed, leaving only basal cells covering the basement membrane. However, repair of the epithelial linings begins by the sixth day of the infection, and normal mucus-excreting columnar-ciliated epithelium is established. In acute influenza virus pneumonia, destruction of respiratory epithelium is more extensive, including alveolar lining cells, resulting in swelling of alveolar walls and in the distended alveolar spaces containing edema fluid, hemorrhagic extravasations, and hyalin membranes. In worse cases, bacterial superinfection occurs because of the edema fluid being used as a rich medium for bacterial growth. Vaccines against influenza A virus is available, which is egg-grown, purified, trivalent, and inactivated virus. The vaccine is valuable in high risk groups such as the elderly (>65) and individuals with cardiorespiratory illness, chronic renal disease, diabetes mellitus, and anemia. Furthermore, amantadine may be used for the prophylaxis and treatment of influenza, while ribavirin is used only for the treatment.

Parainfluenza Viruses

These viruses belong to the paramyxovirus group, along with mumps virus. There are five serotypes of parainfluenza viruses: types 1, 2, 3, 4A, and 4B. Clinically, only types 1, 2, and 3 are important. Type 1 is the major cause of childhood croup; type 2 is similar to type 1 but less virulent; and type 3 is a major cause of bronchiolitis and pneumonia. However, types 1 and 2 also cause bronchitis, pneumonia, and bronchiolitis. The size of parainfluenza viruses is variable, 150 to 520 nm with ovoid shape. Similar to influenza viruses, parainfluenza viruses also have a nucleocapsid and envelope with glycoprotein spikes. The spikes consist of two different glycoproteins; one has a HA and NA function, and the other has membrane fusion capacity. The nucleocapsid consists of a single piece of negative-sense RNA, nucleoprotein (NP), and RNA polymerase. Six structural proteins and one nonstructural protein are expressed from the viral genome. The virus attaches to cells through hemagglutinin-neuraminidase and fuses with the cell membrane through its protease. After entering into the cytoplasm, messages are transcribed from the negative-sense RNA to synthesize viral proteins. Replicated RNA and proteins are assembled and the virions bud off. Vaccines for parainfluenza viruses have not been established. Ribavirin aerosol may be useful for the treatment of severe cases of parainfluenza viral infections.

Respiratory Syncytial Viruses

Respiratory syncytial virus (RSV) belongs to the paramyxovirus group, and one serotype with minor variations is of clinical importance. RSV is recognized as the most important virus inducing respiratory tract infections in infants and young children. RSV is the major cause of bronchiolitis and pneumonia in infants, and causes pneumonia in the elderly. The consequence of the infection is very serious with up to a 35 percent mortality in infants with cyanotic congenital heart disease. The morphology of RSV is similar to parainfluenza virus, but it does not hemagglutinate; nor does it contain neuraminidase. The replicative cycle of RSV is unknown. The viral infection can be diagnosed by identifying the virus or its antigen in the respiratory tract. Though the serological test is specific, it is not very sensitive. Inactivated and live vaccines have been developed without success. Ribavirin aerosol may be effective for the treatment of infections.

Mumps Virus

Mumps virus is also a paramyxovirus, and contains two major antigens: V antigen (envelope lipoprotein) and S antigen (capsid antigen). The virus enters through the upper respiratory tract by the saliva or other secretions. After 16 to 18 days of incubation, clinical swelling of the parotid glands appears. Though the main clinical manifestation of mumps is inflammation of salivary glands, the virus is spread throughout the body. Mumps virus infection can be prevented by immunization with a live attenuated mumps vaccine.

HERPESVIRUSES

Herpesviruses are the most ubiquitous communicable infectious viruses in humans. Herpes virion is enveloped, has double-stranded DNA and icosahedral nucleocapsid, replicates in the cell nucleus, and acquires its envelope from the inner nuclear membrane. The size of naked virion is approximately 110 nm and, with envelopes, 180 to 250 nm. Herpesviruses infections are either productive or nonproductive and result in acute infection or latent and recurrent infection. Some human herpesviruses are oncogenic. There are four known human herpesviruses: herpes simplex virus (HSV) types I and II, cytomegalovirus (CMV), Epstein-Barr virus (EBV), and varicella-zoster virus (VZV).

Herpes Simplex Virus (HSV)

HSV virion consists of four major components: core (DNA), capsid, teguments (fibrillar substance), and envelope. HSV DNA is double stranded with a molecular weight of approximately 100 million daltons. The DNA consists of two unique regions flanked by inverted repeat sequences. Type 1 HSV (HSV-1) and type 2 HSV (HSV-2) share many common antigens and are about 50 percent genetically homologous. Three classes of viral proteins—alpha (immediate early), beta (early), and gamma (late) proteins—are translated in a cascade manner during HSV replication. Alpha proteins are necessary for the synthesis of beta proteins and beta proteins, in turn, are needed for the production of gamma proteins. DNA replication is done in a semiconservative manner (Fig. 22–8).

PATHOGENESIS AND CLINICAL DISEASES CAUSED BY HSV

HSV commonly attacks mucosa, skin, eyes, and the nervous system. In immunocompromised persons and neonates, HSV also involves the liver and lungs. Primary infection may or may not be clinically evident: from 88 to 99 percent of primary oral infections with HSV are asymptomatic. After the primary infection, the virus ascends sensory or autonomic nerves at the site of the primary infection and persists in neuronal ganglia that innervate the site as latent HSV (Fig. 22–9). In response to stimuli such as exposure to ultraviolet light,

trauma, fever, hormonal imbalance, stress, steroids, and cancer chemotherapy, the latent virus is reactivated, grows in the neuron, travels back down the nerves, and causes recurrent viral lesions in the initially infected area. Antibodies and cell-mediated responses may not affect the frequency of recurrences, but do localize subsequent infections.

HSV is the most ubiquitous communicable infectious virus in humans and causes a wide variety of chronically recurring diseases:

1. Recurrent herpes labialis, usually due to HSV-1, afflicts approximately one third of the world's population with one half of them suffering multiple attacks annually (Figs. 22–10 and 22–11).

2. Herpes genitalis, caused by both HSV-1 and HSV-2 although predominated by HSV-2, is the most common genital disease in women, and second only to syphilis as the genital lesion in men. At least 100,000 cases of herpes genitalis are reported each year in the United States.

3. Ocular HSV infection, due primarily to HSV-1 but occasionally to HSV-2, is the leading cause of blindness due to corneal infections in the United States. Approximately 500,000 cases of primary or recurrent ocular herpetic diseases are reported annually in the United States (Fig. 22–12).

4. Herpes encephalitis is the most common acute sporadic viral disease of the brain in the United States. It is a devastating process, with mortality in excess of 50 percent and severe complications in over 80 percent. HSV-1 is the usual culprit in adults and HSV-2 in neonates. HSV-1 appears to spread directly by neural routes and HSV-2 by hematogenous routes.

5. The primary HSV attack in neonates and immunologically compromised patients such as those with leukemia, organ-transplant recipients, and patients with acquired immunodeficiency syndrome (AIDS) is associated with a high degree of mortality and morbidity.

LATENCY AND RECURRENCE OF HSV INFECTIONS

Between episodes of disease, HSV remains in the regional sensory ganglia as latent HSV. Mostly HSV-1 remains in the trigeminal ganglia and HSV-2 remains in the sacral ganglia. Latent virus in the ganglionic cells may exist as nonreplicating, truly latent entities. Therefore, demonstration of the presence of the virus in the ganglia requires organ culture of ganglionic tissue. The presence of viral DNA, virus specific RNA, and some viral proteins, however, is demonstrated in latently infected ganglia. Although the detailed aspects of recurrent HSV infection are relatively unknown, the ganglionic latent HSV serves as the source of virus in the recurrent disease. Recurrent disease can be induced by various stimuli, including fever, men-

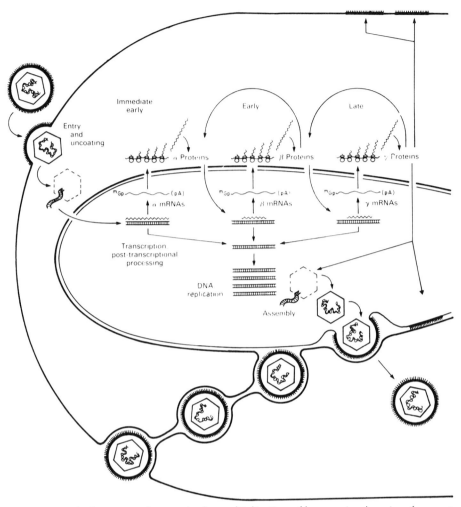

FIGURE 22–8 ✦ Sequence of events in the multiplication of herpes simplex virus from entry of virus into the cell by fusion of the virion envelope with the cell plasma membrane to assembly of virions and their exit from the cell through the endoplasmic reticulum. (From Davis, B. D. et al. (eds): Microbiology. Harper & Row, Philadelphia, 1980, p. 1065, with permission.)

struation, exposure to sunlight, and emotional stress (Fig. 22–11).

LABORATORY DIAGNOSIS OF HSV INFECTIONS

The quickest and most economic test for the diagnosis of HSV infection is to demonstrate multinuclear giant cells, containing intranuclear eosinophilic inclusion bodies, in scrapings from the base of vesicles. However, this procedure does not distinguish HSV from infections caused by cytomegalovirus or varicella zoster virus. Virions can be determined by an electron microscopic examination, and specific HSV antigens can be detected in cells from the lesion by immunofluorescence. Virus can also be isolated by inoculating vesicular fluid or scrapings into susceptible culture cells. Finally,

a rise in HSV antibody can be determined by serologic tests from serum obtained early in the primary disease and again 14 to 21 days after onset (paired sera).

Cytomegalovirus (CMV)

CMV is antigenetically distinct from other herpesviruses and has a very narrow host range, being nearly species-specific. In vitro, CMV grows more readily in fibroblasts than in epithelial or lymphoid cells. Replication of CMV is slow and inefficient. CMV causes latent infections in kidney epithelial cells, salivary glands, and certain leukocytes.

PATHOGENESIS

Transmission of CMV occurs via various routes—through congenital infection, close sexual

FIGURE 22–9 ✦ Electron micrograph of a sectioned trigeminal ganglion from a mouse sacrificed 30 days after oral HSV-1 inoculation. The ganglion was cultured in vitro for 4 days to reactivate latent HSV-1. Typical; HSV particles are seen within nucleus and outside of the cellular membrane *(arrows).* Magnification × 15,700. Complete herpes virion is in inset (Magnification × 47,000). (From Park, N.-H., et al: Oral. Surg. 53:256, 1982, with permission.)

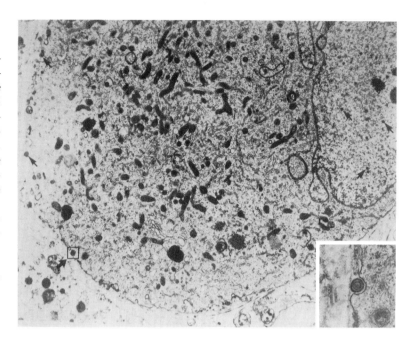

or oral contact, and blood transfusion or organ transplantation. The latent CMV can be reactivated during periods of immunosuppression. Primary infection is usually subclinical, but in fetuses or immunocompromised individuals can cause severe disease. Like HSV, serum antibody is unimportant in preventing reactivation or limiting spread of infection, but cell-mediated immunity may be critical in the latter. CMV also suppresses the cell-mediated immunity of the host, and by so doing may increase the susceptibility of transplant recipients or AIDS patients to infectious and neoplastic complications, i.e., *Pneumocystis carinii* pneumonia and Kaposi's sarcoma.

CLINICAL DISEASES ASSOCIATED WITH CMV

CMV also causes numerous clinical diseases:

1. Congenital CMV infection causes cytomegalic inclusion disease. One out of every 100 neonates in the United States excretes CMV in urine. A small percentage (1 percent) exhibits severe CNS malformation, hepatosplenomegaly, petechiae, or chorioretinitis. Others will exhibit subtle abnor-

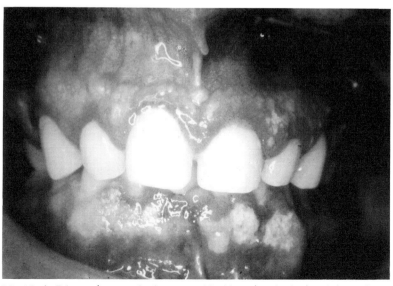

FIGURE 22–10 ✦ Primary herpes gingivostomatitis. Note the gingival vesicles at the attached gingiva. (Courtesy of G. Shklar.)

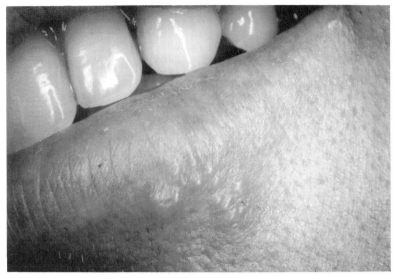

FIGURE 22–11 ✦ Recurrent herpes labialis (RHL). RHL usually occurs at the mucocutaneous junctions and results from the reactivation of latent virus. (Courtesy of L. Gangarosa.)

malities of hearing mentation that may not be appreciated for several years. The majority of infected infants are asymptomatic.

2. CMV mononucleosis results from primary infection by CMV in healthy young adults. This is characterized by prolonged fever, malaise, abnormal liver function, and peripheral blood mononucleosis.

3. Most renal transplant recipients excrete CMV after transplantation. Many have subclinical syndromes, often with leukopenia or pneumonia.

4. Kaposi's sarcoma, a vascular tumor that is observed in AIDS patients, renal transplant recip-

ients, and young male homosexuals, may be associated with CMV.

LABORATORY DIAGNOSIS OF CMV INFECTION

The most sensitive method is virus isolation in human embryonic fibroblast cultures. Characteristic cytomegalic cells with intranuclear and cytoplasmic inclusions can be identified from the urinary sediment or bronchial and gastric washings. Furthermore, CMV antibodies can be determined by immunofluorescence, indirect hemagglutination, and complement fixation.

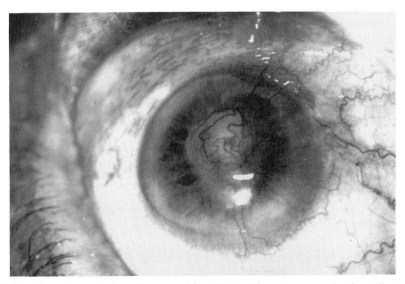

FIGURE 22–12 ✦ Herpetic keratitis caused by HSV-1. There is a growth of capillaries into the cornea (conjunctival injection) and haziness of stoma. (Courtesy of D. Pavan-Langston.)

Epstein-Barr Virus (EBV)

EBV was discovered in 1964 by Epstein, Barr, and Achong in electronmicroscopic examination of lymphoblasts from a patient with Burkitt's lymphoma. EBV was suggested to be the causative agent of infectious mononucleosis in 1968. EBV is antigenically unrelated to other human herpesviruses. It only infects B cells in vitro and also can establish latent infections in B cells. EBV may persist in peripheral blood lymphocytes for years after infection. EBV may also infect certain epithelial cells of the tongue in patients with AIDS or AIDS-related condition (ARC) or the nasopharynx. Infected B cells may undergo blast transformation and go into long-term culture ("immortalization").

PATHOGENESIS

EBV infections are extremely common; over 90 percent of adults have antibody to EBV. Infection is acquired primarily by oral-oral contact (monoculeosis has been called the "kissing disease") and less commonly through blood transfusion. EBV may be excreted into saliva during mononucleosis and for weeks thereafter. Primary infection in children is usually asymptomatic, but in young adults, it often manifests as infectious mononucleosis.

CLINICAL DISEASES ASSOCIATED WITH EBV

EBV induces lymphoproliferative disorders:

1. Infectious mononucleosis is an EBV primary infection in young adults. The virus replicates in the oropharynx for long periods of 4 to 7 weeks while the individual continues to be infectious. The characteristic clinical picture consists of fever, pharyngitis, and cervical lymphadenopathy, accompanied by splenomegaly, swollen eyes, and palatal petechiae. Differentiation of CMV from other causes of mononucleosis are made by the detection of heterophile antibody. Infectious mononucleosis may last for weeks but is usually benign and self-limiting.

2. Seroepidemiologic, molecular biologic, and animal studies have shown that certain cancers (e.g., Burkitt's lymphoma and nasopharyngeal carcinoma) are associated with EBV. EBV may also cause progressive B-cell lymphoproliferative disease in immunocompromised people and may be associated with primary cerebral lymphomas.

3. A number of neurologic syndromes (e.g., Guillian's syndrome, Bell's palsy, meningoencephalitis, and transverse myelitis) may be related to EBV.

4. Recently, some studies have indicated that EBV virions are found in white, hairy tongues of patients with AIDS or healthy homosexuals.

LABORATORY DIAGNOSIS OF EBV INFECTION

Laboratory diagnosis rests upon finding abnormal, large lymphocytes and heterophile antibodies. However, the specific diagnosis can be only made by determination of elevated antibody to early antigens and to the viral capsid proteins.

Varicella-Zoster Virus (VZV)

VZV is relatively unstable and has limited host range but replicates in a variety of human and monkey cells in vitro.

PATHOGENESIS

VZV enters the body via the respiratory route. After a 2-week incubation in which viremia and local replication occur, cutaneous vesicles develop. In a normal host, humoral and cell-mediated immune mechanisms limit the spread of the disease. However, in the immunocompromised, dissemination may continue and visceral organs may become involved. During the primary infection, VZV migrates to the dorsal root ganglia along the sensory nerves and establishes latent infection in the ganglia. In zoster, the latent virus is reactivated and travels down sensory nerves to the skin, where clusters of vesicles occur.

CLINICAL DISEASES CAUSED BY VZV

The primary infection of VZV is called varicella, or chicken pox. Varicella may be preceded by a 1- to 2-day prodrome of fever, headache, malaise, and anorexia. The rash evolves rapidly in crops mainly on the trunk. Primary varicella is more severe in adults where it is frequently accompanied by pneumonia. The infection is highly communicable, and occurs most commonly in winter and spring.

Recurrent infection of VZV is called shingles, or zoster. In contrast to varicella, zoster shows no epidemic or seasonal pattern and is caused by the reactivation of latent virus. It can occur at any age, but the incidence increases sharply in the elderly. The zoster eruption is characteristically unilateral. Patients with decreased immune function are more susceptible to developing zoster.

LABORATORY DIAGNOSIS OF VZV INFECTION

The typical varicella giant cells and cells with characteristic inclusion bodies can be easily and rapidly detected in smears from the base of vesicles. In addition, virus can be detected by electron microscopic examination and culture.

HEPATITIS VIRUSES

Since Voeght, in 1942, found that hepatitis was transmissible, the etiologic agents of hepatitis were subsequently found to be filterable and the disease transmitted in two ways—by the intestinal-oral route (infectious hepatitis) and by the injection of infected blood or its products (serum hepatitis). However, the differences in transmission are not absolute, so that they have now been renamed hepatitis A virus (HAV) for infectious hepatitis and hepatitis B virus (HBV) for serum hepatitis. Furthermore, at least one other hepatitis virus not related to HAV or HBV has been recognized and called hepatitis C virus (or non-A non-B hepatitis virus). The hepatitis C virus is the major cause of hepatitis following transfusions in the United States (Table 22–4; Fig. 22–13).

Hepatitis A Virus (HAV)

HAV virion is similar to picornaviruses and consists of a single-stranded RNA genome and three major polypeptides without envelope. A 27 nm viral particle can be found in stools of patients with hepatitis A.

HAV enters the body mainly through the oral route and grows in the cytoplasm of infected cells in the gastrointestinal tract. After systemic viremia, the virus spreads to the liver, spleen, and kidneys. By this time HAV virions are detected in the feces, duodenal contents, blood, and urine. HAV has an incubation period of 25 to 30 days from the time of exposure. Patients with the disease may be asymptomatic, with only abnormal liver function or seroconversion. Usually children and young adults are susceptible to HAV infection, especially in the autumn and winter. The danger of HAV dissemination from an infected individual is highest during the last stage of incubation. Since the viral shedding in feces is maximal prior to clinical disease, the virus is very contagious. Type A hepatitis may be prevented by passive immunization with pooled adult gamma-globulin. The gamma-globulin must be given no later than 2 weeks after exposure.

Hepatitis B Virus (HBV)

Serum of patients with clinical hepatitis B contains three different structures: the Dane particle, spherical particle, and filamentous form. The Dane particle is 42 nm in diameter with an electrodense nucleocapsid 27 nm in diameter and is the least common form in serum. Spherical particles are 22 nm in diameter and the most abundant. Filamentous particles are also plentiful in serum and are 22 nm in diameter and 50 to 230 nm in length. The Dane particle contains partially double-stranded circular DNA as the genome and two major antigens, the surface antigen (HBsAg) and the core antigen (HBcAg) (Figs. 22–14, 22–15, 22–16, 22–17). Spherical and filamentous particles in

TABLE 22–4 ✦ Comparison of Hepatitis Viruses

CHARACTERISTICS	HAV	HBV	HCV
Size	27 nm	42 nm Dane particle 22 nm surface antigen	Unknown
Nucleic acid	ss RNA	ds DNA	Unknown
Antigen	HA Ag (major antigen)	HBsAg (surface antigen) HBcAg (core antigen) HBeAg (core-related antigen)	Reportedly identified but not confirmed
Antibody	Anti-HA, IgG, IgM	Anti-HBs, anti-HBc, anti-HBe	Reportedly identified but not confirmed
Route of infection	Oral and parenteral	Oral, parenteral, and sexual or maternal-fetal contact	Mainly parenteral
Incubation period	15–45 days (mean 30)	45–150 days (mean 60–90)	15–160 days (mean 50)
Presence of virus in body fluid	Feces, blood, urine	Feces, blood, saliva	Blood
Severity	Mild	Often severe	Moderate
Prognosis	Generally good	Worse with age and debility	Moderate
Immune serum globulin (ISG) prophylaxis	Good	Partial	Unknown
Hepatitis B immune globulin prophylaxis	No	Yes	No
Carrier state	Rare	5–10%	Exists, but prevalence unknown

HAV = hepatitis A virus; HBC = hepatitis B virus; HCV = hepatitis C virus (non-A, non-B hepatitis virus).

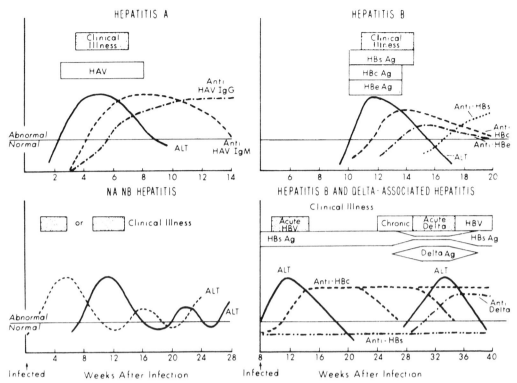

FIGURE 22–13 ✦ The panels illustrate the sequence of development of clinical illness, liver function abnormalities, and hepatitis antigen and antibody for each of the four currently recognized forms of viral hepatitis. (From Jaklik, W. K. (ed.): Virology. Appleton-Century-Crofts, New York, 1985, p. 300, with permission.)

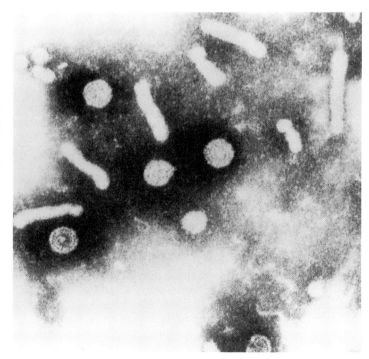

FIGURE 22–14 ✦ Electron micrograph of negatively stained hepatitis B virus Dane particles, filaments, and 22 nm HBsAG particles present in the serum of a patient with active infection. Magnification × 150,000. (Courtesy of J. Gerin, Oak Ridge National Laboratory; from Davis, B. D. et al. (eds.): Microbiology, ed 3. Harper and Row, Philadelphia, 1980, p. 1221, with permission.)

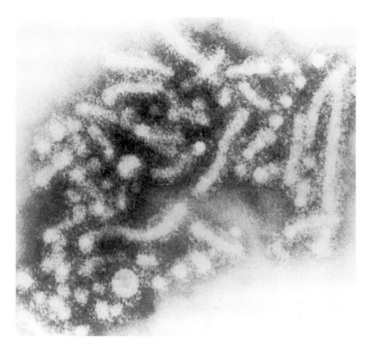

the serum only contain HBsAg. The HBcAg is found only in the core of Dane particles. High antibody titers to HBcAg are detected during the early phase of the disease, and these antibodies are consistently present in chronic carriers of HBsAg.

Although HBV mainly enters via the parenteral route, its primary site of replication is unknown. The disease caused by HBV varies from mild to a severe, prolonged disease. The incubation period also varies from a few weeks to 4 months. The clinical signs and symptoms of hepatitis B are similar to those of hepatitis A: jaundice, fever, headache, malaise, anorexia, abdominal pain, nausea, vomiting, serum-sickness like syndrome with arthralgia, skin rashes and arthritis, periarthritis, glomerulonephritis. Although 10 to 20 percent of adult patients and 35 percent of children show HBsAg for extended periods, less than half of them become chronic HBsAg carriers. More than half the chronic HBsAg carriers continuously manifest chronic liver disease. The risk of persistent infection is highest in infants and decreases with age. Infected males are two to three times more likely to become carriers than infected females. The probability of persistent infection is increased in high-risk groups including male homosexuals and persons with immune defects, on immunosuppressive therapy, or with chronic renal disease. Approximately 5 to 10 percent of persons infected with the disease have circulating HBsAg for prolonged periods of time.

There are a number of tests for detection of HBV antigens, particularly HBsAg. These include ra-

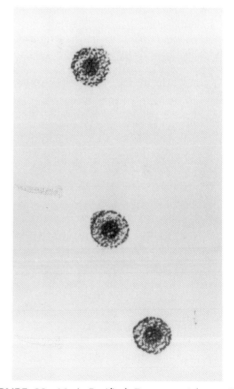

FIGURE 22–16 ✦ Purified Dane particles stained with uranyl acetate to show the DNA core. Magnification × 200,000. (Courtesy of J. Gerin, Oak Ridge National Laboratory; from Davis, B. D. et al. (eds.): Microbiology, ed 3. Harper and Row, Philadelphia, 1980, p. 1221, with permission.)

\1,9,3

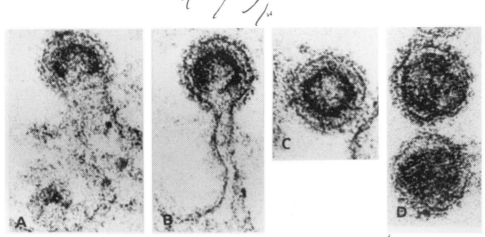

FIGURE 22–17 ✦ Thin sections of type C particles from cells producing a mouse leukosis virus. **A** and **B**, Two phases of budding of the virions at the cell surface. **C**, Detached immature virion, with an electron-lucent nucleoid. **D**, Two mature particles with dense nucleoids. (Courtesy of L. Dmochowski; from Davis, B. D. et al. (eds.): Microbiology, ed. 3. Harper and Row, 1980, p. 1284, with permission.)

dioimmunoassay, complement fixation, immune adherence, and enzyme immunoassays. Although there are sensitive immunologic blood tests for detection of viral carriers, blood transfusions are the major route of viral transmission. Therefore, individuals with a history of jaundice or with detectable HBsAg in the serum should be excluded from being blood donors. HBV is also associated with hepatocarcinoma. The evidence is (1) a close correlation between the geographic distribution of HBV infection and hepatocarcinoma and (2) a high frequency of detection of HBsAg in patients with hepatocarcinoma.

Passive immunization with serum containing high antibody titers to HBs has marginal benefit in high-risk groups. However, inactivated hepatitis B vaccine was effective in a high-risk population of male homosexuals. This was prepared by purification and formalin inactivation of HBsAg collected from the serum of chronic carriers. Following two initial injections one month apart and a booster 6 months later, 96 percent of those vaccinated had acquired anti-HBs and experienced a reduced incidence of hepatitis B greater than 90 percent.

Hepatitis C Virus (Non-A Non-B Hepatitis Virus)

Hepatitis C virus was identified by prospective studies of patients with post-transfusion hepatitis without evidence of hepatitis A or B. The virions of hepatitis C virus are nonenveloped icosahedrons, about 27 nm in diameter, resembling picornaviruses in morphologic and physical characteristics. The hepatitis C virus antigens do not cross-react immunologically with antigens of HAV and HBV.

Recent studies indicate that over 90 percent of post-transfusion hepatitis cases are attributed to hepatitis C virus. Transmission by means other than blood is still unknown since specific viral antigens have not yet been identified. The incubation period of this virus is 6 to 12 weeks. The clinical manifestations of hepatitis C are similar to those of hepatitis A or B. The most important finding in hepatitis C research is a strong association between elevated alanine aminotransferase (ALT) levels in donor blood and appearance of hepatitis C in the blood recipients. The higher the ALT level in the blood, the greater the risk of transmission of the disease.

Hepatitis Viruses and Health Care Professionals

Viral hepatitis is one of the most serious occupational risks of dentists, nurses, physicians, and laboratory technicians who are exposed to patients and their blood. Hepatitis A outbreaks have occurred in hospitals, but the risk in health care professionals is mainly hepatitis B. The transmission of HBV is usually via blood, saliva, and semen of patients. Although chronically infected professionals can transmit the virus to their patients, the risk of patient transmission to health professionals appears much greater than the reverse. Hepatitis B markers are found in 20 to 40 percent of high risk health care worker groups, in contrast to only 5 percent in the members of the general population. Asymptomatic HBsAg-positive carriers represent the greatest risk to health care personnel. Therefore, patients with histories of hepatitis, multiple blood transfusion, parenteral drug abuse, chronic liver disease, chronic renal failure, leukemia, Hodgkin's disease, and Down's syndrome should have routine HBsAg determinations because of the higher frequency of the HBsAg carrier state in those groups. If positive, they must be treated as potentially infectious with appropriate precautions taken.

In treating dental patients with a history of hepatitis B, dentists and assistants should adhere to aseptic techniques and wear masks and gloves (Chapter 32). Although dentists and auxiliaries with a history of hepatitis B have a moral, ethical, and legal obligation to protect their patients, there is insufficient evidence to prevent a health care professional from practicing because of positive antigen-screening tests. However, dentists and assistants must follow aseptic techniques to prevent transmission.

For the prevention and treatment of hepatitis A, immune serum globulin (ISG) containing anti-HAV is administered. When given before exposure or during the early incubation period, ISG is effective in aborting the development of clinical symptoms. For intimate contact with hepatitis A patients, administration of 0.02 ml/kg of ISG is recommended. For travelers to tropical and developing countries, ISG prophylaxis is recommended: 0.02 ml/kg for travel less than 3 months and 0.05 ml/kg every 4 to 6 months for longer travel. For postexposure prophylaxis against hepatitis B, high titer of hepatitis B immune globulin (HBIG) is recommended: 0.05 to 0.07 ml/kg as soon as possible after exposure. Preparations of purified HBsAg have shown to be effective in protecting laboratory animals from hepatitis B infection, but further investigation is needed for use in humans. Two recombinant hepatitis B vaccines, Recombivax (manufactured by Merck) and Engerix-B (manufactured by SmithKline Beecham) are available in the United States. They are produced by a yeast in which the genetic code for HBsAg has been incorporated. Though the vaccines are 80 to 90 percent effective, the duration of their effectiveness is unknown. The vaccine appears to be safe for pregnant women and infants. Table 22–5 shows the recommended dosage of hepatitis B vaccine.

ONCOGENIC VIRUSES

Since Ellerman and Band in 1908 demonstrated development of chicken leukemia by cell-free filtrates from other chickens, viruses have been suspected as causative agents for certain tumors in humans and other mammals. The oncogenic viruses are divided into DNA-containing viruses and RNA-containing viruses. DNA-containing oncogenic viruses include papovaviruses, adenoviruses, and herpesviruses. RNA-containing oncogenic viruses include C-type leukosis-sarcoma viruses and B-type (mammary tumor) virus.

Papovaviruses (Polyoma and Papillomaviruses)

The virions of papovaviruses are naked icosahedrons with a diameter of 45 nm. They contain circular, double-stranded DNA and are resistant to heat and formalin. Infections by these viruses may be either productive or nonproductive. Productive infection leads to production of progeny viruses and the nonproductive infection can lead to abortive transformation of the cells. Cells transformed by papovaviruses express two viral proteins—tumor (T) antigen and tumor-specific transplantation antigen (TSTA). Both T and TST antigens are virus-encoded and appear early in the productive viral infection. These viral proteins are identical in cells of different species transformed by the same virus, but differ in transformed cells or tumors induced in the same species by the two different

TABLE 22–5 ✦ Recommended Dosage of Hepatitis B Vaccine

	RECOMBIVAX HB	ENGERIX-B	SCHEDULE
Infants of HBsAg-negative mothers and children <11 years old	2.5 µg (0.25 ml)	10 µg (0.5 ml)	0, 1–2, 6–8 months or 1–2, 4, 6–18 months old
Infants of HBsAg-positive mothers: prevention of perinatal infection	5 µg (0.5 ml)	10 µg (0.5 ml)	0, 1, 6 months old*
Children and adolescents 11 to 19 years old	5 µg (0.5 ml)	20 µg (1.0 ml)	0, 1, 6 months apart
Adults ≥20 years old	10 µg (1.0 ml)	20 µg (1.0 ml)	0, 1, 6 months apart
Dialysis patients and other immunocompromised persons	40 µg (1.0 ml)	40 µg (2.0 ml)	0, 1, 2, 6 months apart

*First dose within 12 hours of birth; with Enerix-B only, alternative schedule is 0, 1, 2, and 12 to 18 months old.
From Abramowicz M: Drugs for viral infections. Med. Lett. 34:71, 1992.

viruses. Neither of these proteins is a structural protein, or associated with the virion. After the adsorption, penetration, and uncoating, the papovaviral DNA enters the nucleus where it transcribes an early mRNA to synthesize early proteins such as T antigen and TSTA. In a nonproductive infection, the viral DNA is then integrated into the cellular DNA and continuously transcribes early regions of viral DNA to make early proteins. This transformed cell continuously replicates without production of progeny virus. In case of productive infection, late gene products (structural proteins) are produced after early transcription and translation. Virion assembly and cell death then follow within 48 hours after the virus infection.

In general, only a fraction of the viral genome is required for the induction of cellular transformation. Radiation treatment or chemical inactivation of viruses increases the oncogenic capacity of the viruses. In case of papovaviruses, half of the viral genetic material is involved in the process of transformation. This amount of viral DNA is sufficient to code a single frame for only a few discrete proteins.

Among the papovaviruses, papillomaviruses are most closely associated with premalignant and malignant lesions found in the human anal-genital area and oral cavity. Over the past two decades, research with papillomaviruses that induce papillomas in animals has exploded. Papillomaviruses contain circular DNA (approximately 8.0 kilobase pairs in size) as genome, are nonenveloped and replicate in epithelial nuclei. About 66 types of human papillomaviruses (HPVs) have been identified. Several are associated with different human papillomas, premalignant lesions, and malignant cancers. HPV DNA is frequently found in condylomata acuminata of the anal-genital areas such as the cervix, vulva, and anus. High-risk HPVs such as types 16 (HPV-16) and 18 (HPV-18) are most frequently associated with malignant genital lesions, while HPV-6 and HPV-11 are mostly found in benign tumors. Evidence that high-risk HPVs are involved in the genesis of anal-genital cancer is as follows: (1) More than 90 percent of anal-genital cancer tissue contains HPV-16 or 18 DNA. (2) The cancer cells contain an integrated form of viral DNA with disruption of early gene 2 open reading frame (E2 ORF), whereas benign cells contain an episomal form of viral DNA. (3) Most cancer cell lines derived from cervical cancer containing high risk HPVs actively transcribe viral E6 and E7 mRNAs that are able to transform normal cells in vitro. Though the exact role of high-risk HPVs in carcinogenesis is largely speculative, HPV may induce cell transformation by altering the expression pattern of c-*myc* protooncogene. Overexpression of c-*myc* oncogene is frequently found in cancer cells

derived from the cancer tissue containing high-risk HPV DNA. Further evidence of HPV carcinogenicity comes from the in vitro cell transforming capacity of HPV DNA. Transformation of human skin fibroblasts, skin keratinocytes, cervical epithelial cells tranfected with cloned HPV-16 and 18 DNA has been reported. Though the molecular mechanisms of HPV-induced cell transformation are unknown, early viral gene products such as E6 and E7 proteins may play a crucial role in HPV-induced carcinogenesis. Transfection of normal cells with either cloned HPV-16 or 18 E6/E7 gene induces immortalization of the cells. Recently the molecular biological functions of E6 and E7 proteins of high-risk HPVs were partly unveiled. The E6 protein binds and promotes the degradation of wild-type cellular p53, while the E7 protein binds and inactivates the function of retinoblastoma (Rb) tumor suppressor protein.

Benign and malignant oral lesions also appear to be associated with HPV infection. Many studies suggest that HPV is involved in the development of oral squamous-cell papillomas, chondylomas and focal epithelial hyperplasia. DNA hybridization studies and amplification of viral DNA using polymerase chain reaction have shown the presence of viral DNA in premalignant and malignant oral lesions. This association is based on finding HPV DNA in up to 40 to 50 percent of cancer tissues. Inasmuch as oral epithelium is histologically similar to that of the female genital tract with continuous challenge by many environmental factors, close association of HPVs with the development of oral malignancies has been anticipated. In addition, a number of cell lines derived from cervical and oral cancers contain both high-risk HPV DNA and RNA. Normal human oral epithelial cells can be immortalized by transfection with recombinant HPV-16 or HPV-18 DNA. The HPV-immortalized oral epithelial cells are not tumorigenic in vivo, but subsequent exposure of the immortalized, non-tumorigenic cells to chemical carcinogens results in the emergence of tumorigenic cells. These results led to a hypothesis that oral cancer arises by sequential combined effect of high risk HPV and tobacco use in humans.

Retroviruses

Retroviruses are enveloped, ether sensitive, 110 nm in diameter, and contain single-stranded RNA as a genome. The 60 to 70S RNA genome is diploid having two identical molecules of 35S RNA held together near their 5' termini. The most peculiar characteristic of retroviruses is the presence of reverse transcriptase in the virions. Approximately 30 molecules of reverse transcriptase are present in one virion. This enzyme encoded by viral genome is capable of synthesizing complementary DNA (minus strand) from viral RNA and has an exonuclease activity (RNase H) that degrades the RNA strand in RNA-DNA hybrids from the 5′ end of the RNA. Cellular tRNA participates in the synthesis of complementary DNA as a primer. The nucleoprotein core is central in viruses in C type morphology, whereas it is eccentric in viruses with B type morphology.

REPLICATION CYCLE

Less than 1 hour after viral infection, the complementary viral DNA (minus strand) synthesis begins in the cellular cytoplasm; then the synthesis of plus strand (complementary to the minus strand) begins to form linear double-stranded viral DNA. This linear DNA moves into the nucleus, circularizes, and then is incorporated into cellular DNA as proviral DNA. The linear, circular, and proviral forms of DNA contain a complete genome and are infectious. The replication cycle for retroviruses requires 10 to 12 hours under proper conditions. Cells survive by the productive infections of these viruses. Cells may be transformed or nontransformed with or without the production of progeny viruses (Fig. 22–18).

TRANSMISSION

Retroviruses are transmitted by horizontal transmission, congenital transmission, or vertical transmission. Feline leukemia viruses and sarcomaviruses can be transmitted by horizontal transmis-

sion, that is, can be acquired from the outside, as infectious agents. Mammary tumor viruses and avian leukosis viruses are transmitted congenitally. Vertical transmission is unique to endogenous retroviruses and consists of genetic transmission of proviral DNA in the same manner as any other chromosomal gene of the host.

EVIDENCE FOR INVOLVEMENT OF RETROVIRUSES IN HUMAN CANCERS

Human T-cell leukemia, which is endemic to Southeast Japan and West India, is strongly associated with type 1 or 2 human T-cell leukemia virus (HTLV-I or HTLV-II). High antibody titer to HTLV-I or -II is found in all patients with T-cell leukemia, whereas they are absent in healthy individuals. HTLVs are C-type retroviruses. Their viral oncogene has not yet been identified.

AIDS AND HUMAN IMMUNODEFICIENCY VIRUS (HIV)

Since the late 1970s a number of previously healthy male homosexuals have developed various opportunistic infectious diseases or neoplasms, such as Kaposi's sarcoma, complicating an underlying defect in the cellular immune mechanism. Since these diseases had almost never been seen in immunocompetent individuals, extensive effort has been given to find the causes of them. Finally, the Centers for Disease Control (CDC) named this syndrome acquired immunodeficiency syndrome

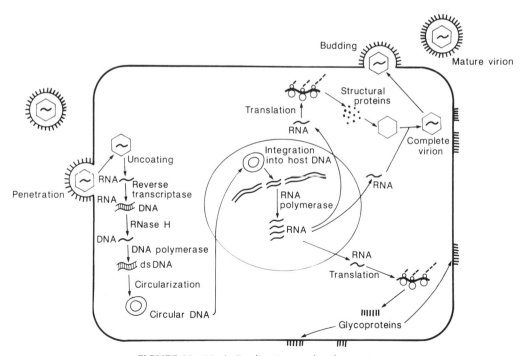

FIGURE 22–18 ✦ Replicative cycle of retrovirus.

(AIDS). AIDS results from the quantitative deficiency of the T-helper cell population.

Clinical Signs and Symptoms of HIV Infection and AIDS

HIV infected individuals are classified into four major groups: Group I, people with acute infection; Group II, people with asymptomatic infection; Group III, people with persistent generalized lymphadenopathy; and Group IV, individuals with constitutional neurologic, secondary or other conditions. The HIV-infected individuals belonging to Group IV are subdivided into five subgroups: Subgroup A, people with constitutional disease; Subgroup B, people with neurologic disorder; Subgroup C, patients with secondary infectious diseases; Subgroup D, patients with secondary cancers; and Subgroup E, people having other conditions. CDC defines AIDS as a disease of life-threatening illness caused by human immunodeficiency virus (HIV) and characterized by HIV encephalopathy, HIV wasting syndrome, or certain diseases due to immunodeficiency in a person with laboratory evidence of HIV infection or without certain other causes of immunodeficiency. There is a great variation in the clinical course of AIDS. Many patients have no prodromal symptoms until they show cutaneous Kaposi's sarcoma, life-threatening *Pneumocystis carinii* pneumonia, or cryptococcal meningitis. Some patients, however, experience malaise, weakness, weight loss, oral candidiasis, oral hairy tongue leukoplakia, and diarrhea for several weeks or months before exhibiting the life-threatening opportunistic infectious diseases. Finally, in some patients, the prodromal malaise, fever, and weight loss may last several months or years before a specific opportunistic infection or Kaposi's sarcoma occurs. Some patients also show generalized lymphade-nopathy for months or years. Opportunistic infectious diseases under the CDC definition include (1) pneumonia, meningitis, or encephalitis due to aspergillosis, candidiasis, cryptococcus, cytomegalovirus (CMV), herpes simplex virus (HSV), or nocardiosis; (2) esophagitis due to candida, HSV, or CMV; (3) extensive mucocutaneous HSV infections; (4) progressive multifocal leukoencephalopathy; (5) Kaposi's sarcoma; (6) lymphoma limited to the brain; (7) chronic enterocolitis; or (8) central nervous system infection due to coccidiomycosis, cryptococcosis, or histoplasmosis. Among these, the most common opportunistic infections in AIDS are *Pneumocystis carinii* pneumonia, disseminated CMV infection, disseminated *Mycobacterium avium-intracellulare,* candidal esophagitis, mucocutaneous HSV infection, cryptococcal meningitis, cerebral toxoplasmosis, and enteric cryptosporidiosis. The most common clinical manifestations in AIDS are fever of unknown origin, weight loss, fatigue, diffuse pneumonia, diarrhea, neurologic disorders, and retinitis (Figs. 22–19, 22–20, and 22–21).

Epidemiologic Studies

The CDC reported 230,179 cases of AIDS in the United States as of June 30, 1992; 226,281 cases of adult/adolescent and 3898 cases of pediatric (<13 years old) AIDS cases. Among the adult/adolescent AIDS cases (1) 58 percent are homosexual men; (2) 23 percent are injecting drug abusers; (3) 6 percent are men who have sex with men and inject drugs; (4) 1 percent are patients with hemophilia coagulation disorder; (5) 6 percent are patients infected by heterosexual contact; (6) 2 percent are recipients of blood transfusion, blood components, or tissue; and (7) 4 percent are patients with undetermined risk factors. Among the pediatric AIDS cases, (1) 85 percent have mothers

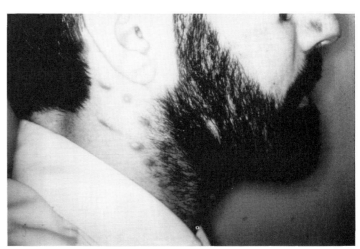

FIGURE 22–19 ✦ Kaposi's sarcoma in the face and neck of an AIDS patient. (Courtesy of F. Lucatorto.)

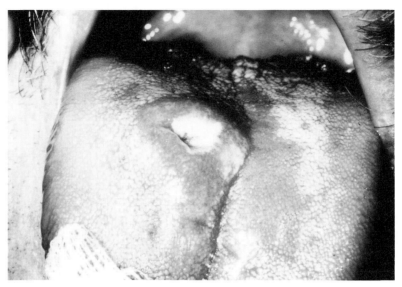

FIGURE 22–20 ✦ Squamous cell carcinoma of tongue in an AIDS patient. (Courtesy of F. Lucatorto.)

with or at risk for HIV infection; (2) 8 percent are recipients of blood transfusion, blood components, or tissue; (3) 5 percent are patients with hemophilia/coagulation disorders; and (4) 3 percent are those with no risk factors. So far, approximately half of the AIDS patients have died. According to the CDC, certain populations are at increased risk of getting AIDS: promiscuous homosexual males, intravenous drug abusers, hemophiliacs, heterosexual contacts of the aforementioned groups, newborns of high-risk mothers, and persons receiving whole blood or blood component transfusion.

Epidemiologic studies have indicated that a transmissible infectious agent must be involved in the development of AIDS. Since a number of viruses capable of suppressing body immune mechanisms, including HSV, CMV, Epstein-Barr virus, hepatitis B virus (HBV), and adenovirus, are frequently found in AIDS patients, these viruses were initially suspected as the causative agents. Recently, human immunodeficiency virus (HIV), a retrovirus, was isolated frequently in AIDS and pre-AIDS patients. Almost 100 percent of all AIDS sera showed antibody to HIV.

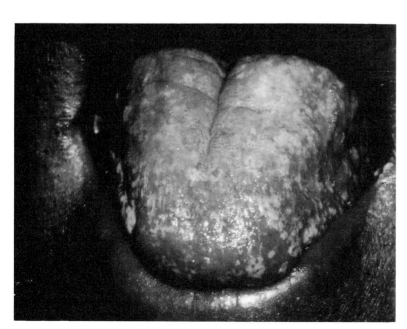

FIGURE 22–21 ✦ Candida albicans of tongue in an AIDS patient. (Courtesy of F. Lucatorto.)

Human Immunodeficiency Virus (HIV)

The etiologic agent for AIDS is human immunodeficiency viruses type 1 (HIV-1) and type 2 (HIV-2). HIV-1 was first isolated in France, and identified as the etiologic agent of AIDS in the United States, Europe, and other countries. HIV-2, mostly restricted to West Africa, is more closely related to the simian immunodeficiency virus (SIV) than HIV-1. Though the genetic and biological features of these two viruses are similar, recent studies show that HIV-1 is a blood-borne virus that transmits through open wound or needle stick, whereas HIV-2 is a mucous membrane-prone virus that can be easily transmitted through heterosexual contact. These differences are the reasons why HIV-1 infection, at least in the United States and Europe, is mostly found in homosexual men and IV drug abusers, while the HIV-1 infection is extremely prevalent in heterosexual men and women in Africa.

Like other retroviruses, HIV-1 and HIV-2 are enveloped viruses and contain single positive-strand RNA as genome. The size of the virion is approximately 110 nm in diameter, and has a dense, cylindrical protein core encasing the viral genome and several viral enzymes such as reverse transcriptase, integrase, and protease. The genome encompasses *gag, pol,* and *env* genes that are normally found in retroviruses, and a number of different regulatory genes, i.e., *sor,* 3'-*orf, tat, art,* and 5'- and 3'-LTR. The *tat* and *art* genes are essential for replication and killing of cells, but *sor* and *orf* genes are not. The major core protein is p24, and the envelope contains viral specific glycoprotein 41 (gp41) and gp120 that are essential for the penetration into cells. The replicative cycle of HIV is well known. First, the virus attaches on the cell surfaces containing CD4 receptors, namely, T4-lymphocytes, macrophages, monocytes, neurons, and Langerhans' cells. Fusion of viral envelope and cell membrane is required for internalization of the virus after the binding of viral gp140 to CD4 receptor. Similar to other retroviruses, complementary DNA (cDNA) is synthesized from the viral genome using the viral reverse transcriptase, and the cDNA is integrated into cellular genome. After certain latency, the virus actively replicates and kills infected cells. HIV shows a tremendous genomic diversity. Not only the isolates from different patients, but also sequential isolates from the same patients over a few months show differences because of point mutation, gene deletions, and insertions. The number of people with HIV infection has significantly increased each year in the United States. So far, no vaccine or treatment measures are available to prevent or treat HIV infections, respectively. The CDC estimates that approximately over 20 million Americans will be infected with HIV by the year 2000 (Fig. 22–22).

Mode of Transmission of HIV

Epidemiological data suggest that HIV is not transmitted by casual contact. It is transmitted by sexual contacts (homosexual contact between men, and heterosexual contact from men to women and women to men), by exposure to blood (use of contaminated needle, transfusion of contaminated blood, plasma, packed cells, platelets and factor concentrates, and occupational needle stick injury), and by the perinatal route (during pregnancy, intrapartum, and postpartum [breastfeeding]). In cases of transmission by sexual contact, HIV and HIV-infected cells in semen and vaginal fluid may play major roles. Earlier reports of HIV in high percentages of saliva specimens from HIV-infected individuals and AIDS patients caused considerable concern regarding a possible oral route of infection and the role of saliva in transmitting HIV. However, recent controlled studies indicate that less than 1 percent of saliva cultures from HIV-infected patients contain cell-free infectious virus particles, while a higher proportion of serum cultures (38 percent) showed cell-free infectious HIV. The low recovery of HIV from the saliva may be due to the lower concentration of HIV in the saliva, or due to factors inhibiting the viral activity in the saliva. These studies indicate that potential transmissibility of HIV infection by saliva is very unlikely.

AIDS and the Dentist

Although HIV is not transmissible through casual contact, occupational exposure of health care workers to HIV has been reported in clinical and laboratory workers. Since dentists and auxiliaries have regular contact with patients' blood and saliva, there is great concern among dental professionals. Furthermore, as of February 1986, the Centers for Disease Control reported that 26 out of 17,115 reported AIDS cases were in dental personnel. However, there is no evidence that health care or laboratory personnel are at significant risk of contracting AIDS as a consequence of their occupation. Precautions for avoiding AIDS closely resemble those recommended for hepatitis B. To minimize the transmission of infection from AIDS patients, dentists must follow recommended procedures (Chapter 32).

Though HIV-1 infection from infected patients to health professionals has been documented, transmission of the virus from the health care workers to patients is rare. Recent epidemiologic and molecular biologic studies showed that five dental patients became infected with HIV-1 from a dentist

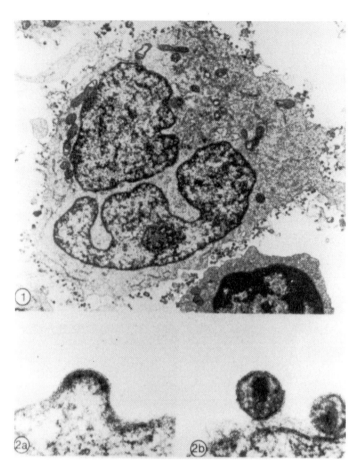

FIGURE 22–22 ✦ Electron micrograph of HIV-infected cells **(1)**, showing the budding virus **(2a)** and mature virion **(2b)**. (From Sarngadharan, M. G., Markham, P. D., and Gallo, R. C.: Human T-cell leukemia viruses. In Fields, B. N., et al. (eds.): Virology. Raven Press, New York, 1985, p. 1360, with permission.)

during invasive dental procedures. Though the exact mode of transmission is unknown, it may be possible that patients can be infected from infected dentists during the invasive dental treatment. This incidence has caused a great deal of concern in the dental community. However, recommended barrier technique procedures during the dental treatment are considered to be effective for preventing the transmission of the virus from the dentist to patients, and vice versa.

ANTIVIRAL THERAPY

During the last two decades, a number of potent and selective antiviral agents have been introduced. Among the viruses, herpesviruses are particularly susceptible to chemotherapeutic agents. Since herpesviruses—especially herpes simplex virus (HSV)—are the most ubiquitous, communicable, and infectious viruses in humans and are the etiologic agents of a wide variety of chronically recurring diseases, herpesviruses are generally among the first to be studied when new antiviral agents are developed.

To date, 12 antiviral agents have been approved for clinical use by the Food and Drug Administra-

tion. Table 22–6 shows the antiviral spectrum, mechanisms of action, and clinical uses of these agents.

Amantadine HCl

Amantadine HCl interferes with the early interaction of influenza viruses with the cell membrane; it blocks the penetration and uncoating processes. Amantadine is approximately 60 percent effective as a prophylactic agent against influenza A strains. Side effects of amantadine include tremor, instability of motion, frank ataxia, inability to concentrate, insomnia, and slurred speech. Amantadine has been used more extensively as an agent in the treatment of Parkinson's disease than in the prophylaxis of influenza A (Fig. 22–23).

Idoxuridine

Idoxuridine is effective in the treatment of superficial herpes keratitis. Recurrences of the disease and drug resistance are problems. The effectiveness of idoxuridine against recurrent herpes labialis and genitalis has not been established. Idoxuridine is possibly mutagenic, teratogenic, and

TABLE 22–6 ✦ Comparison of Antiviral Agents

NAME	ANTIVIRAL SPECTRUM	MECHANISM OF ACTION	CLINICAL USES
Amantadine HCl	Influenza A virus	Blocking the penetration and uncoating process	Prophylaxis of influenza A infection
Idoxuridine	HSV-1 and HSV-2	Inhibition of DNA synthesis	Treatment of herpetic keratitis
Vidarabine	HSV-1 and HSV-2	Inhibition of DNA synthesis	Treatment of herpetic keratitis and encephalitis
Trifluridine	HSV-1 and HSV-2	Inhibition of DNA synthesis	Treatment of herpetic kerato-conjunctivitis
Acyclovir	HSV-1 and HSV-2, and VZV	Inhibition of DNA synthesis	Treatment of primary and recurrent herpes genitalis, herpetic encephalitis, mucocutaneous herpetic infections in immunocompromised patients, and neonatal herpetic infection Varicella, herpes zoster, and varicella and herpes zoster in immunocompromised.
Foscarnet	HSV, VZV, and CMV	Inhibition of DNA synthesis	Treatment of acyclovir-resistant HSV and herpes zoster virus infections, and CMV retinitis
Ganciclovir	CMV	Inhibition of DNA synthesis	Treatment of CMV retinitis
Interferon alfa-2b	Hepatitis B and C virus	Inhibition of protein synthesis	Treatment of chronic hepatitis
Zidovudine	HIV	Inhibition of cDNA synthesis	Treatment of symptomatic, or AIDS or advanced AIDS-related complex (ARC)
Didanosine	HIV	Inhibition of cDNA synthesis	Treatment of AIDS and ARC

HSV-1 = herpes simplex virus type 1; HSV-2 = herpes simplex virus type 2; CMV = cytomegalovirus; VZV = varicella zoster virus; HIV = human immunodeficiency virus; cDNA = complementary DNA.

carcinogenic. In cells, idoxuridine is metabolized to mono-, di-, and triphosphate forms. They competitively inhibit the activity of thymidine kinase, thymidylate kinase, and DNA polymerase. Thus, idoxuridine inhibits the synthesis of viral and cellular DNA. Furthermore, idoxuridine is incorporated into cellular and viral DNA, and makes defective DNA. Therefore, idoxuridine does not specifically attack the infected cells. Idoxuridine is known to increase the replication of retroviruses in transformed cells and to produce toxic effects in

normal cells. Recently idoxuridine was found to activate the latently infected human immunodeficiency virus in vitro (Fig. 22–24).

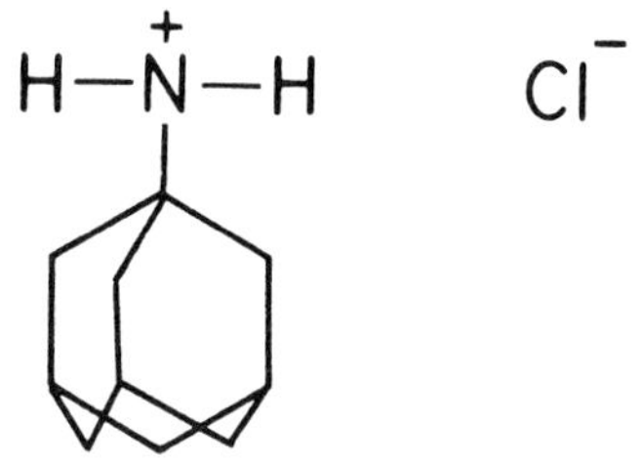

FIGURE 22–23 ✦ Chemical structure of amantadine HCl.

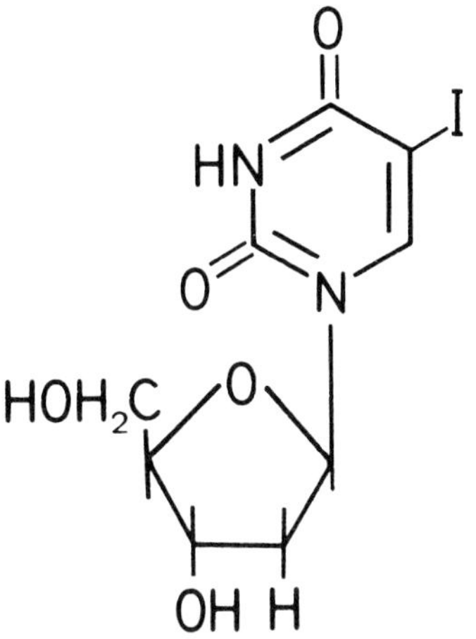

FIGURE 22–24 ✦ Chemical structure of iododeoxyuridine.

Vidarabine

Vidarabine has a broad spectrum of antiviral activity and is active against herpes simplex virus, poxviruses, retroviruses, and rhabdoviruses. Vidarabine is metabolized in cells to vidarabine mono-, di-, and triphosphate. Vidarabine diphosphate and triphosphate provide antiherpes activity by inhibiting the activity of viral and cellular ribonucleotide reductase and DNA polymerase. Thus, vidarabine does not show specific selectivity. It was first approved for the treatment of herpes keratitis. Subsequently, it was shown to improve the mortality and morbidity among patients with herpes encephalitis. Side effects of vidarabine are anorexia, nausea, vomiting, weight loss, weakness, and bone marrow depression (Fig. 22–25).

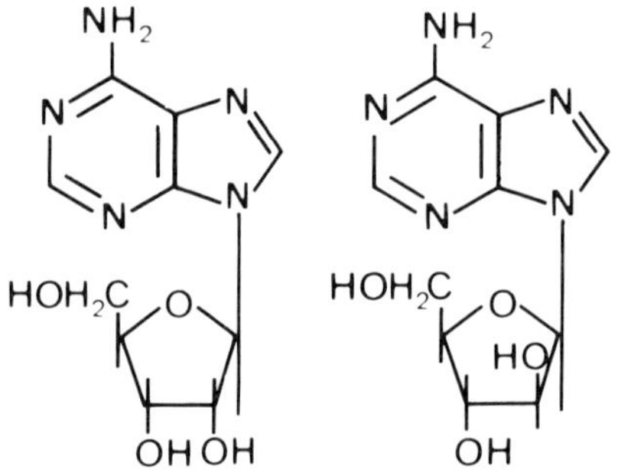

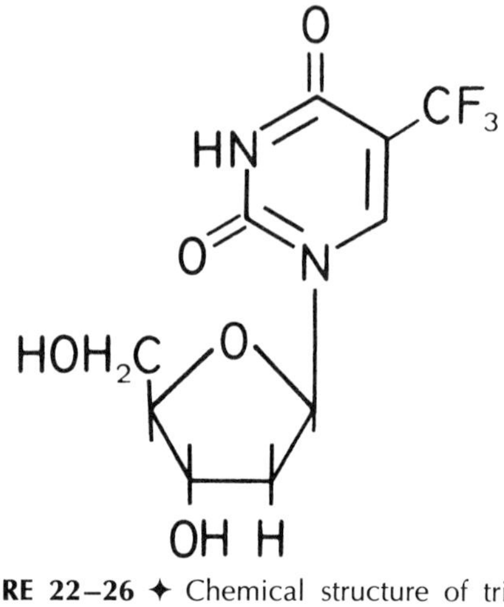

FIGURE 22–26 ✦ Chemical structure of trifluorothymidine.

Trifluridine

Trifluridine is a fluorinated thymidine derivative (Fig. 22–26) and a potent antiherpetic agent. It has an antiviral effect against DNA viruses such as herpes simplex virus types 1 and 2. Trifluridine is phosphorylated to trifluridine monophosphate by thymidine kinase. The monophosphate form is further phosphorylated to di- and triphosphate forms. Trifluridine monophosphate and triphosphate inhibit the activities of thymidylate synthetase and DNA polymerase, respectively. Finally, the synthesis of viral DNA is inhibited by the agent. However, it is not selective and shows significant cytotoxic activity. This drug penetrates into human cornea and aqueous humor after topical instillation. It is useful for the control of superficial herpetic keratitis.

Acyclovir

The major breakthrough in antiviral chemotherapy was the introduction of acyclovir, an analogue of guanosine. It is a potent and selective antiviral agent (Fig. 22–27). Acyclovir is phosphorylated to acyclovir-monophosphate by herpesvirus-encoded thymidine kinase. Then acyclovir-diphosphate and -triphosphate are formed by cellular enzymes. Acyclovir-triphosphate inhibits the viral DNA polymerase and terminates the elongation of the viral DNA chain. Thus, it selectively affects only viral infected cells and leaves uninfected cells essentially untouched (Fig. 22–28). Acyclovir is highly effective in vitro against HSV-1, HSV-2, varicella zoster virus, and cytomegalovirus. Recently, intravenous and oral preparations have been released. The intravenous form is indicated for the treatment of primary and recurrent mucosal and cutaneous herpes simplex infections in immunocompromised patients. It is also used for severe initial episodes of herpes genitalis in patients who are not immunocompromised. Oral administration of acyclovir has recently been approved by FDA for the prevention of recurrent herpes genitalis. Up to 1000 mg of acyclovir per day could be given for a maximum of 6 months. However, the

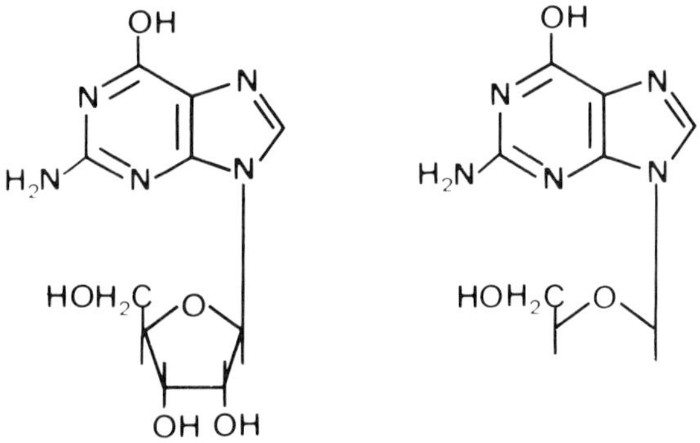

FIGURE 22–25 ✦ Chemical structure of adenosine and vidarabine.

FIGURE 22–27 ✦ Chemical structure of guanosine and acyclovir.

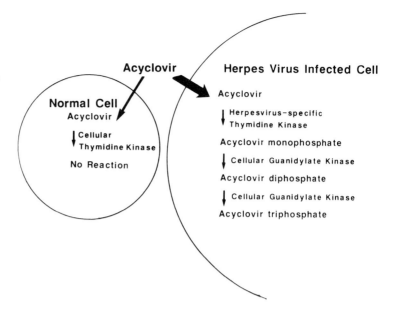

FIGURE 22–28 ✦ Mechanism of action by acyclovir. Acyclovir is activated by herpesvirus thymidine kinase to be acyclovir monophosphate. Acyclovir monophosphate is further phosphorylated to be a triphosphate, which is responsible for the antiherpetic activity by inhibiting viral DNA polymerase and terminating the viral DNA chain elongation.

recurrent herpes disease rebounds when the drug administration is stopped.

Foscarnet

Foscarnet, an analogue of phosphonoacetic acid, is effective against HSV, CMV, and HIV-1. This drug inhibits the cellular and herpetic DNA polymerase, and by so doing inhibits synthesis of HSV and CMV DNA. Foscarnet also inhibits synthesis of cDNA in HIV-1 by suppressing the activity of reverse transcriptase in vitro, but the clinical efficacy is controversial. Though clinical use of foscarnet for HIV-1 has not been approved by the FDA, the drug is effective for the treatment of acyclovir-resistant HSV infections and CMV retinitis when administered parenterally in AIDS patients. Foscarnet can lead to renal toxicity, malaise, nausea, vomiting, fatigue, headache, genital ulcers, CNS disturbances, hypocalcemia or hypercalcemia, hypophosphatemia and hyperphosphatemia, anemia, proteinuria, leukopenia, and liver dysfunction.

Ganciclovir

Systemic ganciclovir is useful for the treatment of life- and sight-threatening CMV infections, especially CMV retinitis in immunocompromised patients. Ganciclovir is a carcinogenic, teratogenic substance, and can cause aspermatogenesis in animals. The most common side effects of ganciclovir are agranulocytopenia and thrombocytopenia, which are not always reversible after the cessation of the drug administration.

Ribavirin

Ribavirin is a synthetic nucleoside with broad spectrum antiviral activity against HSV, HIV-1, and respiratory syncytial virus. Ribavirin inhibits the synthesis of viral DNA, directly inhibiting the function of guanine deaminase and its metabolite, and inosine monophosphate dehydrogenase. Though ribavirin shows broad antiviral spectrum in vitro, it is only useful as an aerosol for the treatment of respiratory syncytial virus bronchitis and pneumonia in children in the U.S. Inasmuch as the agent is a nucleoside analogue and nonselective antiviral agent, it is mutagenic, tumor-promoting, and teratogenic agent. Furthermore, acute deterioration of respiratory function has been reported with ribavirin aerosol use in infants and in adults.

Interferons

Interferons are glycoproteins secreted by virus-infected cells, which promote the establishment of an antiviral state in uninfected cells (Fig. 22–29). Although all cells in the body appear capable of synthesizing interferons, cells derived from the hematopoietic system (e.g., lymphocytes and macrophages) may contribute more to the total interferon synthesis. All DNA or RNA viruses—single- or double-stranded, enveloped or not, with or without virion-associated polymerase, and replicating in the cytoplasm or nucleus—are sensitive to interferon, although differences in the degree of sensitivity exist.

Interferon induces two enzymes: an oligonucleotide polymerase which synthesizes a series of

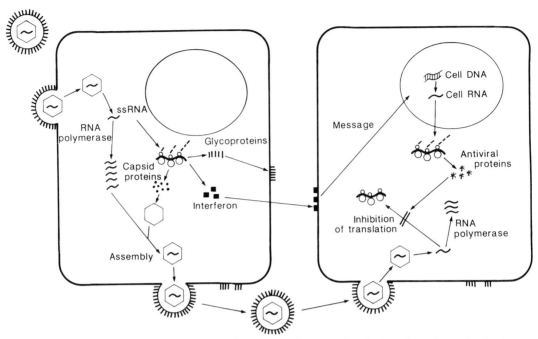

FIGURE 22–29 ✦ Interrelationships of virus, interferon, and cells. Interferon is synthesized in the virus infected cells but shows antiviral activity in the second cell by inhibiting viral translation through the production of antiviral proteins.

oligonucleotide containing 2'5'-phosphodiester bonds from ATP (2'5'-oligo[A]polymerase), and a protein kinase, which phosphorylates the small subunit of initiation factor eIF-2. The product of 2'5'-oligo(A)polymerase pppA(2'p5'A)n is the activator of cellular endonucleases that restrict viral nucleic acids. Its activity depends on the continuous presence of pppA(2'p5'A)n with which it binds. Accumulation of viral RNA is also inhibited in interferon-treated cells that may result from the action of endonucleases (Fig. 22–30). The average half-life of viral mRNA is approximately 12.7 hours in normal cells but only 4.8 hours in interferon-treated cells. The dsRNA-dependent protein kinase phosphorylates the alpha subunit of eIF-2 and subsequently inhibits the binding of initiator tRNA to 40S native ribosomal subunits. Interferon also blocks the proper formation of the viral mRNA cap by inhibiting the process of methylation. Interferon is a macromolecule and must be administered parenterally. It can cause increased pulse rate and temperature, decreased white blood cell counts, headache, and malaise.

For prophylaxis or early treatment, interferons may have advantages over narrow-spectrum antiviral agents. However, under other circumstances, a specific antiviral agent may be preferable to interferons for convenience of administration, quicker onset of antiviral action, and lack of side effects.

Antiviral Agents for AIDS

There are two difficult problems in developing anti-AIDS drugs; (1) HIV eventually becomes part of the cells it infects preventing its removal by antiviral chemotherapy; and (2) the HIV may infect the brain and establish a latent infection, which means antiviral drugs must cross the blood-brain barrier.

Zidovudine, formerly called azidothymidine or AZT, is an analogue of thymidine (Fig. 22–31). Zidovudine is very useful for controlling the replication of HIV-1. The mechanisms of anti-HIV-1 by zidovudine are well known. Zidovudine is phosphorylated by cellular enzymes to zidovudine triphosphate, that is incorporated into viral cDNA by the reverse-transcription of HIV-1. With its incorporation into the viral cDNA, the 3' substitution (3'-azido group) further prevents 5'- to 3'-phosphodiester linkages and terminates chain elongation of viral cDNA (Fig. 22–32). HIV-1 reverse transcriptase is approximately 100 times more susceptible to inhibition by zidovudine than DNA polymerase of mammalian cells. Zidovudine seems not only to block the replication of the virus, but also aids in some regeneration of CD4 lymphocytes. The agent also delays progression of AIDS in HIV-infected individuals with CD4 lymphocyte counts of less than 500 cells/mm^3 and in individuals with no symptoms or early ARC symptoms. Though prophylactic use of zidovudine immedi-

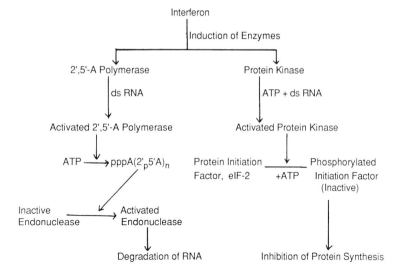

FIGURE 22–30 ✦ Molecular mechanism of antiviral action of interferon.

ately after exposure to HIV-1 has been proposed, the efficacy of zidovudine for post-exposure prophylaxis is uncertain. Zidovudine is administered 200 mg four times a day or 100 mg five or six times a day. For individuals without AIDS or ARC symptoms, zidovudine is given 100 mg every four hours while awake (500 mg/day). Side effects of zidovudine include asthenia, headache, dizziness, insomnia, anorexia, nausea, vomiting, malaise, and myalgia. Long-term use of this drug is infrequently associated with a toxic myopathy. Though this agent induces cell transformation in vitro and tumors in animals, the teratogenicity of this drug in humans is unknown. Recently, many HIV-1 strains resistant to zidovudine were isolated from clinical specimens. Though HIV-1 strains from individuals not receiving zidovudine are very susceptible to zidovudine, the sensitivity of HIV-1 from patients receiving zidovudine for six months is significantly decreased. Zidovudine-resistant HIV-1 strains are susceptible to other anti-HIV-1 agents such as didanosine, dideoxycytidine, and foscarnet in vitro.

Didanosine (DDI) is an investigational drug that is active against HIV-1, including zidoduvine-re-

sistant HIV-1 strains. Similar to zidoduvine, didanosine inhibits the activity of reverse transcriptase of HIV-1, and by doing so inhibits the synthesis of HIV-1 cDNA. Oral didanosine increases the number of CD4 lymphocytes, decreases p24 antigen level, and decreases symptoms in AIDS and severe ARC patients. So far, cross-resistance between didanosine and zidoduvine has not been reported. Importantly, some patients with HIV-1 infection resistant to zidoduvine respond well to didanosine. Daily dose is 12 mg/kg twice a day or 20 mg/kg once daily. Major side effects are peripheral neuropathy and fatal pancreatitis.

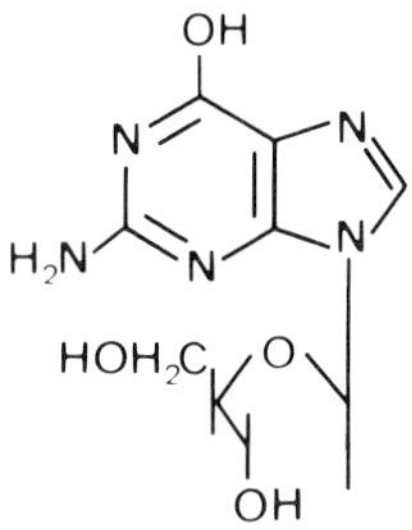

VACCINES

The best way to prevent viral diseases is vaccination. Vaccination induces antibodies in serum and extracellular fluids, which provide the main protection against primary viral infections. There are two types of viral vaccines: inactivated viral vaccines and attenuated viral (living) vaccines (Table 22–7).

Inactivated Viral Vaccines

In these vaccines there is complete inactivation of infectivity without loss of viral antigenicity. Only a few substances and methods are used to inactivate the infectivity by disrupting the viral genomes without affecting the viral proteins, which are a source of antigenicity.

ULTRAVIOLET IRRADIATION

Although ultraviolet (UV) irradiation can destroy the viral genomes without alteration of proteins, this method is not appropriate, because virus is frequently incompletely inactivated. Further-

FIGURE 22–31 ✦ Chemical structure of 5-azidothymidine.

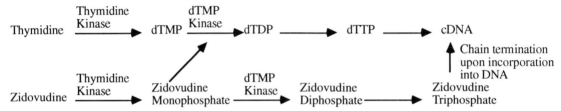

FIGURE 22–32 ✦ Metabolic pathway and mechanisms of anti-HIV action of zidovudine. Zidovudine is phosphorylated to monophosphate form by cellular thymidine kinase, and to diphosphate form by cellular dTMP kinase. It is further phosphorylated to zidovudine triphosphate and is incorporated into HIV-1 cDNA. Upon the incorporation of zidovudine triphosphate into viral cDNA, cDNA chain elongation is terminated because of lack of 3'-OH group in zidovudine. Instead, zidovudine contains azido group at its 3'-carbon. Therefore, 3',5'-phosphodiester linkage is not established with next nucleotide. Furthermore, zidovudine monophosphate inhibits the function of dTMP kinase, and by doing so inhibit the formation of dTDP. dTMP, deoxythymidine monophosphate; dTDP, deoxythymidine diphosphate; dTTP, deoxythymidine triphosphate.

more, the UV inactivated virus such as herpes simplex virus can transform normal cells to be tumorigenic in vitro.

PHOTODYNAMIC INACTIVATION

Photodynamic inactivation refers to the treatment of virus with numerous dyes such as neutral red dyes, which intercalate between viral nucleic acid bases; then the viruses are irradiated with white light to damage the nucleic acid without altering viral proteins. However, photodynamically inactivated virus can transform normal cells into tumorigenic ones.

TREATMENT WITH FORMALDEHYDE

The best means to inactivate the function of the viral genome without damaging the antigenicity of virus is formaldehyde. Formaldehyde reacts with nucleic acid bases containing amino group in its structure. Viruses containing single-strand nucleic acid are more readily inactivated by formaldehyde than ones with double-strand nucleic acid. Formaldehyde also reacts with viral capsid proteins and forms extensive crosslinkage, which prevents the access of formaldehyde to nucleic acid. Therefore, formaldehyde treatment can produce viral mutants with altered capsid and intact nucleic acid, which show resistance to formaldehyde. All formaldehyde-inactivated vaccines must be carefully tested for infectivity before human use to ensure complete inactivation. Formalin-inactivated vaccines are available for the prevention of influenza, poliomyelitis, and rabies. These vaccines are prepared from virus that is grown in eggs (influenza virus types A and B), monkey kidney cell culture (poliovirus types 1, 2, and 3), or human diploid fibroblast cell culture (poliovirus, rabies) and then is inactivated in formaldehyde.

TABLE 22–7 ✦ **Viral Diseases and Currently Available Vaccines**

		VACCINE	
DISEASES	**NAME OF VIRUS**	**INACTIVATED**	**ATTENUATED**
Smallpox	Vaccinia virus		+
Yellow fever	Yellow fever virus		+
Poliomyelitis	Poliovirus	+	+
Measles	Rubeola virus		+
Influenza	Influenza virus	+	+
Mumps	Mumps virus	+	+
Rabies	Rabies virus	+	+
Adenovirus infections	Adenovirus	+	+
Rubella	Rubella virus		+
Viral hepatitis	Hepatitis B virus	Recombinant vaccine	

+ = currently available.

Attenuated Viral Vaccines

Since Jenner successfully demonstrated the prevention of smallpox infection in humans with live cowpox virus vaccine in 1798, numerous attenuated viral vaccines have been developed and used in clinic. These vaccines include the attenuated yellow fever virus, poliovirus, measles, mumps, and rubella virus vaccines. Since the attenuated virus can multiply in the human body, very small amounts of vaccines are needed for the effective induction of humoral and cellular immunity. The Sabin polio vaccine can be given orally to allow the virus to grow locally in the gastrointestinal tissue, which results in the massive production of secretory IgA in the infected local tissue. Since poliovirus is encountered by the fecal-oral route, the local IgA can neutralize the poliovirus in the gastrointestinal tissue and prevent systemic viremia.

Vaccines Produced by Recombinant DNA Technology

Recent advances in molecular biology have led to the use of recombinant DNA techniques in the design of a new generation of vaccines. Many viral genomes are cloned and sequenced: as a result, amino acid sequences of proteins responsible for the production of neutralizing antibodies have become known. These known amino acid sequences of viral proteins will soon allow us to develop certain vaccines against influenza, paramyxovirus, hepatitis B, rotavirus, togavirus, and human immunodeficiency virus. Recently, a new type of recombinant DNA that contains vaccinia virus and herpes simplex virus glycoprotein D gene was introduced as a future vaccine to herpes simplex virus. This recombinant DNA was able to produce IgD against herpes simplex virus glycoprotein D in animals and protected them from the primary infections caused by herpes simplex virus types 1 and 2.

BIBLIOGRAPHY

Abramowicz, M.: Drugs for viral infections. Med. Lett. 34:31, 1992.

Abramowicz, M.: New recommendations for immunization against pertussis and hepatitis B. Med. Lett. 34:69, 1992.

Almeida, J. D., Howaltson, H. F., and Williams, M.: Morphology of varicella (chickenpox) virus. Virology 16:165, 1962.

Baltimore, D.: Expression of animal virus genomes. Bacteriol. Rev. 35:235, 1971.

Baker, L. F., Gerety, R. J., and Tabor, E.: The immunology of the hepatitis viruses. Adv. Med. 23:327, 1978.

Baringer, J. R. and Swoveland, A. J.: Recovery of herpes simplex virus from human trigeminal ganglions. N. Engl. J. Med. 288:648, 1973.

Ben-Porat, T. and Kaplan, A. S.: Studies on the biogenesis of herpesvirus envelope. Nature 235:165, 1972.

Beneson, A. S.: Smallpox. In Evan, A. S. (ed.): Viral Infections of Humans: Epidemiology and Control. New York, Plenum Press, 1976, p. 426.

Berk, A. J. and Sharp, P.A.: Spliced early mRNA of simian virus 40. Proc. Natl. Acad. Sci. U.S.A. 75:1274, 1978.

Bishop, J. M.: Retroviruses. Ann. Rev. Biochem. 47:35, 1978.

Buddingh, G. J., Schrum, D. I., Lanier, J. C., and Guidry, D. J.: Natural history of herpetic infections. Pediatrics 11:595, 1953.

Centers for Disease Control: Hepatitis Surveillance. U.S. Department of Health and Human Services, Public Health Service, Washington, D.C., Report 47, 1981.

Dale, D. and Avers, J.: AIDS: Reference guide for medical professionals. University of California, Los Angeles, 1984.

Epstein, M., Boav, Y., and Achong, B.: Studies with Burkitt's lymphoma. Wistar Inst. Symp. Monogr. 1:69, 1965.

Fields, B. N. and Knipe, D. M.: Fundamental Virology. Raven Press, New York, 1991.

Francis, D. P., Hadler, S. C., and Thompson, S. E.: The prevention of hepatitis B with vaccine: Report of CDC multicenter efficacy trial in homosexual men. Ann. Intern. Med. 97:362, 1982.

Fraenkel-Conrat, H. and Wagner, R. R. (eds.): Regulation and genetics—Genetics of animal viruses. Comp. Virol. Vol. 9, 1977.

Galasso, G. J., Merigan, T. C., and Buchanan, R. A.: Antiviral Agents and Viral Diseases of Man. Raven Press, New York, 1979, pp. 1–38.

Gerety, R. J. (ed.): Non-A, non-B hepatitis. New York, Academic Press, 1981.

Green, M.: Transformation and Oncogenesis: DNA Viruses. In Fields, B. N., Knipe, D. M., Chanock, R. M., Melnick, J. L., Roizman, B., and Shope, R. E. (eds.): Virology. Raven Press, New York, 1985, pp. 183–234.

Grob, P. J. and Jemelka, H.: Fecal SH (Australia) antigen in acute hepatitis. Lancet 1:206, 1971.

Henle, G., Henle, W., and Dieb, V.: Relation of Burkitt's tumor-associated herpes-type virus to infectious mononucleosis. Proc. Natl. Acad. Sci. U.S.A. 59:94, 1968.

Hiatt, H. H., Watson, D. J., and Wistein, J. A.: Origins of Human Cancer. Book B. Mechanisms of Carcinogenesis. Cold Spring Harbor Laboratory, Cold Spring Harbor, New York, 1977.

Hollinger, F. B. and Melnick, J. L.: Features of viral hepatitis. In Fields, B. N., Knipe, D. M., Chanock, R. M., Melnick, J. L., Roizman, B., and Shope, R. E. (eds.): Virology. Raven Press, New York, 1985, pp. 1417–1494.

Holmes, A. W., Wolfe, L., Deinhardt, F., and Conrad, M. E.: Transmission of human hepatitis to marmosets: Further coded studies. J. Infect. Dis. 124:520, 1971.

Hutchinson, M. A., Hunter, T., and Eckhart, W.: Characterization of T antigens in polyoma-infected and transformed cell. Cell 15:65, 1978.

Jenson, A. B., Clifton, C. L. Jr., and Lancaster, W. D.: Papillomavirus Etiology of Oral Cavity Papillomas. In Hooks, J. J., and Jordan, G. W. (eds.): Viral Infections in Oral Medicine. Elsevier/North-Holland, New York, 1982, pp. 133–146.

Johnson, R. T.: Pathogenesis of viral infections. In Hooks, J. J., and Jordan, G. W. (eds.): Viral Infections in Oral Medicine. Elsevier/North-Holland, New York, 1982, pp. 3–12.

Joklik, W. K.: Interferons. In Fields, B. N., Knipe, D. M., Chanock, R. M., Melnick, J. L., Roizman, B., and Shope, R. E. (eds.): Virology. Raven Press, New York, 1985, pp. 281–308.

Kaplan, A. S. (ed.): The Herpesviruses. Academic Press, New York, 1973.

Lane, J. M., Miller, D., and Neff, J. M.: Smallpox and smallpox vaccination policy. Ann. Rev. Med. 22:251, 1971.

Long, W. K. and Francis, R. D.: Structure, replication, and classification of viruses. In McGhee, J. R., Michalek, S. M., and Cassell, G. H. (eds.): Dental Microbiology. Harper & Row, Philadelphia, 1982, pp. 549–575.

Lowy, D. R.: Transformation and Oncogenesis: Retroviruses. In Fields, B. N., Knipe, D. M., Chanock, R. M., Melnick, J. L., Roizman, B., and Shope, R. E. (eds.): Virology. Raven Press, New York, 1985, pp. 235–264.

Luria, S. E., Darnell, J. E. Jr., Baltimore, D., and Campbell, A. (eds.): General Virology, ed. 3. John Wiley and Sons, New York, 1978.

Maynard, J. E.: Hepatitis A. Yale J. Biol. Med. 49:227, 1976.

McDougall, J. K., Crum, C. P., Fenoglio, C. M., Goldstein, L. C., and Galloway, D. A.: Herpesvirus-specific RNA and protein in carcinoma of the uterine cervix. Proc. Natl. Acad. Sci. U.S.A. 79:3853, 1982.

Melnick, J. L., Dreesman, G. R., and Hollinger, F.B.: Approaching the control of viral hepatitis type B. J. Infect. Dis. 133:210, 1976.

Nahmias, A. J. and Roizman, B.: Infection with Herpes Simplex virus 1 and 2. N. Engl. J. Med. 286:667; 719; 781, 1973.

Nathanson, N. and Cole, G. A.: Immunosuppression: A means to assess the role of immune response in acute virus infection. Fed. Proc. 30:1822, 1971.

National Institutes of Health: Workshop on the treatment of herpes simplex virus infection. J. Infect. Dis. 127:117, 1973.

Nichols, W. W.: Virus-induced chromosome abnormalities. Ann. Rev. Microbiol. 24:479, 1970.

Norman, C.: AIDS therapy: New push for clinical trials. Science 230:1355, 1985.

Ou, C.-Y., Ciesielski, C. A., Myers, G., Bandea, C. I., et al.: Molecular epidemiology of HIV transmission in dental practice. Science 256:1165, 1992.

Overall, J. C.: Oral herpes simplex: Pathogenesis, clinical and virologic course, approach to treatment. In Hooks, J. J., and Jordan, G. W. (eds.): Viral Infections in Oral Medicine. Elsevier/North Holland, New York, 1982, pp. 53–78.

Pagano, J. S.: Diseases and mechanisms of persistent DNA virus infection: Latency and cellular transformation. J. Infect. Dis. 132:209, 1975.

Park, N.-H. and Pavan-Langston, D.: Purines. In Came, P. E., and Caliguiri, L. A. (eds.): Chemotherapy of Viral Infections: Handbook of Experimental Pharmacology. Vol. 61. Springer-Verlag, Berlin, 1982, p. 117.

Park, N.-H.: Current aspects of anti-herpes research: Problems, established work, and future goals. California Dental Association Journal, December 1984, pp. 167–169.

Park, N.-H., Pavan-Langston, D., and DeClercq, E.: Effect of acyclovir, bromovinyldeoxyuridine, vidarabine and L-lysine on latent ganglionic herpes simplex virus in vitro. Am. J. Med. 73:151, 1982.

Park, N.-H., Min, B.-M., Li, S.-L., Huang, M. Z., Cherrick, H. M., and Doniger, J.: Immortalization of normal human oral keratinocytes with type 16 human papillomavirus. Carcinogenesis 12:1627, 1991.

Pavan-Langston, D. R.: Ocular viral diseases. In Galasso, G. J., Merigan, T. C., and Buchanan, R. A. (eds.): Antiviral Agents and Viral Diseases of Man. Raven Press, New York, 1979, pp. 253–304.

Pavan-Langston, D. R. (ed.): Ocular viral disease. Int. Ophthalmol. Clin. 15:171, 1975.

Rawls, W. E., Tompkins, W. A., and Melnick, J.L.: The association of herpesvirus type 2 carcinomas of the uterine cervix. Am. J. Epidemiol. 89:547, 1969.

Robinson, W. S., and Lutwick, L. I.: The virus of hepatitis, type B. N. Engl. J. Med. 295:1168; 1232, 1976.

Roizman, B. (ed.): The Herpesviruses. Plenum Publishing, New York, 1985.

Roizman, B. and Furlong, D.: Replication of herpesviruses. Comp. Virol. 3:229, 1974.

Sarngadharan, M. G., Markham, P. D., and Gallo, R. C.: Human T-cell leukemia viruses. In Fields, B. N., Knipe, D. M., Chanock, R. M., Melnick, J. L., Roizman, B., and Shope, R. E. (eds.): Virology. Raven Press, New York, 1985, pp. 1345–1372.

Shillitoe, E. J., Greenspan, D., Greenspan, J. S., and Silverman, S.: Antibody to early and late antigens of herpes simplex virus type 1 in patients with oral cancer. Cancer 54:266, 1984.

Smee, D. F., Martin, J. C., Verhyden, J. P. H., and Matthew, T. R.: Anti-herpesvirus activity of the acyclic nucleosides 9-(1,3-dihydroxy-2-propoxymethyl)-guanine. Antimicrob. Agents Chemother. 23:676, 1983.

Stevens, J. C. and Cook, M. L.: Latent herpes simplex virus in spinal ganglia of mice. Science 173:843, 1971.

Szmuness, W., Stevens, C. E., and Harley, E. J.: Hepatitis B vaccine—Demonstration of efficacy in a controlled clinical trial in a high risk population in the United States. N. Engl. J. Med. 303:8323, 1980.

Szmuness, W., Alter, H. J., and Maynard, J. E. (eds.): Viral Hepatitis. Franklin Institute Press, Philadelphia, 1981.

Tooze, J. (ed.): DNA tumor viruses—Molecular biology of tumor viruses. Cold Spring Harbor Laboratory, Cold Spring Harbor, New York, 1981.

Vilcek, J.: Fundamentals of virus structure and replication. In Galasso, G. J., Merigan, T. C., and

Buchanan, R. A. (eds.): Antiviral Agents and Viral Diseases of Man. Raven Press, New York, 1979, pp. 1–38.

Wadsworth, T. H., Hayward, G. S., and Roizman, B.: Anatomy of herpes simplex virus DNA. V. Terminally repetitive sequences. J. Virol. 17:503, 1975.

Wellere, T. H.: The cytomegaloviruses: Ubiquitous agents with protean clinical manifestation. N. Engl. J. Med. 285:203, 1971.

Whitley, R. J., Ch'ien, L. T., Dolin, R., Galasso, G. L., Alford, C. A., and the Collaborative Study Group: Adenine arabinoside therapy of herpes zoster in the immunocompromised NIAID collaborative antiviral therapy. N. Engl. J. Med. 294:1193, 1976.

23 *Oral Mycology*

Colin K. Franker

CHAPTER OUTLINE

The fungal cell
Vegetative growth in fungi
Sexual reproduction
Classification of fungi
Laboratory identification of fungi
Mycoses with orofacial manifestations

Infections caused by fungi are called *mycoses*. Only a small minority of the 100,000 species are pathogenic in humans, and most of the frequently encountered mycoses are benign. While not as prevalent as bacterial and viral infections, the incidence of superficial as well as invasive mycoses has recently increased. Iatrogenic factors such as immunosuppressive treatments in transplant and oncotherapy, parenteral feeding, and widespread use of antibacterials have accounted for this increment. Most of the fungi associated with human disease are saprophytic members of soil microbial communities. Others exist either as commensals in the alimentary canal or as harmless residents of the skin and only infrequently assume the role of pathogens.

THE FUNGAL CELL

Two major cell morphotypes represent the majority of fungi of medical importance. Oval or spheroidal cell shapes are typical of *yeasts* or *blastospores* and range from 5 to 25 μM in diameter (Fig. 23–1). Tubular or filamentous cells are characteristic of *hyphae,* and a single hyphal cell may range from 5 to 50 μM in length and 2 to 5 μM in diameter (Fig. 23–2). Yeasts usually occur as single cells or as clusters of two or three, with one of the cells distinctly larger than the others. Adjacent hyphal cells may or may not be compartmentalized by cross-wall–like structures called *septa*. A mass of septate hyphal cells constitutes a

mycelium. A similar aggregate of hyphal cells lacking septa is referred to as a *pseudomycelium*. Both mycelia and pseudomycelia represent what is often meant by the term *mold*.

Many fungi can proliferate either as yeasts or as molds. This reversible transition is defined as *dimorphism*. Yeasts can be converted to filamentous hyphal cells by the outgrowth of a cylindrical *germ tube* (Fig. 23–3), and hyphal cells can differentiate during growth into nonfilamentous yeast-like cells. A variety of other cell morphotypes also may be differentiated from hyphal cells, and, as described later in the chapter, a number of these have specialized functions.

VEGETATIVE GROWTH IN FUNGI
Yeasts

A process described as *budding* characterizes the reproduction of most pathogenic yeasts. Simple binary *fission* is another method used by several species, but very few of these yeasts have been implicated in human diseases. As depicted in Figure 23–4, the budding process is initiated by a site-specific outgrowth in a region of the parent cell where curvature is maximal. The *bud initial* then increases in size until it is almost as large as the parental cell from which it was derived. A ring of actin and then chitin is synthesized at the constriction between the mother cell and enlarging bud. After mitotic division and cytoplasmic partitioning of organelles such as mitochondria occurs, a pri-

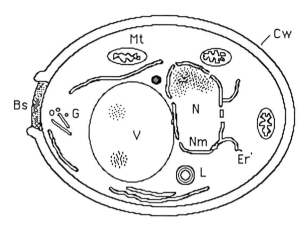

FIGURE 23–1 ✦ Blastospore or yeast cells. Bs, Bud scar; Cw, Mannan-glucan cell wall; Er, endoplasmic reticulum; G, Golgi complex; L, lipid granule; Mt, mitochondria; N, nucleus; Nm, nuclear membrane; V, vacuole.

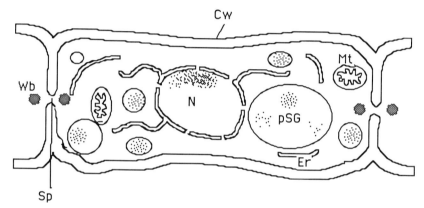

FIGURE 23–2 ✦ Hyphal unit of septate mycelium. pSG, Polysaccharide granule; Sp, septal pore; Wb, Woronin body. See legend of Figure 23–1 for other symbols.

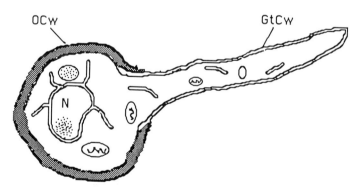

FIGURE 23–3 ✦ Germ tube formation from blastospore. OCw, Old cell wall; GtCw, newly synthesized cell wall delimiting germ tube.

mary septum is formed by the centripetal growth of the chitin ring separating the parent from progeny cells. Secondary septa compositionally similar to the cell wall are then synthesized on both sides of the primary septum. If the cells separate, the primary septum remains with the mother cell and can be identified on the surface as a *bud scar*. In instances in which there is no separation of cells, continuous rounds of budding may give rise to a cell chain or *pseudohypha*.

Mycelial Growth Patterns

Hyphal cells elongate by a process called *apical extension*. If the cells are partitioned by septa, de novo synthesis of cross-wall and nuclear division are coordinated with the growth of the apical tip. Hyphal cells can differentiate into *conidia* (sing. *conidium*) by a diversity of ontogenic processes, which result in the formation of a reproductive unit that, in many instances, is able to survive harsh environmental conditions. Conidiogenesis in fungi

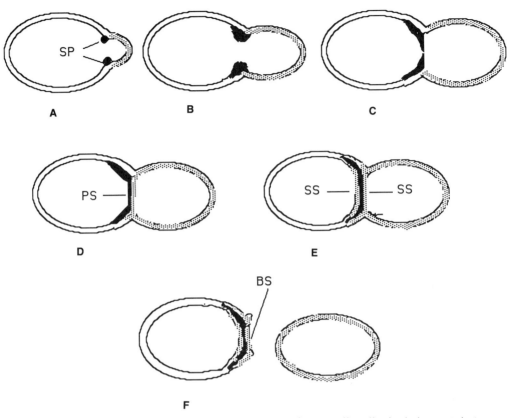

FIGURE 23–4 ✦ Synthesis of chitin *(black areas)* and new cell wall *(shaded areas)* during cell division in budding yeasts. SP, Septal primordia; PS, primary septum; SS, secondary septum; BS, bud scar.

is a highly varied developmental sequence. Some hyphal cells, by a process analogous or identical to bud formation, can give rise to yeastlike *blastospores,* and in some mycelia this type of cell may become the numerically dominant morphotype. When some molds are growing on solid substrate, an elaborate variety of stalklike conidiophoric structures can be observed. Growth on solid substrates can also elicit the differentiation of root-like structures called *haustoria,* which can anchor the mycelium to the underlying surface.

SEXUAL REPRODUCTION

Gametic fusion, a process that defines eukaryotic sex, has only been observed in some of the fungi identified as human pathogens. In the forms with no apparent sexual component in the life cycle *(anamorphs),* genetic variation is sustained by mitotic recombinational mechanisms *(parasexual reproduction).* The basic requirements for the more conventional pattern are fulfilled in a variety of ways. First, two compatible haploid nuclei are juxtaposed in the same cytoplasm *(plasmogamy).* This is followed by nuclear fusion *(karyogamy)* and a meiotic division sequence to yield four or more

haploid progeny nuclei, which can be partitioned into cells that differentiate as *sexual* spores (Fig. 23–5). A number of complex variations of this fundamental sequence have evolved. In some forms there are discernible differences between gametes, while in others any somatic nucleus can assume the role of gamete. In some species, gametic fusion occurs only between cells from distinct organisms *(thalli).* In many of these kinds of situations, specialized structures are available to promote interthallic contact. Temporal phases of sexual cycles are also variable. In many fungi, karyogamy may not immediately follow plasmogamy. In fact, a multinucleate thallus may be produced consisting entirely of binucleate cells *(dikaryons)* and the dikaryophase may be the predominant state in the life cycle of the fungus. In other forms, the thallus may consist of diploid cells resulting from an initial nuclear fusion, but without an ensuing postkaryogamic meiosis. The diplophase is the temporally significant state of the organism.

CLASSIFICATION OF FUNGI

Fungal evolution has appeared to diverge along two distinct phyletic lines, the *Myxomycota,* which

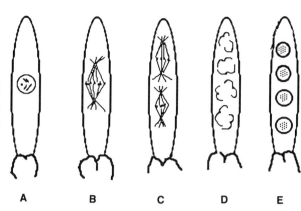

FIGURE 23–5 ✦ Meiotic lineage of sexual spores in ascogenous hypha. **A,** Diploid nucleus in ascus mother cell; **B,** anaphase I; **C,** anaphase II; **D,** initiation of ascospore differentiation; **E,** mature ascus with four ascospores.

A   B   C   D   E

include the slime molds, and the *Eumycota*, which includes all human pathogens and opportunistic fungi. The *Eumycota* can be further resolved into subcategories that reflect basic structural and physiologic disparities that are useful in identification. The *Zygomycetes* represent the simplest forms of the *Eumycota* and are nonseptate filaments that are capable of differentiating into spore bearing sacs, or *sporangia* (Fig. 23–6). The latter house asexual spores, in contrast to the *zygospore,* which in this class of fungi is formed as the result of gametic fusion. The fungi classified as *Ascomycetes* also produce asexual spores known as *conidia* and sexual spores designated *ascospores* because they are products of meiotic divisions that occur in *asci* (sing. *ascus*). Asci are enclosed in complex fruiting body type structures known as *ascocarps* (Fig. 23–7). Another clinically significant group of fungi is the *Basidiomycetes* group, characterized by their septate hyphae and a structure specialized for the formation of sexual spores—the *basidium.*

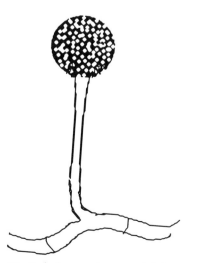

FIGURE 23–6 ✦ Sporangium containing asexual spores in *Rhizopus.*

LABORATORY IDENTIFICATION OF FUNGI

Many mycotic infections are easily diagnosed because the etiologic agents can be readily observed in clinical specimens such as skin scrapings, hair, sputum, and/or tissue biopsies. Hyphal elements and yeast cells can be discerned with simple stains if the clinical material is pretreated with a dilute solution of potassium hydroxide that removes the alkali-soluble debris. Most pathogenic fungi also can be easily propagated on simple selective media, a feature that facilitates their identification. The yeast and mycelial phases of some dimorphic species can be observed by propagating the organism at 23°C and 37°C.

MYCOSES WITH OROFACIAL MANIFESTATIONS

Because some fungal pathogens exhibit distinct histotropisms, mycoses can be classified as *superficial, cutaneous, subcutaneous,* or *systemic.* The latter usually are initiated as pulmonary infections with subsequent dissemination to other sites, which in several instances may include the orofacial region of the body. The major features of the more commonly encountered clinical entities will be outlined here.

Superficial Orofacial Mycoses

A small number of fungi, some commensalistic members of the flora of the skin, can reach population densities that result in chronic but asymptomatic infections. These kinds of mycoses are referred to as superficial, and in most instances these elicit minimal host responses. The affected sites are commonly the outer layers of the stratum corneum and cuticular surfaces of hair shafts. One of the more prevalent examples is *pityriasis versicolor,* a condition that appears as a discolored area of the torso and/or upper limbs, and that is believed to be associated with local overgrowth of either or

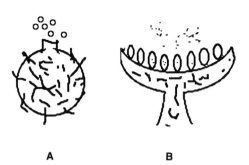

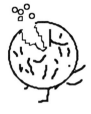

FIGURE 23–7 ✦ Ascocarp types. **A,** Perithecium; **B,** Cleistothecium; **C,** Apothecium.

A **B** **C**

both of two lipophilic yeasts, *Malassezia furfur* and *M. ovalis* (Fig. 23–8). Occasionally, the face, eyelids, and ears may be involved. Depigmentation of the affected area may occur especially in tropical climates. Another superficial infection, in which bearded regions of the face can often be involved, is *white piedra*. This condition represents colonization of hair shafts by *Trichosporon beigelii* (Fig. 23–9) and is distinguishable from *black piedra*, which is a mycosis primarily of scalp hair with a different etiologic agent *(Piedraia hortae)*. Very seldom is there discomfort with these infections and, except for their cosmetic impact, superficial mycoses represent minor clinical problems.

OROFACIAL DERMATOPHYTOSES

Keratinophilic fungi called *dermatophytes* are responsible for another clinical category of mycoses that also involve the skin, hair, and nails. This affinity for keratinized surfaces or structures, or both, reflects a convergent specialization of species from three major genera, *Microsporum, Trichophyton,* and *Epidermophyton,* and includes the elaboration of enzymes that permit the use of epithelial and connective tissue as substrates (e.g., keratinases, elastases, and collagenases). The infections are also referred to as *tineas (ringworm)* and, as might be expected, the one most frequently

encountered on orofacial surfaces is *tinea barbae,* ringworm of the beard. This dermatophytosis is usually associated with tissue colonization by *Trichophyton mentagrophytes* (Fig. 23–10). Deep pustular lesions, characteristic of the more severe form of the infection, are associated with *Trichophyton verrucosum*. Both of these dermatophytes can be identified by their morphologic and physiologic idiosyncrasies. *Microsporum canis* (Fig. 23–11), another significant dermatophyte, is often implicated in tineas of the eyebrow. Children appear to be more susceptible than adults to this form of dermatophytosis. Other dermatophytes, more frequently associated with tineas of other sites of the body, are capable of infecting orofacial tissue. These include *Trichophyton rubrum, Trichophyton concentricum,* and *Microsporum audounii*.

Subcutaneous Mycoses in Orofacial Tissue

Subcutaneous mycosis usually is the sequela of the implantation of fungus-contaminated material beneath the skin, as a result of a puncture wound or deep abrasion. Dissemination beyond the site of inoculation with these infections is rare and, if it does occur, is usually via lymphatic channels as opposed to more conventional hematogenous

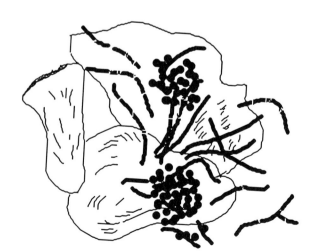

FIGURE 23–8 ✦ Skin scales infected with short-branched mycelia and yeast cells of *Malassezia furfur.*

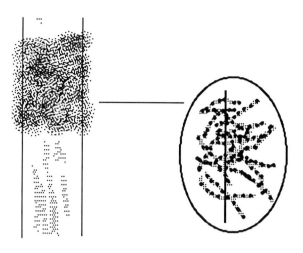

FIGURE 23–9 ✦ Hair shaft infected with arthro-conidia-enriched hyphae of *Trichosporon beigelli*.

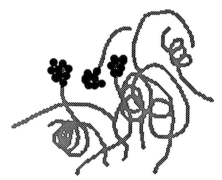

FIGURE 23–10 ✦ Globose microconidia and coiled hyphae of *Trichophyton mentagrophytes*.

routes. Three major pathologic entities frequently involving subcutaneous orofacial sites have been documented—sporotrichosis, entomophthoromycosis conidiobolae, and rhinosporidiosis.

SPOROTRICHOSIS

The etiologic agent for this mycosis is the dimorphic *Sporothrix schenckii* (Fig. 23–12), an organism usually associated with plants and/or plant-derived material such as timber or straw. Most of these orofacial infections result from being scratched by contaminated leaves, thorns, or twigs. The primary signs of infection are the appearance of nodules that become discolored (pink-purple-black) and regional adenopathy. If the lesions break through the overlying skin and become necrotic, they assume the characteristic form of sporotrichotic chancres, which may remain without resolution for weeks or months. Secondary lesions may develop in adjacent areas connected by lymph channels, especially if the primary chancre is not treated. Most infections of the face and neck, however, are of the "fixed" type—that is, they are restricted to the site of inoculation—and these rep-

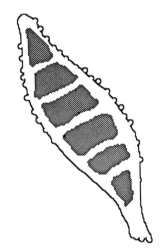

FIGURE 23–11 ✦ Macroconidium of *Microsporum canis*.

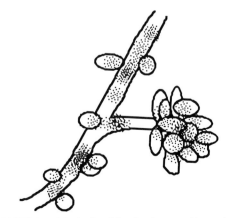

FIGURE 23–12 ✦ Conidiophoric mycelium of *Sporothrix schenkii*.

resent about 25 percent of human infections. Less frequent is involvement of mucous membranes (e.g., the mouth and pharynx), where the lesions may be ulcerative and painful and can be mistaken for aphthous ulcers, lichen planus, or other mycotic infections. All three kinds of infection can be chronic, with intermittent remissions. Spontaneous cure apparently does not occur. Successful treatment has been achieved by oral and/or topical administration of potassium iodide.

ENTOMOPHTHOROMYCOSIS CONIDIOBOLAE

The etiologic agent for this subcutaneous mycosis is a zygomycete, *Conidiobolus coronatus* (Fig. 23–13), which also infects arthropods but in humans exhibits a pronounced affinity for nasal submucosal tissue. The fungus is a soil saprophyte found in tropical and subtropical latitudes. Infection is thought to be initiated by implantation of contaminated insect parts or by abrasion with contaminated fingernails. Growth of the organism elicits a characteristic inflammatory reaction through which hyphal elements are ensheathed by large numbers of eosinophils *(Splendore-Hoeppli phenomenon)*. Macroscopically, a painless swelling develops around the inferior turbinates that can expand to cause occlusion of the nares and severe disfigurement. Overlying tissue may become erythematous and/or acanthotic but remains intact. Except for recalcitrant cases, most infections respond to potassium iodide chemotherapy.

RHINOSPORIDIOSIS

Another mycosis with a decided bias for the submucosa of the nose is rhinosporidiosis. A minority of cases involve the palpebral conjunctiva and constitute the "ocular" form of the disease. The putative causal organism, *Rhinosporidium seeberi*, is thought to be a primitive *Phycomycete* and appears to be an obligate parasite, as it has not been propagated in vitro. The etiologic association is therefore predicated on consistent histologic observations. It is assumed that the infection is initiated by a traumatic event that breaches the mucosal surface. The infectious unit is thought to be a "spore," about 6 to 10 µm in diameter, which enlarges in size to become a 200- to 300-µm sporangium containing numerous endospores generated by successive mitoses (Fig. 23–14). The endospores are believed to escape from mature spherules through a porelike rupture in the sporangial wall and to reinitiate the development cycle in adjacent tissue. Macroscopically a painless, vascularized, papillomatous mass develops as a reaction to the infection and in time can attain a size large enough to obstruct the nasal passage. Ocular lesions have similar histologic lineages and, when sufficiently enlarged, may cause tearing, lid eversion, and secondary conjunctival infections. Nasal infection is noted for its high endemicity in India and Sri Lanka, and this may be attributable to exposure to fungus-containing bodies of water. The ocular form of the disease is more prevalent in arid regions where dust storms occur. Although only partly successful (there is a significant amount of recurrent infection), surgical removal of affected tissue remains the optimal method of control.

Orofacial Complications in Systemic Mycoses

The fungi responsible for systemic infections are usually classified as either "true pathogens," which are inherently virulent, or "opportunistic," that initiate disease in hosts with abrogated defense mechanisms. The group with intrinsic pathogenicity is represented by four species: *Histoplasma capsulatum, Coccidioides immitis, Blastomyces dermatitidis,* and *Paracoccidioides brasiliensis.* The primary infection produced by these pathogens is usually pulmonary, but disseminated forms of the diseases with orofacial involvement are quite common. Species of the genera *Candida, Mucor,* and *Rhizopus* are most frequently implicated in the etiology of mycoses in patients who are immunocompromised and/or debilitated, and in several instances, the primary infection occurs at oropharyngeal sites.

HISTOPLASMOSIS

The causal agent of this mycosis is an ascomycete with a well-documented teleomorphic (sexual) state *(Emmonsiella capsulata),* but it is the conidia from the anamorphic phase *(H. capsulatum)* that are the major vectors in the transmission of this disease. Conidiophoric mycelia (Fig. 23–15) of this organism flourish in nitrogen-enriched soil (especially with bird and bat droppings) and both micro- and macroconidia serve as infectious units because they can be easily aerosolized and inhaled. Inhaled conidia are phagocytosed by al-

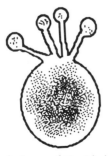

FIGURE 23–13 ✦ Spore of *Conidiobolus coronatus* with papillalike appendages.

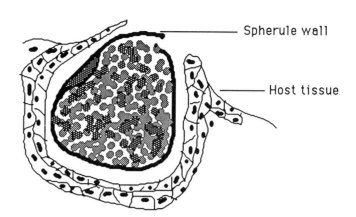

FIGURE 23–14 ✦ Endospore-filled spherule (sporangium) of *Rhinosporidium seeberi*.

veolar macrophages and proliferate as yeasts in host cells. This temperature-dependent, morphologic transition is also observed with some other fungal pathogens when translocated from a saprophytic environment to the cytoplasm of mammalian cells. In a substantial majority of instances, infection elicits a benign, localized, inflammatory reaction that may be roentgenographically discernible because it calcifies upon healing. This type of finding and a positive histoplasmin skin test reaction are usually the only evidence of exposure to the fungus. This is particularly true in endemic areas. On the other hand, if large numbers of conidia are inhaled a more extensive and decidedly symptomatic course may ensue with fever and respiratory impairment *(acute pulmonary histoplasmosis)*. The disease may become chronic and such situations enhance the possibility of dissemination via the reticuloendothelial system. Immunologic insufficiencies also predispose patients to disseminated histoplasmosis. Painful oropharyngeal ulcers appear in many individuals with the disseminated forms of the disease. As is the case with most systemic mycoses, amphotericin B adminis-

tered intravenously in monitored amounts is effective, particularly when there is a potentially fatal fulminating infection in young children.

COCCIDIOIDOMYCOSIS

Endemic in areas characterized by dry alkaline soils (e.g., the desert zones of the Southwest United States), *Coccidioides immitis* is a dimorphic fungus with an arthroconidium (Fig. 23–16) that is easily dispersed and small enough (3 to 6 μm) to be directly deposited onto alveolar surfaces. Postinhalation sequelae include phagocytosis by neutrophils as well as macrophages. The engulfed organism may then differentiate into a thick-walled spherule (30 to 60 μm) in which large numbers of endospores arise by successive cell divisions. The mature endospore (2 to 5 μm) is released by rupture of the spherule. In most individuals the infection is limited at this stage because endospores appear to be quite vulnerable to innate fungicidal mechanisms and the typical histologic response is a granuloma with empty spherules and nonviable endospores surrounded by eosinophilic material. Endospores that survive, however, can perpetuate the

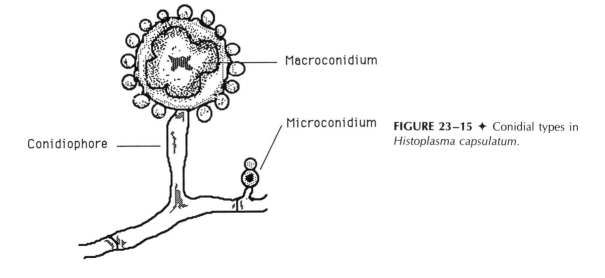

FIGURE 23–15 ✦ Conidial types in *Histoplasma capsulatum*.

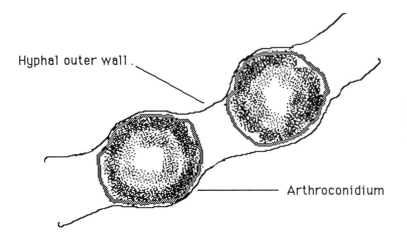

Hyphal outer wall

Arthroconidium

FIGURE 23–16 ✦ Segment arthroconidia-enriched mycelium of *Coccidiodes immitis.*

spherule-endospore cycle. Coccidioidin sensitivity, as revealed by intradermal injection of antigenic extracts, is often the only other indication of exposure to the organism in asymptomatic infections. More extensive involvement is characterized by fever, chest pain, and anorexia. In some individuals, symptomatic infection also elicits erythemas. Affected orofacial tissue indicates disseminated disease, and crusted granulomatous lesions on nose and face are the common manifestations of this advanced stage of the mycosis. Amphotericin B still prevails as the treatment of choice in severe cases.

BLASTOMYCOSIS

All instances of blastomycosis begin as an alveolitis following inhalation of conidia from *Blastomyces dermatitidis* (Fig. 23–17), the anamorph phase of an ascomycete, *Ajellomyces dermatitidis.* The habitat of the conidiogenic morphotype is still not precisely known because it is difficult consistently to isolate the organism from soil and fomites even in highly endemic areas. In vivo the predominant cell types are phagocytosed yeasts. Neutrophils appear to play a growth-promoting role in the course of the infection. The severity of pulmonary involvement can range from a small, well-healed fibrotic scar with mild symptoms to unresolved progressive blastomycosis entailing acute bronchopneumonia and pleuritis. The most common symptom of blastomycosis, however, is the skin lesion, which in turn reflects how easily the organism is disseminated to extrapulmonary sites. In fact, about half of the individuals with discernible symptoms have only cutaneous disease. Foci of organisms first appear in subcutaneous nodules, which become pustular and then ulcerate. The lips, tongue, and buccal mucosa, in addition to facial and nasal areas, are often affected, and in time the lesions evolve into characteristic verrucous granulomas. The latter may persist for months and con-

tain yeast-type cells varying from 8 to 15 μm in diameter. Serologic assays for diagnostic purposes are still equivocal for *B. dermatitidis,* primarily because the organism shares antigens with other pathogenic fungi. Amphotericin B and hydroxystilbamine have been successfully used to treat blastomycoses.

PARACOCCIDIOIDOMYCOSIS

Until recently, paracoccidioidomycosis was restricted to Latin America. Because of the large, recent influx of immigrants from endemic areas, this disease is now appearing in North America. The etiologic organism, *Paracoccidioides brasiliensis,* like other mycopathogens, is thermally dimorphic, with inhaled conidia producing a primary infection in the lungs and then phagocytosed yeast cells disseminating to form secondary infective foci in the mucosa of the mouth and nose. The lesions in these areas initiate in submucosal lymph nodes and extend upward, developing into ulcerative granuloma. The formation of multiple buds (2 to 5 μm) from a single parent cell (15 to 40 μm) is typical of the yeast phase in this fungus (Fig. 23–18). A relatively reliable immunodiffusion assay

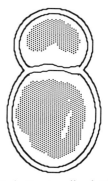

FIGURE 23–17 ✦ Yeast cell of *Blastomyces dermatitidis* with broad-based bud.

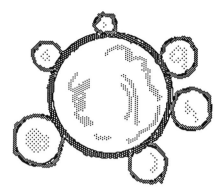

FIGURE 23–18 ✦ Multiple bud formation in *Paracoccidiodes brasiliensis.*

is available for antigens of *P. brasiliensis* and is useful for prognosis. Paracoccidioidomycosis is now treated with ketoconazole, although amphotericin B has been very effective in the past.

Orofacial Mycoses in Compromised Individuals

Endocrinopathy and immunodeficiency constitute physiologic states that are conducive to serious and often life-threatening infections by fungi that either are part of the commensalistic human flora or are ubiquitous members of the human environment. Organisms with this potential have been designated as "opportunistic" pathogens, and two groups of fungi are frequently associated with orofacial infections in this context.

CANDIDIASIS

Several "species" of the unnatural genus *Candida* are responsible for the spectrum of mycoses that can be included in this disease complex. The most frequently implicated representative is *C. albicans,* which has only been found in the anamorphic state and appears to be obligately associated with homeothermic animals. Candidiases attributable to *C. tropicalis, C. parapsilosis, C. pseudotropicalis,* and *C. stellatoidea* have been documented. Ordinarily harmless residents of mucous membranes, most *Candida* cells proliferate as budding yeasts (3 to 6 μM), and hyphae are rare. When the epithelium is breached by trauma or hormonally altered, however, invasion of submucosal tissue can occur, and in many instances there is significant conversion to hyphal growth (Fig. 23–19). In and around the mouth, two major kinds of infection are encountered. The most common of these, *thrush,* presents as a subepithelial invasion of lingual and buccal surfaces by the organism with the formation of a white opaque *pseudomembrane.* In infants the disease is often acquired from mothers with vaginal candidiasis. In older patients contributing circumstances are often intake of broad-spectrum antibiotics or immunosuppressive substances that reduce the level of commensalistic bacteria. Denture stomatitis is often accompanied by increments of oral populations of *Candida,* but a causal relationship has not been unequivocally established. Individuals with some T-cell aberrations are predisposed to *chronic mucocutaneous candidiasis,* characterized by widespread hyperplastic outgrowths that are particularly disfiguring when incurred on the face. Onset of the disease early in life suggests inherited defects in cell-mediated immunity. Thymomas are frequently associated with the condition in older patients. Hypothyroidism and hypovitaminoses have also been linked to susceptibility. An immunodiffusion assay of cytoplasmic antigens has been adopted as a useful serologic tool in candidiasis. Topical application of polyene as well as imidazole antifungal agents has been successful in treatment of thrush. A similar chemotherapeutic record does not exist for the chronic mucocutaneous form, but recent trials with the Lawrence transfer factor administration are promising.

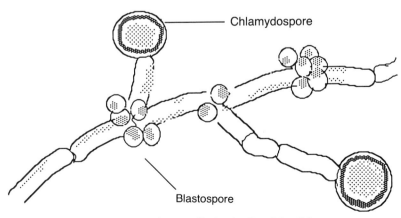

FIGURE 23–19 ✦ Myceliation in *Candida albicans.*

MUCORMYCOSIS

Species of three major genera, *Rhizopus, Absidia,* and *Mucor,* can be responsible for severe and often fatal infections caused by the rapid proliferation and invasion of blood vessels with nonseptate hyphal cells from these types of fungi. Diabetics prone to episodes of ketoacidosis, burn patients, patients with leukemia, and malnourished or immunosuppressed individuals are at greatest risk. The form that involves the nose and palate—rhinocerebral mucormycosis—usually results from the inhalation of sporangiospores that germinate on the nasal epithelium. Mortality approaches 90 percent. The particular susceptibility of patients with diabetes may be related to ability of many of the pathogens (especially *Rhizopus*) to elaborate ketoreductases and grow rapidly in the presence of high levels of glucose. Serologic parameters are of little value in mucormycosis. Intravenous administration of amphotericin B and debridement of infected tissue is currently indicated as a treatment regimen.

BIBLIOGRAPHY
General Mycology

Diamond, R. D.: The growing problem of mycoses in patients infected with human immunodeficiency virus. Rev. Infect. Dis. 13:480, 1991.

Murphy, J. W.: Mechanisms of natural resistance to human pathogenic fungi. Ann. Rev. Microbiol. 45:509, 1991.

Rippon, J. W.: Medical Mycology, ed. 3. W. B. Saunders, Philadelphia, 1988.

Superficial Mycoses

Cohn, M. S.: Superficial fungal infections. Topical and oral treatment of common types. Postgrad. Med. 91:239, 249, 1992.

Dermatophytoses

Calderon, R. A.: Immunoregulation of dermatophytosis. Crit. Rev. Microbiol. 16:339, 1989.

Tagami, H., Kudoh, K., and Takematsu, H.: Inflammation and immunity in dermatophytosis. Crit. Rev. Micriobiol. 16:339, 1989.

Subcutaneous Mycoses

Belknap, B. S.: Sporotrichosis. Dermatol. Clin. 7:193, 1989.

Tnianprasit, M., Thagernpol, K.: Rhinosporidiosis. Curr. Top. Med. Mycol. 3:64, 1989.

Systemic Mycoses

Bronnimann, D. A., Galgiani, N.: Coccidiomycosis. Eur. J. Clin. Microbiol. Infect. Dis. 8:466, 1989.

Davies, S. F. and Sarosi, G. A.: Blastomycosis. Eur. J. Clin. Microbiol. Infect. Dis. 8:474, 1989.

de Almeida, O. P., Jorge, J., Scully, C., and Bozzo, L.: Oral manifestations of paracoccidiomycosis (South American blastomycosis). Oral Surg. Oral Med. Oral Pathol. 72:430, 1991.

de Almeida, O. P. and Scully, C.: Oral lesions in the systemic mycoses. Curr. Opin. Dent. 1:423, 1991.

Eissenberg, L. G. and Goldman, W. E.: *Histoplasma* variation and adaptive strategies for parasitism: New perspectives on histoplasmosis. Clin. Microbiol. Rev. 4:411, 1991.

Odds, F. C.: *Candida* and Candidiasis, ed. 2. University Park Press, Baltimore, 1990.

Rinaldi, M. G.: Zygomycosis. Infect Dis. Clin. North Am. 3:19, 1989.

24 *Parasitology*

Philip T. LoVerde

In this chapter the two organisms that inhabit the oral cavity, *Entamoeba gingivalis* and *Trichomonas tenax,* are presented. In fact, they are not parasites but commensals normally found subgingivally and interproximally in a low percentage of healthy individuals. Most often these two organisms are associated with periodontal disease and caries and thus are an indication of poor oral hygiene.

Another group of organisms is presented in this chapter because it is associated with patients with acquired immune deficiency syndrome (AIDS) and its transmission to humans is through the oral ingestion of fecally contaminated material containing the infective stage of the parasite. In particular, transmission in homosexual males is due to oral-anal contact. An understanding of the biology and pathogenesis of these organisms will allow the dentist to evaluate accurately the risks of treating these patients. It is hoped that this will dispel some unfounded fears associated with treating AIDS patients or homosexual males.

Entamoeba gingivalis inhabits the oral cavity. This ameboid organism is a commensal and is cosmopolitan in distribution. Only the trophozoite stage has been described. Transmission is by direct contact (mouth to mouth). The trophozoite is 10 to 35 μm in diameter. The organism produces pseudopodia and behaves like a phagocyte. It contains a nucleus with a centrally located endosome. *E. gingivalis* is not a pathogen but is associated with periodontal disease, calculus around teeth, and caries. Approximately 10 percent of people with healthy mouths harbor *E. gingivalis,* whereas

more than 90 percent of people with oral disease harbor these organisms.

Trichomonas tenax inhabits the oral cavity. The flagellated organism (7 × 3 μm) is a commensal that appears to have a cosmopolitan distribution. The trophozoite is the only known stage. Transmission is by direct contact (mouth to mouth). The trophozoite has four anterior free flagella of equal length, a relatively short undulating membrane, and a slender axostyle that protrudes a distance beyond the posterior end of the body. The organism is associated with periodontal disease, calculus around teeth, and caries. It is not pathogenic, but its presence indicates poor oral hygiene.

ENTAMOEBA HISTOLYTICA

E. histolytica is the etiologic agent in amebiasis or amebic dysentery. This ameba is one of six species associated with humans. *E. histolytica* and *Dientamoeba fragilis* are pathogenic; the other four species are commensals. With the exception of *E. gingivalis,* which is found in the oral cavity, they all inhabit the intestine.

Morphology and Life Cycle

E. histolytica has two stages in its life cycle: trophozoite and cyst (Fig. 24–1). Both stages are found in the feces; only trophozoites invade the tissues.

The trophozoite (the vegetative stage), which inhabits the large intestine and is capable of invading the tissues of the body, varies from 12 to

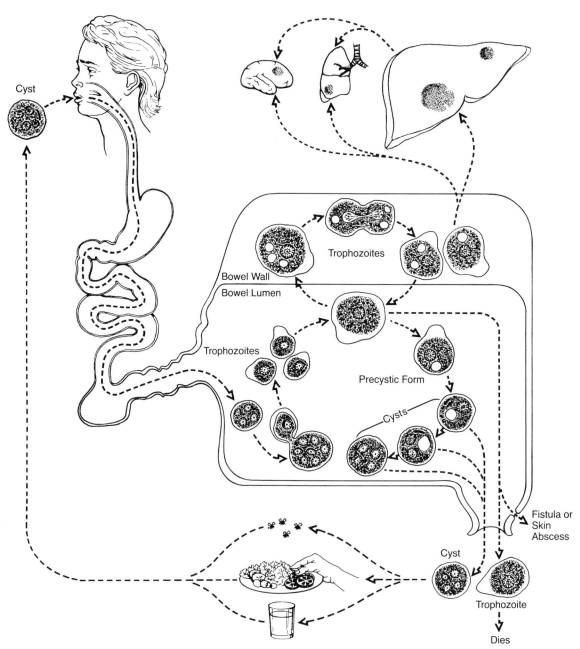

FIGURE 24–1 ✦ Trophozoite and cyst stages of *Entamoeba histolytica*.

30 μm in diameter. It has a finely granular endoplasm that is sharply separated from the clear ectoplasm, and appears with a grayish tinge when observed under the microscope. Pseudopodia can be seen during movement. The single nucleus, which is used in distinguishing one species from the others, is spherical with an evenly distributed chromatin that is finely granular around its periphery and contains a centrally located dense spherical chromatin body, the karyosome. The trophozoite is anaerobic and multiplies by binary fission. The

cytoplasm contains food vacuoles that may contain host cells (e.g., red blood cells). The cyst stage, which is important in transmission, measures 5 to 20 μm in diameter. The mature cyst contains four nuclei, each identical in morphology to the nucleus of the trophozoite. As the cyst forms, the cytoplasm may contain chromatoid bodies that are diagnostically rod-shaped. Chromatoid bodies are not seen in the mature cyst. The mature cyst is the infective stage for humans. The cyst, which is passed in the feces, is surrounded by a protective covering that allows the parasite to resist dehydration, disinfectants, temperature changes, and gastric juices. The ingested cyst passes through the stomach and excysts in the small intestine. The quadrinucleated parasite undergoes nuclear division, giving rise to an eight-nucleated organism. The cytoplasm divides to produce eight uninucleate amebae. Intestinal stasis often enables the amebae to establish the site of infection in the cecal area of the colon. They begin to colonize the intestine by division. As stool containing parasites is passed down the intestine, the absorption of fluid triggers the trophozoite to expel its food vacuoles and undergo cyst formation. As an immature cyst, the nucleus, divides to give rise to a binucleate organism, the rod-shaped chromatoid bodies may appear. Each nucleus divides again, the chromatoid bodies disappear, the cyst wall forms, and the mature infective cyst is passed to the outside environment.

E. histolytica often behaves as a commensal inhabiting the lumen of the colon. The ability of *E. histolytica* to cause disease is, in part, determined by the environment of the gut. Individuals on a low-protein, high-carbohydrate diet have more amebae in the intestine. The species of bacteria present also influences pathogenicity, apparently by creating a reducing environment favorable for amebic growth.

Pathogenesis and Symptomatology

There are two forms of clinical manifestations: intestinal and extraintestinal (Fig. 24–1).

E. histolytica are able to quickly colonize the cecal and sigmoid-rectal areas of the intestine, where the colonic flow is slow. As they divide, the amebae release cytolytic enzymes that cause cell lysis. Cytolysis can also be caused by a cell contact–dependent mechanism. In either instance, release of cell juices induces amebic division. The progeny invade and advance the lesion as they divide. The first lesion appears as a button-hole ulceration (a small nodular elevation with a minute opening) in the intestinal mucosa. The increasing colony of amebae usually proceeds to the base of the more resistant muscularis and then spreads laterally to form a vase-shaped or crateriform ulceration. If this primary lesion is not complicated by accompanying bacteria, there is no host reaction (inflammation) to the invading amebae. Secondary bacterial invasion accounts for most of the clinical symptoms. The intestinal involvement can be localized or extensive and is classified as an ulcerative colitis. Destruction of tissue is followed by regenerative proliferation of connective tissue, which in cases of extensive damage may ultimately cause a fibrous thickening of the intestinal wall. From the submucosa, the amebae can extend into the muscularis and perforate the serosa, resulting in peritonitis. Amebae can extend to the diaphragm and enter the pleural cavity and lungs as well. Cutaneous amebiasis results from invasion of perianal tissue or genitalia. The cecal and sigmoid-rectal areas are those in which a majority of the lesions are found. In any lesion, *E. histolytica* inhabits only the perimeter of the necrotic tissue because the amebae feed only on living tissue.

When they occur, symptoms may be insidious, with vague abdominal discomfort or soft stools for a variable period and constipation alternating with mild diarrhea, or they may be abrupt with cramps, abdominal pain, diarrhea, and fever. There may be as many as 15 to 20 stools per day, resulting in dehydration. Stools are often bloody and contain mucus and sloughed tissue. The patient usually does not suffer the acute systemic intoxication seen in bacillary dysentery.

Extraintestinal amebiasis occurs when amebae invade mesenteric capillaries or venules and metastasize to other parts of the body, usually the liver. The amebae can be carried to any tissue or organ in the body (e.g., heart, lungs, kidneys, brain). The extraintestinal lesion, except in the case of cutaneous spread, is always secondary to intestinal involvement. The extraintestinal amebic lesion is caused by trophozoites that have lodged in a tissue and proceeded to colonize producing necrosis of surrounding host cells manifesting as a sterile abscess.

Patients with hepatic abscesses usually present with fever, an enlarged, tender liver, bulging in the right upper portion of the abdomen, and frequently pain in the right pleura radiating to the right shoulder.

Diagnosis and Treatment

Intestinal amebiasis must always be considered in any patient with protracted diarrhea and in all patients with dysentery. In cases of dysentery, it is important to differentiate bacterial from amebic etiologies because the latter may result in extraintestinal disease.

For intestinal amebiasis, one needs to demonstrate the parasite (trophozoite or cyst stage) in feces. A diagnosis cannot be reliably made on clinical evidence alone.

Identification of parasites in stool specimens requires fresh specimens to be examined by experienced personnel. Often multiple stool examinations are required to make a diagnosis. Purgatives (e.g., phosphate of soda) are used to obtain fresh samples. Typical stool from a patient with amebic dysentery will have exudates, mucus, blood, and cellular debris mixed with the feces. The amebae will most likely be found in the part of the stool containing the exudates, blood, and cellular debris.

Serologic tests such as indirect hemagglutination, ELISA, and countercurrent immunoelectrophoresis are helpful in diagnosis.

Diagnosis of extraintestinal amebiasis is made by a combination of serology and radiology, ultrasound, or radionuclide tests. Biopsy of the edge of the abscess may be helpful. Often patients with extraintestinal abscess show no history suggestive of amebic colitis, which makes the diagnosis more difficult.

The methods of treatment vary with the clinical type of amebiasis. No one treatment is ideal. Each drug carries with it certain contraindications. In severe amebic dysentery, the primary objective in treatment is to stop the dysentery and then to cure the infection. The drug of choice is metronidazole. Emetine hydrochloride and dehydroemetine are also given. With either of the latter two drugs, which arrest the dysentery, an amebicidal drug such as diiodohydroxyquin is also administered. With all treatments, antibiotics are also given to control symptoms due to bacterial invasion of the intestinal lesions. Several drugs, including diloxanide furoate and diiodohydroxyquin, provide good cure rates in nondysenteric intestinal amebiasis.

In the United States all asymptomatic patients should be treated. In endemic countries, usually only symptomatic patients are treated, partially because of the frequency of reinfection and the high incidence of infected patients who are asymptomatic.

For extraintestinal abscesses, metronidazole, emetine, or chloroquine, or a combination of the three, is recommended. Aspiration of the abscess may be necessary for cure.

Epidemiology and Control

E. histolytica has a worldwide distribution. Some 400 million people, approximately 10 percent of the world's population, are afflicted. In the United States there is a 4 percent incidence. Thirty-six million people have severe colitis or extraintestinal involvement. Approximately 75,000 people die each year. Infections are more prevalent and the intensity of infection more severe in tropical and subtropical climates than in temperate zones. People of all races and ages and of both sexes appear to be equally susceptible to infection. In the United States, the high-risk populations include (1) sexually active homosexual males, (2) residents of institutions, (3) travelers to endemic areas, (4) immigrants from endemic areas, (5) migrant workers, and (6) the lower socioeconomic class in the southern United States.

Transmission is fecal-oral. Therefore, food handlers, contaminated food (vegetables), and water with viable cysts and flies as mechanical vectors are common modes of transmission. Among homosexuals, anal-oral sex is the mode of transmission. In homosexuals, lesions occur in the oral cavity and on the genitalia owing to direct transmission of trophozoites. The cyst, however, is normally responsible for transmission.

Control of amebiasis results from improvements in sanitation and hygiene. In particular, the proper treatment of night soil is necessary to destroy cysts before it is used as fertilizer.

GIARDIA LAMBLIA

Giardia lamblia is a flagellated parasite that has a cosmopolitan distribution. It is the most prevalent clinical infection caused by a protozoan in the United States today.

Morphology and Life Cycle

G. lamblia has a trophozoite and cyst stage (Fig. 24–2). The trophozoite measures 9 to 20 μm in length by 7 to 15 μm in width and is 2 to 4 μm thick. The trophozoite appears pear-shaped, broadly rounded anteriorly, and tapered to a point posteriorly. On its ventral surface are two adhesive disks for attachment to epithelial surfaces. The parasite has four pairs of flagella that function in locomotion. In the center of the organism is a rod-shaped organelle, the parabasal body. In the area of each adhesive disk there is a nucleus containing a centrally located karyosome. The trophozoite appears bilaterally symmetrical. Multiplication of this anaerobic organism is by longitudinal binary fission.

The oval cyst, which is important in transmisson, measures 9 to 12 μm long by 7 to 10 μm wide. The mature cyst contains four nuclei.

The cyst stage is ingested and excysts in the small intestine. Each cyst gives rise to two organisms that begin to multiply and colonize the upper two thirds of the small intestine. The trophozoites are not invasive. Instead they attach to the epithelial brush border by their powerful adhesive disks, and in a few days many millions pave the epithelium. As the intestine moves feces containing trophozoites into the large intestine, the parasite forms a cyst that is passed to the outside environment. The cyst is the infective form of the parasite and is seen in formed stools. Trophozoites are observed only in watery stools during diarrhea.

Pathogenesis and Symptomatology

G. lamblia infections are usually asymptomatic but occasionally cause protracted diarrhea or malabsorption. The parasites opposed to the brush border irritate the mucosa causing catarrhal inflam-

Giardiasis

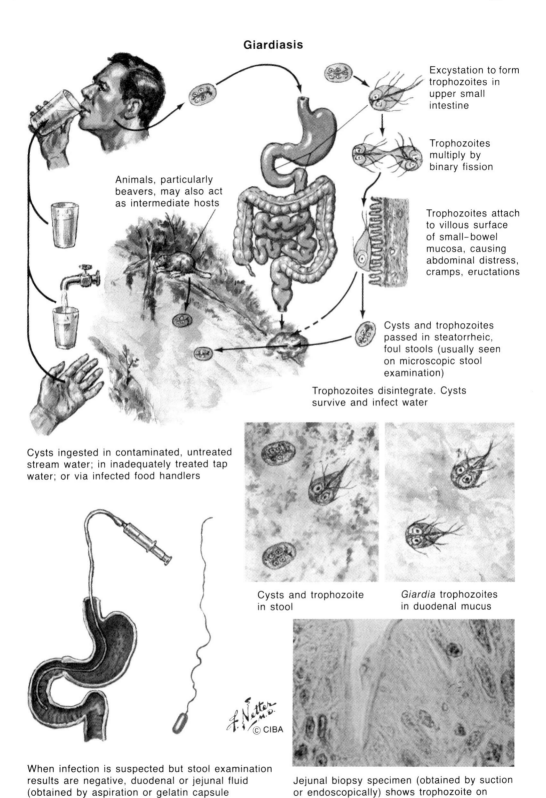

Excystation to form trophozoites in upper small intestine

Trophozoites multiply by binary fission

Trophozoites attach to villous surface of small-bowel mucosa, causing abdominal distress, cramps, eructations

Animals, particularly beavers, may also act as intermediate hosts

Cysts and trophozoites passed in steatorrheic, foul stools (usually seen on microscopic stool examination)

Trophozoites disintegrate. Cysts survive and infect water

Cysts ingested in contaminated, untreated stream water; in inadequately treated tap water; or via infected food handlers

Cysts and trophozoite in stool

Giardia trophozoites in duodenal mucus

When infection is suspected but stool examination results are negative, duodenal or jejunal fluid (obtained by aspiration or gelatin capsule with string) should be examined

Jejunal biopsy specimen (obtained by suction or endoscopically) shows trophozoite on villous surface of mucosa

FIGURE 24–2 ✦ Trophozoite and cyst stages of *Giardia lamblia*. (Copyright 1984. CIBA Pharmaceutical Company, a division of CIBA-GEIGY. Reproduced with permission from Clinical Symposia—by Frank H Netter, M.D. All rights reserved.)

mation. This can lead to diarrhea that can be mild to intensive and debilitating when the stools become watery and voluminous with 40 million parasites passed per day. Untreated, the diarrhea may last for months with exacerbations and remissions occurring. Symptoms consist of epigastric pain, abdominal cramps, flatulence, steatorrhea, and foul-smelling stools containing large amounts of mucus. There may be weight loss, dehydration, and fatigue. In young children a malabsorption syndrome caused by atrophy of microvilli of the brush border and mechanical blockage of absorption of fats may result. Often vitamin A deficiency results. Clinically children are more seriously affected than adults; in adults infections are usually self-limiting. Secretory IgA appears to play an important role in pathogenesis. IgA-deficient patients develop more severe infections.

Diagnosis and Treatment

Diagnosis is based on demonstrating the parasite in stool samples—most often the cyst stage in formed stools, but sometimes the trophozoite stage in liquid stools. It often takes multiple stool examinatons to make a diagnosis. Duodenal aspirates and a string test, a technique for sampling the duodenal mucosal surface, are also used in diagnosis. There are no routine serologic tests available. In the United States today one must consider giardiasis in any case of protracted diarrhea. Treatment is with quinacrine hydrochloride (Atabrine), with metronidazole, or with furazolidone. In severe cases supportive treatment is also recommended. All patients with *Giardia* infection, including asymptomatic carriers, should be treated.

Epidemiology and Control

Infection with *Giardia* results from ingestion of cysts. Reservoir hosts such as dogs, beavers, and muskrats are responsible for contaminating streams and watershed areas. Backpackers drinking from mountain streams often acquire infections. Inhabitants of towns where there was a break in the water purification systems have become infected. Sporadic epidemics have been reported in day care centers, nurseries, and institutions. In homosexual populations, giardiasis is very prevalent. Giardiasis is endemic in certain areas of the United States.

Control is very difficult because *G. lamblia* cysts are very resistant to chlorination. Boiling water for 2 to 5 minutes is recommended. Measures to prevent fecal-oral transmission apply.

TOXOPLASMA GONDII

Toxoplasma gondii is an obligate intracellular parasite that has evolved a very complex life cycle.

It is found in a large number of mammals including humans. The parasite is cosmopolitan in its host range and ubiquitous in its distribution.

Morphology and Life Cycle

In humans, two forms of the parasite are found: The trophozoite (tachyzoite), usually seen during acute proliferative infection, and the pseudocyst (containing bradyzoites), found during chronic or latent infecton (Fig. 24–3). Reproduction is by an asexual process of internal budding termed endodyogeny. The trophozoites measure 3 to 6 μm in length. They are crescent- or banana-shaped, with one end more pointed than the other. The cysts that occur in chronic infection are formed when the parasites multiply and produce a wall within a host cell; hence the term "pseudocyst."

Toxoplasma is a coccidian parasite of the cat family Felidae. The parasite has evolved a life cycle that includes transmission by (1) oocysts shed in cat feces, (2) pseudocysts ingested in improperly cooked meat, and (3) trophozoites involved in congenital transmission.

In the cat, the definitive host, the parasite infects the epithelial cells of the intestine. Here the parasite undergoes asexual reproduction (schizogony) and sexual reproduction (gametogony). The end result of sexual reproduction is the zygote, which protects itself with a resistant cell wall before elimination in the feces as an immature oocyst. Oocysts are approximately 9 μm in diameter. During primary infection, the cat sheds unsporulated oocysts for a period of 2 weeks. The freshly shed oocysts are not infective. However, after 3 to 4 days at 20°C to 22°C the zygote contained within the oocysts divides into two sporocysts, and four sporozoites are contained within each sporocyst. These sporulated oocysts are infective. They are relatively resistant to a variety of chemicals and will remain infective in the soil for at least 1 year.

Oocysts ingested by transport hosts (earthworms, snails, arthropods, birds) are spread throughout the environment. If ingested by humans or other mammals (including herbivores), the oocysts release the sporozoites in the intestine. They rapidly penetrate the intestinal wall, are phagocytized by macrophages, and are distributed throughout the body. Inside the macrophages, the parasites (tachyzoites) reproduce at the expense of the host cell. The parasites are not destroyed by the macrophage microbicidal mechanisms, in part because the parasite is able to prevent the fusion of lysosomes with the vacuole containing them. As the parasite numbers increase, the cell lyses, releasing tachyzoites, which are able to penetrate any cell in the body (including red blood cells). During this acute phase, any tissue or organ in the body can be infected with *Toxoplasma* parasites. With

Toxoplasma gondii

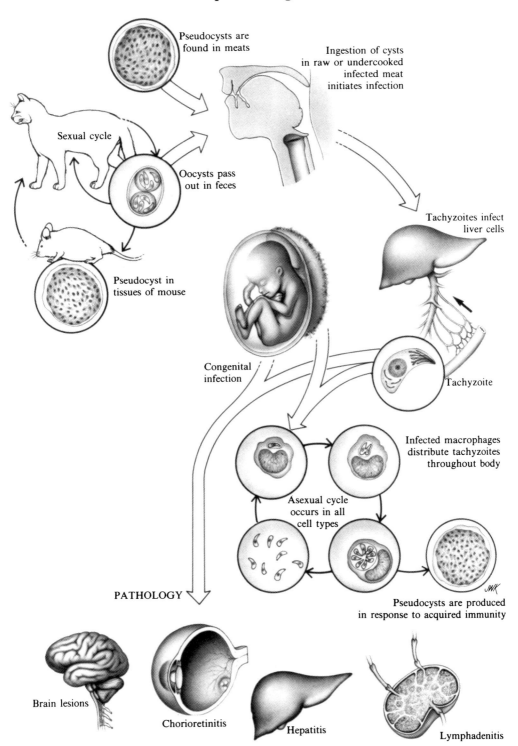

FIGURE 24–3 ✦ Life cycle of *Toxoplasma gondii*. (From Katz, M., Despommier, D. D. and Gwadz, R. W.: Parasitic Diseases. Springer-Verlag, New York, 1982, with permission. Illustration by John W. Karapelou.)

the appearance of antibody, the parasites remain in infected cells, forming pseudocysts. Each pseudocyst contains hundreds of infectious units (bradyzoites) that can be liberated when immunity wanes (e.g., during immunosuppression) or when ingested by a naive host. Humans can acquire *Toxoplasma* infection by ingesting pseudocysts in the flesh of improperly cooked meat. This route of transmission is very common among carnivores. The life cycle in humans is the same as described earlier when oocysts are ingested. A third form of transmission is congenital. If pregnant women in their second or third trimester acquire a primary infection in which there is a parasitemia, parasites can cross the placenta and multiply in the tissues of the fetus, causing serious damage. Infection acquired before pregnancy induces immunity and prevents congenital transmission.

Pathogenesis and Symptomatology

The large numbers of humans with serum antibodies to *Toxoplasma* suggest that most infections are asymptomatic. The most seriously affected are newborns who acquire the infection transplacentally, usually from an asymptomatic mother. Approximately 40 percent of infants born of females acquiring *Toxoplasma* infection during pregnancy show signs of disease. At birth or shortly thereafter, these infants commonly have evidence of retinochoroiditis, cerebral calcification, and occasionally hydrocephalus or microcephaly. Psychomotor disturbances are also common. Severe damage in the central nervous system, stillbirth, and abortion can occur.

Acquired infections are manifested by lymphadenitis, fever, headache, myalgia, and splenomegaly. The symptoms are often confused with those of infectious mononucleosis. However, since during acute infection the parasites can infect any cell in the body, inflammation can occur in any organ, in the form of myocarditis, pneumonitis, or encephalitis. Retinochoroiditis may result in some cases. Recrudescence in toxoplasmosis occurs when a patient with pseudocysts is immunosuppressed or immunocompromised. Clinically, this form of toxoplasmosis is identical to the acquired acute infection. *Toxoplasma* infection (cerebral toxoplasmosis) is a major cause of death in AIDS patients.

Diagnosis and Treatment

Specific diagnosis is made by serologic tests or demonstration of the organisms in tissues. Clinical symptoms alone are not sufficient to make the diagnosis. Serologic tests include the Sabin-Feldman dye test, the indirect fluorescent antibody (IFA) test, the ELISA test, the indirect hemagglutination test, and the complement fixation (CF) test. Serum titers for the Sabrin-Feldman dye test, IFA, and ELISA tests appear early in infection, reach a higher level, and drop much later than those obtained with the CF test. Occasionally diagnosis can be made from smears of biopsy material. However, in certain laboratories body fluids or ground tissue are inoculated into mice free of *Toxoplasma* and 7 to 10 days later their tissues examined for the proliferating parasite.

Patients with acute toxoplasmosis who appear normal may not require treatment. When treatment is required clindomycin plus sulfadiazine and pyrimethamine are recommended drugs; the last drug causes side effects.

In pregnant women with acute toxoplasmosis, the possibility of congenital infection must be considered; in some cases chemotherapy that is teratogenic or therapeutic abortion may be recommended.

Epidemiology and Control

The high prevalence of *Toxoplasma* in the human population (approximately half of the population in the United States) can be explained by the continuous exposure to the risk of infection by ingesting improperly cooked meat and ingestion of oocysts introduced in the environment by cats. As expected, prevalence of infection increases with age.

Congenital transmission accounts for relatively little of the high prevalence observed in humans. However, toxoplasmosis acquired by the mother during pregnancy (two to six cases per 1000 pregnancies in the United States) may result in severe or fatal damage to the fetus.

Immunocompromised individuals such as transplant patients and those with debilitating disease such as AIDS also account for those with serious disease.

Control measures are to cook meat (from sheep, cattle, and swine) properly. Freezing is not as dependable as adequate heating to destroy infectivity. The principal mode of transmission is by ingestion of oocysts shed into the environment in the feces of cats. These stages remain viable for 1 year and are a source of infection for mice, birds, and other prey that return the infections to cats. Protection of sandboxes where children play is advisable. A vaccine for cats, which has recently become available, has shown some success.

PNEUMOCYSTIS CARINII

Pneumocystis carinii is a ubiquitous parasite found in many species of mammals including humans. The organism maintains itself in an immune population, and clinical disease presents itself in those few who are immunosuppressed or immunologically compromised. *Pneumocystis* causes an interstitial plasma cell pneumonia. At one time, pneumocystis pneumonia was associated with newborns or individuals who were immunosuppressed by underlying disease or chemotherapy. Today, it is a well-known disease because of its association with acquired immune deficiency syndrome (AIDS).

Morphology and Life Cycle

P. carinii inhabits the lungs, where it is found in either the alveoli or the alveolar walls. The organism exists in two forms: as trophozoites and as cysts. The trophozoites, which are ameboid, range from 1 to 5 μm in size. They consist of a small nucleus surrounded by a mass of protoplasm, enclosed in a double-layered pellicle. Fine filopodia project from the trophozoite, apparently functioning like pili to facilitate attachment to one another and to the alveolar walls of the lungs. The cysts are 3.5 to 5 μm in diameter, with a thick wall. Within the cyst are typically found eight trophozoites, each 1 to 2 μm in size. The life cycle is unknown. It is thought that the cyst is the infective form and that transmission is more likely from human to human than from animal to human.

Pathogenesis and Symptomatology

The lungs, which appear grayish to tan, are firm and airless. Microscopically the alveoli are filled with a foamy, honeycomb material. Within this exudate are found various stages of parasite, histiocytes, lymphocytes, plasma cells, and cellular debris. In advanced cases, most of the alveoli are filled and the alveolar septa are thickened. The material in the alveoli persist with little phagocytosis or other inflammation, and expectoration is deficient. At autopsy the thickened alveolar septa are infiltrated with plasma cells; hence the name "interstitial plasma cell pneumonia." The infiltrate also consists of lymphocytes and histiocytes. Parasites may not be numerous in the thickened septa, even though many are in the alveoli.

Dyspnea is the most common symptom observed, followed by fever and a nonproductive cough. *Pneumocystis* infection may be suspected in any patient with a diffuse or nodular bilateral pulmonary infiltrate that is disproportionate with the minimal physical findings consisting of malaise, anorexia, slight fever, dyspnea, or nonproductive cough, with lungs clear to percussion and auscultation except for scattered rales. Patients with *P. carinii* pneumonia but no immunodeficiency disease show normal serum immunoglobulin levels.

The incubation period is 6 to 8 weeks. Death, almost always occurring in untreated cases, is usually by asphyxia.

Diagnosis and Treatment

Clinical signs and symptoms have been used to make a diagnosis, especially when immunosuppressed or immunocompromised individuals develop a pneumonitis that cannot otherwise be explained. However, the demonstration of the parasite in affected lung tissue or secretions is necessary to confirm the diagnosis. Transbronchial lung biopsy via fiberoptic bronchoscopy is safer than open lung biopsy and more effective than brush-biopsy by bronchoscopy. Staining tissue imprints or tissue sections with methenamine-silver is useful for screening purposes. To differentiate the thick-walled cysts from yeast cells, a follow-up stain with Gram's, Giemsa's, or trichrome is necessary. Serologic tests are not satisfactory and still need development.

Drug treatment is available. The drug of choice for adults and children is the fixed combination of trimethoprim-sulfamethoxazole. Supportive measures such as administering antibiotics and oxygen are also important. Recurrent infection in immunosuppressed individuals is a problem.

Epidemiology and Control

Pneumocystis is a very common parasite of humans and numerous species of mammals. Overt disease is rare except in immunocompromised individuals. Clinical infections occur usually in infants who are premature or malnourished; in older children and adults, the disease is associated with hypogammaglobulinemia, debilitating diseases such as malignancies (e.g., leukemia), or the administration of immunosuppressive drugs such as corticosteroids. AIDS patients are particularly prone to this opportunistic infection.

At present no preventative measures are available. Infection should be anticipated in immunocompromised individuals (e.g., AIDS patients) so that treatment can be given early.

CRYPTOSPORIDIUM

Cryptosporidium is a cosmopolitan parasite that inhabits the human intestinal tract. In the gastrointestinal tract of immunocompromised individuals, *Cryptosporidium* causes a severe diarrheal disease known as cryptosporidiosis.

Morphology and Life Cycle

Cryptosporidium is a coccidian parasite, with a life cycle similar to that of *Toxoplasma,* except that the sexual and asexual developmental stages occur in the same host. There appears to be no obligate intermediate host. All known stages of this parasite are found in the brush border of the mucosal epithelium of the stomach and intestine. The oocysts (4 to 5 µm in diameter), which are passed in the feces, represent the infective stage for humans. The freshly passed oocyst contains four sporozoites. Infection begins when sporozoites released from ingested oocysts enter the brush border of the mucosal epithelium. The sporozoite grows into a trophozoite and then undergoes asexual division (schizogony) to produce a schizont (2 to 5 µm in diameter) that contains eight crescent-shaped merizoites that are released to repeat the schizogonic cycle. Some may form macro- and microgametocytes that mature and by fertilization produce a zygote. The zygote will eventually develop into the oocyte, the transmission stage. The wall of the oocyte protects the parasite from environmental stresses.

Pathogenesis and Symptomatology

In immunocompetent individuals, *Cryptosporidium* causes a short-term flulike, gastrointestinal illness with minimal histologic changes. Illness results in self-limiting (1 to 2 weeks) episodes of watery diarrhea. Parasite multiplication is interrupted by T-cell–dependent immune mechanisms.

In immunocompromised individuals (e.g., AIDS patients) the unchecked cycle of multiplication of the parasite results in heavy parasite burdens producing a chronic infection with profuse debilitating diarrhea, malabsorption syndrome, anorexia, weight loss, and signs of cachexia.

The incubation period ranges from one to several weeks. Onset of illness may be accompanied by fever, malaise, nausea, and vomiting; this is followed by abdominal cramps and diarrhea.

Diagnosis and Treatment

Diagnosis is made by demonstrating the oocysts in the feces. They are usually present in sufficient numbers for a direct fecal smear. However, standard concentration methods are employed as well. Biopsy specimens of intestinal mucosa have also been used to detect *Cryptosporidium*.

No good treatment has been identified for immunocompromised individuals. In immunocompetent individuals the disease is self-limiting and therefore only supportive treatment is necessary.

Epidemiology and Control

Cryptosporidium is a cosmopolitan parasite found in many mammals including humans. Infection is acquired through the ingestion of oocysts from human or animal feces. Oocysts are infective when passed and are resistant to ordinary disinfectants. Control measures include those for all fecal-orally transmitted diseases. Immunocompromised patients are at risk. As of April 1986, 19,182 persons with AIDS had been reported to the CDC. Of these 697 (3.6 percent) had confirmed cases of cryptosporidiosis. The reported case fatality rate for this group of patients was 61 percent. The case fatality rate for AIDS patients without reported cryptosporidiosis was slightly but significantly lower than that for patients with this disease. The high incidence of *Cryptosporidium* in homosexual males compared with other groups (e.g., heterosexuals) is consistent with the hypothesis that oral-anal contact contributes to the transmission of *Cryptosporidium*.

BIBLIOGRAPHY

Beaver, P. C., and Jung, R. C.: Animal Agents and Vectors of Human Disease. Lea and Febiger, Philadelphia, 1985.

Beck, J. W., and Davies, J. E.: Medical Parasitology. C. V. Mosby, St. Louis, 1981.

Brown, H. W., and Neva, F. A.: Basic Clinical Parasitology. Appleton-Century-Crofts, Norwalk, CT, 1983.

Cook, C. G.: Parasitic Disease in Clinical Practice. Springer-Verlag, New York, 1990.

Katz, M., Despommier, D. D., and Gwardz, R.: Parasitic Diseases, ed. 2. Springer-Verlag, New York, 1989.

Martinez-Paloma, A.: Human Parasitic Diseases. Vol. 2, Amebiasis. Elsevier, New York, 1986.

25

Ecology of the Oral Flora

Walter J. Loesche

CHAPTER OUTLINE

Bacterial populations on the surfaces of animals
The oral flora
Host-bacteria inter-relationships
Germ-free animals
Selection forces operating on the oral flora
Anaerobiosis
Nutrient sources in the oral cavity
Ecologic niches
Summary

The mucous membranes of animals are normally colonized by a large and diverse microbial flora. These bacteria are constantly interacting with the host and with each other in competition for survival. In this chapter some of the parameters of these interactions will be discussed.

BACTERIAL POPULATIONS ON THE SURFACES OF ANIMALS

Bacteria colonize all animal surfaces, particularly the oral cavity and lower gastrointestinal tract, where they achieve high densities of 100 million bacteria per milligram plaque wet weight or fecal wet weight. These bacterial populations can fluctuate with environmental changes. Thus, considerable investigation is necessary before even simple statements can be made about the flora of the surfaces.

Researchers define the flora in terms of numerical dominance of various organisms in certain sites, under certain well-recognized conditions. The best examples of this approach are found in the study of the rumen flora present in various grazing animals exposed to a standard dietary regimen. Information and concepts obtained from these studies have been transposed to the human situation, particularly to the oral flora. It should be remembered, that it has not been possible to study the oral flora under standard conditions of diet and frequency of eating. Thus, the following discussions about indigenous, transient, and supplemental flora, are attempts of imposing a modicum of order on a system about which we have only fragmentary knowledge.

THE ORAL FLORA

Bowden and colleagues identified about 21 genera of bacteria comprising about 60 species, from the oral cavity. This was an underestimation, as it is now estimated that there may be over 200 different species that can be isolated from dental plaque alone. Some such as *Actinomyces, Bacterionema, Rothia,* and *Leptotrichia* (all gram-positive rods or filaments) appear to be autochthonous genera, as they have not been isolated from any other habitat. Others, like *Actinobacillus actinomycetemcomitans* and *Streptococcus mutans,* are species described 60 to 70 years ago but more recently have been reisolated and associated with dental pathology.

To deal with this degree of taxonomic diversity, many bacteriologists recognize a normal and a transient bacterial species simply on the basis of prevalence. A normal species is almost always present, whereas a transient species is only occasionally present. A normal species present in numerically dominant numbers is defined as an indigenous species, or it can be present in low numbers and called a supplemental species. The distinction between an indigenous and a supplemental species can change with the environment, as will be illustrated with *S. mutans* and the *Lactobacillus* species.

The Indigenous Flora

The indigenous flora comprise those species that are almost always present in high numbers (greater than 1 percent) in a particular site, such as the supragingival plaque or the surface of the tongue. Their numerical dominance implies that they are compatible with the host and have entered into a stable relationship with the host. They do not compromise the host's survival.

The environments found in the oral cavity of various animals must share some similarities, as the indigenous oral flora of these animals bear some resemblances to each other. Thus, the oral flora is dominated by anaerobic and facultative bacteria, which exhibit optimal growth at about body temperature (37°C). Also, many of these organisms have complex nutritional requirements only met in a rich organic milieu such as exists in or on animal surfaces. Beyond these similarities, however, there are apparently pressures that select for a characteristic oral flora. Thus, certain genera, such as the *Streptococcus, Actinomyces,* and *Neisseria,* appear to be found in the oral cavity of all animals tested (Table 25–1), whereas other genera, such as the *Bacteroides* and the *Enterobacteriaceae,* are characteristically intestinal organisms and are only occasionally isolated from the oral cavity.

Supplemental Flora

The supplemental flora comprise species that are nearly always present, but in low numbers (less than 1 percent). These organisms may become indigenous if the environment changes. For example,

Lactobacillus species normally are found in low levels in plaque (i.e., 0.00001 to 0.001 percent of the viable flora). If a carious lesion develops under this plaque, the plaque pH will become acidic. In this new environment the lactobacilli, which are acid tolerant, will be selected for and can become numerically dominant in the carious lesion. In this case one may consider the lactobacilli as being indigenous to the carious lesion, a finding that has pathologic significance.

A single bacterial species can be an indigenous species in one mouth and a supplemental species in another. This is often the case with *S. mutans.* For example, in an epidemiologic investigation involving 500 first-grade students, *S. mutans* was found in the occlusal fissure plaque of all children. In this sense it was a normal organism in these children. In most subjects, *S. mutans* was a member of the supplemental flora. Statistical analysis revealed that *S. mutans* was a member of the indigenous plaque flora when decay was present.

Thus, as with the lactobacilli, the transition of *S. mutans* from the supplemental flora into the indigenous flora was associated with dental pathology. This pattern is repeated in periodontal disease where increased levels of spirochetes, *Porphyromonas gingivalis,* and *Actinobacillus actinomycetemcomitans* in the subgingival plaque are associated with inflammation and bone loss. From this we may deduce that the supplemental flora contains most of the potential dental pathogens found in the plaque. When we speak of dental decay and periodontal disease as endogenous infections, we concede that some new factor(s) have imposed themselves into the microbial ecosystem on the dentogingival surfaces, which allow the emergence of the odontopathogens.

Transient Flora

Transient flora comprise organisms "just passing through" a host. At any given time a particular

TABLE 25–1 ✦ Genera That Appears to be Indigenous to the Tooth Surfaces

ANIMAL	GENERA			
	STREPTOCOCCUS	*ACTINOMYCES*	*NEISSERIA*	*BACTEROIDES*
Humans	+ +*	+ +	+	+
Primates	+ +	+ +	+	+
Herbivores	+ +	+ +	+	0
Carnivores	+ +	+ +	±	0
Others†	+	+	±	0

*+ + = present in all animals examined; + = usually isolated; ± = occasionally isolated; 0 = not isolated.
†Others include Indian fruit bat, spinny tenrec, bushbaby, and red mantled tamarin.
Adapted from Bowden et al.: Microbial ecology of the oral cavity. In Alexander, M. (ed.): Advances in Microbiol Ecology. Plenum Publishing, New York, 1979.

species may or may not be represented in the flora. Bacteria present in food or drink may be temporarily established in the mouth. However, as these transients normally do not have mechanisms for persisting in the crowded oral environment, they quickly disappear. Overt pathogens of the type that are medically important are exceptions to this general concept, in that under certain circumstances they appear to quickly pass from a transient stage to a predominant stage on the mucous membrane. These medically important pathogens do not dominate in plaque, but often can be isolated in high numbers from many periapical, pericoronal, and periodontal abscesses.

HOST-BACTERIA INTER-RELATIONSHIPS

The preceding discussion described the quantitative nature of the mucous membrane flora. However, this flora cannot be adequately understood independent of its host environment. The relationship of a host to its flora can be described in one of three ways.

Symbiosis

When both the host and the bacteria benefit from their inter-relationship, it is termed "symbiotic." A classic example of symbiosis is found in the digestive tract of ruminants and termites. These two hosts subsist on diets containing a large proportion of cellulose, yet lack the enzyme to degrade the cellulose. This enzyme is supplied by the gut bacteria that breaks down the cellulose to residues that can be absorbed by the host. In return, the bacteria receive a supportive environment with optimal temperature, nutrients, water, and the absence of inhibiting agents. This relationship is extremely stable, as the survival of both members is dependent upon it. In fact, from an evolutionary standpoint this has been a very stable solution, as evidenced by the universal success of grazing animals.

Antibiosis

An antibiotic relationship is the opposite of a symbiotic relationship. Instead of helping each other, the bacteria and the host are antagonistic to each other. When bacteria cause an infection that is combatted by the defense systems of the host, the relationship is said to be antibiotic.

This antibiotic relationship is very unstable for both the host and the pathogenic bacteria. If the host is killed by the pathogen, the pathogen also dies unless it is able to make its way to another host. If the pathogen can be passed from host to host, killing as it goes, it will eventually eliminate

its host populations, which again results in death for the pathogen. On the other hand, if the pathogen is not virulent enough to withstand the host's defense systems, such as antibodies and phagocytic cells, it will be eliminated. Thus, an antibiotic relationship will not be a permanent one.

In some instances a balance is struck between the virulence of a pathogen and the ability of the host population to contend with the organisms. An example of such a balance is the measles virus, which causes a mild illness in the inhabitants of most industrialized nations. Hosts in which this balance has not been achieved are readily susceptible to the viral pathogen. When the American Indians were first exposed to the measles virus by European colonists, they had no defense systems prepared. As a result, the same pathogen that caused a relatively minor illness in the colonists decimated the Indian populations. This problem is seen today, as humans living in isolated communities succumb readily to what are mild infectious diseases in westernized humans.

Amphibiosis

The new relationship described between the measles virus and the host appears to be a general rule in biology. An unstable relationship, such as the antibiotic one, will clearly be discriminated against by the evolutionary selection process. Recent medical history has shown a decreased virulence for all the classic pathogens, such as the *tubercle bacillus, Treponema pallidum,* and others. This means that these organisms have entered into a new, more stable relationship with the host. Rosebury introduced the term "amphibiotic" to describe an intermediate state in which the host and its flora exist in a form of stable balance with each other. Most of the oral flora are thought to exist in an amphibiotic relationship with their host, as there has been no demonstration, yet, of their being harmful or beneficial.

This balance can change, as when *S. mutans* or *P. gingivalis* increases proportionately in the plaque, causing evidence of dental pathology. This overgrowth does not compromise the survival of the host, so that from an evolutionary perspective this type of lowgrade infection is inconsequential.

In many instances, members of the indigenous flora are related to overt pathogens. For example, the indigenous oral spirochetes resemble morphologically and serologically the virulent spirochete, *T. pallidum,* the causative agent of syphilis. The bacteria, now recognized as indigenous varieties, probably evolved from more virulent species. Organisms would be selected on the basis of reduced virulence. Eventually the species that came to dominate on a mucous membrane would be those with minimal, if any, virulence for the host. Later, some of these bacteria might become beneficial to the host.

Such symbiotic interactions undoubtedly have occurred but, except for the cellulase-producing bacteria in the rumen, little is known about them, because in nature the host and its flora cannot be separated. However, a unique research animal, the germ-free animal, has recently become available to aid in this type of research. It now is possible to raise a large number of mammalian species in the absence of detectable bacteria permitting the study of a host in the presence of one or more known organisms.

GERM-FREE ANIMALS

The fetus grows and matures in a bacteria-free uterus. Contamination of the fetus occurs during passage through the birth canal, subsequent handling by hospital personnel and family, and exposure to atmospheric and surface bacteria. If these sources of contamination can be avoided, the neonate should remain bacteria- or germ-free. A germ-free animal is obtained by a cesarean section in which the neonate is delivered and placed aseptically into a sterile chamber. Once obtained, a newborn can be kept sterile by preventing any contact with environmental contaminants.

The air, food, water, and other objects are sterilized before being placed in the chamber and given to the animal. All research animals can be raised for at least one generation in such a sterile environment. The rat and mouse are the only germ-free species that can be bred, for reasons to be discussed shortly. The germ-free animal requires the introduction of new definitions. The normal animal, harboring an unknown flora, is referred to as a conventional animal. Animals that have a known flora are called gnotobiotic animals. Gnotobiotic animals may be germ-free or colonized with one or more known bacterial species.

Defense Systems

Germ-free animals have several significant differences from conventional animals. Lymphoid tissue, particularly along the gastrointestinal tract, is poorly developed, antibody levels to bacteria are significantly depressed, and the rate of antibody synthesis is reduced. The reduction of lymphoid tissue and antibody levels was predictable, as the normal flora and environment provide the host with a considerable amount of antigenic stimulation. Germ-free animals are somewhat sluggish in their response to antigens but, if suitably challenged, make antibody in a normal manner. They clearly are not immunologically incompetent.

In germ-free animals, the lining of the lower portion of the small intestine also is atrophied, with a significant reduction in the total mucosal surface area. But, the most obvious change is the greatly enlarged cecum that lies at the junction of the large and small intestines. It is about 1 percent of the body weight in a conventional animal, and may exceed 18 percent of the animal's body weight in the germ-free animal. This greatly enlarged cecum prevents normal gestation in all germ-free animals except the rat and mouse, which explains why these two are the only animals capable of breeding in a sterile environment.

The enlargement of the germ-free cecum is a direct result of the disruption of normal digestive mechanisms by the lack of appropriate flora. In conventional animals, the large quantities of proteins and glycoproteins present in the secretions and surface cell sloughings from the duodenum and jejunum are degraded by the gut flora into a form that can be absorbed in the ileum and reused by the animal. Without this degradation, the animal loses the protein equivalent of a diet that contains 15 percent protein. This endogenous protein accumulates in the cecum of the germ-free animal, where it is further degraded by endogenous proteolytic enzymes, such as trypsin and chymotrypsin, to osmotically active, low molecular weight compounds that retain water. The failure to reabsorb this endogenous protein forces the germ-free animal to eat more dietary protein in order to remain in nitrogen balance.

This demonstrated a symbiotic relationship between the host and the intestinal flora that was not identified until the flora was eliminated.

Dental Disease

Germ-free animals do not develop dental decay despite the ingestion of high sucrose diets. This observation confirmed the essential role of bacteria in the decay process. Germ-free animals also have reduced inflammation in the periodontal tissues. However, germ-free animals will form calculus and may exhibit what appears to be genetically related patterns of bone loss. The germ-free rat and mouse have been successfully utilized to test the virulence of odontopathic organisms such as *S. mutans, A. viscosus, A. naeslundii, A. actinomycetemcomitans,* and *Capnocytophaga* strains. Potentially periodontopathic organisms such as *P. gingivalis* and various spirochetes cannot be evaluated in these animals because of their inability to grow on the aerobic mucous membranes of these animals.

The demonstration of dental pathology in a germ-free animal, infected with a single species, should be interpreted with some caution given the peculiarities of the germ-free animal. First, the germ-free animal's immune system would be hypofunctional at the time of the initial colonization. Second, all the available sites on the dentogingival surfaces are unoccupied, so that the introduced species would have exclusive access to those niches which, in the conventional animal, would already be occupied by an established bacterial community. Third, the introduced species would not have to contend with the competition and antagonisms related to survival, which exist in any densely and diversely populated microbial community. Fourth, the altered metabolism and eating patterns of the host that are secondary to cecal enlargement could introduce various factors that would not be operable in conventional animals. Even after these peculiarities are accounted for, the germ-free animal has proved to be an invaluable animal model for the demonstration of the virulence of *S. mutans.*

SELECTION FORCES OPERATING ON THE ORAL FLORA

Until the mid-1960s the oral flora had been regarded as a homogeneous bacterial community that was accurately represented by the bacteria found in the saliva. However, salivary cultures reflect the flora found on the oral soft tissues and, only minimally, the flora found on the teeth. First, however, the main environmental selection forces, which serve to shape the normal oral flora into distinct ecosystems—namely, the anaerobic nature of the oral mucous membranes and the available nutrient sources must be considered.

ANAEROBIOSIS

The transit of air through the mouth would seem to preclude any possibility that the oral cavity contained niches where anaerobes could thrive. However, when quantitative culturing procedures were first employed, about 10 percent of the organisms observed microscopically could be cultured aerobically, whereas about 20 percent could be cultured when anaerobic jars were used. These recoveries increased to about 50 to 70 percent when investigators used procedures such as the roll tube or anaerobic chamber in which oxygen was eliminated from the gas atmosphere. The conclusion was obvious. If anaerobes dominated in the flora, the oral mucous membranes must constitute an anaerobic environment.

Oxygen Tensions in the Mouth

Little attention had been given to the oxygen tension of the oral cavity as an ecologic determinant. The oxygen tension, which is a measure of the amount of oxygen in a gas, is about 21 percent

(160 mm Hg) for air. When an oxygen electrode was placed in the mouth and then the lips were closed so as to provide a seal, the gas space over the tongue had an oxygen tension of 12 to 14 percent. When a miniaturized electrode was placed into a periodontal pocket, the oxygen tension was about 1 to 2 percent oxygen.

These data indicate that the gaseous atmosphere over the dentogingival surfaces is mainly anaerobic, particularly in the sites where subgingival plaques would form. The oxygen tensions in the atmosphere over supragingival plaques, especially those on the labial, lingual, and occlusal surfaces, could range from 1 to about 20 percent. Thus, it should come as no surprise that anaerobic species are found primarily in subgingival plaques, while facultative and microaerophilic species dominate in supragingival plaques.

Oxidation-Reduction Potential (Eh)

Another measure of anaerobiosis is the level of the electrical potential of a site relative to a standard hydrogen electrode. This potential, called the Eh, is the tendency for a medium or compound to oxidize or reduce an introduced molecule by the removal or addition of electrons. Tissues or microbes that need a positive Eh for viability are termed "aerobes," and those that need a negative Eh are "anaerobes."

Experience has shown that media that are "prereduced" with sulfhydryl compounds so as to have a negative Eh, permit the reliable growth of anaerobes, and yield the highest recoveries of viable bacteria from plaque samples. If a low Eh is beneficial for the in vitro growth of these organisms, then it is likely that similar low Ehs exist in their "in vivo" habitat. Such Ehs would be expected in any crowded microbial community that performs a fermentative metabolism, as fermentation results in the formation of reduced end products. Thus, one could conclude that the Eh in oral sites where microbes accumulate would eventually become negative. This was verified by the in vivo measurement of Eh in plaque in which subjects wore artificial teeth containing Eh electrodes (a platinum wire) for several days. On the first day, the potential was much the same as saliva, +200 millivolts (mv). As the plaque got older, the Eh dropped to −112 mv and eventually, in some, reached an Eh of −141 mv.

The study indicated that portions of plaque are indeed changing over time from an aerobic to an anaerobic environment, with a corresponding drop in Eh. This change in Eh in undisturbed plaque coincides with a shift in the flora from entirely facultative microaerophilic bacteria to one in which anaerobes such as spirochetes can be detected. Indeed, in subgingival plaques associated with periodontitis, these anaerobic spirochetes can account for half of the flora (see Chapter 19).

Superoxide Radical

Some mention should be made about how oxygen kills a cell and how aerobic cells avoid this fate. First, oxygen can react with the double bonds in lipids, forming peroxides that irreversibly alter the lipids. Since lipids are found in membranes, their oxidation would destroy the integrity of the cell. Second, oxygen can react with sulfhydryl groups of enzymes, forming a disulfide bond. This oxidation of an enzyme may inactivate the enzyme, shutting down the related metabolic pathways, and resulting in cell death. These effects have not been proved in cells but have been observed using pure enzymes and lipid membranes.

Recent evidence indicates that molecular oxygen reacts with reduced flavoprotein to form a superoxide radical. This superoxide radical rapidly destroys the lipids and enzymes of living cells. Oxygen by itself, as well as hydrogen peroxide, reacts with lipids and enzymes, but at such low rates that the superoxide radical appears to be the actual lethal form of oxygen in biologic systems.

Superoxide Dismutase

How do bacteria and other organisms, including tissue cells exposed to oxygen, protect themselves against this superoxide radical? Humans have a copper-containing blood protein, hemocuprine, which removes the superoxide radical. Hemocuprine (or, as called by its enzymatic function, superoxide dismutase) converts the superoxide radical to hydrogen peroxide, which in turn is reduced to water by the cell in a reaction involving gluta-

thione. The oxidized glutathione is subsequently reduced by a reaction involving NADPH.

Bacteria normally exposed to oxygen (facultative aerobes), also have a superoxide dismutase that destroys the superoxide radical. Anaerobes generally do not have a superoxide dismutase and are killed by oxygen via the superoxide radical. In fact, the absence of this enzyme may be the functional definition of an anaerobe. Several investigators have surveyed various fermentative bacteria for the presence of superoxide dismutase and found a significant positive relationship between the absence of this enzyme and the inability to grow in the presence of oxygen.

Biologic Significance of an Anaerobic Flora

Anaerobes dominate in the mucous membrane flora of all animals from insects to humans. The universality of this occurrence suggest an unequivocal advantage to both the host and flora in this arrangement. The host advantage is so obvious that it is amazing that it has been unrecognized for so long. Anaerobes cannot survive in aerobic tissues because they lack enzymes such as superoxide dismutase. If anaerobes penetrate the physical barrier of the mucous membrane epithelium, as shown for the periodontium, they are quickly killed by the molecular oxygen present in the aerobic host tissue, before they can propagate. This would imply that an anaerobic mucous membrane flora should be nonpathogenic and thus selected for by the host during evolutionary time. The universal success of anaerobes on the mucous membranes indicates that this relationship is so stable that it should be considered a symbiotic relationship.

But why symbiotic? The defense mechanisms of the host include the physical barrier of the lining epithelial cells, the phagocytic actions of the white

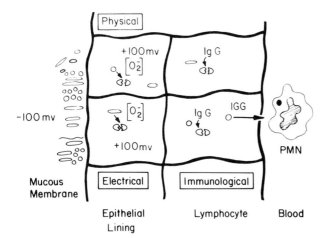

FIGURE 25–1 ✦ Barrier systems in the host against bacterial invasion include the physical barrier composed of the surface epithelium, the electrical barrier that reflects the Eh difference between the host cell and the microbial layer, the immunologic barrier composed of the antibody-forming cells, and the reticuloendothelial system. (From Loesche, W. J. L.: Dental Caries: A Treatable Infection. University of Michigan, 1986, with permission.)

blood cells, and the finely tuned response of the immune system (Fig. 25–1). The last two mechanisms respond to those organisms capable of both invading and propagating in the host tissue. When an anaerobe moves from a mucous membrane locale where the Eh is about − 100 mv to an oxidized host cell environment where the Eh is about + 100 mv, its enzymes are quickly inactivated and its lipid membranes are disrupted. Thus, when the host is colonized by an anaerobic flora, an electrical potential of about 200 mv difference is created between the mucous membranes and the underlying, highly vascularized host tissues. Electrical barriers of this magnitude ensure that the anaerobic bacteria and the aerobic host cells remain physically separated. In this manner the host benefits from its anaerobic flora and provides, in exchange, the nutrient base essential to the survival of the normal flora.

The importance of Eh in regard to the growth of anaerobes is demonstrated by the difficulty of anaerobes to establish on the mucous membranes of germ-free animals. This is because the Eh of the sterile secretions is positive, resembling that of the host tissues. Anaerobes cannot grow at these Ehs and, therefore, do not colonize the mucous membranes. A similar situation occurs each time a newborn confronts the environment. In this case, the sterile mucous membranes are first colonized by facultative organisms. The metabolism of these organisms lowers the Eh to negative values that permit the establishment and eventual domination of the anaerobic flora.

Thus, nature exploits the incompatibility of anaerobic and aerobic forms of life to establish a stable symbiotic relationship between the host and its flora.

NUTRIENT SOURCES IN THE ORAL CAVITY

The host contributes to this symbiotic relationship by providing a ready supply of usable nutrients for the normal flora. In this regard the oral flora has access to a wider range of nutrients than perhaps the normal flora in any other mucous membrane niche. Nutrients are derived from at least five sources. The ingested food is probably quantitatively the most important nutrient source for the oral flora. Nutrients also are present in saliva and the gingival crevice fluid. Epithelial cells are shed from the oral surfaces and some cells lyse in the hypotonic saliva, thereby releasing nutrients into the saliva. In some cases, the bacteria themselves add nutrients to their surrounding environment, which in turn are used by other organisms (Table 25–2).

TABLE 25–2 ✦ Nutrient Sources Available to the Oral Microbial Ecosystems

NUTRIENT SOURCE	MICROBIAL ECOSYSTEMS ON OR IN
Diet	Tongue
	Soft tissue
	Supragingival plaque
Saliva	Tongue
	Soft tissue
	Supragingival plaque
Gingival crevicular fluid	Subgingival plaque
	Supragingival plaque
Microbial products	Subgingival plaque
	Supragingival plaque
	Soft tissue
	Tongue
Host products	Subgingival plaque
	Supragingival plaque
	Soft tissue
	Tongue

Magnitude of Microbial Nutrient Needs

These nutrients must provide an energy source, such as fermentable carbohydrates or amino acids as well as biosynthetic compounds necessary for the growth and maintenance of the various organisms. The quantitative nutrient daily needs for the entire oral flora can be estimated. The number of organisms swallowed per milliliter of saliva is approximately 100 million, which corresponds to 1 mg wet weight of bacteria. If about 1 liter of saliva is swallowed per day, then 100 billion bacteria, corresponding to 1 g wet weight, exit from the oral cavity per day. In order to keep the oral bacteria mass constant, enough nutrients must be consumed to replace this 1 g wet weight bacteria. Studies with *Escherichia coli* show that 80 percent of a nutrient source is expended in energy metabolism and 20 percent is converted to bacterial mass. If this 4:1 ratio holds for the oral flora, then 1 g wet weight of cell mass would require 5 g wet weight of nutrients. This is a small amount, which can easily be met in the oral environment.

Growth Rate(s) of the Oral Flora

The 100 billion bacteria that are shed into the saliva daily come from all the oral surfaces. The teeth constitute a relatively small surface area for washoff and, accordingly, their flora are poorly represented in the saliva. Studies in which volunteers rinsed with a mouth rinse containing radioactive carbon-14–labeled chlorhexidine before and after extraction of diseased teeth indicated that the tooth surfaces composed about 5 percent of the surface area of the mouth. From this it can be estimated that if shed rates from hard and soft surfaces are similar, the total plaque flora constitutes about 5 percent of the salivary flora. This value allows calculation of the approximate growth rate of the oral flora, if this flora is considered a single entity, and the weight of the plaque present at any given time on the teeth is known.

If plaque on all the teeth weighs 10 mg wet weight, the amount found on teeth subjected to reasonable levels of oral hygiene, then the biomass of the oral flora would be about 200 mg wet weight (10 mg plaque = 5 percent of the salivary flora; therefore, 100 percent of the salivary flora = 200 mg). If this biomass remains constant, then in order for 1 g wet weight of bacteria to be shed daily into the saliva, the oral bacteria must divide about five times per day, i.e., 5×200 mg = 1 g that is shed.

According to this calculation the generation, or doubling time, of the oral flora in vivo is just under 5 hours, considerably slower than the 30- to 50-minute generation times that pure cultures of oral bacteria, such as the streptococci, exhibit in vitro. Therefore, the oral flora is growing at a relatively slow rate in vivo. The rate limiting step(s) could be either a nutrient deficiency or an inhibitory environment. Whenever a new site becomes available for colonization, such as a clean tooth surface or a new epithelial cell surface, it seems to be populated rapidly by the oral flora. This suggests that the overall growth rate of the oral flora is regulated by physiochemical considerations, such as pH, Eh, or accumulations of toxic products, rather than by nutrient needs.

These considerations suggest that although the oral flora is not growing rapidly in vivo, it does have the potential to do so (at least some of its members have this potential) and that it is able to utilize nutrients rapidly once they are sequestered. This latter capability may be of great survival value, as it enables the oral flora to remove the maximal amount of nutrients from a flowing stream, such as the saliva or the gingival crevicular fluid.

Diet as a Nutrient Source

Three factors influence the effectiveness of the diet as a microbial nutrient source: the chemical composition of the diet, the physical consistency of its components, and the frequency of its presentation. The macromolecular nutrients such as starches, proteins, and lipids are normally not available to the oral flora, as their transit time through the oral cavity is too short for them to be degraded to usable nutrients. However, if the phys-

ical consistency of the foods that contain them permits retention, such as fibrous foods between the teeth or sticky foods in fissures, pits, and contact points, then some starch and protein utilization could occur. Low molecular weight, soluble carbohydrates such as sucrose (sugar) and lactose (milk sugar) are readily metabolized by the oral flora. It is this bioavailability of these simple sugars that make them cariogenic.

In dental decay the consistency of the diet and the frequency of ingestion may be more important than diet composition. Both consistency and frequency influence the length of time that food remains in contact with plaque and thus is available for bacterial use. The longer bacteria have food available, the more they can grow, the more acid they will produce, and the greater the plaque mass that will accumulate. When snacks are interspersed between meals, they augment the time of nutrient availability, allowing further growth of the plaque organisms. If the plaque is only partially debrided by toothbrushing prior to retiring, the plaque mass remaining on the teeth of the snackers may metabolize stored polysaccharides and produce an appreciable pH drop on the tooth surfaces during sleep. In experimental animals and in clinical studies, frequent eating of a high sucrose diet is associated with high caries activity.

The consistency of food also influences the plaque flora. Liquid foods, such as fruit juices and tonics, are usually swallowed quickly, and are therefore not readily available to the oral flora. Sticky and fibrous foods, however, are retained in those areas that trap food (e.g., fissures, missing contacts, pockets, and cavities) and can be used by the flora in these areas for extended periods of time. It is no mere coincidence that these sites usually are associated with dental pathology. Hard candy, in this context, would be an exceptionally cariogenic foodstuff. The sucrose that is slowly released would bathe the supragingival plaque and lead to the selection of organisms, such as *S. mutans,* which can efficiently utilize sucrose.

The importance of between-meal eating of sucrose and the consistency of sucrose-containing foods in dental disease was unequivocally demonstrated by a clinical study conducted in adult residents of a mental hospital in Vipeholm, Sweden. The 5-year caries attack rate in these subjects on the institutionalized diet—that is, the control group—was about 0.2 DMF (decayed-missing-filled) teeth per year. The addition of about one-half pound of sucrose per day in the form of toffees, caramels, chocolates, or bread at meal times caused less than one decayed tooth per year. However, the ingestion of the same forms of sucrose between meals led to an explosive increase in DMF teeth, in that five to seven newly decayed teeth were observed per year. The frequent ingestion of sucrose was shown to cause an elevation in the levels of salivary sugars and in the length of time that sugars could be detected in the saliva.

Thus, for those subjects who ate between meals, sugar could be detected in their salivas during most of the day. This meant that some microbial fermentation was ongoing in the plaque for most of the day and accordingly, the pH at the plaque-enamel interface probably was below pH 5.5, the critical pH for enamel demineralization. This long exposure of the tooth surface to an acidic pH could easily account for the increased decay rate observed in these adults.

Diet is the single most important nutrient source for the plaque found on the coronal surfaces of teeth. Dietary restriction of carbohydrates, especially sucrose, should profoundly influence the composition of the supragingival microbial flora. The salivary lactobacilli levels and the plaque levels of intracellular polysaccharide-forming bacteria decrease appreciably on low-carbohydrate diets. These low-carbohydrate diets are difficult for patients to maintain and are therefore essentially impractical for caries control.

However, dietary reduction of caries by replacement of sucrose with noncariogenic sugar substitutes, such as xylitol, or sorbitol, may be possible. Xylitol, in particular, has been shown in human studies to reduce caries either when a total substitution for sucrose was made or when chewing gum sweetened with xylitol was taken between meals. The xylitol either is not fermented by the plaque flora or, if fermented, does not lower the pH. The use of such a sucrose substitute should change the microbial composition of plaque, and indeed the proportions of efficient sucrose-fermenting organisms such as *S. mutans* decline in the plaque when xylitol is substituted for sucrose.

Saliva as a Nutrient Source

Saliva is a homeostatic fluid that buffers the plaque. However, saliva can provide nutrients to the flora that resides on the surface it bathes. Saliva contains about 1 percent solids, which include glycoproteins, inorganic salts, and most importantly for the plaque flora, milligram amounts of amino acids and glucose, and microgram amounts of certain vitamins. These quantities are sufficient to sustain some bacterial growth during periods when a person does not eat, such as between meals and overnight during sleep. The glycoproteins present in saliva could also serve as nutrient sources, if they are trapped in plaque. Some plaque bacteria possess neuraminidases, which break down the terminal sugar residues on certain glycoproteins, but no evidence exists that shows that the neuraminic

acid (sialic acid), which is released, can be used by the plaque flora. Those bacteria that can utilize and have access to the salivary nutrients always have a good source available. The bacteria that reside in the gingival crevices and periodontal pockets have limited access to salivary nutrients and do not appear to be influenced by them.

Gingival Crevice Fluid

The gingival crevice is bathed by microliter amounts of a serum transudate that contains tissue and serum proteins, as well as free amino acids, vitamins, glucose, and so forth. Under healthy gingival conditions, this gingival crevice fluid is protective, flushing out nonadherent plaque from the sulcus and bringing phagocytic cells and antibodies into the area. The presence of certain serum components may act as a strong selection factor for some of the gingival crevice microbes such as the spirochetes and black-pigmented bacteroides (see section on Nutrient Needs later in this chapter).

Shed Cells

The epithelial surfaces of the oral cavity undergo a turnover, shedding their surface cells; also, phagocytic cells enter the oral cavity from the gingival crevice area. These mammalian cells can be lysed by the hypotonicity of saliva and their contents are then available for microbial nutrition. The magnitude of this food source for microbial metabolism is not known.

Bacteria

The bacteria themselves can provide nutrients for each other. In a dense microbial population such as plaque, one would expect considerable microbial interactions. One well-documented interaction is the relationship between lactic-acid–producing bacteria such as the streptococci and a lactate-utilizing species such as *Veillonella alkalescens*. *V. alkalescens* has lost the enzyme, hexose kinase, so it cannot phosphorylate glucose. Under most conditions that would be a lethal mutation and the mutant never observed. However, if this mutation occurred in the presence of lactic acid, the mutant could survive because this acid is absorbed by *V. alkalescens* and fermented so as to yield ATP.

Many organisms in plaque, including the streptococci, form lactic acid. This would suggest that the *Veillonella* parasitize the lactate producers. However, the relationship between the *Veillonella* and organisms such as streptococci may be symbiotic, as the lactic acid is converted to propionate, acetate, and carbon dioxide, with a resultant elevation in pH. This shift away from low pHs would be beneficial for acid-sensitive streptococci such as *S. sanguis*. Other examples of plaque-microbial interactions exist. *Treponema denticola* is dependent on cohabitant plaque species for isobutyrate and spermine. *Prevotella melaninogenicus'* requirement for vitamin K can be provided by a variety of other oral bacteria, such as *Campylobacter sputorum* and *Bacteroides oralis*.

These microbial interactions indicate that some of the oral flora are microbe dependent—that is, they will not grow in the absence of the provident microbes. This is indeed the case, as none of the cited organisms will easily establish in pure cultures in germ-free animals. *Veillonella* can be grown in germ-free animals after prior establishment of a streptococcus.

ECOLOGIC NICHES

Thus far we have discussed the oral flora as if it were a single entity. It is known that microorganisms that live on the tongue are not necessarily the same organisms that are found in the plaque. Moreover, organisms like spirochetes and gram-negative anaerobic rods inhabit the subgingival plaque but are rarely found in supragingival plaque or in high numbers in the saliva. Clearly, there is some heterogeneity within the "oral" flora.

Prior to 1963 most bacteriologists had considered the "oral" flora to be uniformly distributed throughout the mouth, and they concentrated their efforts on the culturing of saliva on the assumption that the saliva reliably reflected the "oral" flora. This approach ignored the unique contributions to the saliva of the bacteria shed from the different anatomic sites within the mouth and, accordingly, delayed the understanding of the role of specific microbes in both dental caries and in periodontal disease. For example, if an organism such as *S. mutans* composed less than 1 percent of the salivary flora, it is difficult to conceive how it could be a cariogenic organism. However, if *S. mutans* constituted 25 percent of the flora in an occlusal fissure, then its role as a cariogenic organism is plausible.

Plaque

In the late 1950s and early 1960s quantitative culturing procedures were introduced in which plaques and saliva were dispersed, serially diluted, and cultured under an anaerobic atmosphere. Gibbons, Socransky, and their colleagues collected plaque from either the coronal or subgingival surfaces of all the teeth in a mouth and pooled them so as to give a single sample for each subject. The pooled plaques from the coronal surfaces contained mainly gram-positive saccharolytic organisms (carbohydrate fermenters), whereas the pooled plaques from the subgingival surfaces contained, in addition, gram-negative saccharolytic and asaccharolytic (proteolytic) organisms. Neither plaque contained *S. salivarius,* although this organism had until this time been considered to be the numerically dominant streptococcus in the oral cavity because of its prominence in the saliva.

When Krasse, in the early 1950s, reported that *S. salivarius* was not present in plaque, he said that a discrepancy must exist between salivary sampling techniques and the technique of sampling material from the tooth surface. This discrepancy is now known to be the incorrect assumption that plaque and saliva are bacteriologically identical. The washoff of bacteria from all the surfaces in the oral cavity are found in the saliva. Since the tongue and cheeks constitute most of the mouth's surface areas, the flora shed from their surfaces is highly prominent in the salivary flora. As *S. salivarius* is the predominant streptococcus on these surfaces, it becomes also the predominant streptococcus in the saliva.

These quantitative culturing studies were extended to look at other sites in the mouth and to look for specific bacterial types, so that eventually the geographic localization of many oral species was determined (Table 25–3). The flora on the tongue, on the buccal mucosa, and in the saliva are similar, whereas the plaque flora differs by having almost undetectable levels of *S. salivarius* and appreciable levels of *Actinomyces* and gram-negative species. The gram-negative species are mainly confined to the subgingival plaque so that it is not even valid to think of plaque as a homogeneous entity.

Not only do microbial populations differ from location to location in the mouth, but the plaque flora in the same location also may show definitive changes over time. For example, following cleaning of the teeth, the plaque that initially forms at the dentogingival margin after 1 day is made up primarily of cocci. If the plaque remains undisturbed for a few weeks, some gram-negative, motile species are observed (see section on Plaque Formation in Chapter 26).

These studies with pooled plaques demonstrated the differences between subgingival and supragingival flora and their respective differences from salivary flora. However, they did not demonstrate appreciable differences between patients with and without dental diseases. This is because the pooled plaques contained mostly plaque from nondiseased sites, which would dilute out the plaque obtained from single sites that were diseased. It is only in the last few years that plaques from single diseased pockets or single carious fissures have been cultured and compared with plaques from nondiseased sulci or fissures.

TABLE 25–3 ✦ Intraoral Site Distribution of Various Indigenous and Supplemental Members of the Oral Flora

| SPECIES | SALIVA | TONGUE | PLAQUE | |
			SUPRAGINGIVAL	SUBGINGIVAL
Streptococcus salivarius	+ + +	+ + +		
S. sanguis	+ +	+ +	+ + +	+
S. mitior	+ +	+ +	+ +	+ +
S. milleri	±	±	+ to + + +	0
S. mutans	± to +	±	+ to + + +	0
Lactobacillus sp.	± to +	+	+	±
Actinomyces sp.	+	+	+ +	± to + +
Fusobacterium sp.	0	0	±	± to + +
Capnocytophaga	0	0	±	± to +
Treponema sp.	0	0	±	± to + + +
Prevotella melaninogenicus	0	0	±	± to +
Porphyromonas gingivalis	0	0	0	0 to +
Actinobacillus actinomyce-temcomitans	0	0	±	0 to +
Veillonella	+	+	+ +	+ +

0 = not usually detected; ± = rarely present; + = usually present in low proportions; + + = usually present in moderate proportions; + + + = usually present in high proportions.
Data from following sources: Gibbons, R. J. and van Houte, J.: J. Periodontol. 44:347, 1973; Loesche, W. J.: J. Periodontol. 6:245, 1968; Mejare, B. and Edwardsson, S.: Arch. Oral Biol. 20:757, 1975; Slots, et al.: Infect. Immunol. 29:1013, 1980; Loesche, W. J., and Syed, S. A., unpublished data.

Ecologic Determinants

What phenomena can explain the microbial diversity that exists in different anatomic sites in the mouth? Bacteria establish themselves in sites where they can obtain their nutrient requirements and do not encounter inhibitory or adverse conditions for growth. Could these factors be the determinants responsible for the different microbial ecosystems?

Nutrient Needs

The nutrient sources in the mouth are diverse and should provide a wide variety of organic compounds capable of supporting the growth of the most fastidious organisms, yet it is possible that some unique growth factor needed by *S. salivarius*, for instance, is not present in the plaque microenvironment. Carlsson explored this by developing chemically defined media for *S. salivarius*, *S. sanguis*, and *S. mutans*. These species had similar nutrient requirements except for differences in single amino acids. Thus, nutrient needs could not account for the absence of *S. salivarius* in the plaque.

Nutrient availability, however, could explain the localization of certain gram-negative species to the subgingival plaque. *P. melaninogenicus*, *P. gingivalis*, and *Capnocytophaga* either have a requirement for or are stimulated by hemin. Many isolates of the black-pigmented bacteroides also are stim-

ulated by vitamin K, estradiol, and progesterone. *T. denticola* has a requirement for spermine.

The only site in the mouth where microbes would have access to these nutrients would be in the flow bed of the gingival crevicular fluid. Thus, the aforementioned species could thrive only in subgingival plaque. If gingival pathology occurs and the transudate increases in volume, a proliferation of these organisms might occur. In fact, when gingivitis has progressed to the point when bleeding occurs, these organisms can be found among the indigenous flora of the site. This can be documented in pregnancy gingivitis, where a specific increase in *P. intermedia* was found after bleeding occurred. The specificity of this increase was correlated with the ability of this organism to utilize estradiol and progesterone, both increased in the gingival crevice fluid during pregnancy. Thus, in the case of the spirochetes and the black-pigmented bacteroides, nutrient supply appears to be of paramount importance in their localization and actual levels in the plaque.

Inhibitory Factors

A variety of inhibitory host or microbial factors could be responsible for the distinct ecosystems observed in plaque and soft tissues. The host factors would include specific antibodies, lysozymes, lactoperoxidase, lactoferrin, and high molecular weight adhesins—all of which are present in the saliva. These host antibacterial mechanisms do not appear to be responsible for the establishment or maintenance of the various oral ecosystems.

Bacteria produce factors such as organic acids, which lower the pH; reduced end products, which lower the Eh; hydrogen peroxide, which oxidizes certain enzymes and membranes; and fatty acids and bacteriocins, which prevent the growth of certain species. All of these could shape the microbial composition in a niche. The role of these factors in regulating microbial populations in vivo has not been adequately investigated.

Acidic pHs. Members of the oral flora grow best in vitro at about pH 7.0. This is the level found in saliva and maintained by the carbonate buffer in the saliva. However, the plaque pH can drop to below 5.0 during eating. This low pH could select for aciduric organisms, which could account for the absence of species such as *S. salivarius* in the plaque. This possibility was investigated by observing the relative abilities of several oral species, including *S. salivarius,* to initite growth in media with acid pHs.

All tested species grew luxuriantly when the initial pH was 7.0 but exhibited diminished growth when the initial pH was 5.5 (Table 25-4). When the pH dropped to 5.0, only *S. mutans* and *L. casei* were capable of growth. There was no difference in acid tolerance between *S. salivarius* and such prominent plaque organisms as *S. sanguis, S. mitis,* and *A. viscosus.* Thus, the absence of *S. salivarius* from the plaque could not be related to its being more sensitive to low pH than *S. sanguis* or *S. mitis.* Tolerance of low pH can explain the selection of *S. mutans* and *L. casei* in the cariogenic plaques and lesions, and this trait, known as aciduricity, may be the single most important determinant in the cariogenicity of these organisms.

The absence of *S. salivarius* from the plaque is best explained by its inability to attach to the tooth and plaque-covered surface. The importance of adherence to attachment in oral microbial ecology is covered elsewhere in this volume.

SUMMARY

The host supports a large and diverse bacterial population on its surfaces. Powerful selection pressure such as anaerobiosis, temperature, and nutrient availability shape this flora into distinct microbial communities on the various anatomic surfaces and orifices of the body. Each community contains, as its characteristic members, those species that have no, or low, virulence for the host. This so-called normal flora separates out into those species that are numerically dominant, or the indigenous flora, and those that persist in low num-

TABLE 25-4 ✦ Effect of Initial pH of Broth Media on Growth of Various Plaque Bacteria

BACTERIA	INITIAL pH OF MEDIA		
	7.0	5.5	5.0
Streptococcus salivarius	0.9	0.20	NG†
S. sanguis	0.9	0.40	NG
S. mitis	0.7	0.04	NG
Actinomyces viscosus	1.3	0.20	NG
S. mutans	1.1	0.50	0.2
Lactobacillus casei	0.8	0.70	0.6

*Terminal optical density after 53 hours of anaerobic incubation.
†NG = no growth.
Adapted from Harper, D. S., and Loesche, W. J.: Arch. Oral Biol. 29:843, 1984.

bers and are known as the supplemental flora. The indigenous flora probably interacts with the host in a symbiotic fashion, whereas some members of the supplemental flora interact in an amphibiotic or unstable fashion. In the oral cavity, overgrowth of certain members of the supplemental flora can be associated with either dental caries or periodontal disease. These common dental afflictions appear then to be specific, albeit chronic, endogenous infections.

Nutritional and inhibitory factors, to the extent that they could be identified, can explain the localization of anaerobic and certain fastidious organisms to the subgingival plaque. They explain why saccharolytic-microaerophilic organisms dominate in the supragingival and soft-tissue sites. They do not explain why certain organisms such as *S. salivarius* dominate in the soft tissue but are absent from the plaque. Clearly, other ecologic determinants are operative. One of these, the ability of an organism to adhere to a surface, will be described in Chapter 26.

BIBLIOGRAPHY

Alexander, M.: Microbial Ecology. John Wiley and Sons, New York, 1971.
Bonesvoll, P., and Olson, I.: Influence of teeth, plaque and dentures on the retention of chlorhexidine in the human oral cavity. J. Clin. Periodontol. 1:214, 1974.
Bowden, G. H. W., Ellwood, D. C., and Hamilton, I. E.: Microbial ecology of the oral cavity. In Alexander, M. (ed.): Advances in Microbial Ecology. Plenum Publishing, New York, 1979, pp. 135-217.
Burnett, M. and White, D. O.: Natural History of Infectious Disease, ed 4. Cambridge University Press, Cambridge, 1972.
Carlsson, J.: Nutritional requirements of *Streptococcus sanguis*. Arch. Oral Biol. 17:1327, 1972.

Gibbons, R. J. and van Houte, J.: On the formation of dental plaque. J. Periodont. 44:347, 1973.

Gustafsson, B. E., Quensel, C. E., Lanke, L. S., Lundquist, C., Grahnen, H., Bonow, B. E., and Krasse, B.: The Vipeholm dental caries study. The effect of different levels of carbohydrate intake on caries activity in 436 individuals observed for five years. Acta Odontol. Scand. 11:232, 1954.

Harper, D. S. and Loesche, W. J.: Growth and acid tolerance of dental plaque bacteria. Arch. Oral Biol. 29:843, 1984.

Hungate, R. E.: The Rumen and its Microbes. Academic Press, New York, 1966.

Kenney, E. B., and Ash, M. M.: Oxidation reduction potential of developing plaque, periodontal pockets and gingival sulci. J. Periodont. 40:630, 1969.

Kornman, K. S., and Loesche, W. J.: Effects of estradiol and progesterone on *Bacteroides melaninogenicus* and *Bacteroides gingivalis*. Infect. Immunol. 35:256, 1982.

Krasse, B.: The proportional distribution of *Streptococcus salivarius* and other streptococci in various parts of the mouth. Odont. Rev. 5:203, 1954.

Loesche, W. J.: The rationale for caries prevention through the use of sugar substitutes. Int. Dent. J. 35:1, 1985.

Loesche, W. J., Eklund, S., Earnest, R., and Burt, B.: Longitudinal investigation of human fissure decay: Epidemiological studies in molars shortly after eruption. Infect. Immun. 46:765, 1984.

Luckey, T. D.: Germfree Life and Gnotobiology. Academic Press, New York, 1963.

Minah, G. E. and Loesche, W. J.: Sucrose metabolism in resting-cell suspensions of caries-associated and non-caries-associated dental plaque. Infect. Immunol. 17:43, 1977.

Morris, J. G.: Oxygen and growth of the oral bacteria. In Kleinberg, I., Ellison, S. A., and Mandel, I. D. (eds.): Proceedings of Saliva and Dental Caries. Sp. Supp. Microbiol. Abstr. pp. 293–306, 1979.

Rogosa, M., Krichevsky, M. I., and Bishop, F. S.: Truncated glycolytic system in *Veillonella*. J. Bacteriol. 90:164, 1965.

Rosebury, T.: Microorganisms Indigenous to Man. McGraw-Hill, New York, 1962.

Tally, F. P., Stewart, P. R., Sutter, V. L., and Rosenblatt, J. E.: Oxygen tolerance of fresh clinical anaerobic bacteria. J. Clin Microbiol. 1:161, 1975.

26 *Dental Plaque and Calculus*

Mariano Sanz and Michael G. Newman

CHAPTER OUTLINE

Dental plaque
Dental calculus

DENTAL PLAQUE

The importance of bacteria in dental plaque and its key role in the etiology of both dental caries and periodontal diseases has been clarified in the last 20 years. In 1963, Socransky and colleagues demonstrated that human dental plaque contains 1.7×10^{11} organisms per wet weight per gram, showing that plaque consists predominantly of bacteria rather than food remnants as had been previously thought. At the same time, several longitudinal studies conclusively showed that plaque control can arrest and prevent dental caries and periodontal diseases. Evidence also has shown that in compromised patients, poor plaque control and dental pathology may have even more serious local and systemic consequences.

Therefore, a thorough understanding of the structure and composition of dental plaque is required to fully understand dental caries and periodontal diseases.

Definition

After tooth eruption, several organic deposits may form on the surfaces of teeth. These deposits include dental plaque, materia alba, pellicle, and calculus. Dental *plaque* is defined as bacterial aggregations that are attached to the teeth or other solid oral structures. *Materia alba* describes bacterial aggregations, leukocytes, and desquamated oral epithelial cells accumulating at the surface of plaque and teeth, but lacking the regular internal structure observed in dental plaque. Both deposits are functionally differentiated by the strength of their adherence. Deposits removed by the mechanical action of a strong water spray are termed "materia alba," but if it withstands the water spray, it is called "dental plaque."

Pellicle is an organic film derived mainly from the saliva and deposited on the tooth surface. Pellicle in its early stages contains no bacteria; however, it is soon colonized by bacteria and then is part of the dental plaque. *Calculus* represents calcified dental plaque, but it is always covered with a superficial layer of noncalcified plaque.

Based on plaque's relationship to the gingival margin, it is differentiated into two categories: *supragingival* and *subgingival* plaque. Supragingival plaque is sometimes further differentiated into *coronal plaque*, or plaque in contact only with the tooth surface, and *marginal plaque*, in association with both tooth surface and gingival margin.

Physical and Clinical Description

Small amounts of plaque are only clinically visible when there are naturally occurring pigments; it is stained by disclosing solutions such as erythrosin or can be scraped off the tooth surface with a probe or scaler (Fig. 26–1). Supragingival plaque becomes clinically detectable once it has reached a certain thickness. As plaque develops and accumulates, it becomes a visible globular mass with a nodular surface and a whitish to yellowish color (Fig. 26–2).

Dental plaque also can grow on other hard oral surfaces, mainly if the site is protected from the normal mechanical cleansing action of the tongue, cheeks, and lips. Therefore, plaque deposits regularly occur in pits and fissures of occlusal surfaces, on restorations and artificial crowns, orthodontic bands, dental implants, removable orthodontic appliances, and dentures.

Measurable amounts of supergingival plaque may form within 1 hour after the teeth have been cleaned, with maximum accumulation in about 30 days. The rate of formation and location vary among individuals and is influenced by diet, age, salivary factors, oral hygiene, tooth alignment, systemic disease, and host factors.

320

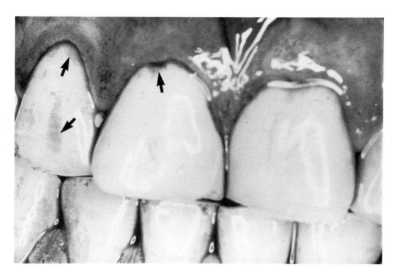

FIGURE 26-1 ✦ Small amounts of dental plaque can only be seen if stained with a disclosing solution *(arrows)*.

Subgingival plaque is usually thin, contained within the gingival sulci or periodontal pocket, and thus cannot be detected by direct observation. Its presence can be identified only by running the end of a probe around the gingival margin. Several sampling techniques have been used to collect subgingival plaque and assess its microbial composition. These sampling techniques use mainly absorbent paper points or scalers.

Clinical Importance

The relationships among improper oral hygiene, formation of dental deposits, and development of dental diseases have been recognized for centuries. Substantial scientific evidence implicates dental plaque as the most important factor in the development of periodontal diseases (Table 26-1).

1. In the middle of this century, well-designed epidemiologic studies examined the effects of several factors on periodontal disease. Oral hygiene and age were the only variables significantly related to the prevalence and severity of periodontal disease. An almost linear relationship exists between severity of periodontal disease and lack of oral hygiene and accumulation of dental deposits.
2. In germ-free animals, periodontal tissue loss accelerated after infection with microorganisms.
3. Final evidence was gathered when gingivitis was experimentally induced in humans when

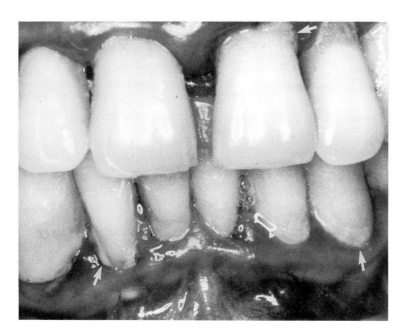

FIGURE 26-2 ✦ Gross accumulations of plaque can be seen forming globular masses of white-yellow color *(arrows)*.

TABLE 26–1 ✦ Etiologic Importance of Dental Plaque: Scientific Evidence

1. Epidemiologic studies—poor oral hygiene increases prevalence and severity of periodontal disease
2. Experimental studies in germ-free animals—monoinfection with suspected pathogen: signs of periodontal disease
3. Experimental gingivitis in humans (Löe 1965); experimental periodontitis in dogs (Lindhe 1976)
4. Longitudinal clinical studies—oral hygiene + mechanical or chemical plaque control therapy arrest and/or prevent the progression of periodontal disease

oral hygiene measures were purposely abolished. When oral hygiene was reinstituted, gingivitis resolved within a week with restoration of gingival health.

4. The transition from gingivitis to periodontitis has not been demonstrated experimentally in humans because of ethical considerations. However, in dogs, plaque accumulation leads to gingivitis which, if allowed to continue, causes loss of attachment and destruction of the supporting tissues of the teeth, similar to typical human periodontal disease (periodontitis).

5. Additional evidence for the role of dental deposits in human periodontal disease comes from studies where the progression of periodontal disease has been retarded by improved oral hygiene and with the use of antimicrobials such as chlorhexidine. These measures inhibited plaque formation and prevented development of experimental gingivitis.

Composition of Dental Plaque—Microbiology

Dental plaque consists primarily of proliferating microorganisms along with a scattering of epithelial cells, leukocytes, and macrophages, in an adherent intercellular matrix. Bacteria make up approximately 70 to 80 percent of this material. One cubic millimeter of dental plaque weighing about 1 mg contains more than 10^8 bacteria. These bacteria exist in an extremely complex arrangement. There may be as many as 200 to 400 different species in one site with some species not currently identified. Dental plaque may contain microorganisms other than bacteria; *Mycoplasma*, fungi, protozoa, and viruses have been demonstrated in different proportions.

Improved bacteriologic sampling techniques, anaerobic culturing, and complex species identification matrices have identified several patterns of dental plaque composition.

Supragingival Plaque
FORMATION AND BIOCHEMISTRY

Supragingival plaque has been examined in multiple studies with different microscopic techniques.

Pellicle is the initial organic structure on the surfaces of teeth and/or artificial splints that forms prior to colonization by bacteria. After bacterial colonization, the pellicle is regarded as part of the dental plaque, which then consists of pellicle, bacteria, and intercellular matrix. The composition of pellicle is dependent on the surface where it forms. Therefore, in vitro pellicle formation on glass or plastic surfaces may differ from formation on hydroxyapatite matrices.

The first stage in pellicle formation involves adsorption of salivary proteins to apatite surfaces. This results from the electrostatic ionic interaction between calcium ions and phosphate groups in the enamel surface and opposite-charged groups in the salivary macromolecules. The structure of the pellicle is heterogeneous. The mean pellicle thickness ranges from about 100 nm at 2 hours to 500 to 1000 nm at 24 to 48 hours.

This structural heterogeneity reflects a complex composition, consisting mainly of high molecular weight blood group reactive glycoproteins, immunoglobulins, virus hemagglutination inhibition factors, and different carbohydrates. Recent studies, however, suggest the main proteins are low molecular weight phosphoproteins and sulphoglycopeptides. These phosphate and sulphate groups may attach to the apatite surface by ion displacement through direct ionic and hydrophobic interaction. In a second stage, the remaining salivary glycoproteins are adsorbed through different intermolecular interactions including ionic, hydrogen-bonding, hydrophobic, and van der Waal's.

The transition between pellicle and dental plaque is extremely rapid. The first constituents include mainly cocci with small numbers of epithelial cells and polymorphonuclear leukocytes. The individual bacteria initially adhere to small irregularities, fissures, or areas with imperfections (roughness, cracks) that are relatively sheltered from oral cleansing forces.

Generally, the first organisms form a cellular monolayer, either singly or in small groups. Bacterial growth extends beyond surface defects and increases in volume. At the periphery the growth continues, eventually coalescing with neighboring patches of plaque. During the first few hours, the attached bacteria proliferate and form small colonies of cocci. With time, other types of microorganisms proliferate, giving rise to different micro-

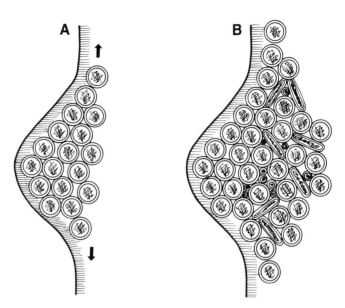

FIGURE 26–3 ✦ Initial colonization of bacteria in dental plaque. **A,** Gram-positive cocci are able to adhere to irregularities in pellicle covered enamel sheltered from oral cleansing mechanisms. **B,** Once adherent, subsequent bacterial colonization (rods) is facilitated in the direction of the arrows and becomes part of the plaque mass. (Adapted from Lie, T.: J. Periodont. Res. 12;73, 1977. © 1977 Munksgaard International Publishers Ltd., Copenhagen.)

colonies. Eventually, dental plaque becomes characteristically complex (Fig. 26–3).

The material among bacteria in dental plaque is termed *intermicrobial matrix* and accounts for approximately 25 percent of plaque volume. Its composition includes microbial substances, salivary material, and gingival exudate. The organic matrix is mainly a polysaccharide-protein complex produced by plaque microorganisms. Several oral streptococci synthesize levans (fructans) and glucans (mainly dextran) from dietary sucrose (see Chapter 6). The levans provide mainly energy, while the glucans provide not only energy, but also act as the organic skeleton of plaque, playing a role in bacterial adhesion and interbacterial coaggregation reactions. Other matrix carbohydrates are galactose and methylpentose in the form of rhamnose. The small amount of lipids present in the plaque matrix is mainly composed of small extracellular trilaminar vesicles from gram-negative microorganisms, representing lipopolysaccharide endotoxins. The matrix protein component is provided by salivary glycoproteins, which both promote bacterial adherence if adsorbed to the tooth surface and agglutinate other bacteria. Other proteins are also provided by lysed bacteria.

This intermicrobial or extracellular matrix not only serves as a framework to bind the microorganisms with a coherent mass and as an extracellular storage of bacterial nutrients, but also contains numerous inflammation-inducing and other toxic substances, such as proteolytic enzymes, antigenic substances, endotoxin, and low–molecular-weight metabolites.

Inorganic components of supragingival plaque matrix include primarily calcium and phosphorus, with small amounts of magnesium, potassium, and sodium. The inorganic early plaque content is very low but greatly increases as plaque transforms into calculus.

Dental plaque formation involves two major processes: (1) initial adherence and subsequent proliferation of salivary organisms to the acquired pellicle, and (2) further aggregation of bacteria to already attached cells. In both processes, the two primary ecologic determinants are bacterial adherence and growth.

BACTERIAL ADHERENCE

Oral bacteria vary markedly in their ability to attach to different surfaces which is not due to differences in growth rate. *Streptococcus mutans, S. sanguis, Lactobacillus* sp., and *Actinomyces viscosus* preferentially colonize tooth surfaces; *S. salivarius* and *A. naeslundii* the dorsum of the tongue; and black-pigmenting bacteria and spirochetes the gingival crevice or periodontal pocket.

In dental plaque development, two adhesive processes are required. First, bacteria must adhere to the pellicle surface and become sufficiently attached to withstand oral cleansing forces. Second, they must grow and adhere to each other to allow plaque accumulation.

During initial adherence, interactions occur mainly between specific bacteria and the pellicle. In subsequent phases of plaque formation, bacteria, bacterial products, interbacterial matrix, host, and dietary factors are involved.

Electrostatic Forces

Oral bacteria bear an overall net negative charge, probably from the outward orientation of cell wall components such as anionic residues on surface glycoproteins (see Chapter 3). Bacterial attachment to the enamel pellicle may occur via electrostatic attractions in which the negatively charged bacterial cell surfaces and negatively charged tooth surface constituents link via cations such as calcium. The electrostatic repulsive forces are overcome by bacterial appendages such as fimbriae and flagella that extend approximately 10 to 20 nm from the bacterial cell wall, permitting cation bridging or other adhesive mechanisms to take place (Fig. 26–4).

Bacterial adhesion is a very complex process. Conditions such as pH and ionic strength have variable effects on bacterial adhesion. Studies of zeta potentials of different oral bacteria show that species such as *S. sanguis* and *S. salivarius*, differing only slightly in zeta potential, are able to elicit a completely different pattern of bacterial adhesion.

Hydrophobic Interactions

The hydrophobic association is based on a close structural fit between molecules. The nature of bacterial cell wall constituents contributing to the hydrophobicity of the cell is not clearly known, although several oral bacteria have hydrophobic surface properties. A contributing factor might be the lipoteichic acid (LTA), with its hydrophilic linear polymer of glycerophosphate and a nonpolar tail of fatty acids that provide a long hydrophobic area (Fig. 26–5).

Organic Components

The organic components in saliva and other tissue fluids profoundly influence adhesion and colonization. Depending on the bacterial species, salivary proteins may either inhibit or promote adhesion. As a general rule, salivary proteins inhibit adhesion through interactions with the bacterial and tooth surfaces or through alterations in the ionic or hydrophobic/hydrophilic balance of both surfaces.

However, in some bacteria, saliva promotes bacterial adherence by a specific reaction between the bacterial surface and the salivary-derived organic pellicle on the tooth. This specificity has been suggested as an explanation for the selective nature of the bacterial attachment to oral surfaces. In competitive binding studies between streptococci and saliva-coated hydroxyapatite, no competition was evident among strains of *S. mutans*, *S. sanguis*, *S. mitis*, and *S. salivarius*, which suggests that these organisms interact with different pellicle receptor sites. The interactions between different bacteria involved in coaggregation are also highly specific; the aggregation of *S. sanguis* with *A. naeslundii* is strain specific. The receptors responsible for these highly specific interactions are associated with the fibrillar coating or fimbriae on the bacterial cell surface.

Recently, different binding sites or biochemical bonds have been identified, which allow interaction of molecules on the bacterial cell surface with specific receptors on the pellicle-covered tooth surface. These molecules are termed *adhesins*. These biochemical bonds, as demonstrated in vitro, are inhibited by certain sugars, which suggests the presence of *lectinlike* substances in oral bacteria. These lectins (proteins) would recognize specific carbohydrate structures in the pellicle (carbohydrate groups of glycoproteins). Lectinlike interactions have been demonstrated by selective inhibition of adherence with the addition of sugars. The adherence of *S. mutans* to saliva coated hydroxyapatite is strongly inhibited by galactose but not by lactose, galactosamine, and mannosamine. *S. mutans* binds to α-galactoside residues of pellicle salivary glycoprotein, whereas *S. sanguis* requires sialic acid residues. Lactinlike interactions also are important in bacterial coaggregations.

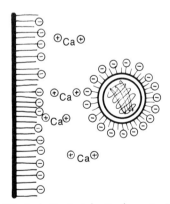

FIGURE 26–4 ✦ Bacterial attachment via electrostatic interactions. Negatively charged components of the bacterial surface and pellicle become linked by cations, such as calcium.

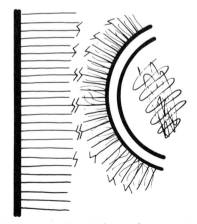

FIGURE 26–5 ✦ Bacterial attachment via hydrophobic interactions. These interactions are based on the close structural fit between molecules on the pellicle (⌐) and bacterial surfaces (⌐).

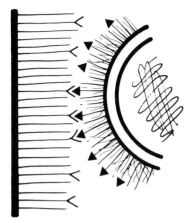

FIGURE 26–6 ✦ Bacterial attachment via specific lectinlike interactions. Lectins (proteins) (▶) in the bacterial surface recognize specific carbohydrate structures in the pellicle (<) and become linked.

Strains of *A. viscosus* and of *S. sanguis* coaggregate through a β-galactose–specific lectin, as well as *S. salivarius* and *Veillonella* (Fig. 26–6).

In 1984, Rolla and associates proposed another specific mechanism for adherence of *S. mutans*. The adhesion of this bacteria involves the production of glycosyltransferase (GTF) by the bacteria. GTF is adhesive and adsorbs to tooth surfaces, where it produces glucans when exposed to sucrose. The interaction between the rigid α-1-3 glucans and adsorbed GTF on the surface may thus cause a strong, specific, sucrose-dependent colonization of *S. mutans*.

Multiple Binding Sites

Evidence suggests that each oral bacteria possesses different cell surface-binding sites responsible for their attachment and accumulation on oral surfaces. *S. mutans* cells react with high molecular weight salivary glycoproteins, which adsorb selectively to hydroxyapatite and which may be responsible for the direct attachment of the bacteria

to the pellicle. This process is very inefficient, probably owing to a low number of binding sites in the pellicle for this organism. *S. mutans* cells also possess other binding sites such as GTF and nonenzyme glucan-binding proteins, which are responsible for their attachment to glucans bound to the tooth surface.

Multiple binding sites involved in interactions with salivary glycoproteins, extracellular polysaccharides, and direct cell-to-cell adhesion are probably necessary for the survival of these organisms in such a complex environment.

GROWTH AND ACCUMULATION OF SUPRAGINGIVAL PLAQUE

Bacteria from saliva or contiguous surfaces adhere to the pellicle saturating the bacterial binding sites. Subsequent growth leads to bacterial accumulation and increased plaque mass. Although adhesion processes dominate in the initial phase of plaque formation, the plaque mass that develops is mainly determined by bacterial multiplication. The relative contributions of adhesion and multiplication to plaque has been demonstrated experimentally where antibacterial treatments have no or negligible effects on adhesion. Plaque accumulation, however, is almost negligible in the absence of cell division (Fig. 26–7).

Accumulation of dental plaque also requires cohesion of bacterial cells. This is accomplished by the formation of plaque matrix, which is dependent on bacterial metabolic activities and salivary and host-derived components. Therefore, factors influencing the ultimate composition and pathogenicity of dental plaque depend on (1) bacterial factors and (2) host and environmental factors (Table 26–2).

Bacterial Factors

Apart from bacterial adhesive mechanisms, already discussed, other bacterial mechanisms play

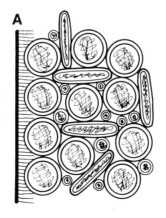
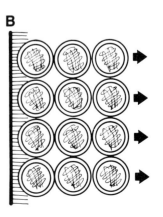

FIGURE 26–7 ✦ Dental plaque growth depends on **(A)** growth via adhesion of new bacteria, and **(B)** growth via multiplication of attached bacteria.

TABLE 26–2 ✦ Factors Influencing the Composition and Maturation of Dental Plaque

I. *Factors of Bacterial Origin*
  A. Extracellular Products:
      Glucans (skeleton of plaque)
      Fructans (energy resources)
  B. Bacterial Interactions: Coaggregation reactions
  C. Plaque Ecology:
      Dietary changes: Sucrose intake—aciduric bacteria
      Oxygen environment—anaerobic bacteria
      Nutritional interactions—bacterial succession
      Bacteriocin production
II. *Host-Derived Factors*
  A. Mechanical Oral Cleansing Mechanisms
  B. Saliva:
      pH, lactoperoxidase, lactoferrin, lysozyme
      Salivary glycoproteins: adhesion mechanisms
  C. Host-Immune Responses:
      Oral secretions—IgA
      Crevicular fluid: leukocytes, IgG, IgM, complement, etc.

TABLE 26–3 ✦ Coaggregation Reactions Between Oral Bacteria

Gram-Positive	Gram-Positive
Streptococcus sp.	*Actinomyces viscosus*
	Actinomyces naeslundii
or	*Actinomyces odontolyticus*
Actinomyces sp.	*Bacterionema matruchottii*
	Propionibacterium acnes
	Gram-Negative
	Bacteroides sp.
	Capnocytophaga sp.
	Fusobacterium nucleatum
	Eikenella corrodens
	Veillonella sp.
Gram-Negative	
Prevotella melaninogenicus	*Fusobacterium nucleatum*
	Capnocytophaga

Adapted from Cisar J. O.: Coaggregation reactions between oral bacteria. In Genco, R. J., and Mergenhagen, S. E. (eds): Host-Parasite Interactions in Periodontal Diseases. ASM, Washington, D.C., 1982.

an important role in plaque growth and accumulation.

Role of Extracellular Products. A variety of oral microorganisms such as *S. mutans, S. sanguis, S. mitis, S. salivarius,* and *Lactobacillus* species can form extracellular polymers from sucrose. The role of these extracellular polysaccharides has been most intensively studied with *S. mutans,* because of its importance in dental caries (see Chapter 27). This microorganism synthesizes large amounts of extracellular glucans (dextran or mutan) from sucrose and forms extracellular enzyme complexes, glucosyltransferases (GTF).

These extracellular glucans are insoluble and result in increased bacterial adhesion. Generally, glucan-induced aggregation does not occur with other streptococcal species, even though they may synthesize glucans. However, *S. mutans* has the capacity to bind glucan molecules, resulting in aggregation and accumulation of these organisms. Furthermore, synthesis of sticky insoluble glucans by *S. mutans* may mediate nonspecific entrapment of other oral microorganisms, promoting the accumulation of bacteria other than *S. mutans. Actinomyces* species can also form copious amounts of plaque in the presence of a variety of carbohydrates. *A. viscosus* synthesizes an extracellular heteropolysaccharide composed of *N*-acetylglucosamine, glucose, and galactose.

Role of Bacterial Interactions. Electron microscopic studies have shown direct interactions between bacteria, with the surface attachment of one species to others. This may have special importance for organisms incapable of attaching *directly* to the tooth surface. *Veillonella,* for example, is unable to attach to glass surfaces in vitro, but adheres and accumulates on preformed plaque of *A. viscosus.* Certain *Actinomyces* species aggregate specifically with *S. sanguis* through β-galactosil residues. The presence of dental plaque containing *Actinomyces* or other gram-positive bacteria may be beneficial for the attachment and colonization of some black-pigmented *Bacteroides* species (Table 26–3).

Plaque Ecology. Changes in dietary carbohydrate alter the microbial composition of dental plaque. Carbohydrate fermentation produces a low pH and an aciduric environment. Among the oral bacteria that grow in this aciduric environment are lactobacilli and certain streptococcal species, mainly *S. mutans.*

Certain bacteria also store intracellular glycogenlike materials known as IPS. These bacteria exhibit prolonged acid production when exogenous carbohydrates are depleted, giving them a better chance of survival. Other exogenous factors, such as ammonia production from urea provoked by bacterial ureases and the presence of lactic acid–fermenting organisms such as *Veillonella* and *Neisseria* also modify the final plaque pH and consequently its pathogenicity.

Oxygen and oxygen products are very important

ecologic determinants because they influence the ability of plaque bacteria to grow and multiply. Streptococci and lactobacilli can grow under facultative conditions, consuming large quantities of oxygen and producing highly reactive and potentially destructive products. Superoxide anions (O_2), hydrogen peroxide (H_2O_2), and hydroxyl radicals (OH^-) that are formed may damage cell membranes and enzyme systems. In order to survive, bacteria must have enzymatic systems that inactivate these oxygen products. The presence of these oxygen products is bactericidal for several oral bacteria and may affect the ultimate bacterial composition of plaque. When there is a heavy accumulation of bacteria, as in mature plaque, the oxygen level and the redox potential are especially low, allowing the growth of obligate anaerobes, unable to survive in an aerobic environment.

For growth, bacteria must be supplied with sources of nutrients and energy. In the formation of supragingival plaque, most nutrients are provided by saliva. Once established, specific members of the supragingival ecosystem produce compounds that are essential nutrients and growth factors for other microorganisms. Lactate, formate, and hydrogen excreted from carbohydrate fermentation by streptococci and *Actinomyces* species are used by *Veillonella* as an energy source. In the catabolism of lactate by *Veillonella*, hydrogen gas is formed, which is used by a number of other organisms such as *Campylobacter, Wolinella,* and black-pigmenting bacteria. Some oral spirochetes require spermine, spermidine, or putrescine, which can be provided by gram-positive rods and fusobacteria. *Veillonella* and other gram-positive rods are able to produce vitamin K, which, together with

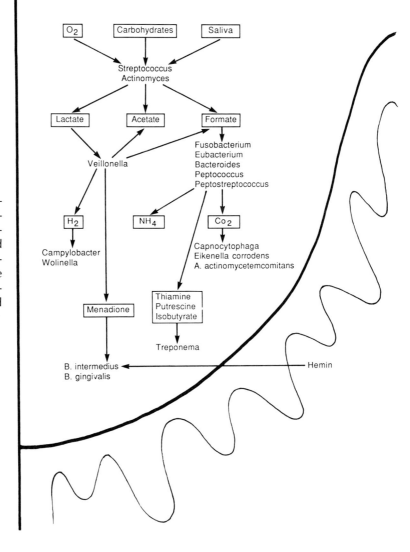

FIGURE 26–8 ✦ Interbacterial and host nutritional interactions influence the maturation of dental plaque. (Adapted from Carlsson, J.: The microbiology of plaque. In J. Lindhe (ed.): Text of Clinical Periodontology. © 1984 Munksgaard Publishers Ltd., Copenhagen.)

hemin, is an essential requirement for the growth of some black-pigmenting bacterial species.

The nutritional interactions among bacteria are thus essential for the microbial succession that takes place in the maturation of supragingival plaque (Fig. 26–8).

Another bacterial factor is bacteriocin. Animal experiments have shown that strains of *S. mutans* are capable of producing bacteriocins that prevent the establishment of *A. viscosus,* but the corresponding nonbacteriocin-producing mutant does not. Therefore, bacteriocin production may influence the microbial ecology by promoting colonization of the bacteriocin-producing bacteria that replace the indigenous flora or prevent accumulation of other bacteria.

Role of Host Factors

Oral cleansing mechanisms such as salivary flow, mastication, and movements of the tongue and cheek are very important in controlling the rate of supragingival plaque formation. Furthermore, the saliva affects the metabolism and microbial composition of this dental plaque.

Saliva influences the plaque pH through several mechanisms, including clearance of carbohydrates, neutralization of plaque acids by salivary buffers, and supply of essential nutrients for specific bacteria such as salivary oxygen, carbon dioxide, and carbohydrates.

Several salivary bacterial inhibitory substances have been identified. Saliva contains the enzyme lactoperoxidase (LPO), which, in combination with a salivary cofactor (salivary thiocyanate-SCN^-) and H_2O_2, generates hypothiocyanate (OSCN), which is much less toxic to the cells than hydrogen peroxide but is a potent inhibitor of bacterial glycolytic enzymes, mainly streptococcal.

Iron is another essential nutrient for bacterial growth. Lactoferrin is an iron-binding protein present in saliva and in other exocrine secretions. The high iron-binding ability of this compound may deprive plaque organisms of iron and thus affect their growth.

Lysozyme, like lactoferrin, is found in saliva. This enzyme splits the bond between *N*-acetylglucosamine and *N*-acetyl muramic acid in the bacterial cell wall.

As mentioned earlier, salivary components including high molecular weight glycoproteins and immunoglobulins can bind to bacterial surfaces and induce their aggregation. This would limit initial bacterial attachment to tooth surfaces or to previously attached bacteria. But the same salivary components are also involved in initial attachment and aggregation of bacteria to saliva-coated oral surfaces. Salivary effects on bacterial adsorption and desorption appear to occur continuously during

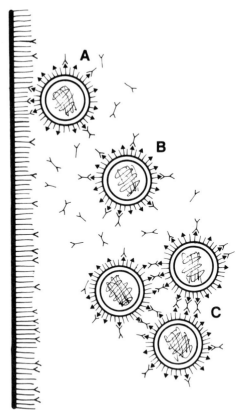

FIGURE 26–9 ✦ Role of saliva in the development and maturation of dental plaque. **A,** Promoting adherence between bacteria and the tooth surface; **B,** inhibiting bacterial adherence by coating their surface receptors; **C,** inhibiting adherence by promoting bacterial agglutination.

plaque formation. Glycoproteins adsorbed to oral surfaces or to firmly attached bacteria in the periphery of plaque may protrude and promote the specific attachment of selected species and prevent adherence of others. On the other hand, salivary polymers adsorbed to bacteria may also promote or inhibit attachment to preexisting plaque (Fig. 26–9).

Finally, the host immune responses also affect the composition of dental plaque. There are two main sources of immune components in the oral cavity: those present in oral secretions and those derived from gingival crevicular fluid. The first category involves antibodies, predominantly IgA, secreted by the salivary glands that act mainly in supragingival plaque by coating bacterial surfaces. This promotes their aggregation and thus prevents their attachment. By interacting with specific receptors on oral surfaces and on bacteria, the antibodies compete with their adherence. Antibodies in the crevicular fluid, in combination with leukocytes and other immune components, such as complement, function predominantly in subgingival areas as a response to the large antigenic challenge in this microenvironment (see Chapter 2).

CLINICAL SIGNIFICANCE

The ecologic mechanisms previously discussed permit the colonization of oral bacteria in a predictable succession. Prevention of the maturation of the microbial community on tooth surfaces may maintain gingival health. However, if plaque is allowed to grow and mature, it usually produces inflammatory changes characteristic of gingivitis.

Clear evidence that supragingival plaque growth and maturation is the direct cause of gingivitis was derived from the experimental gingivitis model (Fig. 26–10). When specific bacteria were studied during the development of gingivitis, young plaque revealed almost entirely gram-positive cocci and rods. By the third day of plaque accumulation, gram-negative cocci and rods, as well as filaments and fusobacteria, began to appear. By day 9, there was a further increase in gram-negative forms, and spiral forms and spirochetes were also detected. Subsequent cultural studies have confirmed these early reports.

At clinically healthy sites, streptococci and facultative species of *Actinomyces,* especially *A. viscosus* and *A. naeslundii,* account for up to 85 percent of the total cultivable flora. During 3 weeks of plaque accumulation, there is an increase of gram-positive rods, especially *A. israelii,* and also of *Fusobacterium, Veillonella,* and *Treponema*

species. At this stage, bacterial species directly associated with periodontitis lesions can be identified in sites with gingivitis. *Eikenella corrodens, Fusobacterium,* and *Capnocytophaga gingivalis* also are elevated in sites with gingivitis. These cultural studies indicate that gingivitis development is not just a mere increase in the amount of plaque, but also requires a sequential colonization of additional specific species. Thus, the bacterial succession in the development of supragingival plaque is ultimately responsible for the inflammatory changes associated with gingivitis.

Subgingival Plaque
STRUCTURE AND DEVELOPMENT

Supragingival plaque directly and indirectly influences the establishment and relative proportions of subgingival microorganisms.

In association with supragingival plaque maturation and accumulation, there are inflammatory changes that modify the anatomic relationships of the gingival margin and the tooth surface (see Chapter 28). When this inflammatory change occurs edema causes gingival enlargement which increases the capacity of the subgingival area for bacterial colonization. This enlarged space protects bacteria from normal oral cleansing mechanisms. At the same time, there is a concomitant increase in the crevicular fluid flow and in pocket epithelial cell turnover. The end result is a new ecologic environment protected from the supragingival mi-

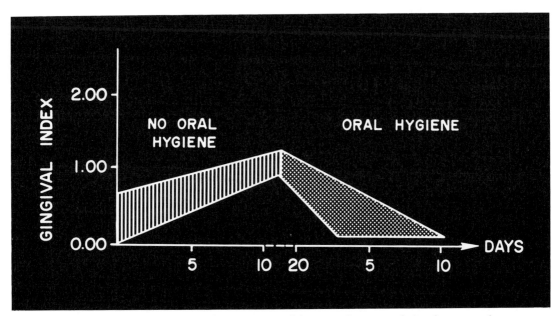

FIGURE 26–10 ✦ Experimental gingivitis model. Note direct correlation between plaque accumulation and gingival inflammation. (Adapted from Löe, H. et al.: Experimental gingivitis in man. J. Periodontal. 36:177, 1965.)

lieu and bathed with gingival crevicular fluid, desquamated epithelial cells, and bacterial end products, which subsequently influence the establishment and relative proportions of subgingival microorganisms. Many of these microorganisms lack the adherence ability to be first colonizers and have evolved mechanisms that can utilize supragingival bacteria as a means of colonization of the subgingival area. Other bacteria, such as certain *Capnocytophaga* species, bind selectively to root cementum and *Eikenella corrodens* binds specifically to epithelial cells, thus demonstrating high specificity to colonize subgingival areas.

Once these microorganisms have colonized the subgingival area, they have access to nutrients (mainly proteins) present in the gingival fluid. This environment has a low oxidation-reduction potential, which allows the most fastidious anaerobic bacteria to become established. Under these conditions, local environmental changes and local host defense reactions allow specific subgingival microorganisms to increase or decrease to a point where they can elicit pathology.

Light and electron microscopic studies of extracted teeth and adjacent tissues from humans have provided information about the internal structure of subgingival plaque. These studies have separated plaque into tooth-associated, epithelium-associated, and connective tissue-associated plaque.

TOOTH-ASSOCIATED SUBGINGIVAL PLAQUE

The structure of this portion of the subgingival plaque is very similar to the supragingival plaque. Bacteria are densely packed, adjacent to the cuticular material covering the root surface. In the inner layers, close to the root surface, the flora is dominated by gram-positive filamentous bacteria. Gram-positive cocci and rods are also present, and some gram-negative cocci and rods can always be found (Fig. 26–11).

This flora is associated with calculus formation, root caries, and root resorption areas in animal models. The apical border of tooth-associated plaque is always found some distance away from the junctional epithelium, and leukocytes are regularly interposed between the plaque and the epithelial surface. In this apical portion, the filamentous organisms are fewer and the bacterial deposit is dominated by gram-negative rods, without a particular orientation.

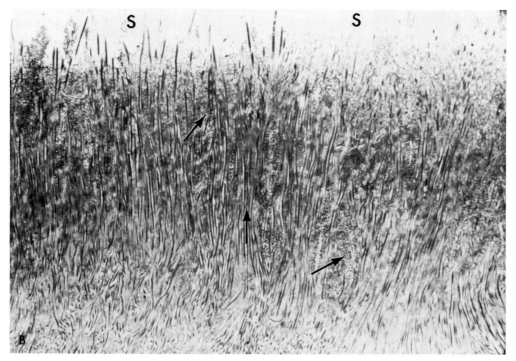

FIGURE 26–11 ✦ Tooth-associated 1-day-old supragingival plaque, dominated by gram-positive cocci microcolonies *(arrows)* and gram-positive filamentous bacteria extending perpendicularly away from the tooth surface. S = surface bathed with saliva. (Courtesy of Dr. Max Listgarten. From Carranza, F. A. Jr.: Glickman's Clinical Periodontology, ed. 6. W. B. Saunders, Philadelphia, 1984, with permission.)

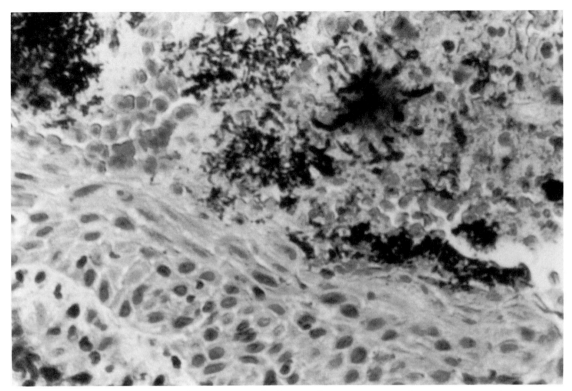

FIGURE 26–12 ✦ Epithelium-associated plaque, showing no specific orientation and organization, being loosely adherent to the epithelial cells.

EPITHELIUM-ASSOCIATED SUBGINGIVAL PLAQUE

This loosely adherent component of subgingival plaque is in direct association with the gingival epithelium, extending from the gingival margin to the junctional epithelium. It contains one layer in contact with the epithelial cells and another loose in the sulcular or pocket lumen.

This plaque contains predominantly gram-negative rods and cocci, as well as a large number of flagellated bacteria and spirochetes. The organisms are not oriented in any specific manner, and they are very loosely adherent due to the absence of a definite intermicrobial matrix (Fig. 26–12).

The relative proportions of the subgingival plaque components appear to be related to the nature and activity of the periodontal condition (see Chapter 28). In rapidly advancing lesions, such as localized juvenile periodontitis, the tooth associated component of the subgingival plaque appears to be minimal. These periodontal pockets contain almost exclusively gram-negative, motile organisms (Fig. 26–13). A similar pattern of subgingival bacterial colonization occurs in rapidly progressing periodontitis. It has been suggested that plaque adjacent to the *junctional epithelium* may be the *"advancing front"* of the periodontal lesion. Recent morphologic data from advanced periodontitis

cases suggests a direct relationship between the bacteria in this "advancing front" and connective tissue–associated bacteria within the gingival tissue (Fig. 26–14).

Electron microscopic studies of the soft tissue wall of periodontal pockets have revealed distinct areas of heavy bacterial accumulation. Other areas along the epithelium exhibit evidence of a strong host response consisting of the emergence of leukocytes and leukocyte-bacterial interactions. Areas of tissue destruction as evidenced by hemorrhage and ulceration can also be seen. The presence of these distinct areas suggests that the pocket wall is constantly changing as a result of the interaction between the epithelium, the epithelium-associated bacteria, and host factors. These different microenvironments may be important in allowing colonization and growth of specific bacteria and, most likely, allowing bacterial penetration into the tissues by some of the subgingival bacteria (Fig. 26–15).

CONNECTIVE TISSUE-ASSOCIATED SUBGINGIVAL PLAQUE

Microscopic studies have shown the presence of subgingival bacteria within gingival connective tissue in different periodontal conditions (see Chap-

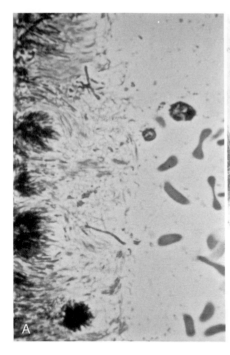

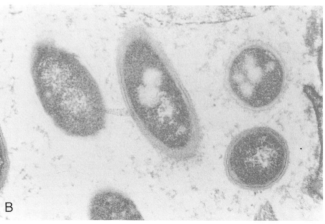

FIGURE 26–13 ✦ Subgingival plaque in juvenile periodontitis. **A,** The tooth-associated component is scarce. It is dominated by loosely adherent plaque. (Courtesy of Dr. Max Listgarten.) **B,** Detail of this subgingival microbiota showing gram-negative rods and cocci as the dominant bacteria.

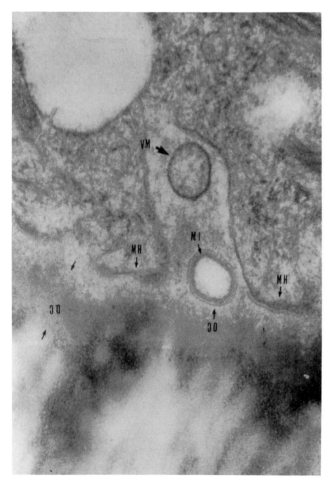

FIGURE 26–14 ✦ Apical progression of subgingival bacteria in advanced periodontitis. In this micrograph a typical gram-negative bacterium is seen penetrating between junctional epithelial cells and the tooth surface. MV = microvilli; OC = outer coat; IM = inner membrane; HM = hemidesmosome; DC = dental cuticle.

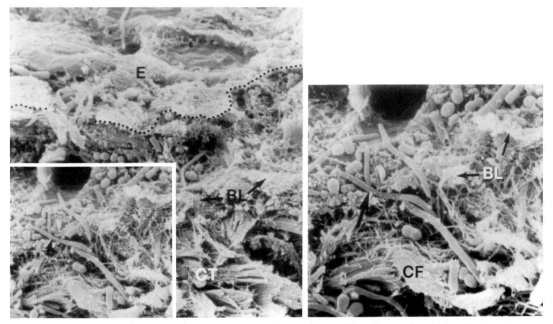

FIGURE 26–15 ✦ Bacterial penetration into the pocket wall in advanced periodontitis. Note the penetration through the pocket epithelium and basement lamina into the connective tissue *(arrows)*. E = epithelium; BL = basement lamina; CT = connective tissue; CF = collagen fibers. (Courtesy of Dr. R. Saglie.)

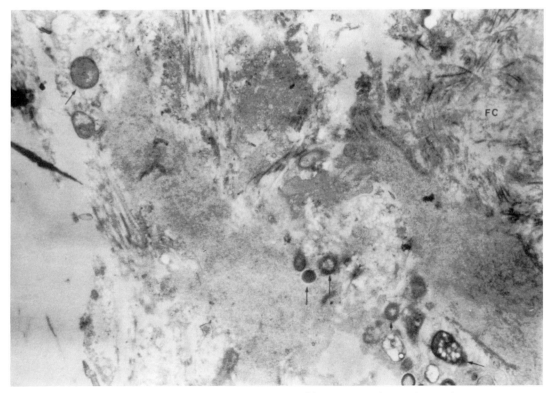

FIGURE 26–16 ✦ Connective tissue associated bacteria in advanced periodontitis.

ter 28). This bacterial presence, has been demonstrated in acute ulcerative gingivitis, advanced periodontitis, and localized juvenile periodontitis (Fig. 26–16). The clinical significance is unclear (see Chapter 28).

DENTAL CALCULUS

Since ancient times, calculus has been etiologically linked with periodontal diseases. In the last 25 years it has clearly been demonstrated that calculus per se does not have *direct* etiologic significance in periodontal disease and only acts to favor plaque accumulation. However, it may play a major role in *maintaining* and *accentuating* periodontal disease by keeping plaque in close contact with the gingival tissue and creating areas where plaque removal is impossible. Subgingival calculus may also facilitate ulceration of the periodontal pocket wall in periodontitis.

The etiologic role of calculus has become clear mainly through two lines of research:

1. Experimental and electron microscopic studies of developing plaque and calculus have demonstrated that supragingival and subgingival calculus consisted of mineralized plaque always covered by an unmineralized bacterial layer.

2. Epidemiologic studies showed a strong correlation between calculus and periodontal disease.

Definition and Classification

Dental calculus may be defined as adherent calcified or calcifying deposits on teeth and other solid structures in the oral cavity. Ordinarily in humans it consists of mineralized bacterial plaque, although in germ-free animals, calcified tooth deposits occur in the absence of bacteria, probably as a result of mineralization of organic films or food derivatives.

Calculus is classified according to its relation to the gingival margin. *Supragingival calculus* refers to calculus coronal to the gingival margin and visible in the oral cavity. It is usually white or whitish yellow, although the color may change to brown as a result of secondary staining. It may localize on a single tooth or a group of teeth or be generalized throughout the mouth forming bridge-like structures along adjacent teeth (Fig. 26–17). Supragingival calculus occurs more frequently and in greatest quantity on the buccal surfaces of the maxillary molars opposite Stensen's duct, and on the lingual surfaces of the mandibular anterior teeth opposite Warton's duct of the submandibular and Bartholin's duct of the sublingual salivary glands (Fig. 26–18). Poor oral hygiene, lack of adequate masticatory function, and tooth malposition can contribute to an increased rate and quantity of calculus.

Subgingival calculus refers to calculus that forms below the gingival margin, usually in periodontal pockets, therefore, it is not visible upon oral examination. It is usually dense and hard, dark-brown or greenish-black, flintlike in consistency, and firmly attached to the tooth surface. Subgingival calculus is more evenly distributed on teeth than supragingival calculus, but on the individual tooth subgingival calculus is more prevalent on the approximal and lingual tooth surfaces than on the buccal surfaces. It is often difficult to detect by visual inspection. It may be seen by detachment of the gingival margin from the tooth by air blast or with an instrument (Fig. 26–19). It can also be detected by tactile detection with a periodontal probe or a fine explorer, although this method has proved inefficient.

Gross deposits of calculus on the approximal surfaces of teeth can also be visible on radiographs, although its appearance is dependent on its density and radiographic technique (Fig. 26–20).

Supragingival and subgingival calculus generally occur together, but one may be present without the other. Microscopic studies have demonstrated that the calcified deposits usually extend near but

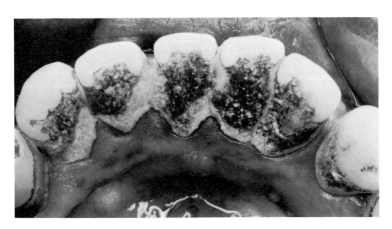

FIGURE 26–17 ✦ Calculus forming a bridge-like structure on the lingual surface of the mandibular anterior teeth. (From Carranza, F. A. Jr.: Glickman's Clinical Periodontology, ed. 6. W. B. Saunders, Philadelphia, 1984, with permission.)

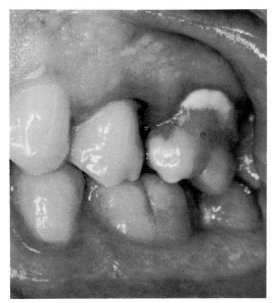

FIGURE 26–18 ✦ Calculus on a molar opposite to the Stensen's duct. (From Carranza, F. A. Jr.: Glickman's Clinical Periodontology, ed. 6. W. B. Saunders, Philadelphia, 1984, with permission.)

do not reach the base of periodontal pockets in chronic periodontal lesions.

Composition

Calculus is a mineralized deposit with an inorganic content similar to bone, dentin, or cementum.

Supragingival calculus consists of 70 to 90 percent inorganic salts, with calcium and phosphorus the major constituents, mainly in the form of calcium phosphate ($Ca_3(PO_4)_2$); although calcium carbonate ($CaCO_3$) and magnesium phosphate ($Mg_3(PO_4)_2$) also occur. At least two thirds of the inorganic component is crystalline in structure, with four main crystal forms: hydroxyapatite [Ca_{10} (PO_4)$_6$ (OH)$_2$] approximately in 58 percent; magnesium whitlockite [Ca_9 (PO_4)$_6$ $\times$ PO_7] and octacalcium phosphate [Ca_4H (PO_4)$_3$ $\times$ $2H_2O$] approximately 21 percent each; and brushite [Ca-$OHP_4 \cdot 2H_2O$] approximately 9 percent.

Generally two or more crystal forms occur in calculus, and their incidence varies according to the age and location of calculus. Brushite is more common in supragingival calculus and in the mandibular anterior region, while magnesium whitlockite is present particularly in the subgingival variety and in the posterior areas. It appears that brushite appears first, then octacalcium phosphate, and as the calculus matures, whitlockite and hydroxyapatite predominate.

The organic component of calculus consists of a mixture of protein-polysaccharide complexes, desquamated epithelial cells, leukocytes, and various types of microorganisms and is comparable to that of dental plaque.

The composition of subgingival and supragingival calculus differ. Subgingival calculus has similar hydroxyapatite content, but more magnesium whitlockite and less brushite and octacalcium phosphate, as well as a higher ratio of calcium to phosphate.

Structure

A clearer understanding of the structure of calculus is provided by electron microscopy. Calculus is a layered structure in which the degree of calcification varies among the different layers (Fig. 26–21). Its structure is dominated by small, needle-shaped, inorganic crystals that, by electron diffraction, show a pattern of apatite. These crystals

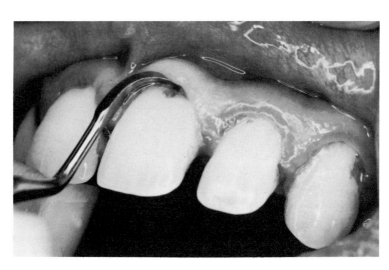

FIGURE 26–19 ✦ Subgingival calculus seen by detachment of the gingival margin. (From Carranza, F. A. Jr.: Glickman's Clinical Periodontology, ed. 6. W. B. Saunders, Philadelphia, 1984, with permission.)

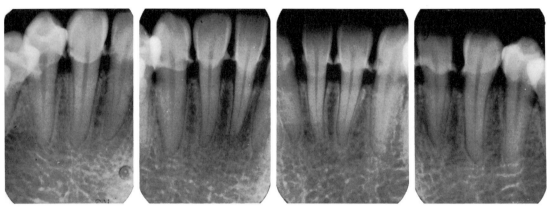

FIGURE 26–20 ✦ Gross deposits of calculus can be seen interproximally on radiographs. Buccally and lingually, their image is superimposed on teeth. (From Carranza, F. A. Jr.: Glickman's Clinical Periodontology, ed. 6. W. B. Saunders, Philadelphia, 1984, with permission.)

are randomly oriented and contain outlines of calcified microorganisms.

Both scanning and transmission electron microscopic studies have shown that its surface is very rough and is covered by a layer of unmineralized bacterial plaque (Fig. 26–22). This bacterial covering is different between supragingival and subgingival calculus. On supragingival calculus, filamentous organisms oriented at right angles to the surface usually dominate. Subgingival calculus is usually covered by cocci, rods, and filamentous organisms, with no distinct pattern of orientation.

The porous nature of calculus is also observed with tubular holes or orifices usually representing areas of uncalcified bacteria surrounded by calcified matrix.

Different experimental studies have also proved its porous nature. In 1970, Baumhammers showed

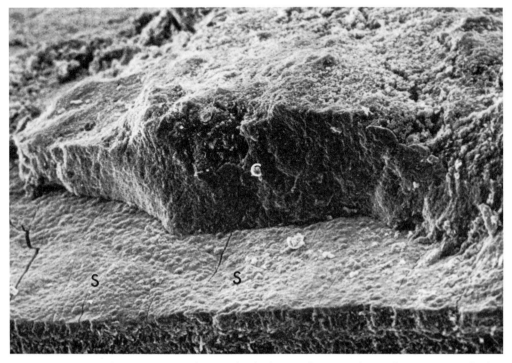

FIGURE 26–21 ✦ Cross-sectional view of calculus (C) showing a layered structure attached to the cementum surface (S). (Courtesy of Dr. Sottosanti.) (From Carranza, F. A. Jr.: Glickman's Clinical Periodontology, ed. 6. W. B. Saunders, Philadelphia, 1984, with permission.)

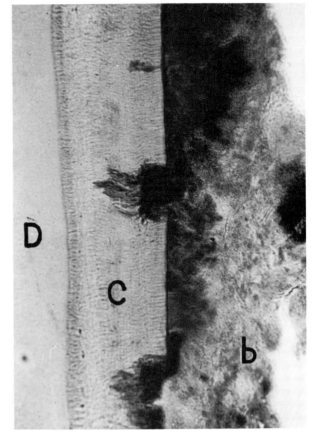

FIGURE 26–22 ✦ Subgingival calculus attached to the cementum surface. Note that its surface is covered by a layer of nonmineralized bacterial plaque. (From Carranza, F. A. Jr.: Glickman's Clinical Periodontology, ed. 6. W. B. Saunders, Philadelphia, 1984, with permission.)

that calculus can be completely permeated by dyes within 24 hours. Therefore, it has been hypothesized that dental calculus acts as a reservoir for irritating substances from microbial plaque and tissue lysis. Patters and coworkers showed a higher bone resorption activity and higher *Porphyromonas gingivalis* antigen in samples from calculus than from cementum. These studies suggested an intrinsic pathogenic potential of dental calculus.

Calculus Formation

As described earlier, calculus is dental plaque that has undergone mineralization. The plaque accumulation serves as an organic matrix for the subsequent mineralization. The precipitation of mineral salts usually begins in 1 to 14 days after plaque formation.

All plaque does not necessarily undergo calcification, and microorganisms are not always essential in calculus formation. The mineral source for supragingival calculus is saliva and for subgingival calculus, gingival fluid, or exudates. Biochemical studies show that plaque from heavy calculus formers contains three times more phosphorus and less potassium than from minimal calculus formers.

Calcification begins by the binding of calcium ions to the carbohydrate-protein complexes of the organic matrix and the subsequent precipitation of crystalline calcium phosphate salts. Crystals form initially in the intercellular matrix and on bacterial surfaces and finally within the bacteria (i.e., *Bacterionema*). Calcification begins as foci along the inner surface of the supragingival plaque and in the attached component of the subgingival plaque adjacent to the tooth. It increases in size and coalescences to form solid masses of calculus.

Calculus is formed in layers, often separated by a thin cuticle that becomes embedded within the calculus as calcification progresses.

Supragingival calculus sometimes forms in less than 2 weeks. However, the development of a hard deposit with a crystal composition characteristic of old calculus may require months.

Different theories have been proposed to explain the mechanisms of calculus calcification, and probably all explain some part of the calcification process. According to the *epitaxic theory*, through a nucleation process an initial crystal or nucleus is formed where subsequent ectopic calcification takes place. According to the *booster mechanism theory*, calcification will occur when the local pH and calcium and phosphorus are high enough to allow for precipitation. Finally, according to the *transformation theory,* amorphous, noncrystalline deposits and brushite are transformed to octocalcium phosphate and then to hydroxyapatite.

Etiologic Significance of Calculus

Although calculus is invariably associated with periodontal disease, it is difficult to separate the effects of calculus from those of plaque because calculus is always covered by a nonmineralized layer of plaque.

From epidemiologic data, there is a positive correlation between calculus and the prevalence of gingivitis, although the correlation between plaque and gingivitis is much stronger. Therefore, it is assumed that the nonmineralized plaque on the calculus surface is the primary irritant, although the underlying calcifying portion may be a contributing factor because its rough surface provides a fixed nidus for the continuous accumulation of plaque and a means to hold this plaque against the gingiva. However, it has been clearly demonstrated that roughness per se does not cause gingivitis, and calculus without bacteria may permit an epithelial attachment to form. Calculus may also become encapsulated in connective tissue without causing a marked inflammatory reaction.

BIBLIOGRAPHY

Ainamo, J.: Concomitant periodontal disease and dental caries in young adult males. Soumen Hammaslaakariseuran Tomituksia 66:301, 1970.

Allen, D. L. and Kerr, D. A.: Tissue response in the guinea pig to sterile and non-sterile calculus. J. Periodontol. 36:121, 1965.

Axelsson, P. and Lindhe, J.: The effect of a preventive programme on dental plaque, gingivitis, caries in schoolchildren. Results after one and two years. J. Clin. Peridontol. 1:126, 1974.

Baer P. and Newton W. L.: The occurrence of periodontal disease in germ-free mice, J. Dent. Res. 38:1238, 1959.

Baumhammers, A. and Rohrbaugh, E. A.: Permeability of human and rat dental calculus. J. Periodontol. 41:39, 1970.

Bladen, H., Hageage, G., Pollock, F., and Harr, R.: Plaque formation in vitro on wires by Gram negative oral microorganisms *(Veillonella).* Arch. Oral Biol. 15:127, 1970.

Boskey A. L.: Current concepts of the physiology and biochemistry of calcification. Clin. Orthop. 157:225, 1981.

Bowden, G. H., Mulnes, A. R., and Boyar, R.: *Streptococcus mutans* and caries. In Guggehein, B. (ed.): Cariology Today. Karger, Basel, 1984, pp. 173–181.

Brecx, M., Ronstrom, A., Theilade, J., and Attstrom, R.: Early plaque formation of dental plaque on plastic films. J. Periodont. Res. 16:213, 1981.

Carranza, F. A., Saglie, F. R., Newman, M. G., and Valentin, P.: Scanning and transmission electron microscopic study of tissue invading microorganisms in localized juvenile periodontitis. J. Periodontol. 54:598, 1983.

Celesk, R. A., McCabe, R. M., and London, J.: Colonization of the cementum surface of teeth by oral gram-negative bacteria. Infect. Immun. 26:15, 1979.

Cisar, J. O.: Coaggregation reactions between oral bacteria. In Genco, R. J., and Mergenhagen, S. E. (eds.): Host-Parasite Interactions in Periodontal Diseases. ASM, Washington, D.C., 1982, pp. 121–131.

Eanes E. D.: An electron microscopic study of the formation of amorphous calcium phosphate and its transformation to crystalline apatite. Calcif. Tissue Res. 6:32, 1970.

Egelberg, J.: Local effect of diet on plaque formation and development of gingivitis in dogs. Odontologysk Revy 16:31, 1965.

Eide, B., Lie, T., and Selvig, K. A.: Surface coatings on dental cementum incident to periodontal disease. I. A scanning electron microscopic study. J. Clin. Periodontol. 10:157, 1983.

Ellen, R. P. and Balcerzak-Raczkowski, I. B.: Interbacterial aggregation of *Actinomyces naeslundii* and dental plaque streptococci. J. Periodont. Res. 12:11, 1973.

Embery, G., Hogg, S. D., Heaney, T. G., Stanbury, J. B., and Green, D. R. J.: Some considerations on dental pellicle formation and early bacterial colonization. In Ten Cate, J. M., Arens J., and Leach, S. A. (eds.): Bacterial Adhesion and Preventive Dentistry. IRL, Oxford, 1984, pp. 73–84.

Frank, R. M. and Houver, G.: An ultrastructural study of human supragingival dental plaque formation. In McHugh, W. D. (ed.): Dental Plaque. Churchill-Livingstone, Edinburgh, 1970, pp. 85–108.

Frank, R. M.: Bacterial penetration in the apical pocket wall of advanced human periodontitis, J. Periodont. Res. 15:563, 1980.

Friskopp, J.: Ultrastructure of noncalcified supragingival and subgingival calculus. J. Periodontol. 54:542, 1983.

Friskopp, J. and Hammarstrom, L.: A comparative, scanning electron microscopic study of supragingival and subgingival calculus. J. Periodontol. 51:553, 1980.

Gibbons, R. J. and Engle, L. P.: Vitamin K compounds in bacteria that are obligate anaerobes. Science 146:1307, 1964.

Gibbons, R. J. and Qureshi, J. V.: Inhibition of adsorption of *Streptococcus mutans* strains to saliva treated hydroxyapatite by galactose and certain amines. Infect. Immunol. 26:1214, 1979.

Gillet, R. and Johnson, N. W.: Bacterial invasion of the periodontium in a case of juvenile periodontitis. J. Clin. Periodontol. 9:93, 1982.

Gonzalez, F. and Sognnaes, R. F.: Electron-microscopy of dental calculus. Science 131:156, 1960.

Gustafsson, B. E. and Krasse, B.: Dental calculus in germ free rats. Acta Odontol. Scand. 20:135, 1962.

Huis in't Veld, J. H. J.: Ecological aspects of dental plaque development. In Leach, S. A. (ed.): Dental

Plaque and Surface Interactions in the Oral Cavity. IRL, London, 1980, pp. 123–143.

Jordan, H. V. and Keyes, P. H.: Aerobic gram positive filamentous bacteria as etiologic agent of experimental periodontal disease in hamsters. Arch. Oral Biol. 9:401, 1964.

Kleingerg, I., Kanapka, J. A., and Craw, D.: Effect of saliva and salivary factors on the metabolism of the mixed oral flora. In Stiles, Loesche, and O'Brien (eds.): Microbial Aspects of Dental Caries. Microbiology Abstr. (Suppl.) Vol. 11, 1976, pp. 433–464.

Kolenbrohder, P. E., Andersen, R. N., and Holdeman, L. V.: Coaggregation of oral bacteroides species with other bacteria. Infect. Immunol. 48:741, 1985.

Leach, S. A. and Agalamany, E. A.: Hydrophobic interactions that may be involved in the formation of dental plaque. In Ten Cate, J. M., Leach, S. M., and Arens, J. (eds.): Bacterial Adhesion and Preventive Dentistry. IRL, Oxford, 1984, pp. 43–49.

Lie, T.: Early dental plaque morphogenesis. J. Periodont. Res. 12:73, 1977.

Lie, T.: Ultrastructural study of early dental plaque formation. J. Periodont. Res. 13:391, 1978.

Liljemark, W. F. and Schauer, S. V.: Competitive binding among oral streptococci to hydroxyapatite. J. Dent. Res. 56:157, 1977.

Lindhe, J., Hamp, S.-E., and Loe, H.: Experimental periodontitis in the Beagle dog. J. Periodont. Res. 8:1, 1973.

Lindhe, J., Haffajjee, A. D., and Socransky, S. S.: Progression of periodontal disease in adult subjects in the absence of periodontal therapy. J. Clin. Periodontol. 10:433, 1983.

Lindhe, J. and Nyman, S.: Long-term maintenance of patients treated for advanced periodontal disease. J. Clin. Periodontol. 11:504, 1984.

Listgarten, M. A.: Electron microscopic observations on the bacterial flora of acute necrotizing ulcerative gingivitis. J. Periodontol. 36:328, 1965.

Listgarten, M. A.: Structure of the microbial flora associated with periodontal health and disease in man. A light and electron microscope study. J. Periodontol. 47:1, 1976.

Listgarten, M. A. and Ellegard, B.: Electron microscopic evidence of a cellular attachment between junctional epithelium and dental calculus. J. Periodont. Res. 8:143, 1973.

Listgarten, M. A., Mayo, H., and Amsterdam, M.: Ultrastructure of the attachment device between coccal and filamentous microorganisms in corn cob formations in dental plaque. Arch. Oral Biol. 8:651, 1973.

Listgarten, M. A., Mayo, H., and Tremblay, R.: Development of dental plaque on epoxy resin crowns in man. A light and electron microscope study. J. Periodontol. 46:10, 1975.

Little, M. F. and Hazen, S. P.: Dental calculus composition. II. Subgingival calculus: ash, calcium, phosphorus and sodium. J. Dent. Res. 43:645, 1964.

Loe, H.: Epidemiology of periodontal disease, and evaluation of the relative significance of the etiologic factors in light of recent epidemiological research. Odontologisk Tidskrift 71:479, 1963.

Loe, H. E., Theilade, E., and Jensen, S. B.: Experimental gingivitis in man. J. Periodontol. 36:177, 1965.

Loesche, W. J. and Syed, S. A.: The bacteriology of human experimental gingivitis. Infect. Immunol. 21:830, 1978.

Lovdal, A., Arno, A., and Waehaug, J.: Incidence of clinical manifestations of periodontal disease in light of oral hygiene and calculus formation. J. Am. Dent. Assoc. 56:21, 1958.

Mandel, I. D.: Histochemical and biochemical aspects of calculus formation. Periodontics 1:43, 1963.

Mandel I. D. and Gaffar A.: Calculus revisited: A review. J. Clin. Periodontol. 13:249, 1986.

Moore, W. E., Holdeman, L. V., Smibert, R. M., Good, I. J., Burmeister, J. A., Palcanis, K., and Ranney, R. R.: Bacteriology of experimental gingivitis in young adult humans. Infect. Immun. 38:651, 1982.

Newman, H. N.: Ultrastructure of the apical border of dental plaque. In Lehner, T. (ed.): The Borderland Between Caries and Periodontal Disease. Academic Press, London, 1977, pp. 78–103.

Olsson, J., Glantz, P.-O., and Krasse, B.: Surface potential and adherence of oral streptococci to solid surfaces. Scand. J. Dent. Res. 84:240, 1976.

Oste, R., Ronstrom, A., Birkhed, D., Edwardsson, S., and Stemberg, M.: Gas-liquid chromatographic analysis of aminoacids in pellicle formed on tooth surface and plastic film in vitro. Arch. Oral Biol. 26:635, 1981.

Østravik, D.: Initial bacterial adhesion to surfaces: ecological implications in dental plaque formation. In Ten Cate, J. M., Leach, S. A., and Arens, J. (eds.): Bacterial Adhesion and Preventive Dentistry. IRL, Oxford, 1984, pp. 153–166.

Patters, M. R., Landersberg, R. L., Johansson, L. A., Trummel, C. L., and Robertson, P. B.: *Bacteroides gingivalis* antigens and bone resorption activity in root surface fractions of periodontally involved teeth. J. Periodont. Res. 17:122, 1982.

Pollock, J. J., Iacono, V. J., Goodman Bicker, H., McKay, B., Katona, L. I., Taichman, L. B., and Thomas, E.: The binding, aggregation and lytic properties of lysozyme. In Stiles, Loesche, and O'Brien (eds.): Microbial Aspects of Dental Caries. Microbiol. Abstr. 11(Suppl.):325, 1976.

Ramfjord, S. P.: The periodontal status of boys 11–17 years old in Bombay, India. J. Periodontol. 32:237, 1961.

Ramfjord, S. P., Knowles, J. W., Nissle, R. R., Schick, R. A., and Burgett, F. G.: Longitudinal study of periodontal therapy. J. Periodontol. 46:66, 1973.

Rogers, A. H., van der Hoeven, J. S., and Mikx, F.: Effect of bacteriocin production by *Streptococcus mutans* on the plaque of gnotobiotic rats. Infect. Immun. 23:571, 1979.

Rolla, G.: Formation of dental integuments—Some basic chemical considerations. Swed. Dent. J. 1:241, 1977.

Rolla, G., Bonesvoll, P., and Opermann, T.: Interaction between oral streptococci and salivary proteins. In Kleinberg, Ellison, and Mandel (eds.): Proceedings of Saliva and Dental Caries (sp. supp.) Microbiology Abstr. 1979, pp. 227–241.

Rolla, G., Ciardi, J. E., Deas, M., Lau, A., and Bowen, W. H.: Adherence of active glycosyltransferase from *Streptococcus mutans* to ionic, hydrophobic and dextran surfaces. In Ten Cate, J. M., Leach, S. A., and Arens, J. (eds.): Bacterial Adhesion and Preventive Dentistry. IRL, Oxford, 1984, pp. 133–142.

Rowles, S. L.: The inorganic composition of dental calculus. In Blackwood, H. J. J. (ed.): Bone and Tooth. Pergamon Press, Oxford, 1964, pp. 175–183.

Saglie, R., Newman, M. G., Carranza, F. A., and Pattison, G. L.: Bacterial invasion of gingiva in advanced periodontitis in humans. J. Periodontol. 53:217, 1982.

Sanz, M., Herrera, I., Bascones, A., Newman, M. G., and Saglie, R.: Association of bacterial invasion with the advancing front of the periodontitis lesion. J. Dent. Res. 65, Spec Iss. AADR A#116, 1986.

Schroeder, H. E.: Inorganic content and histology of early calculus content in man. Helv. Odontol. Acta 7:17, 1963.

Schroeder, H. E. and Baumbauer, H. U.: Stages of calcium phosphate crystallization during calculus formation. Arch. Oral Biol. 11:1, 1966.

Schroeder, H. E.: Formation and inhibition of dental calculus. Bern, Switzerland, Hans Huber Publishers, 1969.

Silverman, G. and Kleinberg, I.: Fractionation of human dental plaque and the characterization of its cellular and acellular components. Arch. Oral Biol. 12:1387, 1967.

Slots, J. and Gibbons, R. J.: Attachment of *Bacteroides melaninogenicus* subsp. *asaccharolyticus* to oral surfaces and its possible role in colonization of the mouth and of periodontal pockets. Infect. Immunol. 19:254, 1978.

Socransky, S. S., Gibbons, R. J., Dale, A. C., Bortnick, L., Rosenthal, E., and McDonald, J. B.: The microbiota of the gingival crevice in man. Arch. Oral Biol. 8:275, 1963.

Sonju, T. and Glantz, P.-O.: Chemical composition of salivary integuments formed in vivo on solids with some established surface characteristics. Arch. Oral Biol. 20:687, 1975.

Tanner, A. C. R., Haffer, C., Brathall, G. T., Visconti, R. A., and Socransky, S. S.: *Wolinella* gen. nov., *Wolinella succinogenes* comb. nov. and description of *Bacteroides gracilis* sp. nov., *Wolinella recta* sp.

nov., and *Eikenella corrodens* from humans with periodontal disease. Int. J. Syst. Bacteriol. 31:432, 1981.

Theilade, E., Wright, W. H., Jensen, S. B., and Loe, H.: Experimental gingivitis in man. II. A longitudinal clinical and bacteriological investigation. J. Periodont. Res. 1:1, 1966.

Theilade, J.: The microscopic structure of dental calculus. Thesis. University of Rochester, Rochester, NY, 1960.

Theilade, J.: Development of bacterial plaque in the oral cavity. J. Clin. Periodontol. 4 (extra issue No. 5):1, 1977.

Turesky, S., Renstrup, G., and Glickman, I.: Histologic and histochemical observations regarding early calculus formation in children and adults. J. Periodontol. 32:7, 1961.

van Houte, J.: Bacterial adhesion in the mouth. In Leach, S. A. (ed.): Dental Plaque and Surface Interactions in the Oral Cavity. IRL, London, 1980, pp. 69–99.

van Houte, J.: Colonization mechanisms involved in the development of the oral flora. In Genco, R. J., and Mergenhagen, S. E. (eds.): Host-Parasite Interactions in Periodontal Diseases. ASM, Washington, DC, 1982, pp. 86–97.

Waerhaug, J.: Healing of dento-epithelial junction following subgingival plaque control. II. As observed on extracted teeth. J. Periodontol. 49:119, 1978.

Waerhaug, J.: The infrabony pocket and its relationship to trauma from occlusion and subgingival plaque. J. Periodontol. 50:355, 1979.

Warl, W.: Role of oral hygiene practices in oral health and general health. In Loe, H., and Kleinman, D. (eds.): Dental plaque—control measures and oral hygiene practices, IRL, Oxford, 1986.

Weerkamp, A. H., van der Mei, H. C., Engelen, D. P. E., and de Windt, C. A. E.: Adhesion receptors (adhesins) of oral streptococci. In Ten Cate, J. M., Leach, S.A., and Arens, J. (eds.): Bacterial Adhesion and Preventive Dentistry. IRL, London, 1984.

Westergaard, J., Frandsen, A., and Slots, J.: Ultrastructure of the subgingival flora in juvenile periodontitis. Scand. J. Dent. Res. 86:421, 1978.

World Health Organization (WHO): Periodontal Disease. Geneva WHO Technical Report Series No. 207, 1961.

Yawazaki, Y., Ebisu, S., and Okada, H: *Eikenella corrodens* adherence to buccal epithelial cells. Infect. Immunol. 31:21, 1981.

27 *Caries and Cariology*

Lawrence E. Wolinsky

CHAPTER OUTLINE

Caries microbiology

Caries physiology

Caries theories

Caries histopathology

Plaque formation

Plaque biochemistry

Host factors and caries

Caries control and prevention

Root caries

Dental caries is a slow decomposition of teeth resulting from the loss of hydroxyapatite crystals. This mineralized matrix dissolution reduces the structural integrity of the teeth. The bacterial nature of this process may result in a chronic infection of the tooth, eventual loss of teeth and supporting alveolar bone. Current understanding supports the "plaque-host-substrate" theory, whereby caries has a bacterial etiology interdependent on (1) the host defense systems, (2) dietary factors, and (3) time. Caries occurs when all these factors are operating together (Fig. 27–1). This chapter will consider the microbiology, physiology, and immunology of dental caries. In addition, an examination of recent developments in the treatment of caries will be presented.

CARIES MICROBIOLOGY

A large body of in vitro and in vivo data supports the belief that caries only occurs in the presence of microorganisms. First, germ-free animals only develop caries in the presence of bacteria. Second, oral bacteria can cause demineralization of enamel in vivo. Third, histologic studies have shown bacteria within the enamel and dentin of carious lesions. However, which bacteria are the primary etiologic agents in various types of dental caries is not completely clear.

To examine this question, one must realize there are three types of caries: enamel, dentin, and root

surface caries. Enamel surface caries can be further divided into smooth surface and pit and fissure caries. The smooth-surface lesion has a well-characterized microbiology (Table 27–1). The most consistently found organisms in this lesion are gram-positive facultative cocci, specifically *Streptococcus mutans* and *S. salivarius*. *S. mutans* is the primary etiologic organism for this type of carious lesion based upon several observations. It ferments sugars to lactic acid which is thought responsible for dissolution of the enamel matrix. *S. mutans* also is a prolific producer of insoluble extracellular dextrans, which allow bacteria to stick to the tooth surface. Furthermore, it is highly selective for the pellicle-coated enamel surface. While *S. mutans* is a minor smooth-surface plaque component (2 to 7 percent of the total), it is considered the primary etiologic organism because of its caries producing potential. *S. salivarius,* also present in smooth surface caries, has been shown to produce caries in animals. However, its role in the production of the carious lesion is not yet fully known. Although the facultative streptococci are the predominant organisms, the microbial ecology of smooth-surface plaque is quite complex. The microbial population of plaque changes dramatically with time. During the early stages of plaque development, the gram-positive cocci predominate, owing to their preferential affinity for pellicle-bound salivary components of the tooth. During this early period the environment is fairly rich in

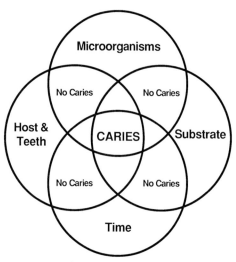

FIGURE 27–1 ✦ Diagrammatic representation of the parameters involved in the development of human caries. All individual factors must be present before caries can occur.

Pit and fissure caries are the most common human lesions. However, much less is known about its microbiology compared to smooth surface caries. In addition, a good model for this lesion is not available. One would expect to find a wide variety of bacterial types because of the varied environment. However, the microbiology has remained elusive, owing to difficulties in accurately sampling these areas. "Artificial fissures" have been created by folding mylar strips and inserting them into the mouth for subsequent bacterial sampling. Coccoid forms constituted 75 to 95 percent of the organisms, with *S. sanguis* being the predominant bacteria. As the plaque aged, the relative numbers of *S. mutans* and lactobacilli increased. The validity of the mylar strip model for pit and fissure plaque formation is questionable since the mylar surface characteristics are very different from those of enamel. Of the several species of bacteria isolated from these lesions *S. mutans* and lactobacilli are suspected as etiologic organisms.

Dentinal caries exhibit a somewhat different microbial ecology related to its location. Organisms growing here must be more anaerobic and derive most of their food from the tooth itself. The most commonly found pathogens in this region are lactobacilli. However, other gram-positive anaerobic rods and filaments such as *Bifidobacterium, Eubacterium,* and *Propionbacterium* have been identified. In addition *Actinomyces* and *Bacillus* species have been noted at the invasive front of the deep dentinal lesion.

The root surface lesion is also initiated on pellicle-coated cementum by different flora than in the

oxygen. However, as the plaque matures a phenomenon of bacterial succession is seen (see Chapter 26). The relative percentage of cocci decreases and after approximately 7 days, filaments and rods constitute about 50 percent of the total bacterial counts. The coccal organisms have thus changed the local environment to allow growth of other organisms. The rapid growth of the streptococci alters the pH, nutrients, and oxidation-reduction potentials in the deepest portions of the plaque matrix favoring growth of other organisms.

TABLE 27–1 ✦ **Bacteria Associated with Caries Type**

CARIES TYPE	ORGANISMS ISOLATED	POSSIBLE SIGNIFICANCE IN CARIES
Pit and fissure	*Streptococcus mutans*	Highly significant
	S. sanguis	Slight significance
	S. mitis	No significance
	Lactobacillus sp.	Highly significant
	Actinomyces sp.	May be significant
Smooth-surface	*S. mutans*	Highly significant
	S. salivarius	Little significance
Dentinal caries	*Lactobacillus* sp.	Highly significant
	Actinomyces viscosus	Significant
	A. naeslundii	Highly significant
	S. mutans	May be significant
	Filamentous rods	Significant
Root caries	*A. viscosus*	Highly significant
	A. naeslundii	Highly significant
	S. mutans	Some significance
	S. sanguis	Significance unclear
	S. salivarius	No clear significance
	Filamentous rods	Highly significant

From Newbrun, Cariology, ed 2, p. 52, 1983, with permission.

smooth surface lesions. Bacterial sampling of plaque from cemental caries reveals high numbers of *Actinomyces* sp. including *A. viscosus*, *A. naeslundii*, and *A. odontolyticus*. Other organisms including *Nocardia* and *S. mutans* also have been identified (Table 27–1).

The *Streptococcus mutans* Group

Studies performed in the 1960s indicated that *S. mutans* consists of a heterogeneous family of bacteria (see Chapter 6). The identification of four genetically distinct groups by DNA analysis has resulted in the reclassification of *S. mutans* (Table 27–2). Each group is given an individual species name: *S. cricetus*, *S. mutans*, *S. rattus*, and *S. sobrinus*. In addition other species of *S. mutans* have been identified. Two species named *S. macacae* and *S. downeii* were identified in a monkey host. *S. ferus* has been isolated in a rat. Among the *S. mutans* bacterial group *S. mutans* (serotypes *c*, *e*, and *f*) and *S. sobrinus* (serotypes *d*, *g*, and *h*) are the most commonly isolated in humans from westernized cultures. Both *S. mutans* and *S. sobrinus* have been isolated from human carious lesions and cause caries in various animal models. *S. rattus* has been identified from humans in Africa.

Lactobacillus

Bacteria of the genus *Lactobacillus* comprise another group of microorganisms that may have an etiologic role in the progression of human dental caries. This areo-tolerant anaerobe is represented in the oral cavity by several species which most commonly include *L. plantarium*, *L. salivarius*, and *L. oris*. Other species have been known to colonize the mouth; they include *L. acidophilus*, *L. grasseri*, *L. casei*, *L. brevis*, and *L. fermentum*.

Lactobacillus species grow most readily in an anaerobic environment, however, they will grow under a low oxygen tension supplemented with 5 to 10 percent carbon dioxide. They can undergo both fermentative and oxidative metabolism. Depending on the primary fermentation product derived from glycolysis, these bacteria can be further classified into three types: (1) **homolactic fermenters,** which primarily convert hexoses to lactic acid; (2) **heterolactic fermenters,** which produce ethanol, carbon dioxide, acetic acid as well as lactic acid; and (3) **facultative heterofermenters,** which primarily produce lactic acid, but which have inducible enzymes able to produce other fermentation products.

An important ecological feature of this bacteria is their ability to produce lactic acid and grow in the relatively acidic environment created by their fermentation. Due to these characteristics, *Lacto-*

TABLE 27–2 ✦ Classification of the Human *Streptococcus mutans* Group

SPECIES	SEROTYPE†	DNA HOMOLOGY MOLES % G + C*
S. mutans	c, E, f	36–38
S. sobrinus	d, g, SL	44–46
S. rattus	b	41–43
S. cricetus	a	42–44

*G + C = guanosine plus cytosine.
†Brathall/Perch serotyping.
Adapted from Slots and Taubman, Contemporary Oral Microbiology and Immunology, p. 395, 1992, with permission.

bacillus are respectively termed acidogenic and acidophilic. These features may be important to their association with some carious lesions.

The role of *Lactobacillus* in the development and progression of dental caries is still unclear. Bacteriological studies to identify cultivable isolates from carious lesions have shown that lactobacilli represent a relatively small percentage of the total bacteria found in most carious sites. There have been some studies that have reported significant correlation of lactobacilli in root-surface plaques and root-caries lesions, however, their low relative numbers are suggestive of possible salivary contamination. Histological analyses of deep dentinal caries also have shown the presence of lactobacilli. This observation has led to the suggestion that lactobacilli may play an active role in the progression of dentinal caries. This is not too surprising since these opportunistic bacteria are well-suited to an anaerobic environment and are acidophilic, however, this is inconclusive at present.

CARIES PHYSIOLOGY

Dental caries has been a prevalent disease since the first recorded history of mankind. Observations of "demons" and "tooth worms" can be found in ancient writings at about the time of Christ. Although the existence of this malady was well documented, the basic understanding of the disease process was not understood until the end of the 18th century. Dr. W. D. Miller (1890) first described dental caries as the action of organic acids upon the calcium phosphate of the teeth. He showed that after teeth were incubated with saliva and carbohydrates, acids formed that dissolved the mineralized portion of the teeth. He concluded that acid formed by bacteria in the saliva resulted in the breakdown of the teeth. From this he formulated the "chemo-parasitic" theory of dental caries.

Since then, further experimental data substantiated that lowering the pH by bacterial acid production causes dissolution of the enamel. Dr. Miller's work has formed the basis for the modern "plaque-host-substrate" theory of caries formation.

To understand why acidity adjacent to the enamel is so important to the carious process, the structure of enamel must be considered. Enamel, which is 95 percent calcified, is the most highly mineralized structure in the human body. The majority of the mineral is hydroxyapatite, a large family of calcium phosphate salts. The commonly represented formula for hydroxyapatite is $Ca_{10}(PO_4)_6OH_2$. Pure hydroxyapatite has a unique structure (Fig. 27–2). There is a sixfold axis of symmetry surrounding a threefold axis of symmetry. The crystals are arranged in a hexagonal configuration with calcium and phosphorus atoms placed on the outer crystal. In the center of the crystal, hydroxyl groups are surrounded by three calcium atoms. The relationship of each hydroxyl group in the crystal plays an important role in the crystal stability. In fact, replacement of some hydroxyl groups with fluoride results in increased crystal stability. The hexagonal crystals are grouped together into rods constituting the enamel (Fig. 27–3). These rods extend from the surface of the enamel to the dental junction. Density measurements on the enamel show that the outer surface has a slightly greater density than the remaining structure. This may result from the lower carbonate concentration or the higher fluoride concentration of the surface enamel. Interspaced between each enamel rod is an organic matrix. Although the enamel appears extremely hard and well mineralized, its surface is porous to small ions including sodium, potassium, magnesium, and flu-

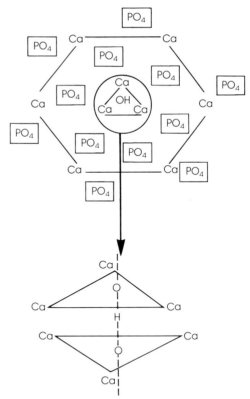

FIGURE 27–2 ✦ Crystal structure diagram of pure hydroxyapatite found in enamel.

oride. These interprismatic spaces may explain the observed permeability of the enamel.

Hydroxyapatite has a finite solubility constant dependent upon the temperature, pH, and ionic strength of the solvent surrounding the crystal. Alterations in these parameters can result in a solu-

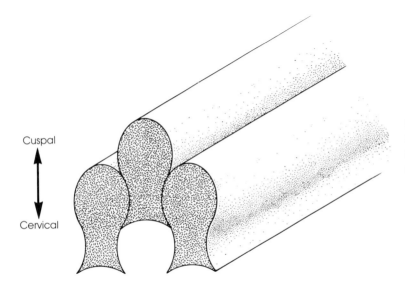

FIGURE 27–3 ✦ Diagrammatic representation of a microscopic cross section of enamel showing some enamel rods.

Cuspal

Cervical

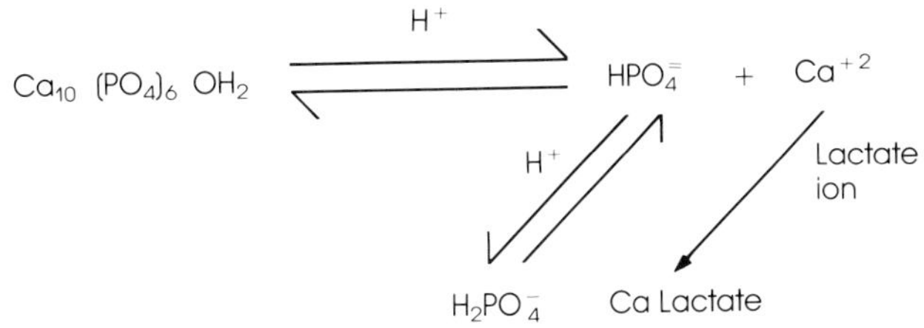

FIGURE 27–4 ✦ The chemical equation for the acid catalyzed demineralization of hydroxyapatite.

$$Ca_{10}(PO_4)_6 OH_2 \rightleftharpoons HPO_4^= + Ca^{+2}$$

$$H^+ \qquad H^+ \qquad Lactate \ ion$$

$$H_2PO_4^- \qquad Ca \ Lactate$$

bilization of the crystals. For example, a tooth placed in a container of distilled water would eventually undergo a finite dissolution of the hydroxyapatite until the ionic strength of the solution reached a favorable equilibrium. In the oral cavity, saliva is supersaturated with respect to calcium and phosphate which favors the crystalline state of enamel. As a result, the teeth do not dissolve. Because of the nature of the equilibrium reaction in the oral cavity, enamel is under a constant state of mineralization and demineralization at physiologic conditions (saturated Ca^{+2}, PO_4, pH 6.8). At this pH, the solubility is extremely small and, for practical purposes, insignificant; however, if the pH is lowered approximately 1.3 log units to 5.5, the solubility is then increased to the point where dissolution occurs. At this "critical" pH, hydroxyapatite is destabilized by the acid effect on the hydroxyl groups in the center of the crystal resulting in the formation of water (Fig. 27–4). The dissociated form of calcium phosphate then becomes favored and the crystal dissolves. Like all acid-base reactions, the dissolution of the hydroxyapatite is an equilibrium process, so that the deformation of the crystal can occur with the resultant precipitation of hydroxyapatite. For example, if the local calcium concentration is increased and/or the pH increases the hydroxyapatite could be reformed.

CARIES THEORIES

The Acid Theory

Since Dr. Miller's observations, considerable experimental evidence has supported the acid theory that acids produced by plaque bacteria result in the demineralization of enamel. This includes:

1. Plaque pH can drop below 5.5 for extended periods following the production of bacterial organic acids.
2. pH measurements in carious lesions are lower than in surrounding tissues.
3. Caries incidence correlates with the presence of *S. mutans* and *Lactobacillus,* both capable of producing organic acids on consumption of fermentable sugars.

4. In germ-free rats, oral bacteria capable of producing acid without proteolytic capacity can induce caries.

Other hypotheses have been proposed for enamel breakdown by plaque bacteria.

The Proteolysis-Chelation Theory

This theory is based on the concept that enamel demineralization occurs without acid if complexing agents such as lactate decrease calcium ions surrounding the enamel crystal shift the equilibrium toward dissolution. If this is true, demineralization could occur at neutral or even alkaline pH. Although there is some experimental support for this theory, the overwhelming evidence supports the acid theory.

The Proteolytic Theory

This theory assumes that caries are initiated by plaque proteolytic enzymes which destroy the inter-rod organic material and destabilize the enamel crystals. There is not much support for this theory.

The Phosphoprotein Theory

This theory is based on a rat experiment that showed that plaque bacteria produce enzymes capable of removing phosphate from enamel phosphoproteins. The removal of these proteins is thought to destabilize the enamel matrix leading to enamel breakdown. However, phosphoprotein concentrations in human enamel are not high enough to play a role in caries formation.

CARIES HISTOPATHOLOGY

Macroscopic examination of initial enamel caries usually reveals a white-chalky area with an intact surface. In general, bacterial plaque will be present over this lesion. Microscopic examination of ground sections reveals a relatively intact enamel surface with an area of subsurface demineralization. The lesion can be characterized by four microscopic zones (Fig. 27–5): the innermost translucent zone representing approximately 1.2 percent mineral loss; a dark zone with 6 percent mineral loss; the body of the lesion, with about 24 percent mineral loss; and the surface layer which appears

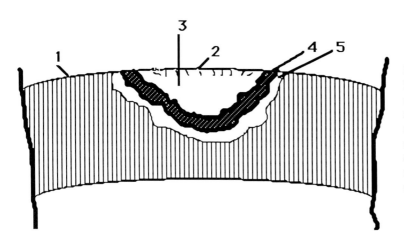

FIGURE 27–5 ✦ Diagrammatic representation of a microscopic thin ground section showing enamel caries. Major zones are (1) sound enamel, (2) surface enamel slightly demineralized, (3) body of the lesion, (4) dark zone, and (5) translucent zone.

intact. In actuality, the surface has some demineralization which appears as pitting. Radiographically, the smooth-surface lesion appears as a cone with its tip pointing toward the dentin. Photodensity tracings of microradiographic sections of sound and carious enamel support the observations of a relatively intact surface and demineralized subsurface (Fig. 27–6).

It is thought that non-ionized acid diffuses through the porous interprismatic junctions of the enamel surface where it dissociates and interacts with the subsurface hydroxyapatite crystals at the rod surface. In time, small gaps develop between the enamel rods. As the number of dissolved hydroxyapatite crystals increases, the lesion becomes progressively more porous. These porous spaces become filled with fluid leading to clinical translucency of the enamel. As the destruction of the subsurface hydroxyapatite advances, the surface enamel becomes weakened and breaks down leading to bacterial ingression. Since early enamel caries is aseptic and simply the results of the action of acids on the hydroxyapatite, it has a high potential for remineralization. Once the bacteria have entered the lesion, treatment must be through mechanical means.

When the caries reaches the dentin, the lesion rapidly spreads laterally along the dentin-enamel junction and radiographically appears as a less well-defined hemispherical lucency. This rapid dentinal spread is related to several factors. First, dentin is less mineralized than enamel, so acids will destroy more of the mineralized matrix. Second, dentin is cellular, which allows easy bacterial movement into the deeper portions of the lesion. Microscopically, the dentin lesion reveals several distinct zones described by Newbrun (1983) (Fig. 27–7). The innermost zone (first) contains retreating odontoblasts. The second zone contains fatty degeneration. The next zone (third) consists of dentinal sclerosis where peritubular dentin formation blocks the bacterial insult. The fourth zone is the area of demineralization, similar to the "body of the lesion" zone in enamel caries. The most superficial zone (fifth) is an area of bacterial invasion and this is followed by the zone of bacterial necrosis (sixth).

The next logical step in understanding the physiology of dental caries is to examine bacterial plaque formation, since without bacterial plaque, the typical carious lesion can not exist.

FIGURE 27–6 ✦ Photodensity tracing of microradiographs of sound enamel (—) and initial enamel caries (- - - -). (From Newbrun's Cariology, ed. 2, p. 240, Williams and Wilkins, Baltimore, 1983, with permission.)

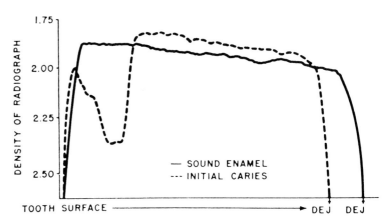

PULP   DEJ

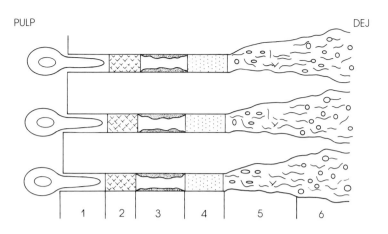

FIGURE 27–7 ✦ Diagrammatic illustration of Newbrun's six zones seen in microscopic sections of dentinal caries. Zone 1, retreating odontoblastic process; zone 2, fatty degeneration; zone 3, dentinal sclerosis; zone 4, dentinal demineralization; zone 5, bacterial invasion; and zone 6, necrotic dentin.

PLAQUE FORMATION

The production of acids from plaque bacteria and subsequent formation of dental caries is the culmination of a highly selective process of bacterial adherence and colonization on the tooth surface. For oral bacteria to survive in the mouth they must be able to firmly attach and colonize a host surface.

Research has shown a high degree of selectivity in plaque formation (see Chapter 26). Despite the relatively wide variety of oral flora, only select organisms colonize a particular oral surface (Table 27–3). This bacterial selectivity seems related to the salivary pellicle absorbed onto the enamel surface. The enamel pellicle, an acellular material derived from specific salivary components, which consists of highly charged proteins and glycoproteins that rapidly adsorbs on the tooth. A strong absorption occurs through electrostatic interactions between the highly charged surface of the enamel and the charged proteins (Fig. 27–8) with a pellicle forming within minutes of enamel exposure to the oral cavity. Salivary pellicle is believed directly responsible for the subsequent adherence of oral bacteria. There are two major theories for how this occurs. The first, supported by Rølla (1979), proposes that the interaction of bacteria with the pellicle-coated tooth occurs through electrostatic charges (Fig. 27–9). The highly negative surface of most oral bacteria can interact with calcium ions complexed to the surface of the pellicle. There is some experimental support for such a theory. Most streptococci possess highly anionic outer cell walls. The surface of the enamel pellicle also carries a negative charge density from the selective adsorption of anionic salivary glycoproteins. Interaction of the oral streptococci with the pellicle happens in much the same fashion as the binding of salivary components to the enamel; that is, bridging cations such as calcium support the interaction and allow initial adherence to occur. This theory has drawbacks. First, it does not explain the varying selectivity among several strains of streptococci which possess similar anionic surface charges. Second, some strains of oral bacteria without negatively charged cell wall components still bind to the

TABLE 27–3 ✦ Percentage Distribution of Bacteria in Different Sites in the Oral Cavity

	LOCATION				
BACTERIUM	**TONGUE**	**GINGIVAL CREVICE**	**SALIVA**	**CHEEK**	**SUPRAGINGIVAL PLAQUE**
Streptococcus mutans	0.3	—	0.2	0.5	3.9
*S. sanguis**	9.0	—	47.0	29.0	75.0
*S. salivarius**	55.0	0.5	47.4	10.7	0.7
Provotella melaninogenicus†	0.4	4.5	0.4	0.3	0.3
Treponema sp.‡	—	1.5	—	—	>0.1
Lactobacillus sp.	—	—	0.01	—	>0.01

Data from Socransky and Manganiello: J. Periodontol. 42:486, 1971.
*% of facultative streptococci.
†% of total cultivable flora.
‡% of microscopic counts.

PELLICLE FORMATION

CHARGED SALIVARY
GLYCOPROTEINS

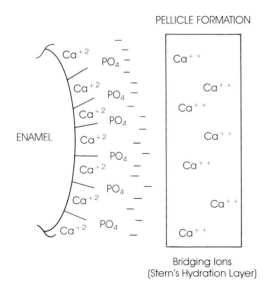

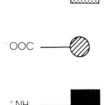

Bridging Ions
(Stern's Hydration Layer)

FIGURE 27–8 ✦ The interaction of host-derived salivary glycoproteins with the charged surface of enamel. This electrostatic interaction is believed to occur through bridging calcium ions found in the "Stern hydration layer."

enamel surface. An alternative hypothesis proposed by Gibbons (1977) is that bacterial attachment occurs through a "lectinlike" interaction of specific bacterial surface receptors with pellicle-bound glycoproteins (Fig. 27–9). This theory is also supported by experimental evidence. The adsorption of oral bacteria to saliva-treated hydroxyapatite is inhibited by specific sugars suggesting sugar-protein interactions. In vitro studies have shown that the number of binding sites for bacterial strains on saliva-treated hydroxyapatite differs markedly. In addition, more than one bacterial strain can bind to the surface of the hydroxyapatite without competing for the same binding sites. In general, recent opinion favors the Gibbons hypothesis.

Once initial bacterial attachment and colonization have occurred, secondary adherence processes begin. This involves production of extracellular bacterial products which act as intracellular glue to protect the bacteria and supply them with a food source. These polymeric sugars are commonly known as glucans and levans.

Dental plaque has three phases of development as described by Newbrun: (1) initial colonization, (2) rapid bacterial growth, and (3) remodeling. Enamel pellicle forms within minutes after exposure to saliva followed within a few hours by the initial stages of bacterial adherence. The streptococci, the first bacterial colonizers, have a short doubling time of approximately 2 hours. Therefore, within 12 to 24 hours after initial adherence, a well-defined bacterial colonization as a thin plaque mass covers the exposed enamel surface. During this time the bacteria, with appropriate substrate, produce copious amounts of extracellular glucans adding to the overall plaque matrix. With time, the plaque forms up to the height of contour of the

tooth and fills the interproximal areas. Growth above these areas is somewhat limited by mastication. The consumption of fibrous foods can effect the overall distribution of plaque, but chewing these foods has little if any effect on plaque growth in the cervical and interproximal areas of the teeth. Unfortunately, these are the areas of high caries prevalence. After 2 to 3 days, if left undisturbed, the plaque begins to change. The innermost environment of the plaque becomes more anaerobic and other bacterial forms begin to appear. The plaque mass has increased by 10 to 200 percent and appears as a thick jelly-like mass on the enamel (Fig. 27–10). If allowed to remain on the tooth surface, calcium phosphate deposition can occur, leading to the transformation of plaque into calculus.

PLAQUE BIOCHEMISTRY

The single most important feature of dental plaque is its unique ability to selectively utilize fermentable sugars in the diet and rapidly convert them to destructive organic acids and sticky insoluble dextrans. Focusing on this concept, let us examine some chemical aspects of the process.

Like all living organisms, bacteria must produce energy by various biochemical processes. Humans and other higher organisms use a complex biochemical pathway to first breakdown molecules into pyruvate anion. Pyruvate is then converted enzymatically to acetate, which serves as the primary substrate for the pathway known as the tricarboxcylic acid cycle. This biochemical pathway produces high energy molecules to power the individual cells. Bacteria also have energy-producing pathways, the most common of which is glycolysis (see Chapter 3). By this process, glucose is enzymatically broken down into two molecules of

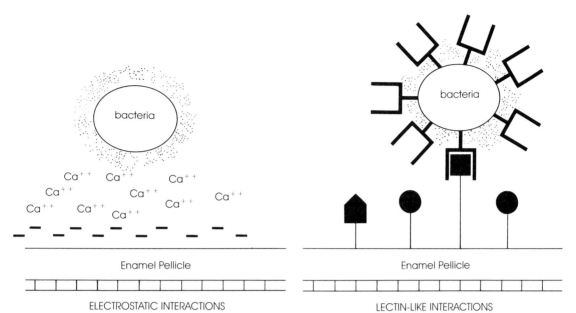

FIGURE 27–9 ✦ The diagrammatic representation of the proposed interaction of oral bacteria with pellicle-coated enamel surfaces. The upper figure illustrates the electrostatic hypothesis, while the lower shows the "lectinlike" interactions.

lactate making glucose a very important substrate for the maintenance and growth of common oral bacteria. The bacteria possess enzymes capable of breaking down and transporting sugars into the cell cytoplasm. Obviously, production of small organic acids from glucose fermentation plays a key role in the development of dental caries. However, the ability of oral bacteria to produce extracellular polysaccharides is probably the single most important feature in plaque development and the caries process. Oral bacteria, specifically streptococci,

possess a unique family of enzymes called transferases which are capable of rapidly converting disaccharides, particularly *sucrose,* into long-chain polysaccharides. They produce glucans, composed of glucose units, and levans, composed of fructose moieties (Fig. 27–11). The glucans, specifically the water-insoluble fraction, serve as a structural component in the plaque matrix. More simply, they are a "biologic glue" holding the plaque mass together and allowing the adherence of plaque to the tooth surface. The soluble levans and glucans

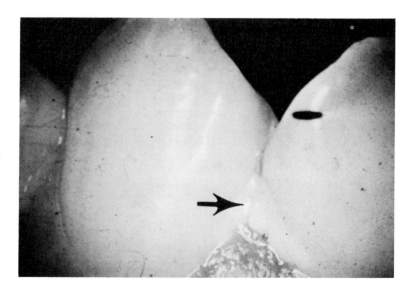

FIGURE 27–10 ✦ Clinical photograph of supragingival plaque formed on the cervical area of the teeth. Note the white "gelatinous" appearance.

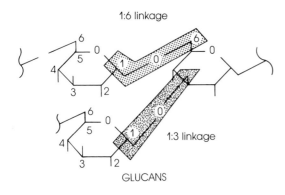

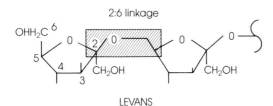

FIGURE 27–11 ✦ Molecular diagrams of bacterial dextrans and levans, two common types of polysaccharides produced by oral plaque-producing streptococci.

also serve as a carbohydrate food reserve, which is readily available in times of carbohydrate deprivation. These enzymes are primarily cell-membrane bound and show a high specificity for sucrose. They function by binding sucrose and cleaving the high-energy dihemiacetal linkage resulting in the formation of one glucose and one fructose molecule. The glucose molecule is then transferred to a previously bound glucose moiety to yield a dextran primer. Sequential addition of glucose residues then yields long-chain glucans. Other glucosyl-bearing disaccharides such as maltose and lactose are not utilized by these enzymes and therefore don't produce dextrans. This can be explained by examining the high-energy bond in the sucrose molecule. The glucose and fructose moieties are linked together by a dihemiacetal bond, which has a very high free energy of hydrolysis (Fig. 27–12). When this bond is broken, a significant amount of energy is released to the environment (Table 27–4). This energy may be con-

served by the oral bacteria through enzymatic coupling reactions and used to power the transferase enzyme systems.

HOST FACTORS AND CARIES

Another important factor in caries formation is the host. Caries, which is selective for humans, occurs relatively slowly, requiring 1 to 2 years for progression through the enamel. There appear to be host factors that favor caries and host mechanisms that inhibit the development of caries.

The first human host factors that favor caries are the **dental anatomic contours** and **arch form.** In humans, the height of contour of teeth is above the gingival margin, which lends itself to bacterial growth as a result of stagnation. The molar teeth also frequently contain deep pits and fissures favoring plaque development. The evolutionary development of the human arch form has led to the proximal contact of the teeth and the appearance of tooth crowding. Each of these features favors plaque formation as a result of stasis.

The second and most obvious host factor that affects caries is **saliva.** This unique secretion contains a wide variety of substances acting in unison as the host's primary defense against dental caries. In fact, rampant caries occurs when saliva production ceases. The important role of saliva in the host defense mechanisms has led to the isolation and identification of many unique chemical components. For discussion purposes these defense components will be divided into two types: (1) active defense molecules and (2) passive defense agents (Table 27–5). Active agents, similar to antibiotics, are bacteriocidal or bacteriostatic for oral flora. The passive defense agents disrupt or prevent plaque formation by modifying the microbial environment rather than actually destroying the bacteria.

Active Salivary Components

Several enzymes isolated from saliva are antibacterial. **Lysozyme,** isolated from parotid saliva, is effective in killing several types of gram-positive bacteria by promoting cell wall disruption and subsequent cell lysis. While lysozyme was first believed to play a key role in bacterial destruction, recent microbiologic studies with isolates of

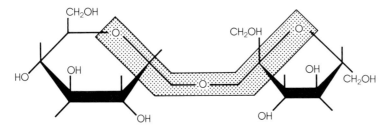

FIGURE   27–12 ✦ Molecular structure of sucrose. *Shaded area* indicates the high-energy di-hemiacetal bond thought to be important to the production of extracellular glucans.

TABLE 27–4 ✦ Free Energy of Hydrolysis of Glucosyl Donors and Some Polysaccharide

COMPOUND	STANDARD FREE ENERGY OF HYDROLYSIS (ΔG_H, cal/mole)
Glucose 1-phosphate	−5000
UDP-glucose*	−7600
Sucrose	−6600
Maltose	−3000
Lactose	−3000
Glycogen	−4300
Dextran	−2000
Levan	−4600

*UDP = uridine diphosphate.
From Newbrun, Cariology, ed. 2, Williams & Wilkins, p. 105, 1983, with permission.

TABLE 27–5 ✦ Proposed Salivary Bacterial Defense Components

COMPONENT	MODE OF ACTION
Active	
Lysozyme	Bacterial cell wall lysis
Lactoperoxidase	Catalyzes OSCN⁻ formation, which disrupts bacterial proteins
Lactoferrin	Binds up Fe leading to cell growth inhibition
Passive	
Secretory IgA	Interferes with bacterial attachment
Salivary glycoproteins	Can act as specific bacterial agglutinins
Salivary bicarbonate	Can buffer organic acids produced during sugar fermentation

plaque-producing bacteria have shown that lysozyme is not that effective and is probably of lesser importance. Two other enzymes have been identified and characterized from saliva—lactoperoxidase and lactoferrin. **Lactoperoxidase,** in the presence of hydrogen peroxide and thiocyanate ion, catalyzes the formation of hypothiocyanate ion (OSCN⁻). This compound reacts rapidly with sulfhydryl groups within proteins, leading to disruption of bacterial metabolic systems. **Lactoferrin,** a sulfur-containing enzyme, binds iron that is essential for bacterial growth. Therefore, the presence of this compound inhibits bacterial growth.

Passive Salivary Components

SALIVARY BUFFERS

Saliva is important as a buffer and for the passive host defense against caries. The major buffer system found in saliva is bicarbonate-carbonate, which rapidly neutralizes strong acids at a pH of 6.1 or lower. Therefore, it efficiently handles lactic and acetic acids produced by plaque bacteria and reduces enamel demineralization. Although phosphate is also present in the saliva which can act as a buffer, bicarbonate appears to be of greater importance. There are several explanations for this:

1. Bicarbonate buffers react rapidly by losing CO_2.
2. It has a dissociation constant (pK) effective in the range at which plaque acids are produced.
3. As salivary flow increases, the bicarbonate concentration also increases. This is in contrast to phosphate, which falls slightly.

PELLICLE COMPONENTS

The salivary pellicle proteins also may serve a protective function for the host. Surface enamel is more resistant to bacterial acids than the subsurface mineral. It is thought that surface salivary pellicle may stabilize the surface hydroxyapatite, increasing its acid resistance. This hypothesis is supported by the observation that acid demineralization of hydroxyapatite in vitro does not produce the same carious lesion as seen in vivo unless bacterial plaque and salivary pellicle are both present on the tooth surface.

IMMUNOGLOBULINS

Like most other glandular excretions, saliva contains immunoglobulins. The major immunoglobulin found in saliva is secretory IgA (see Chapter 2). This molecule differs from serum IgA in both structure and stability. Serum IgA is found as a monomer, whereas secretory IgA is a dimer consisting of two IgA monomers connected by a protein "J" chain. The secretory IgA also contains a secretory associated protein. The secretory unit is thought to facilitate transport of immunoglobulin into the saliva. In addition, it makes the immunoglobulin resistant to the oral proteolytic enzymes. It has been suggested that salivary IgA may protect the host from oral pathogens by acting as a specific agglutinin. As mentioned earlier, the ability of bacteria and other pathogens to survive in the oral cavity is dependent on their ability to adhere to an oral surface. Secretory IgA binds and agglutinates specific oral bacteria, blocking their binding to host tissues, resulting in their removal from the mouth.

The host has a wide variety of oral defense mechanisms. However, protection from localized oral infections is dependent upon all these systems acting in unison to achieve a balance.

No single mechanism effectively protects the host.

Diet, Nutrition, and Dental Caries

Diet also is important in the etiology of dental caries. Consumption of foods has a local effect on the oral structures rather than a systemic one, as in the case of nutrition. Nutrition is the process by which foods are assimilated and metabolized in the body. Nutritional effects on the teeth are greatest during development. Systemic incorporation of fluoride during tooth formation results in a more caries-resistant tooth. Other nutritional factors including calcium and phosphorus would be expected to play an important role in tooth development. However, the present evidence is inconclusive about their effects.

Dietary factors, on the other hand, have dramatic effects on caries. The role of dietary sugars, particularly sucrose, in the prevalence of dental caries has been extensively studied. One of the earliest experiments with sugars was performed by Stephan (1940). Within 2 to 3 minutes following a sugar rinse, the plaque pH rapidly fell from about 6.8 to 5.0. This drop lasted 20 minutes and took about 40 minutes to return to the original, "resting pH" (Fig. 27–13). Similar experiments with repeated sucrose rinses showed that multiple sugar exposures have an additive effect upon plaque acid production (Fig. 27–14). Animal studies in rodents to assess the relative cariogenicity of human foods and drinks have shown a direct relationship between sucrose concentration and caries scores. Several human studies also have examined the relationship of diet to caries. In one of the first controlled studies, Sognnaes (1948) examined the caries incidence among European schoolchildren during World War II. During sugar rationing, caries scores significantly decreased. When rationing ceased the caries scores increased to prewar levels. Although this work is widely quoted, there are questions concerning the validity of the conclusions drawn from the experimental design. The Sognnaes study was based on routine examinations rather than research surveys and were relatively crude. It is believed that the reduced caries rate noted by Sognnaes would not have occurred until several years after rationing had been present. Therefore, the lowered caries score would be delayed until after rationing had begun. Some scientists have suggested that the observed lowered caries rate was due instead to an increased consumption of unrefined carbohydrates and fibrous foods.

The Vipeholm study (Gustafsson et al., 1954) examined institutionalized patients in Sweden. The investigators studied the effects of frequency and form of carbohydrate consumed upon caries. Caries increased significantly with increased consumption of sucrose-containing food. It also was observed that sticky or adhesive forms of carbohydrates delayed the clearance time from the mouth and increased the caries risk.

Another human study examined children in an Australian orphanage who were on restricted diets that did not contain processed sugar. Their caries experience was significantly lower (about 10 percent) than other children. However, after the children left the orphanage and were no longer under strict dietary control, their DMFT (decayed, missing, and filled permanent teeth) approximated that of the general population. This implied that the teeth are always susceptible to caries and do not acquire permanent resistance. Another study examined individuals with hereditary fructose intolerance, in which there is a reduced enzymatic ac-

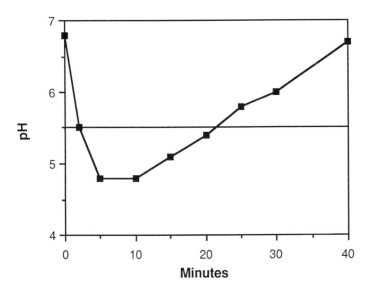

FIGURE   27–13 ✦ The pH of plaque after rinsing the mouth with 10 percent glucose solution. The line at pH 5.5 is the value at which decalcification of enamel will occur. This is termed the "critical pH." The curve is commonly called a *Stephan curve.*

FIGURE 27–14 ✦ The effect of plaque pH following the application of repeated ingestion of 0.5 percent glucose solutions at 2 minute intervals. Note the additive effects of repetitive glucose applications which results in an overall drop in plaque pH to well below the "critical pH" of 5.5. *One addition 0.06 ml of 0.5 percent glucose; **0.06 of 0.5 percent glucose per 2 minute intervals; ***5 percent glucose added similarly.

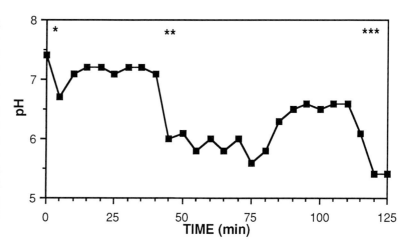

tivity of fructose 1-phosphate aldolase, resulting in an inability to metabolize fructose. These individuals become very sick upon ingestion of foods containing fructose or sucrose, forcing them to restrict their sugar intake. An examination of the DMFS caries score of 17 individuals with hereditary fructose intolerance showed a greater than 90 percent reduction in caries incidence when compared with a control group.

Several other epidemiologic studies have examined isolated human populations such as Eskimos, Aborigines, and the Bantu tribes in Africa with generally low sucrose diets. When their diets were modified to contain more refined carbohydrate, their DMFS scores increased proportionately. Thus, the type and amount of carbohydrate exposure directly effects the caries experience.

Other dietary components have also been thought to play a role in caries. The phosphates are thought to have some anticaries activity because animals on diets supplemented with inorganic phosphates have reduced caries. Organic phosphates have also been suggested as having some cariostatic properties. While the mechanism of this anticaries activity is unknown, the effects are local rather than systemic. Several mechanisms for this activity have been proposed:

1. Increased phosphate ions in the saliva may shift the equilibrium dissociation of hydroxyapatite to favor the mineralized salt in the presence of acids.
2. Phosphate could act as a buffer to the bacterial acids.
3. Phosphate ions can desorb pellicle proteins, which may alter bacterial adherence.

Although the results in the animal models are encouraging, similar human studies have been inconclusive. The anticaries potential of phosphates must be more fully investigated.

Another anticaries dietary component is lipid. Addition of lipids to a cariogenic diet reduces den-

tal caries in animals. Medium-chain fatty acids and their salts also have some antibacterial properties in vitro and in animal models. Whether these materials would work in humans has not been established. Studies by Gibbons and Dankers (1981), Wolinsky and Sote (1984), and Staat and associates (1978) have reported that some plant extracts act as specific bacterial agglutinins. These studies suggest that "lectinlike" components in specific foods may affect plaque formation and alter caries susceptibility. Wolinsky and Sote have found that natural plant polyphenolic compounds known as *tannins* are quite effective bacterial agglutinins.

The last areas of consideration in dietary factors that may affect dental caries are trace elements including barium, vanadium, strontium, selenium, and molybdenum, which may influence dental caries. Enamel is permeable to small ions, which can change the surface composition. The adsorption of these ions may alter the surface characteristics of the enamel and cause changes in the pellicle. This in turn may alter plaque formation.

CARIES CONTROL AND PREVENTION

Despite our knowledge of dental caries and its prevention, a large portion of the general population still suffers from dental caries. There have been great strides in the prevention of the disease, notable with water fluoridation. More recently, attention has focused upon the possibility of a caries vaccine. In this section we will examine several approaches for control of dental caries, including chemotherapeutic agents that are effective.

Immunologic Control of Caries

The development of vaccines has resulted in the control of many viral and bacterial diseases. These past successes have generated much interest in the concept of a caries vaccine. As mentioned earlier, the saliva is known to contain immunoglobulins. The concentration of immunoglobulins in saliva is approximately 1 to 3 percent. The major source of these immunoglobulins is the salivary secretions which product secretory IgA. However, saliva also contains the humoral IgG and IgM from the gingival sulcular fluid. In addition, cellular components of the immune system such as lymphocytes, macrophages, and neutrophils occur in the gingival sulcus (Fig. 27–15). The immunoglobulin host defense system is not totally understood. However, it is believed that the control of cariogenic bacteria by these molecules does play an important role in the overall maintenance of oral health. There are two possible ways antibodies might control bacterial growth:

1. The salivary immunoglobulins may act as specific agglutinins interacting with bacterial surface receptors and inhibiting colonization and subsequent caries formation. They might also inactivate surface glucosyltransferases, which would then reduce the synthesis of extracellular glucans resulting in reduced plaque formation.

2. The antibodies might also increase opsonization leading to phagocytosis by lymphocytes and PMNs.

The stimulation of salivary immunoglobulins generally occurs through the small intestine where Peyer's patches populating the lamina propria contain B cells. These B cells can be stimulated by the common swallowing of oral bacteria and the sensitized plasma cells produced can migrate to the excretory glands. The plasma cells in the salivary glands produce S-IgA to specific bacteria. The current basis for a caries vaccine suggests stimulation of secretory IgA via the gut. The question arises,

how can IgA stimulation be maintained when there are low levels of a particular bacteria? Animal and human studies have examined the use of salivary immunoglobulins for control of caries incidence.

ANIMAL STUDIES

In gnotobiotic rats, ingestion of whole *Streptococcus mutans* selectively produces S-IgA, which correlates with reduced caries. In another study, hamsters fed bacterial surface proteins from *S. mutans* developed antibodies and had a lowered incidence of caries when fed high-sucrose diets. The effects of serum antibodies on caries was also studied. Animals injected with high doses of streptococci had elevated serum IgG, however, the incidence of caries was not consistently reduced. This may indicate that serum antibodies are at insufficient levels in the saliva to have an effect. In addition, serum antibodies excreted into the oral cavity through the gingival sulcus do not have a secretory associated protein. Therefore, their activity is rapidly destroyed by oral proteolytic enzymes. Lehner and coworkers do not agree with this view and feel that serum IgG probably accounts for most of the caries reduction noted in immunized animals. This is based upon the fact that IgG levels are quite high in plaque—about three times the IgA levels.

HUMAN STUDIES

Currently, clinical trials are underway to test a "pill" of *S. mutans* for control of caries. There have been some conflicting results thus far in human studies. Some workers have actually reported a negative correlation between S-IgA and caries prevalence. However, this result could be the result of the experimental design. It has been shown that

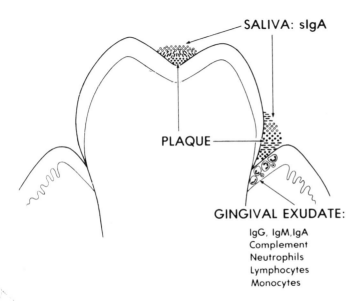

SALIVA: sIgA

PLAQUE

GINGIVAL EXUDATE:

IgG, IgM, IgA
Complement
Neutrophils
Lymphocytes
Monocytes

FIGURE 27–15 ✦ Illustration of the sources of immunoglobulins in the oral cavity. (From Newbrun's Cariology, ed. 2, p. 31, 1983, Williams and Wilkins, Baltimore, with permission.)

ingestion of capsules containing *S. mutans* stimulates the production of S-IgA. In a study of individuals who could not produce any salivary immunoglobulins, the caries rates were much higher than in the normal control group. Stimulation of serum immunoglobulins in humans also has produced mixed results and no correlation could be made between caries experience and serum immunoglobulin stimulation.

The idea of a caries vaccine is valid. However, several problems must be resolved. First, bacteria have the ability to rapidly change antigenic properties, which could render the immunity ineffective. In addition, the removal of a particular strain of oral flora will not ensure against the repopulation with another equally or more virulent organism. One must be certain that the antigens injected don't induce cross-reacting antibodies that can also react with other body tissues. For example, it is thought that *S. mutans* possess antigenic components shared with heart muscle. Induction of these antibodies could be disastrous leading to heart damage. Last, if a vaccine were developed, would it be necessary to remove most of the oral flora and then allow for a repopulation to occur following antibody stimulation? How long would the immunity last? These are questions still to be answered.

Fluorides

The routine use of fluorides in the maintenance of oral hygiene remains the most effective chemotherapeutic method currently used in the United States. Extensive data show significant reduction in enamel caries when fluoride is used topically or systemically. As a result of its widespread use in drinking water and home dentrifices, there has been a 50 to 60 percent reduction of the DMFS in children and teenagers. Several mechanisms have been proposed to explain the anticaries effects of the fluoride ion (Table 27–6). The first and most widely accepted concept is that the incorporation of fluoride ions into the developing enamel increases its acid resistance. Experiments have shown that systemic incorporation of fluoride in developing hydroxyapatite crystals occurs readily leading to the formation of a mixed fluorhydroxyapatite. The fluoride ion is thought to replace hydroxyl groups or fill voids found in the center of the crystal structure (see Fig. 27–2). This results in a more stable crystal structure which results in a less soluble crystal. An alternative explanation has been proposed by Simmons (1972). He believes that the incorporation of fluoride into the hydroxyapatite crystal changes the crystal surface pH. This in turn reduces the rate of growth of the crystal. The slower the rate of crystal formation, the more

TABLE 27–6 ✦ Proposed Hypotheses for the Anticaries Effects of Fluoride

1. Substitution of fluoride for hydroxyl ion in apatite makes the crystal less soluble at low pH, therefore, making the enamel more resistant to bacterial demineralization. Fluoride occupies some of the voids created by improper stacking of the hydroxyl groups resulting in stabilization of the lattice.
2. Fluoride in the developing hydroxyapatite influences the solubility of the enamel matrix proteins. This results in a slower crystal formation and an increased stability of the hydroxyapatite.
3. Fluoride may compete for carbonate ion which makes the apatite crystals smaller and may provide "seed" sites for dissolution.
4. Fluoride can act as an effective antibacterial agent. Concentrations of 30 ppm and greater have been shown to inhibit glycolytic enzymes in plaque bacteria.
5. Systemic fluoride during tooth formation can result in altered tooth formation. The teeth can be smaller and the pit and fissures of the posterior teeth may be more coalesced. This may increase their resistance to caries.

stable the fluorhydroxyapatite crystal. Elemental analysis of enamel has shown that the outermost surface of the enamel contains higher levels of fluoride than the remaining crystal. It has been proposed that this changes the surface charge characteristics influencing the nature of the salivary pellicle. This in turn may alter the plaque.

Another property of fluoride is its antibacterial activity. Fluoride ion is a potent inhibitor of many bacterial enzymes including enolase, which is required for bacterial metabolism of sugars. Concentrations of 10 ppm or greater in the plaque reduces plaque acid. These levels of fluoride can easily be attained in plaque because the ion accumulates following repeated exposures. Therefore, very high levels of fluoride in the plaque can result from a daily application of topical gel, rinse or use of a fluoridated dentrifice.

One other important anticaries property of fluoride may be its ability to cause remineralization of incipient enamel caries. The fluoride ion is rapidly converted orally to calcium fluoride. This salt is not soluble and precipitates out onto the tooth surface. If enamel demineralization occurs, the calcium fluoride can act as a reservoir releasing fluoride ion which can react with the dehydroxyapatite. This will result in a remineralization of the enamel. Some researchers believe that acid demineralization microscopically occurs frequently at the tooth-plaque interface but remineralization lowers the rate of caries. Therefore, topical fluorides are extremely important in a caries prevention pro-

TABLE 27–7 ✦ Recommended Fluoride Supplementation Dosage Schedule*

AGE (yr)	CONCENTRATION OF FLUORIDE IN WATER (ppm)		
	0–0.3	0.3–0.7	0.7–1.0
0 to 2	0.25	0.0	0.0
2 to 3	0.50	0.25	0.0
3 to adult	1.00	0.50	0.0

*Adjusted allowance in mg of fluoride/day; 2.2 mg sodium fluoride contains 1 mg F^-
From Newbrun, Cariology, ed. 2, Williams & Wilkins, p. 312, 1983, with permission.

gram and should be emphasized for routine home care. The recommended fluoride supplementation dosage is given in Table 27–7.

Other Chemotherapeutic Anticaries Agents

Other chemical agents have recently appeared that are potentially effective anticaries agents. These agents are antibacterial and reduce plaque formation (see Chapter 29). The most widely known agents in present use in Europe are chlorhexidine at a 2 percent concentration and its chemical analogue alexidine (Fig. 27–16). These bisguinide aromatic compounds are excellent antimicrobial agents for gram-positive streptococci. These cationic compounds are believed to bind to the negatively charged surfaces of gram-positive bacteria, resulting in a disruption of the cell membrane leading to cytoplasmic leakage and cell death. The bisguinides also have the interesting property of being substantive; that is, they bind to tooth pellicle where they act as a chemical reservoir where they are slowly released, extending their plaque-inhibiting properties. The disadvantage of these agents is that they stain the teeth over time, are also bitter tasting, and may sometimes alter taste perception. Chlorhexidine (Peridex) also is available in the United States as a prescription mouthwash at 0.12 percent concentration. This concentration minimizes the staining effects.

There are many other agents that have produced some antiplaque activity. These include the phenolic compounds, Sanguinarine, and mixtures of povidone-iodine/hydrogen peroxide. Each of these agents has been shown to be somewhat effective as oral antibacterial agents when studied in both in vitro and in vivo environments. However, their long-term anti-caries effects are not totally clear. Most recently, dentrifices and mouth rinses containing the antibacterial agent Triclosan have been introduced in Europe. This agent also has been

Structure of Chlorhexidine

Bis-Biguanide

FIGURE 27–16 ✦ Chemical structural illustrations of chlorhexidine and its chemical analogue alexidine. The microbiologic activity of these molecules is related to the presence of the vicinal guanidine moieties giving this molecule a highly cationic nature.

shown to be effective at reducing the numbers of plaque-producing bacteria in the mouth and reducing the severity of gingivitis. However, the value of Triclosan in caries prevention has not yet been clarified. This along with its long-term safety in the mouth are being investigated in the United States before its introduction in this country. As yet, none of the agents replace the need for judicious oral hygiene with mechanical devices. However, the daily use of antimicrobial agents in conjunction with mechanical debridement and fluoride may prove to be the most effective means of controlling this dental disease.

Caries Activity Tests

Knowledge of caries etiology has led to the development of tests which attempt to measure a patients' individual susceptibility to dental caries. Although a multitude of tests are described in the literature, none is presently thought an ideal indicator of disease activity. This is due to the multifactorial nature of the disease. All the current assay methods focus on one feature of the caries process and attempt to draw strong positive correlations to actual caries experience. This approach precludes many other variables which may affect the overall caries experience of an individual. Perhaps it may be necessary to use several tests simultaneously to provide the high degree of correlation necessary to give a valid indication of caries prediction. However, these assays can act as a valuable aid for patient motivation in a well-designed plaque control program.

An ideal caries test should have the following characteristics: validity, reliability, and feasibility. **Validity** simply means that the test accurately measures what it says it does. In order to measure test validity properly a prediction of caries experience must be made in a group of test patients. The patients must then be followed for some period of time—perhaps 1 or 2 years—and the caries occurrence must be recorded. If a high percentage of positive test responders develops caries, the test is then said to exhibit validity.

Reliability is a second characteristic necessary for a good predictive test. Reliability means that the test will yield the same results under varied conditions and among several independent observers.

Finally, **feasibility** of the assay must also be considered. The ease and costs of performing the test are important to the overall acceptance of the method to clinical situations. Ideally, a test that is noninvasive, inexpensive, and easily run is desired.

Among the large number of caries tests that have been developed, several have gained some clinical acceptance. The first group of tests are based upon the microbiologic vector. These tests attempt to correlate oral bacteria and/or their metabolic products to caries incidence. The older test of this type is the lactobacillus colony count, in which salivary samples are obtained and incubated in selective media for lactobacilli. The numbers of lactobacillus colonies per milliliter of saliva are quantitated and related to caries activity. Although this test has been used as a standard assay for many years it has some drawbacks, including a relatively high cost per test. This method also requires several days to run and requires tedious counting of bacterial colonies. A newer, more convenient method for estimating oral lactobacilli is now available.* This test measures lactobacilli present by comparison to a standard optical density chart that has been correlated to the number of organisms per milliliter. This method is relatively simple and can be adapted to most dental offices. However, once again this method requires several days to complete.

The Snyder test is another caries prediction test. It measures the salivary acid production over a 3-day period. The test uses pH color indicators, which make it quite easy to determine bacterial acid production. Snyder and others who have used this assay report a strong correlation between clinical caries activity and a positive test result. Table 27–8 indicates how the results of the Snyder test may be interpreted. Although this test is relatively

*Orion Diagnostica (Helsinki, Finland).

TABLE 27–8 ✦ Interpretation of Snyder Caries Test Results

	TIME (hr)		
	24	48	72
Color	Yellow	Yellow	Yellow
Caries activity	High	Definite	Limited
Color	Green	Green	Green
Caries activity	Continue test	Continue test	Inactive

From Newbrun, Cariology, ed. 2, Williams & Wilkins, p. 259, 1983, with permission.

inexpensive to run, it also requires 3 days to obtain the results and is therefore somewhat time-inefficient for the clinical dental setting.

The reductase test, a colorimetric assay that measures the activity of the salivary enzyme reductase, has also been used as a caries predictive test with some success. It has the advantage of giving results in the relatively short time of 15 minutes. However, the validity of this test has been questioned, since results have not been confirmed by several independent investigators.

The buffering capacity of whole saliva has also been used as a means of predicting caries experience. This method measures the ability of a salivary sample to neutralize a standard acid solution. It is based upon the hypothesis that increased acid production by plaque bacteria leads to increased enamel demineralization and caries. Therefore, an inverse relationship between buffering capacity of the saliva and caries activity should exist. Although there is some validity to this test, the results obtained cannot be adequately correlated to caries activity. Table 27–9 conveniently lists these and other proposed caries predictive tests that are based upon chemical or bacteriologic assays.

Another approach to predicting caries activity is to examine an individual's previous caries experience and try to formulate future trends. This type of method has been successfully applied to groups of children and was shown to be a predictable means of identifying children with high and low caries activity.

The role of dietary carbohydrate in the carious process has been clearly established. Furthermore, sucrose is implicated as the key substrate for caries-producing bacteria and the relationship of the percent of sucrose in foods and their caries-producing activity is shown in Table 27–10. Therefore, the correlation of sucrose ingestion to caries experience may be another method for predicting caries potential. The variability of caries among individuals raises the question of what differences, if any, exist between caries-prone and caries-resistant individ-

TABLE 27–9 ✦ Caries Activity Tests: Basis, Method, and Clinical Correlation

TEST	BASIS	METHOD	CLINICAL CORRELATION
Lactobacillus count	Aciduric bacteria (saliva)	Quantitative counts/ml	Group correlation only
Snyder	Aciduric bacteria (saliva)	Qualitative colorimetric	Group correlation only
Swab	Aciduric bacteria (plaque)	Qualitative colorimetric	Unsatisfactory
Fosdick	Total bacteria (saliva)	Quantitative Ca demin. of enamel	None established
Dewar	Total bacteria (saliva)	Quantitative modified Fosdick	Unsatisfactory
Rickles	Total bacteria (saliva)	Quantitative buffering capacity	Unsatisfactory
Reductase	Total bacteria (saliva)	Qualitative color indicator	Group correlation only
Amylase	Starch hydrolysis (saliva)	Qual./Quant. color indicator	Unsatisfactory
Buffer capacity	Buffer capacity (saliva)	Quantitative titration	Some extreme deviations
Streptococcus mutans screening	*S. mutans* (plaque)	Semiquantitative	Best correlation for high caries group

From Newbrun, Cariology, ed. 2, Williams & Wilkins, p. 266, 1983, with permission.

uals. Early studies focused upon the saliva, since its protective role in caries was somewhat understood. Researchers looked at calcium-to-phosphate ratios in caries-resistant humans. Although some caries-resistant individuals did show higher calcium-to-phosphate ratios, no definite conclusions could be made. Investigators also looked at the resting salivary pH and found the pH to be significantly higher in people who were caries free. Other

TABLE 27–10 ✦ Correlation of Sucrose Content of Selected Foods to Caries Score in Rats*

FOOD*	SUCROSE CONC. (%)	CARIES SCORE
Sucrose	99.5	62
Milk chocolate	42	34
Dates	47	33
10% sucrose/water	10	32
Raisins	14	31
Candy mints	78	25
Bananas	9	21
Apples	3	19
Figs	0.1	10
Milk	0	0
Soda crackers	0	0

*Rats fed a noncariogenic diet for 1 hour twice a day. Test food was continuously available.
Data adapted from Table 4–3 in Newbrun, Cariology, ed. 2, Williams & Wilkins, p. 99, 1983, with permission.

studies examining specific salivary components such as salivary IgA, lysozyme, amylase, and lactoperoxidase have shown some differences among caries-free and caries-prone humans. Still other studies have focused upon plaque in these two groups, supporting the concept that caries occurs at the enamel-plaque interface and that examination of saliva may not be as useful for comparison. Examination of plaque samples from caries-resistant and -susceptible groups was shown generally to produce equivalent amounts of lactic acid after sucrose ingestion. Therefore, the basic nature of the plaque is the same. However, plaque from caries-free individuals was shown to contain lower numbers of *S. mutans* and *L. acidophilus*. The variability in the results of these and other studies supports the concept that no single factor is common to all caries-free humans. It seems likely that in some caries-free individuals, salivary antibodies may be inhibiting cariogenic bacteria; however, this single effect is not enough to totally eliminate caries, and other salivary and host factors must work in unison to afford the individual overall caries protection. Furthermore, clinical observations suggest that different combinations of factors operate in each person resulting in a specific caries risk.

ROOT CARIES

Root caries comprise the group of carious lesions that affect the cementum and dentin of the root surface. Many lesions are associated with gingival recession. It is a lesion generally found in adults. The prevalence of root caries increases significantly after the age of 35 and has been noted in more than 50 percent of the population between the ages of 40 and 50. The nature of root caries is somewhat different from that of enamel caries. It is a soft progressive lesion of the root surface, which is associated with microbial plaque. It differs from abrasion, erosion, and idiopathic resorption. Caries on the root surface usually appears as a shallow, ill-defined area, often discolored, and quite soft. Lesions are thought to start at the cemental-enamel junction. The progression of this lesion usually extends laterally rather than in depth. However, lesions can spread rather rapidly with pulpal involvement within a few months. Diagnosis of root caries is based upon the clinical features of location, color, surface roughness, softness of the root, and/or obvious cavitation. As yet, no clear diagnostic tests are available for root caries detection.

The etiology of root caries is primarily microbial. Plaque-sampling studies have identified gram-positive filamentous *Actinomyces* species as a predominant bacteria. Animal studies in rodents have supported this finding and bacteria such as *A. viscosus* were shown to be essential for the development of cemental caries in these animals. Other microorganisms such as *A. naeslundii, S. mutans, S. salivarius, S. sanguis,* and *B. cereus* have all been shown to produce root caries in animal models. Although *A. viscosus* remains a favored etiologic bacteria in this lesion, no specific microorganism or particular group of oral flora has been clearly associated with the initiation or progression of root caries.

As with other caries, the role of the host is important in the overall development and progression of root caries. Specifically, decreased salivary function (xerostomia) can dramatically increase root surface caries. Xerostomia can be associated with individuals undergoing head and neck radiation therapy, patients taking a variety of medications, and those suffering from Sjögren's syndrome. Therefore, persons with reduced salivary function must be carefully watched and maintained in order to prevent the rapid occurrence of root caries. Probably the most effective means of reducing root caries is by dietary control, strict oral hygiene, and the daily use of topical fluorides. The consumption of fermentable carbohydrates should be closely monitored. These patients should be given repeated home care instruction to ensure excellent plaque control. Fluoride therapy will usually consist of a daily application of a fluoride gel using a custom-fitted stent. The most common formulations are a 0.4 percent stannous fluoride gel, which provides about 1000 ppm of fluoride ion, or a 1.1 percent neutral sodium fluoride gel which yields about 5000 ppm of fluoride ion.

BIBLIOGRAPHY

Gibbons, R. J.: Adherence of bacteria to host tissue. In Schlessinger, D. (ed.): Microbiology. A series of monographs. ASM, Washington, D.C., 1977, p. 395.

Gibbons R. J. and Dankers, I.: Patterns of lectin-like reactivity of selected oral bacteria. J. Dent. Res. (spec. iss. A), 547, 1981.

Gustafsson, B. E., Quensel, C. E., Lanke, L. S., Lundqvist, C., Grahnen, H., Bonow, B. E., and Krasse, B.: The Vipeholm dental caries study. The effect of different levels of carbohydrate intake on caries activity in 436 individuals observed for five years. Acta. Odontol. Scand. 11:232, 1954.

Miller, W. D.: The microorganisms of the human mouth, edited by K. Konig. S. Karger, Basel, p. 205, 1890 (reprinted 1973).

Newbrun, E.: Cariology, ed 2. Williams and Wilkins, Baltimore, p. 246, 1983.

Rolla, S., Bonesvoll, P., and Opermann, R.: Interactions between oral streptococci and salivary proteins. In Kleinberg, Ellison, and Mandel (eds.): Saliva and Dental Caries. (sp. suppl.) Microbiology Abstr. 1979, p. 227.

Simmons, N. S.: Extraction of enamel rods and apatite ribbons from embryo teeth. J. Dent. Res. 51(sp. iss.):252, 1972.

Sognnaes, R. F.: Analysis of war-time caries reduction in European children, with special regard to observations in Norway. Am. J. Dis. Child 75:795, 1948.

Staat, R. H., Doyle, R. J., Langley, S. D., and Studdick, R. P.: Modification of in vitro adherence of Streptococcus mutans by plant lectins. Adv. Exp. Med. Biol. 107:639, 1978.

Stephan, R. M.: Changes in the hydrogen ion concentration on tooth surfaces and in carious lesions. J. Am. Dent. Assoc. 27:718, 1940.

Wolinksy, L. E. and Sote, E. O.: Isolation of natural plaque-inhibiting substances from "Nigerian Chewing Sticks." Caries Res. 18:216, 1984.

28 *Periodontal Disease*

Russell J. Nisengard, Michael G. Newman, and
Joseph J. Zambon

CHAPTER OUTLINE

Microbiology of periodontal disease—general aspects
Immunology of periodontal disease—general aspects
Gingival health
Specific diseases
Diagnostic tests for periodontal disease

The term *periodontal disease* describes a number of distinct clinical entities that affect the periodontium including the gingiva, gingival attachment, periodontal ligament, cementum, and supporting alveolar bone.

The most common periodontal diseases, gingivitis and periodontitis, as well as many other less common periodontal diseases, usually are chronic bacterial infections. Like other infections, the bacterial-host interactions determine the nature of the resulting disease. The pathologic microorganisms may produce disease indirectly (e.g., through the effects of toxins), or by direct invasion of the tissues. The host response to microorganisms may be protective or destructive or both, which accounts for the wide variety of patterns of tissue changes observed in patients. Periodontal diseases may be generalized or site-specific (affecting isolated areas) and may contribute to the development and course of certain systemic disease.

Gingivitis, or inflammation of the gingiva, is characterized clinically by gingival changes in color, form, position (see pocket formation further on), and surface appearance. Bleeding and exudate from the gingival crevice are also sometimes apparent.

Periodontitis occurs by the extension of inflammation into the deeper structures of the periodontium. Pocket formation, bone loss, and mobility are usual clinical features. Periodontitis may be generalized or localized. It is classified into adult forms and juvenile forms depending on the specific clinical, microbiologic, and host factors that are present at the time of diagnosis (Table 28–1).

TABLE 28–1 ✦ Classification of Periodontal Diseases

  I. Gingival Disease
   A. Gingivitis
      1. Nonspecific gingivitis
      2. Acute necrotizing ulcerative gingivitis (ANUG)
   B. Manifestations of systemic diseases and hormonal disturbances—e.g., desquamative gingivitis, primary herpetic gingivostomatitis, "pregnancy gingivitis" and other hormonally mediated changes, diabetes and other metabolic diseases
   C. Drug-associated gingival inflammation—e.g., dilantin hyperplasia
 II. Mucogingival conditions—e.g., gingival recession and aberrant frena and/or muscle attachment
III. Periodontitis
   A. Adult Periodontitis
      1. Slight
      2. Moderate
      3. Advanced
      4. Refractory and rapidly progressive
   B. Juvenile Periodontitis (JP)
      1. Prepubertal
      2. Generalized juvenile periodontitis (GJP)
      3. Localized juvenile periodontitis (LJP)
   C. Periodontal abscess
 IV. Pathology Associated With Occlusion
  V. Other Conditions—Miscellaneous (e.g., infection, trauma)

Adapted from Current Procedural Terminology for Periodontics, ed. 5., Am. Acad. Periodontol. 1986.

A periodontal pocket is a pathologically deepened gingival sulcus and it is one of the key clinical features of periodontitis (Fig. 28–1). Pocket formation occurs by the apical migration of the junctional epithelium along the root. Destruction of the periodontal ligament and alveolar bone occurs as a result of bacterial and host factors described later in this chapter.

Classification

The classification of periodontal disease is based on clinical, bacterial, host, and environmental factors. The contribution of each factor determines the course and treatment of the particular disease. With the discovery of new bacterial etiologic agents, more specific diagnoses will permit further refinement of the present classification and treatments (Table 28–1). In the future, some descriptive clinical names for periodontal diseases may be supplanted by bacterial names in recognition of their role in the etiology of the diseases.

Among the periodontal diseases, several are considered "aggressive" forms (Table 28–2). These forms of periodontitis frequently demonstrate rapid bone loss, sometimes measured in millimeters per year. This contrasts with adult periodontitis in which bone loss usually is in tenths of a millimeter per year.

Prevalence of Periodontal Disease

The most common inflammatory periodontal diseases, nonspecific gingivitis and periodontitis, occur worldwide. Gingivitis involving at least one site per patient affects more than 80 percent of the population and in some instances nearly 100 per-

TABLE 28–2 ✦ "Aggressive" Periodontal Diseases

Localized juvenile periodontitis
Generalized juvenile periodontitis
Prepubertal periodontitis
Rapidly progressive periodontitis
Refractory periodontitis

cent. It is seen in all age groups. Similarly, periodontitis affects approximately 75 percent of the adult American population. Alveolar bone loss associated with periodontitis may start as early as the teen years, although it usually begins in adulthood, and progresses with age. Sex, socioeconomic factors, race, and the methods of detection all contribute to the reported prevalence. The other forms of periodontal disease, including periodontal abscesses, acute necrotizing ulcerative gingivitis, prepubertal periodontitis, herpetic gingivostomatitis, juvenile periodontitis, rapidly progressive adult periodontitis, and drug or systemic-induced gingival conditions, are considerably less common and account for less than 10 percent of all periodontal disease.

Concept as an Infection

The primary cause of the most common forms of gingivitis and periodontitis are bacteria. Plaque, an organized bacterial mass, attaches to the tooth surface above and below the gingival margin and is necessary to initiate these diseases (see Chapter 26). The pathogenic potential of the particular bacteria within the plaque varies from individual to individual and from one gingival site to another

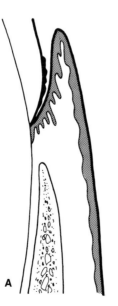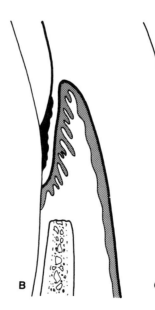

FIGURE 28–1 ✦ Types of periodontal pockets. **A,** Normal gingival sulcus, where there is only soft tissue inflammation associated with plaque. **B,** Suprabony pocket. The base of the pocket is coronal to the alveolar bone. The alveolar bone loss is horizontal in nature. **C,** Infrabony pocket. The base of the pocket is apical to the level of the alveolar bone. The alveolar bone loss is vertical in nature. (From Carranza, F. A., Jr.: Glickman's Clinical Periodontology, ed 6. W. B. Saunders Co., Philadelphia, 1984.)

A   B   C

within the same mouth. A small but varying amount of plaque can be controlled or tolerated without causing periodontal disease probably as a result of host defense mechanisms. When specific bacteria within the plaque increase to significant numbers or produce virulence factors or both, the "controlled environment" or balance shifts toward the development of disease. Disease also occurs by a reduction in the host defensive capacity. These host factors can be local or systemic (see further on).

Early theories regarding the role of dental plaque in periodontal disease suggested that there was only a quantitative change resulting from increased numbers rather than an alteration in the types of bacteria. It was later discovered that bacterial plaque associated with gingival health differed from that seen in periodontal disease and most periodontal diseases had their own characteristic flora (Table 28–3). In general, gram-negative, anaerobic microorganisms are the principal bacteria associated with most bacterial caused periodontal diseases. *Porphyromonas gingivalis, Prevotella intermedia, Bacteroides forsythus, Campylobacter rectus* (formally *Wolinella recta*) and *Actinobacillus actinomycetemcomitans* are the most common bacteria identified to date. These are thought to be important because of their pathogenic capabilities and the increased numbers associated with disease states. Other bacteria found in lower numbers may also be important but have not been studied to the same extent as the principal bacteria.

At present, the etiologic relationship of bacteria to different periodontal diseases is based on several factors, as summarized in Table 28–4:

1. An organism thought to be important in the disease process should be commonly found in high numbers and absent or infrequently found in health.

TABLE 28–3 ✦ Principal Bacteria Associated with Periodontal Disease

Adult periodontitis	*Porphyromonas gingivalis, Prevotella intermedia, B. forsythus, Campylobacter rectus*
Refractory periodontitis	*Bacteroides forsythus, P. gingivalis, Campylobacter rectus, P. intermedia*
Localized juvenile periodontitis (LJP)	*Actinobacillus actinomycetemcomitans, Capnocytophaga*
Periodontitis in juvenile diabetics	*Capnocytophaga, A. actinomycetemcomitans*
Pregnancy gingivitis	*P. intermedia*
ANUG	*P. intermedia,* intermediate-sized-spirochetes

TABLE 28–4 ✦ Identification of the Bacterial Etiology in Periodontal Disease

1. Large numbers of the bacteria are *associated* with the disease state and absence or reduced numbers associated with health
2. *Elimination* or suppression of the organism reverses or reduces the disease
3. Elevated *host responses* are associated with the disease
4. *Animal pathogenicity* similar to periodontal disease occurs upon implantation of the organism(s) into germ-free animals
5. The bacteria possess potentially *pathogenic mediators* that could contribute to the disease process

2. Elimination or suppression of the organism by treatment should have a positive influence.
3. There should usually be an elevated immune (humoral or cellular) response to the organism.
4. Experimental implantation of the organism into the gingival crevice of an animal should induce some characteristics of the naturally occurring disease (e.g., inflammation, connective tissue disruption, and bone loss).
5. The purported pathogen should possess pathogenic or virulent factors.

Treatment of Periodontal Disease

The rationale for treatment depends upon the identification of as many environmental and host factors as possible.

Control of environmental or local factors is the major emphasis of current periodontal treatment. Bacterial plaque is the primary etiologic agent while calculus and other factors are secondary local factors. These components elicit and perpetuate the vast majority of pathologic changes in the periodontium. Therapy is aimed at first identifying, removing, and controlling the etiologic factors and then correcting the defects these pathogens have created. Therapy for many periodontal diseases caused by bacterial plaque includes oral hygiene education and instruction, instrumentation for removal of calculus (scaling) and toxic root substances (root planing), chemotherapy (see Chapter 29), periodontal surgery (if pockets remain), and periodic maintenance therapy.

Other environmental and local factors such as occlusion and iatrogenic factors can modify the progression of the local disease state. Diagnosis, detection, and treatment of each of these factors includes occlusal analysis and therapy, control of temporomandibular joint (TMJ) factors, orthodontics, repair or replacement of existing restorations or prosthesis, and replacement of implanted materials.

Host Factors

Alterations in the periodontium and other oral tissues are caused or influenced by a variety of systemically-associated conditions. Factors such as age, occurrence of systemic disease, immune status, and stress greatly influence the nature of periodontal pathology. For example, infection with human immunodeficiency virus (HIV-1) is associated with two forms of periodontal disease, HIV-gingivitis and HIV-periodontitis. Assessment of these contributing factors significantly influences the therapeutic regimen. Physiologic and psychologic factors, chemotherapy, and hormones influence both the observed periodontal pathology and the associated therapy. Often, control of systemic etiologic factors greatly improves periodontal health. Similarly, periodontal pathology, especially acute gingivitis and periodontitis, affects the patient's general health. In some systemically compromised patients, periodontal disease can be a source of systemic infections. The control of metabolic diseases, such as diabetes, may also be adversely affected by periodontal disease.

Hereditary, genetic, and developmental factors influence every aspect of the periodontal tissues. Recognition and detection of contributing factors are essential to successful maintenance of periodontal health and prevention of disease.

MICROBIOLOGY OF PERIODONTAL DISEASE—GENERAL ASPECTS

Bacterial infectious diseases are a result of one or more mechanisms (Table 28–5). The direct effects include invasion, exotoxins, cell constituents, and enzymes, which can affect the growth and function of fibroblasts, epithelial cells, endothelial cells, and inflammatory cells, will be considered in the section on the microbiology of periodontal disease. The indirect response to the bacteria including immunologic and other host responses are considered subsequently in the section on the immunologic aspects of periodontal disease.

TABLE 28–5 ✦ Potential Bacterial Mechanisms in Periodontal Disease

1. Invasion
2. Exotoxins
3. Cell constituents (such as endotoxins)
4. Enzymes
5. Immunologic—host responses

TABLE 28–6 ✦ Bacterial Factors Important in Direct Tissue Damage

Enzymes
Collagenase
Hyaluronidase
Phospholipase
Phosphatases
Endotoxin
Cell inhibitors
Ammonia

Periodontal microbiology has been examined by several approaches: cultural, taxonomy, microscopy, and immunodiagnosis. All these methods have led to an improved understanding of the etiology and pathogenesis of periodontal disease as well as further clarification of periods of disease activity. These studies also have extended periodontal therapy to include modifying the subgingival flora to one more associated with disease inactivity.

One of the important advances in the field of periodontal microbiology is the concept of specificity. Periodontal disease is now considered to be a group of diseases or infections. Each disease has its own associated group of microorganisms. The concept of bacterial specificity first was developed with the advent of anaerobic microbiology techniques and their application in identifying "unusual" gram-negative rods associated with localized juvenile periodontitis. Since then, characteristic microfloras have been associated with the different periodontal diseases and stages of disease.

The mechanisms by which subgingival bacteria may contribute to the pathogenesis of periodontal disease is varied. These include factors influencing colonization (adhesions, coaggregation, multiplication, interbacterial relationships, and host factors) and tissue damage. The periodontopathogens possess numerous factors that permit them to directly damage the periodontium (Table 28–6) or indirectly compromise the host response (Table 28–7).

TABLE 28–7 ✦ Bacterial Factors Important in Evasion of Host Defenses

Inhibition of PMN
Leukotoxin
Chemotaxis inhibitors
Decreased phagocytosis and intracellular killing
Resistance to C-mediated killing
Lymphocyte alterations
Endotoxicity
IgA, IgG proteases
Fibrinolysin
Superoxide dismutase
Catalase

Disruption of collagen seen in periodontal disease, while mainly a result of release of tissue collagenase, can also result from bacterial collagenase. *Porphyromonas gingivalis* and some strains of *A. actinomycetemcomitans* produce collagenase and can degrade fibrinogen.

Other bacterial enzymes of suspected periodontal pathogens that may cause periodontal destruction include gelatinase, aminopeptidases, phospholipase A, alkaline phosphatase, acid phosphatase, hemolysin, keratinase, arylsulfatase, neuraminidase, DNase, and RNase. Phospholipase A may initiate alveolar bone resorption as a precursor for prostaglandin. Alkaline and acid phosphatases may also cause alveolar bone loss.

Bacterial factors also aid in evasion of host defenses, as previously discussed (Table 28–7). These factors influence both the cellular and humoral responses. Polymorphonuclear leukocytes, for example, are influenced by leukotoxins, chemotactic factors, and inhibitors. Immunoglobulins and complement components are inactivated or destroyed by bacteria such as *Porphyromonas gingivalis* and *Prevotella intermedia,* which adversely affect the bacteriocidal activity of serum. The combination of direct effects of the bacteria on the periodontal tissues and indirect effects achieved by influencing host responses both influence the response of the periodontium to the periodontal pathogens.

IMMUNOLOGY OF PERIODONTAL DISEASE—GENERAL ASPECTS

Host responses play an important role in the pathogenesis of many types of periodontal diseases (Table 28–8). In the bacterial- or plaque-associated diseases, they may contribute to the disease process or modulate the effects of the bacteria. In desquamative gingivitis, they are either the cause or the result of the disease.

In the bacterial-associated periodontal diseases, immune responses may be both beneficial (protective) and detrimental (destructive). Several components of the immune system are active in periodontal disease (Table 28–9). The neutrophils, lymphocytes, plasma cells, and macrophages vary in number depending on the disease status of the tissues. Localized and systemic antibodies to the oral bacteria and complement also are of significance. These functions are thought to influence (1) bacterial colonization, (2) bacterial invasion, (3) tissue destruction, and (4) healing and fibrosis (Table 28–10).

Bacterial Colonization

Antibodies to bacteria confer protection in many bacterial diseases. This results from bacterial destruction by lysis or phagocytosis or both. Antibody interactions with bacteria also prevent the initial bacterial attachment or colonization. In periodontal disease, the subgingival area is the major environment of concern. In contrast to supragingival sites where secretory IgA (S-IgA) from saliva can reduce or inhibit specific bacteria within plaque, there is little if any subgingival S-IgA. Subgingivally, the major source for immunoglobulins and complement is gingival or crevicular fluid, which contains systemically and locally produced antibodies. These could modulate the types and numbers of microorganisms through inhibition

TABLE 28–8 ✦ Significant Immune Findings in Periodontal Diseases

DISEASE	FINDING
ANUG	PMN chemotactic defect
	Elevated antibody titers to *Prevotella intermedius* and intermediate-sized spirochetes
Pregnancy gingivitis	No significant findings reported
Adult periodontitis	Elevated antibody titers to *P. gingivalis* and other periodontopathogens
	Occurrence of immune complexes in tissues
	Immediate hypersensitivity to gingival bacteria
	Cell-mediated immunity to gingival bacteria
Juvenile periodontitis	
LJP	PMN chemotactic defect and depressed phagocytosis
	Elevated antibody levels to *A. actinomycetemcomitans*
GJP	PMN chemotactic defect and depressed phagocytosis
	Elevated antibody levels to *Porphyromonas gingivalis*
Prepubertal	PMN and monocyte chemotactic defects
Rapid periodontitis	Suppressed or enhanced PMN or monocyte chemotaxis
	Elevated antibody levels to several gram-negative bacteria
Refractory periodontitis	Reduced PMN chemotaxis
Desquamative gingivitis	Diagnostic or characteristic immunopathology in two thirds of cases
	Autoimmune etiology in cases resulting from pemphigus and pemphigoid

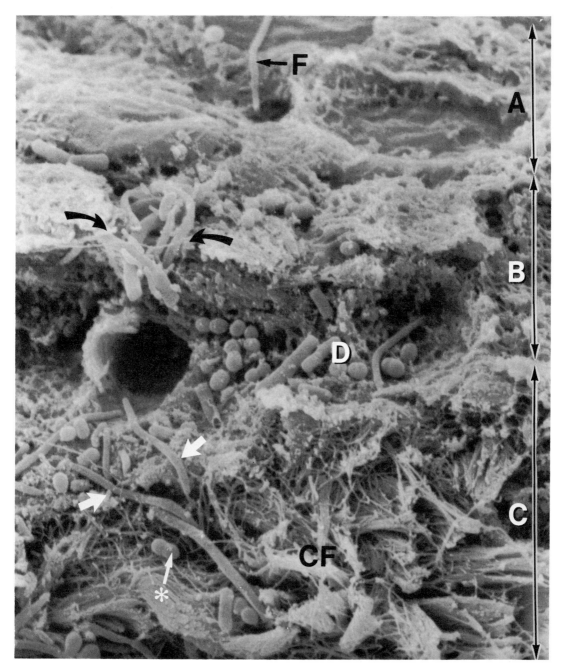

FIGURE 28–2 ✦ Cross-sectional electron micrograph of pocket wall from a patient with advanced periodontitis. View of surface of pocket wall **(A)**, sectioned epithelium **(B)**, and sectioned connective tissue **(C)**. *Curved arrows* point to areas of bacterial penetration into the epithelium. *Thick white arrows* point to bacterial penetration into the connective tissue through a break in the continuity of the basal lamina. F, filamentous organism on surface of epithelium; D, accumulation of bacteria (rods, cocci, filaments) on basal lamina; CF = connective tissue fibers. Asterisk points to coccobacillus in connective tissue. (From Carranza, F. A., Jr: Glickman's Clinical Periodontology, ed 6. W. B. Saunders Co., Philadelphia, 1984.)

demonstrated that topical application of hyaluronidase to gingival epithelium leads to widening of the intercellular spaces and increased permeability. Injection of hyaluronidase into the gingiva causes disruption of gingival connective tissue and apical migration of the gingival epithelium along the cementum, features of the initial phases of pocket formation.

Bacterial Invasion

Studies of acute necrotizing ulcerative gingivitis have clearly demonstrated the invasive nature of spirochetes and *P. intermedia* in this disease. It is thought that this invasion contributes to the disease in a similar fashion to spirochetal invasion in syphilis.

Our concepts of periodontitis are changing. Originally it was thought that bacteria did not actively invade the periodontium. Instead, they were thought to infiltrate passively following routine, mild gingival trauma such as toothbrushing, chewing hard substances, and subgingival scaling.

Recently, more sophisticated techniques including immunofluorescence, anaerobic culture, and electron microscopy have led to a reconsideration of the idea that bacteria can routinely be identified in gingival tissues in periodontal disease.

Bacteria were identified within the gingival tissues and close to resorbing bone surfaces in over half of the cases of advanced human periodontitis. Bacteria-leukocyte interactions on the surface of pocket epithelium, bacteria between junctional epithelial cells and the epithelium lining the lateral wall of pockets, as well as within the connective tissue are also observed (Fig. 28–2). Some of the bacteria observed within the gingival tissues in periodontitis have been identified. Along with the bacterial invasion, alteration in the epithelial basement membrane of the pocket epithelium can be observed with a discontinuous absence of basement membrane antigen. This suggests basement membrane disruption associated with bacterial invasion.

In localized juvenile periodontitis, bacteria, particularly *Actinobacillus actinomycetemcomitans*, have been identified within the gingival connective tissue. The presence of this organism within the tissues may explain why the disease is more resistant to treatment and requires antibiotic therapy.

Exotoxins

Many bacteria, such as *Corynebacterium diphtheriae* and *C. botulinum,* produce exotoxins, which contribute to the pathogenesis of their respective diseases. Production of exotoxins by subgingival bacteria is rare. Those bacteria that produce exotoxins are only transiently found subgingivally at the time of a systemic infection. Exotoxins are therefore not normally considered important in the pathogenesis of periodontal disease. However, one type of exotoxin directed toward human polymorphonuclear leukocytes is produced by *Actinobacillus actinomycetemcomitans*. This leukotoxin may enable *A. actinomycetemcomitans* to destroy leukocytes in the gingival crevice, which assists the microorganism in its ability to colonize and invade the gingival tissues.

Cell Constituents

Cellular constituents of both gram-positive and gram-negative bacteria also may play a role in periodontal disease. These include endotoxins, bacterial surface components, and capsular components.

The predominance of gram-negative bacteria within pockets in periodontal disease leads to high concentrations of endotoxin, a constituent of cell walls of gram-negative bacteria. Endotoxin, a lipopolysaccharide complex commonly shared by all gram-negative bacteria, is released upon cell disintegration. Endotoxins are highly potent, toxic substances affecting tissues directly and through activation of host responses. Important in considering their role in periodontal disease is their ability to (1) produce leukopenia; (2) activate factor XII or Hageman factor, which affects the clotting system by leading to intravascular coagulation; (3) activate the complement system by the alternate pathway which begins with C3 activation and bypasses C1, 4, and 2; (4) lead to a localized Shwartzman phenomenon with tissue necrosis following multiple exposures to endotoxin; (5) produce cytotoxic effects on cells such as fibroblasts; (6) induce bone resorption in organ culture; and (7) activate macrophages to synthesize IL-1, TNF-α, PGE$_2$, and hydrolytic enzymes. Endotoxins penetrate the gingival epithelium into the underlying tissue where their full pathogenic potential can be manifested.

Both gram-positive and -negative subgingival bacteria produce a variety of toxic end products that are also capable of tissue destruction. These include fatty and organic acids such as butyric and propionic acids, amines, volatile sulfur compounds, indole, ammonia, and glycans.

Peptidoglycan, a cell wall component of gram-positive bacteria, affects the host in a variety of ways including complement activation, immunosuppressive activity, stimulation of the reticuloendothelial system, and immunopotentiating properties. Peptidoglycans also appear capable of stimulating bone resorption and stimulating macrophages to produce prostaglandin and collagenases.

Capsular material and slime constituents also are capable of tissue destruction.

Enzymes

Some of the enzymes produced by oral bacteria such as hyaluronidase are capable of influencing gingival permeability and allowing apical proliferation of the junctional epithelium along the root surfaces.

Hyaluronidase occurs in higher concentrations in periodontal pockets than in normal sulci. In addition, a greater number of isolates from pockets produce hyaluronidase. Experimental studies have

TABLE 28–9 ✦ Components of Immune System Affecting Periodontal Disease

SYSTEM	FUNCTION
Secretory immune system	Decreases bacterial colonization on surfaces exposed to saliva
Neutrophil, antibody, complement	Bacteriocidal
Lymphocyte, macrophage, lymphokine	Tissue destruction
Immunoregulatory	Controls immune responses to bacteria

Adapted from Genco and Slots: J. Dent. Res. 63:441, 1984.

of colonization or lysis or both. However, in bacterial-associated periodontal disease, there is an "explosion" in the numbers of subgingival bacteria compared with the situation in gingival health. This heavy antigen load in an "external" environment may overwhelm the immune system, distorting or obviating any apparent positive effects.

Bacterial Invasion

As indicated earlier, invasion of the tissue occurs by whole bacterial cells and products in bacterial-associated periodontal diseases. In contrast to the large numbers of bacteria within the gingival crevice/pocket, few reach beneath the epithelium. This reduction probably is a combination of the physical barrier provided by the junctional epithelium and the host protective responses. The gingival tissues are bathed with both antibodies to the oral bacteria and complement, which enhance bacterial lysis. In addition, chemotactic factors could lead to polymorphonuclear leukocyte and monocyte infiltration with phagocytosis and lysis.

The importance of polymorphonuclear leukocytes and macrophages as phagocytes in defense against periodontopathic microorganisms is evident. In clinically normal gingiva, small numbers

of neutrophils are seen in the gingival crevice. With periodontal disease, increasing numbers of neutrophils infiltrate within and directly below the dentogingival epithelium. Phagocytes are usually chemotactically attracted to invading bacteria where they attach to the bacteria via C3b and other receptors. Following phagocytosis, the bacteria are usually lysed. Functional neutrophil or macrophage chemotactic defects predispose to periodontal disease. Patients with systemic diseases with associated chemotactic defects frequently have severe periodontitis (Table 28–11). Similarly, several periodontal diseases not associated with systemic disease have characteristic chemotactic defects (Table 28–12). Certain bacteria such as *Porphyromonas gingivalis* inhibit the function of leukocytes as a result of porinlike activity that depolarize PMN membranes.

Tissue Destruction

Several bacterial mechanisms could contribute to the pathogenesis of periodontal disease. These include anaphylactic or reagin-dependent reactions, cytotoxic reactions, immune complex or Arthus reactions, and cell-mediated or delayed hypersensitivity reactions (see Chapter 2). While host mechanisms leading to tissue destruction could be activated in any of the bacterial-associated periodontal diseases, most research has focused on gingivitis and periodontitis. Details will therefore be considered later in the section on gingivitis and periodontitis.

Healing and Fibrosis

Macrophages influence fibroblast activity and therefore healing through their release of fibronectin which is chemotactic for fibroblasts and other factors that influence fibroblast function and fibroblast activation. Lymphocytes also release cytokines capable of activating and recruiting fibroblasts.

Immunoregulation appears to play a role in periodontal disease. One important immune mediator

TABLE 28–10 ✦ Influence of Host Responses on Periodontal Disease

ASPECT OF DISEASE	HOST FACTORS
Bacterial colonization	Subgingivally, antibody-C' in crevicular fluid inhibits adherence and coaggregation of bacteria and potentially reduces their numbers by lysis
Bacterial invasion	Antibody-C' mediated lysis reduces bacterial counts; neutrophils as a consequence of chemotaxis, phagocytosis, and lysis reduces bacterial counts
Tissue destruction	Antibody-mediated hypersensitivity; cell-mediated immune responses; activation of tissue factors such as collagenase
Healing and fibrosis	Lymphocytes and macrophage-produced chemotactic factors for fibroblasts; fibroblast-activating factors

TABLE 28–11 ✦ Neutrophil Disorders Associated with Periodontal Disease

Diabetes mellitus
Papillon-LeFevre syndrome
Down's syndrome
Chédiak-Higashi syndrome
Drug-induced agranulocytosis
Cyclic neutropenia

TABLE 28–12 ✦ Periodontal Diseases with Neutrophil Disorders

Acute necrotizing ulcerative gingivitis
Localized juvenile periodontitis
Prepubertal periodontitis
Rapid periodontitis
Refractory periodontitis

is interleukin-1 (IL-1), a cytokine produced by macrophages, B cells, and squamous epithelial cells. IL-1 release is stimulated from these cells by lipopolysaccharides of periodontal pathogens such as *P. gingivalis*. It influences thymocytes, T cells, B cells, and fibroblasts, as well as other cells. IL-1 induces the proliferation of thymocytes, T cells, B cells, and fibroblasts. It also enhances the production of lymphokines including T-cell growth factor (IL-2). In addition, it induces prostaglandin E synthesis and formation of osteoclasts with resultant bone resorption. Furthermore, IL-1 enhances antibody production by B cells and production of collagenase and prostaglandin by fibroblasts. IL-1 particularly IL-1α is found in gingival fluid in greater amounts in inflamed sites and during experimental gingivitis, suggesting it may play a role in periodontal disease by influencing the host immunologic and inflammatory responses to bacterial antigens and mitogens. Lymphocytes from chronically inflamed gingival tissues have also been shown to be capable of producing IL-2, which may affect antibody synthesis, induce cytotoxic cells and bone destruction. However, no relationship has been shown between IL-2 and severity of periodontal disease.

The role of bacteria in modulating the immune response and connective tissue function has also been demonstrated. Leukocyte activity can be affected by the subgingival bacteria. For example, *P. gingivalis, Prevotella intermedia, Actinobacillus actinomycetemcomitans,* and *Campylobacter rectus* lead to increased release of prostaglandin. *P. gingivalis, A. actinomycetemcomitans, C. rectus,* and *Fusobacterium nucleatum* lead to increased release of IL-1. Some periodontopathogens chemotactically attract leukocytes, reduce che-

motactic ability, elaborate leukotoxins, resist phagocytosis, inhibit their own phagocytic killing, and interfere with fibroblast proliferation. For example, lipopolysaccharide from *Porphyromonas* species and other gram-negative bacteria activate the complement system by the classical and alternate pathways inducing PMN chemotaxis. However, soluble products of *Porphyromonas* can also block receptors on leukocytes, reducing the chemotactic response. Pathogenic strains of *Porphyromonas* are more resistant to phagocytosis than less pathogenic strains. Resistance to PMN killing appears to derive from capsular material, an unknown mechanism dependent on serum and ability to split PMN-derived hydrogen peroxide and superoxide dismutase.

The humoral response to subgingival bacteria can be nonspecifically altered by the bacterial production of IgG, IgA, IgM, C3, and C5 proteases. Enzymes to some or all of the humoral components are elaborated by black-pigmented *Porphyromonas* and *Capnocytophaga*. The *Porphyromonas* species completely degrade the immunoglobulins, while *Capnocytophaga* splits the immunoglobulin into Fab and Fc fragments, which may still have some biologic activity. This protease activity may inhibit the local host response, allowing bacterial penetration and spread within the tissues.

Subgingival bacteria also affect the humoral immune response by polyclonal B-cell activation. Bacteria nonspecifically induce multiple clones of B lymphocytes to produce immunoglobulins so that B cells stimulated by one microorganism produce antibodies to other microorganisms. The immunoglobulin production by B cells is under the regulatory control of T cells. Extracts of *P. gingivalis, Prevotella intermedia, Bacteroides melaninogenicus, Fusobacterium nucleatum, Actinobacillus actinomycetemcomitans, Actinomyces viscosus, A. naeslundii,* and *Capnocytophaga ochracea* stimulate polyclonal antibody responses and osteoclast-activating factors in cultures of normal human peripheral blood lymphocytes. These bacterial activators may play a role in the pathogenesis of periodontal disease.

Bacterial factors affect lymphocytes and other cellular constituents via suppression, activation, and mitogenicity. A factor from *A. actinomycetemcomitans* selectively activates human T suppressor cells. Sonic extracts of *F. nucleatum* lead to immunosuppression either by altering T-helper cell activity or by direct effects on the effector or responding cell population. *F. nucleatum* also suppresses mitogen activation of peripheral leukocytes. Extracellular polysaccharide from *C. ochracea* exerts immunosuppressive activity through macrophages, possibly with the participation of T-suppressor cells.

GINGIVAL HEALTH

Gingival health is defined clinically and histologically. Clinically, the gingival tissues are usually pale pink, firm, and scalloped with knife-edged margins and stippling on the surface. Histologically, health is characterized by an absence of an inflammatory infiltrate. It is common to observe clinical health even when there is histologically a minimal inflammatory infiltrate. Histologic health is usually achieved in "supernormals" in whom there is repeated scaling and root planing as well as heavy emphasis on patient home-care plaque control.

Gingival health usually is maintained when there is a balance between the subgingival microflora and host resistance factors active in the gingival crevice and tissues.

Microbiology

The gingival crevice harbors a microbial flora both in health and in disease. During health, the flora is relatively simple and sparse (Tables 28–13 and 28–14). It tends to reflect the bacterial types found in the early stages of plaque formation (see Chapter 26).

In healthy sulci from young adults, gram-positive cocci are the major morphotype and compose almost two thirds of the total flora. Filamentous forms, small spirochetes, fusiforms, and motile rods are also identified. In general, gram-negative species and motile forms are considerably less frequent and in smaller numbers. Similar bacterial findings occur in aged subjects with healthy gingival sulci. However, gram-negative bacteria may be slightly more common.

TABLE 28–13 ✦ Predominant Subgingival Bacteria Associated with Gingival Health

Streptococcus mitis
Streptococcus sanguis
Staphylococcus epidermidis
Rothia dentocariosa
Actinomyces viscosus
Actinomyces naeslundii
Small spirochetes

Immunology

Except in "supernormal" individuals where the gingival tissues exhibit maximum health as a result of comprehensive, ideal plaque control and frequent professional cleaning, the gingival tissues are usually infiltrated by chronic inflammatory cells, primarily lymphocytes. Leukocytes are also common within the junctional epithelium and in the gingival crevice. This cellular infiltrate, part of the host defense, is thought to be a direct response to the plaque. In "supernormals," in whom there is essentially no plaque, the cellular infiltrate is absent.

Serum antibodies to the microbial flora also occur. The titers to many oral bacteria usually are low in health, reflecting the minimal antigenic stimulation of plaque via the gingival tissues. When antibody titers are higher to some organisms, it is thought to reflect extragingival sites of antigenic stimulation in addition to the gingival tissues.

SPECIFIC DISEASES
Gingivitis and Periodontitis

Gingivitis, or inflammation of the gingiva, affects virtually the entire population to some degree.

TABLE 28–14 ✦ Bacterial Types in Health, Gingivitis, and Periodontitis

	HEALTH		GINGIVITIS		PERIODONTITIS	
	FREQ*	PROP*	FREQ	PROP	FREQ	PROP
Small spirochetes	25%	2%	82%	13%	100%	32%
Medium spirochetes	0	0	41	3	100	8
Large spirochetes	0	0	24	1	38	2
Small motile rods	13	1	12	1	75	7
Large motile rods	6	1	47	2	50	3
Curved motile rods	19	1	71	5	94	16
Filaments	31	4	53	4	63	2
Fusiforms	44	7	94	17	81	9
Small nonmotile rods	69	18	100	38	94	13
Cocci	94	66	92	15	50	4
Other nonmotile rods	5	2	3	2	4	7

*Freq = frequency (percent) of detection in sites by dark-field microscopy; Prop = proportion (mean percent) of dark-field groups per site.

Adapted from Savitt, E.D. and Socransky, S. S.: J. Periodontol. Res. 19:111, 1984. © 1984 Munksgaard Publishers Ltd., Copenhagen.

It is primarily a response to the bacteria in plaque. The earliest clinical signs of gingivitis are usually color and texture changes accompanied by slight enlargement of the tissues with some loss of firmness and adaptation to the teeth. The tissues often appear red, glossy, and edematous. The disease may remain in this state or, with continued presence of pathogenic plaque bacteria, progress to a loss of attachment of the gingiva to the tooth and the formation of periodontal pockets. This is termed periodontitis. However, it is important to stress that not all gingivitis conditions proceed to periodontitis.

Periodontitis, the major cause of tooth loss in adults, is the usual sequela to untreated gingivitis. It is an extension of the inflammatory process into the periodontal ligament, cementum, and the alveolar bone surrounding the teeth, leading to progressive destruction of these tissues and loss of teeth. The critical "last step" that permits this transition is currently unknown but appears to involve bacteria and host interactions.

When microorganisms proliferate adjacent to the gingiva, they elicit gingival inflammation. Clinically this may not be initially apparent, but histologically there is a vascular response consisting of capillary dilation and increased blood flow. Pocket formation starts as an inflammatory change in the connective tissue wall of the gingival sulcus caused by bacteria of the epithelial-associated subgingival plaque (Chapter 26) and may be exacerbated by the presence of subgingival calculus. The resulting cellular and fluid exudate causes further breakdown of the adjacent connective tissue, epithelium, and the gingival fibers. In the early stages of gingivitis, the inflammatory infiltrate is mostly lymphocytic with T cells predominating. In advanced gingivitis and periodontitis, the plasma cells are the most common inflammatory cells. Lymphocytes found in periodontitis are predominantly B cells with T cells comprising less than 6 percent. The helper-to-suppressor T-cell ratio in naturally occurring gingivitis in children and in experimental gingivitis is approximately 2:1. In contrast, the ratio in periodontitis with a GI of 1 or 2 is lower, approximately 1:1. In periodontitis with a GI of 3, the ratio increases to 2:1. This suggests a local alteration in the immunoregulatory mechanisms. The organisms present in the pocket are capable of synthesizing an array of products that can cause *direct* tissue damage. In some periodontitis lesions, bacteria can be found within the lateral wall of the periodontal pocket, the junctional epithelium, and periodontal ligament (see Fig. 28–2). As a result of the host-bacterial interactions, the periodontal pocket is formed. Once formed, this deepened area provides a specialized "protected" environment for further disease and diminishes the ability of the patient to cleanse the area.

The perpetuation of the periodontal lesion is controlled by both local and systemic factors. The significant feature associated with progressive periodontitis is the continued loss of periodontal ligament and bone support referred to as periodontal attachment loss. Attachment loss, an indication of disease "activity," may occur rapidly and last for days, weeks, or months. Active disease is associated with increased proportions of pathogenic bacteria, changes in the host response and possibly bacterial invasion within the tissues. The exact triggering mechanisms are not known. Periodontal disease is no longer thought to be a continuously progressive disease. Instead, there appears to be bursts of active periodontal destruction followed by periods of slower activity or quiescence. The periods of activity, which are additive, result in irreversible periodontal destruction—periodontitis. This ultimately causes loss of teeth.

MICROBIOLOGIC FINDINGS

The role of bacteria in the etiology of gingivitis and periodontitis has been well established on the basis of multiple factors.

Epidemiologic Studies

Numerous epidemiologic studies throughout the world have established that plaque is the primary etiologic factor in both gingivitis and periodontitis. Cross-sectional studies demonstrate that with increasing plaque scores, there is increasing severity of periodontal disease. In longitudinal studies of several years' duration, poor plaque control leads to increased severity of periodontal disease. In contrast, good plaque control prevents such periodontal breakdown.

Antimicrobial Studies

Antimicrobial agents including antibiotics, disinfectants, and antiseptics directly affect microorganisms, with minimal effects if any on host tissue. Penicillin, tetracyclines, and other antibiotics, while not usually clinically recommended as the sole means of treatment, significantly reduce gingival inflammation. Antimicrobials such as chlorhexidine in mouthwash are also very effective and are used clinically for control of gingival inflammation.

Oral Hygiene Studies

The classic experimental gingivitis model demonstrates the direct relationship between gingivitis and plaque accumulations. When all forms of plaque control are stopped, plaque rapidly forms and reaches a plateau. Within 7 to 9 days, early gingivitis occurs. When oral hygiene is again instituted and plaque removed, the gingivitis disappears within 3 days. Thus, by simply controlling plaque, gingivitis can be induced or eliminated. When plaque is allowed to accumulate for an extended period of years in dogs, periodontitis can also be induced. Along with the development of human experimental gingivitis, three phases are observed in plaque composition (Table 28–15). The initial phase, from 0 to 2 days after ending plaque control, is characterized by a flora of gram-positive cocci. The second phase from 2 to 4 days is one with increased filaments and fusiform bacilli. The third phase from 4 to 9 days when gingivitis is seen is characterized by increased vibrios and spirochetes.

Pathogenicity Studies

Numerous subgingival bacteria can induce one or more aspects of periodontal disease when orally implanted into germ-free and conventional animals or injected subcutaneously. The pathology observed includes inflammation, destruction of connective tissue, vasculitis, osteoclastic bone resorption, and apical migration of the junctional epithelium. These responses often can be induced by a culture of a single organism such as *A. actinomycetemcomitans,* which leads to rapid bone loss in a germ-free animal within a few months or by *P. gingivalis,* which can cause connective tissue attachment loss and alveolar bone resorption when utilized in the "monkey ligature" model. Selected "mixed cultures" can also induce rapid tissue destruction and periodontitis. However, models of experimental periodontal disease in germ-free animals or soft tissue abscesses must be carefully interpreted and only considered as pathogenic potential. Bacterial interactions in the complex subgingival flora as well as environmental and host factors in the pocket can either inhibit or stimulate bacterial growth.

Viable bacteria appear necessary for such responses. When freshly collected plaque is injected subcutaneously, transmissible, sometimes fulminating, abscesses occur. If the plaque is first autoclaved to prevent bacterial growth, subcutaneous

injection only induces a mild inflammatory response.

Scaling and Root Planing Experience

Clinical experience and studies have demonstrated the efficacy of scaling and root planing in periodontal therapy. Thorough removal of the bacterial deposits quickly and effectively reduces gingival inflammation. This coupled with plaque control at home can completely reverse gingivitis to the healthy state.

With development of gingivitis, there is both a quantitative and a qualitative change in plaque. There is a shift from gram-positive cocci seen in health to increased numbers of filamentous bacteria, gram-negative rods, and spirochetes (see Table 28–13). In the earlier stages of gingivitis, *Actinomyces* species are common. In longstanding gingivitis, gram-negative bacteria including *Veillonella* and *Fusobacterium* increase until they constitute approximately 25 percent of the flora.

In periodontitis, there is a continued change in the flora to one increasingly characterized by gram-negative, anaerobic rods (see Table 28–13). The flora is much more varied and complex than seen in health or gingivitis.

Recent studies have demonstrated qualitative differences in the subgingival flora in "active" sites, defined on the basis of recent loss of alveolar bone or attachment, compared with "inactive" sites, with no recent bone or attachment loss. Active sites usually have elevated numbers of *P. gingivalis, P. intermedia, A. actinomycetemcomitans,* "fusiform" black-pigmented bacteria, *Campylobacter rectus,* and small spirochetes. Conversely, successfully treated sites have small numbers of *P. gingivalis, P. intermedia,* and *A. actinomycetemcomitans.*

IMMUNOLOGIC FINDINGS

The continued exposure to bacterial antigens in the gingival crevice and within the gingival tissues induces systemic and local host responses. In gingivitis and adult-onset periodontitis, these immune responses have both protective and destructive functions (Fig. 28–3). The mechanisms summarized in this figure are potentially active in periodontitis. Their relative importance may vary from patient to patient and from site to site.

Protection

There is little evidence to demonstrate a significant protective immune function, since plaque accumulation inevitably leads to gingivitis. However, crevicular fluid contains immunoglobulins and complement, which constantly bathe the subgingival bacteria. Antibodies in the crevicular fluid are reactive with some of the bacteria and also bind to

TABLE 28–15 ✦ Phases Associated with Experimental Gingivitis

PHASE	TIME PERIOD	CHARACTERISTIC BACTERIAL FLORA
1	0-2 days	Predominantly gram-positive cocci
2	2-4 days	Increased filaments and fusiform bacilli
3	4-9 days	Increased vibrios and spirochetes

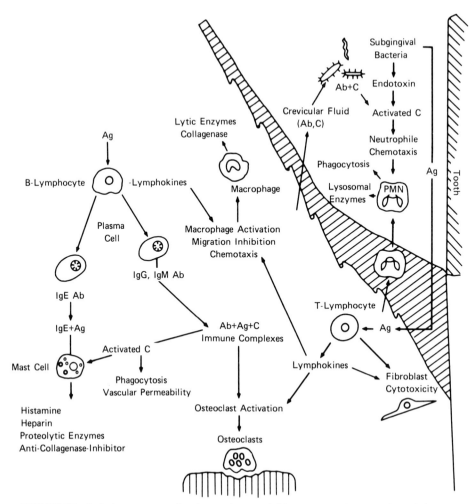

FIGURE 28–3 ✦ Immune mechanisms of potential importance in periodontal disease.

the subgingival bacteria in vivo along with complement. This reactivity may modulate or alter the composition of the subgingival microflora. The bacterial masses could be reduced via antibody-antigen reactions with complement activation leading to bacterial cytolysis and phagocytosis. The important role of the neutrophil in control of the periodontopathogens is evident in systemic diseases with reduced neutrophil function where there usually is severe periodontal disease.

Humoral Responses

The importance of B-cell responses in the pathogenesis of periodontal disease has been demonstrated experimentally in athymic rats devoid of T cells. Athymic rats with predominantly B cells in their gingival tissues show increased bone loss. In contrast, when T cells predominate in athymic rats reconstituted by injection of T cells, or in normal animals, there is less bone loss. Progressive periodontal disease, therefore, appears to be associated with B-cell lesions.

The immunopathology of gingivitis and periodontitis indicates that the gingival tissues contain the necessary elements for humoral responses. IgG-, IgA-, IgM-, and IgE-containing plasma cells are found in the inflammatory infiltrate where IgG and IgM predominate.

It is clear that local and systemic antibody responses to the crevicular microflora commonly occur. Early animal experiments demonstrated that with minimal antigenic stimulation, there is only a local plasma cell infiltration and antibody response at the site of injection. Higher antigen levels induce both a local and a systemic response.

As a measure of local antibody response, antibody levels from crevicular fluid and gingival explant supernates have been compared with serum antibody levels. Frequently, higher levels of antibodies to periodontopathogens occurred locally, suggesting local antibody production in response to local challenge. Local production of antibodies to *A. actinomycetemcomitans, P. gingivalis, F. nucleatum,* and *Campylobacter rectus* has been demonstrated. Indirect evidence for a local antibody response is further provided by the finding that many subgingival bacteria are "coated" in vivo with immunoglobulins and complement.

Because of the ease of assay, systemic serum responses to oral bacteria have been extensively studied. Serum antibody levels to some organisms are uniformly high, and to others, uniformly low, regardless of periodontal status. Antibody levels to most periodontopathogens are usually high, often correlating with the severity or type of periodontal disease. For example, patients with adult periodontitis usually have high numbers of *P. gingivalis* and significantly elevated antibody levels to this organism compared with subjects with healthy gingiva. Similarly, higher antibody levels also occur in periodontitis patients to *Capnocytophaga ochracea,* other gram-negative anaerobic bacteria, *A. naeslundii, Fusobacterium,* and *Leptotrichia buccalis,* which often occur in high numbers.

Dental treatment such as scaling and root planing commonly elicits a humoral response to some, but not all the subgingival bacteria. The serum antibody response generally peaks 2 to 4 months after scaling and root planing and gradually decreases to the prescaling level within 8 to 12 months. After scaling and root planing, elevated antibody levels occur to black-pigmenting bacteria including *P. gingivalis* and *P. intermedia,* as well as *Eikenella corrodens, Campylobacter concisus,* and *A. actinomycetemcomitans.* It has been suggested that this elevated humoral response may play a role in the success of therapy.

Many responses to antigen-antibody interactions are complement dependent. Complement activation is important in bacterial lysis, phagocytosis, bone resorption, chemotaxis, and other biologically significant events. Thoroughly washed gingival tissues from patients with periodontitis reveal significantly reduced complement within the tissues, compared with unwashed samples, suggesting that most of the complement represents extravasated serum rather than immune precipitates. The small amount of C3 and C4 remaining after washing is frequently located in foci, suggesting that while most complement is soluble, small amounts may be tissue bound in immune complexes. Quantitative studies of gingival fluid from periodontitis patients demonstrate significantly reduced C3 levels and marked depression of C4 in comparison to serum. This may indicate complement activation by the classical pathway; however, the role of the complement system is not well established.

The immunopathology of periodontal disease may result from anaphylactic reactions, cytotoxic reaction, immune complex reactions, and cell-mediated reactions playing a role in the pathogenesis.

Anaphylactic Reactions

Anaphylactic or immediate hypersensitivity reactions occur when IgE fixed to mast cells or basophils reacts with antigens and leads to the release of histamine and other mediators. The necessary components for such reactions are all associated with periodontitis.

IgE-containing plasma cells occur in the gingival tissues, though in fewer numbers than IgG-, IgA-, and IgM-containing cells. Mast cell numbers increase from gingival health to moderate periodontitis and then decrease in advanced periodontitis. It has been suggested that the decrease is a result of anaphylactic reactions leading to the degranulation of mast cells. Histamine levels in chronically inflamed gingivae are significantly higher than in normal tissues, and in vitro challenge of inflamed gingival tissues with anti-IgE leads to histamine release, suggesting IgE is already fixed to gingival mast cells.

The traditional method of identifying immediate hypersensitivity with skin tests has been applied to studies of periodontal disease. Intradermal skin tests with extracts of *Actinomyces* have revealed immediate and, less commonly, delayed reactions in humans. There is a significant correlation between the incidence of immediate hypersensitivity to this organism and severity of periodontal disease. The greatest incidence occurs in periodontitis. Similar immediate skin test responses have been demonstrated to *Bacterionema matruchotii, Bacteroides melaninogenicus,* and *Fusobacterium nucleatum.*

Repetitive challenge of the gingival tissues to induce immediate hypersensitivity reactions in monkeys experimentally evokes an inflammatory response. It is characterized by a chronic inflammatory infiltrate of plasma cells and lymphocytes along with connective tissue breakdown. Osteoclastic bone loss is not apparent.

The role of anaphylactic reactions in the pathogenesis of gingivitis and periodontitis has not been definitively shown. While the potential for this mechanism exists, it is not thought to be a major factor, because of the small numbers of IgE-containing cells in the gingival tissues.

Cytotoxic Reactions

Cytotoxic reactions occur when antibodies react with cell or tissue antigens, activating complement. The antigens can be either host cell constituents or bacterial antigens attached to host cells via receptor sites. An example of cytotoxic reactions is humoral autoimmune disease. There is no evidence, however, for considering cytotoxic reactions in the pathogenesis of plaque-associated gingivitis and periodontitis.

Immune Complex Reactions

Immune complex or Arthus reactions occur when antigen forms microprecipitates with IgG or IgM antibodies, or both, in or around blood vessels in tissues. Microcomplexes in moderate antigen excess activate the complement system, leading to hormonal, vascular, and cytotoxic reactions depending on where the complexes lodge.

The elements for immune complex disease are present in the gingival tissues: bacterial antigen, antibodies to the bacteria, and complement activation. The constant shower of bacterial antigens within inflamed gingival tissues, as seen by bacteremias resulting from gingival manipulation and by bacterial invasion, serves to both sensitize and subsequently challenge the host. These bacterial antigens encounter tissue fluids containing bacterial antibodies, permitting immune complex formation. Studies with the Raji cell assay have shown immune complexes commonly occur in soluble extracts of human gingival tissue from patients with periodontitis.

Experimental Arthus reactions in monkey gingivae are similar to those found in human periodontitis. Repetitive reactions lead to chronic inflammatory infiltrates of macrophages, lymphocytes, and plasma cells. Accompanying this is collagen breakdown and osteoclastic bone loss.

Cell-Mediated Reactions

Cell-mediated reactions or delayed hypersensitivity are dependent on T lymphocytes and the release of lymphokines. Numerous studies have demonstrated that peripheral leukocytes from patients with periodontitis blast or proliferate in response to some oral bacteria.

There are three basic types of responses. One pattern is characterized by a low blastogenic response in normal, healthy persons and a uniformly strong blastogenic response in gingivitis and periodontitis, which does not discriminate between the severity of disease. An example is the response to *Actinomyces* antigens. The second pattern is characterized by infrequent blastogenic response upon stimulation, which does not relate to disease severity. This pattern occurs with *Streptococcus sanguis* and *Eikenella corrodens*. The third pattern is one in which blastogenic responses are significantly greater in patients with destructive periodontitis than in individuals with healthy gums or gingivitis. Such responses occur in association with *P. gingivalis* and *Treponema denticola*. This last pattern suggests that pa-

tients with periodontitis are specifically immune to these organisms as a result of the periodontal infection.

The lymphoproliferative response in the gingival tissues is thought to release potent lymphokines including those capable of bone destruction. Gingival lymphocytes isolated from nondiseased gingiva produce low levels of the lymphokines including chemotactic factor, leukocyte migration inhibition factor, and mitogenic factor in response to plaque and specific plaque bacteria. In contrast, lymphocytes from gingivitis and periodontitis tissues produce more lymphokines upon challenge with plaque and specific plaque bacteria suggesting the lymphocytes are sensitized to the bacterial antigens.

Experimental induction of cell-mediated immunity in the periodontium of monkeys is characterized by massive tissue destruction including marked bone loss, reduced fibroblasts, and collagen breakdown. It has been suggested that the bone loss in cell-mediated immune responses results directly from T-cell effects or enhanced B-cell activation.

Experimental depression of cell-mediated immunity with antithymocyte globulin, however, does not influence development of gingivitis or alter existing gingivitis. In addition, patients receiving immunosuppressive therapy, such as transplant patients, have been evaluated for periodontal status. Most longitudinal studies indicate no difference in the rate of periodontitis between immunosuppressed patients and normal controls.

The contribution of cell-mediated immunity to the immunopathology of gingivitis and periodontitis is unknown; however, with the relatively low numbers of T cells in the tissue, it is not thought to be a major contributor.

Pregnancy Gingivitis and Hormonally Related Gingivitis

An increased incidence of gingivitis sometimes occurs during pregnancy, puberty, menstruation, postmenopause, and oral contraceptive use.

CLINICAL FINDINGS

In pregnancy gingivitis, there is erythema, edema, and increased gingival bleeding when a patient brushes and flosses or a dentist probes. The inflammation is a heightened or exacerbated response to plaque during periods of progesterone and estrogen imbalance. The degree of inflammation peaks in the second trimester and decreases following parturition. When there is no plaque-associated gingivitis prior to pregnancy and plaque control is maintained, the gingivitis does not develop. As a consequence, preventive measures are directed toward meticulous plaque control.

During puberty, menstruation, and oral contraceptive use, gingival inflammation is a hyper-response to plaque, just as occurs during pregnancy. Postmenopausal women sometimes exhibit shiny, red gingivae that can be irritated by spicy food.

MICROBIOLOGIC FINDINGS

Bacteriologically, during pregnancy, the changes in hormone levels influence the composition of the plaque. There is a shift toward a greater percentage of anaerobic bacteria, particularly *Prevotella intermedia*. It appears that *P. intermedia* can substitute progesterone or estradiol for vitamin K as a growth factor. Steroid hormones occur in crevicular fluid and may parallel serum concentrations which dramatically change during pregnancy, puberty, and menstruation, and after menopause.

IMMUNOLOGIC FINDINGS

Changes in the immune responses to the oral flora during pregnancy have not been evaluated.

Periodontitis in Juvenile Diabetics
CLINICAL FINDINGS

Patients with insulin-dependent diabetes mellitus (IDDM), or juvenile diabetes, frequently have more severe periodontal disease than the general population. This is related to the degree of metabolic control and plaque factors. Periodontitis begins near puberty with a prevalence of 9.8 percent in 13- to 18-year-old diabetics and increases to 39 percent in IDDM patients 19 years of age or older. IDDM patients may have more severe bone loss. Also, patients with uncontrolled or undiagnosed diabetes who have periodontitis often have multiple periodontal abscesses.

MICROBIOLOGIC FINDINGS

In IDDM associated gingivitis, the predominant cultivable organisms include *Actinomyces* (33 percent), streptococci (36 percent), *Veillonella parvula* (12 percent), and *Fusobacterium* (10 percent).

The predominant cultivable flora in IDDM-associated periodontitis includes *Capnocytophaga* and anaerobic vibrios averaging 24 percent and 13 percent of the cultivable flora respectively. This pattern differs from adult periodontitis, in which *P. gingivalis* frequently predominates and localized juvenile periodontitis (LJP), in which *A. actinomycetemcomitans* usually predominates.

IMMUNOLOGIC FINDINGS

As in other aggressive forms of periodontal disease, IDDM diabetics frequently have a leukocyte chemotactic defect (Table 28–10). This deficiency is thought to contribute directly to the pathogenesis of the disease.

Periodontal Abscesses
CLINICAL FINDINGS

Periodontal abscesses occur with pre-existing periodontitis. This acute infection occurs in the walls of periodontal pockets as a result of the invasion of bacteria into the periodontal tissues. While abscesses usually spontaneously occur in patients with untreated periodontitis, it is more common in periodontitis patients with a systemic disease such as diabetes, in which there is a reduced ability to combat infections. In some cases an abscess can even occur within a few days after a dental cleaning as a result of mechanical disruption of junctional epithelium, allowing the bacteria to gain entrance into the tissues.

MICROBIOLOGIC FINDINGS

Early animal studies demonstrated that fulminating, transferrable abscesses could be induced by subcutaneous injections of plaque. A limited number of bacteria were necessary for this and the abscesses were termed "mixed anaerobic infections." Black-pigmenting bacterial species, probably *P. gingivalis*, were necessary constituents.

Cultural examination of human abscesses reveal a similar microbiota with gram-negative anaerobic rods predominating. *P. gingivalis*, *Fusobacterium* species, *Capnocytophaga,* and *Vibrio* species were the most common gram-negative isolates, making up over 30 percent of the total cultivable microbiota.

Localized Juvenile Periodontitis (LJP)
CLINICAL FINDINGS

LJP occurs in patients approximately 12 to 20 years of age. Clinically, there is usually little gingival inflammation and minimal supragingival plaque. The hallmark of the disease is marked, localized, alveolar bone loss involving the permanent first molars and often the incisors. The bone loss is so discrete that the distal aspect of a second bicuspid may have no bone loss while the adjacent mesial aspect of a first molar can have several millimeters of loss (Fig. 28–4). LJP has a genetic component in that there is a familial inheritance and it is more common in females. The incidence of this disease has been estimated to be approximately 0.1 percent of the United States population, although in certain groups it has been found in up to 10 percent of the population. Prior to recognition of the bacterial factors, the affected teeth were usually extracted. Now the prognosis is greatly improved by scaling, root planing, surgery, and antibiotic therapy.

MICROBIOLOGIC FINDINGS

Early anaerobic cultural studies of first molar sites exhibiting localized bone loss in LJP patients

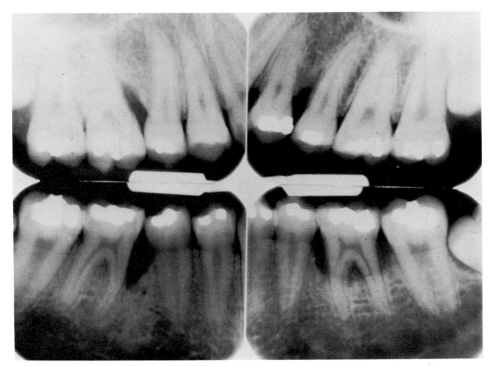

FIGURE 28–4 ✦ Radiographs of teenage female patient with localized juvenile periodontitis. Alveolar bone loss is typically localized to the first molars or incisors or both.

characterized a unique bacterial flora consisting of gram-negative anaerobic rods. These organisms were less frequently isolated and in significantly lower numbers in healthy subgingival sites in LJP patients and their non-LJP siblings or other adolescents. These organisms have been identified as *Actinobacillus actinomycetemcomitans* (Table 28–3, see also Chapter 17).

A. actinomycetemcomitans has been implicated in the etiology of LJP as a result of several factors.

1. The prevalence and the humoral immune response to this organism are elevated in patients with LJP. *A. actinomycetemcomitans* has been isolated in up to 97 percent of LJP patients, compared with 21 percent of adult periodontitis patients and 17 percent of healthy individuals. Not only is the prevalence of this organism six times greater in LJP than in health, but their proportion of the cultivable subgingival flora is also elevated. Among the serotypes, serotype B is the most common, followed by serotype A.

2. The incidence of *A. actinomycetemcomitans* is greater in younger LJP patients than in older LJP patients. If the age is considered representative of the duration of the disease, the younger patients had destructive disease within a short period. This suggests that this organism correlates with disease activity.

3. Large numbers of *A. actinomycetemcomitans* occur in lesions in LJP patients but are absent or found in small numbers in healthy sites.

4. *A. actinomycetemcomitans* can be identified by electron microscopy and immunofluorescence, and can be cultured from the gingival connective tissues of LJP lesions.

5. The organism is quite virulent, producing a leukotoxin, collagenase, phosphatases, and bone-resorbing factors, as well as other factors important in evasion of host defenses and destruction of periodontal tissues.

6. There is a positive correlation between the elimination of this organism from the subgingival flora and the successful clinical treatment of LJP.

The source of *A. actinomycetemcomitans* in LJP has not been well studied. It is known that early bacterial colonizers are derived maternally and from other family members. An intrafamily transmission of *A. actinomycetemcomitans* also is suggested by observations that the same biotype and serotype of *A. actinomycetemcomitans* can be isolated in family members of LJP patients, though in smaller numbers. This may explain the apparent familial tendency for this disease. It appears that the transmissibility of this organism is difficult and probably requires extended exposure. Periodontal probes contaminated with *A. actinomycetemcomitans* from LJP lesions during routine examinations can transfer the organism from infected to healthy, noninfected sulci. However, the organism does not permanently colonize the healthy sites and is eliminated within a matter of weeks.

It has been suggested that development of LJP is dependent on both bacterial and host factors. An explanation for primary involvement of first molars and incisors is not clear. The time of eruption of these teeth, coupled with hormonal factors, host immune factors, and colonization by this organism, are all believed to play a role.

Before recognizing the role of *A. actinomycetemcomitans* in LJP, there was usually a poor response to periodontal therapy. Home care procedures for plaque control, scaling and root planing followed by surgery for pocket elimination which usually were successful in treating adult periodontitis rarely achieved beneficial results in LJP. It is now understood that this organism cannot be eradicated by mechanical methods alone, as it occurs not only in the pocket but also within the gingival tissues. This intragingival location allows rapid repopulation of the pocket. Thus, clinical studies suggest that the best therapeutic approach is a combination of surgery to eliminate the pocket and antibiotic therapy to suppress the organism. The antibiotic of choice is tetracycline (250 mg qid for 3 weeks). Tetracycline can suppress *A. actinomycetemcomitans* for periods of 6 to 18 months.

IMMUNOLOGIC FINDINGS

Studies of LJP were the first to demonstrate the importance of neutrophils in periodontal disease. Approximately 75 percent of patients with LJP exhibit a polymorphonuclear neutrophil chemotactic defect and depressed phagocytosis in peripheral blood. The chemotactic defect is a cellular abnormality that is not associated with serum factors or neutrophil ability for random migration, deformation, or adherence. The demonstration of reduced receptor sites for chemotactic peptides and C5a in patients with LJP futher points to a genetic factor in this disease. In addition to altered systemic neutrophil function, neutrophil migration into the gingival crevice is slower in response to in vivo casein challenge than in healthy individuals. The gingival crevicular neutrophils also appear to have grossly altered morphology and diminished phagocytosis. It is not clear if this altered phagocytosis is inherent or reflects blockage of C3 receptors by surface C3 or they already contain a high amount of previously phagocytosed material.

The role of the neutrophil chemotactic defect in LJP has been clarified by studying families of patients with LJP. In many cases, brothers and sisters of patients with LJP may also exhibit a chemotactic defect without clinical signs of LJP. This has led to the conclusion that the chemotactic defect is a predisposing factor in LJP. The failure in neutrophil chemotactic responsiveness diminishes the host's ability to ward off the effects of periodontopathogens associated with LJP. Coupled with the chemotactic defect, the leukotoxin produced by *A.*

actinomycetemcomitans which destroys the reduced numbers of neutrophils that are chemotactically attracted into the gingiva further complicates the situation.

Associated with the high numbers of *A. actinomycetemcomitans* in LJP, the serum, crevicular fluid, and saliva from LJP patients have elevated antibody levels to this organism. Nearly 60 to 90 percent of patients have serum IgG antibodies and to a lesser extent IgM, IgA, and IgE antibodies particularly to the bacterial leukotoxin, outer membrane proteins and lipopolysaccharide. The response to lipopolysaccharide is primarily of the IgG2 subclass, a subclass less potent in complement activation and binding to phagocytic cells, which may limit the antibody mediated host defense. While the antibody levels in serum and crevicular fluid are usually similar, crevicular fluid antibody levels may exceed serum levels during periods of ongoing attachment loss. This suggests local antibody production within the gingival tissues. As expected, scaling patients with *A. actinomycetemcomitans* introduces bacterial antigens into tissues, leading to a hyperimmune response. Within 2 to 3 months after scaling, IgG serum and salivary antibodies increase.

Capnocytophaga species also are common inhabitants of the subgingival flora in LJP. In contrast to the immune response to *A. actinomycetemcomitans*, the level of antibodies to this organism is low, possibly because of suppressor cell activation or tolerance to the *Capnocytophaga* antigens.

Generalized Juvenile Periodontitis (GJP)

CLINICAL FINDINGS

Patients with GJP have clinical findings similar to those of patients with LJP, except that in GJP the bone loss is generalized rather than localized.

MICROBIOLOGIC FINDINGS

The predominant cultivable microorganisms in GJP differ from those in LJP. *P. gingivalis* is the most common isolate, constituting 13 to 20 percent of the total cell counts. Other common isolates include *Eikenella corrodens*, *P. intermedia*, *Capnocytophaga*, and *Neisseria*. In contrast to LJP, *A. actinomycetemcomitans* is present only in low numbers.

IMMUNOLOGIC FINDINGS

Similar to LJP patients, GJP patients frequently have a neutrophil chemotactic defect and reduced phagocytosis. The chemotactic defect is cellular in nature but the neutrophils have normal random migration and oxidative metabolic activity. While the incidence of chemotactic defects is similar but somewhat less in GJP than in LJP, GJP patients are less likely to exhibit decreased phagocytosis. Twenty-nine percent of GJP patients and 62 percent of LJP patients have decreased phagocytosis, compared with healthy control subjects.

Reflecting the high incidence and numbers of *P. gingivalis* in GJP, patients exhibit high IgG antibody titers to this organism. Approximately two thirds of GJP patients have elevated antibody levels. Antibodies to *A. actinomycetemcomitans* are less frequent in GJP than in LJP, with low titers to serotypes A and B and unexpectedly high titers to serotype C, approximating levels in LJP patients.

Rapid Periodontitis
CLINICAL FINDINGS

Rapid periodontitis, sometimes termed rapidly progressive periodontitis (RPP) or early-onset periodontitis, is a rare form of periodontitis. Frequently, patients have a history of LJP. This disease is clinically similar to adult-onset periodontitis but occurs in a younger age group, usually from post-pubertal to 35 years of age. During the active phase, patients exhibit severe alveolar bone loss, and gingival bleeding with acutely inflamed, pro-

liferative gingival tissue (Fig. 28–5). The disease may become inactive with no signs of clinical inflammation in spite of severe bone loss as a result of spontaneous regression or therapy. Treatment usually consists of thorough scaling and root planing, surgery, and antibiotic therapy.

MICROBIOLOGIC FINDINGS

Limited microbiologic examination has been performed on the subgingival flora in pockets from patients with rapid periodontitis. *P. gingivalis*, *P. intermedia*, and spirochetes—particularly small spirochetes—are major subgingival components in this disease.

IMMUNOLOGIC FINDINGS

The majority of patients with rapid periodontitis have functional defects in either neutrophils or monocytes. This manifests as either a suppression or an enhancement of chemotaxis. Neutrophils and, to a lesser extent, monocytes may play a role in the adverse response to the associated microflora.

While the exact significance of antibodies to oral bacteria is not known, elevated antibody titers occur to *P. gingivalis*, *A. actinomycetemcomitans*,

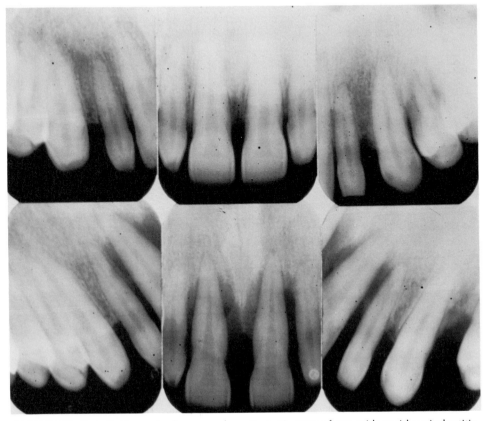

FIGURE 28–5 ✦ Radiographs from a male patient 40 years of age with rapid periodontitis. The lower set of three radiographs taken 15 months after the upper set demonstrate rapid progressive bone loss.

Campylobacter sputigena, C. rectus, Eubacterium brachy, Fusobacterium nucleatum, and *Peptostreptococcus micros.* In RPP, antibodies to *P. gingivalis* are of low avidity and are predominantly IgG2, which lacks strong complement fixation and opsonic activity. This would make control of this organism more difficult.

Prepuberty Periodontitis
CLINICAL FINDINGS

Prepuberty periodontitis, a rare form of periodontal disease, occurs during or immediately after the eruption of the primary teeth. In addition to bacterial and immunologic factors, there appears to be a genetic component, since family members may have the diseases and females are more commonly involved than males. There are generalized and localized forms of the disease.

In the generalized form, the gingiva is intensely red, often with proliferation and cleft formation. Accompanying this is very rapid destruction of alveolar bone and, in some cases, root resorption. While all the deciduous teeth are usually involved, the permanent teeth may not be affected. These children frequently have skin and upper respiratory infections as well as otitis media (middle ear infections). Because only a few cases have been well characterized, treatment is not adequately documented. It appears that the generalized form of the disease is resistant to antibiotic treatment.

In the localized form, a limited number of teeth are involved with minimal gingival inflammation. Frequent systemic infections are not common, as they are in patients with the generalized form. Although reports on treatment are scanty, curettage with antibiotic therapy appears beneficial.

MICROBIOLOGIC FINDINGS

The microflora seen in prepubertal periodontitis differs from that seen in juvenile periodontitis and rapid periodontitis. Species of *Fusobacterium, Selenomonas, Campylobacter, Prevotella,* and *Capnocytophaga* are frequently found in prepubertal periodontitis, while *A. actinomycetemcomitans, Haemophilus aphrophilus,* and *P. gingivalis* are infrequent subgingival inhabitants.

IMMUNOLOGIC FINDINGS
Generalized Form

Although the peripheral white cell counts are elevated, these patients suffer from pronounced depression in neutrophil and monocyte chemotaxis and ability to adhere to surfaces. Whereas gingival biopsies from adult periodontitis usually reveal inflammation including extravascular leukocytes, leukocytes are rare in patients with generalized prepubertal periodontitis. It is thought that these func-

tional defects play a role in the pathogenesis of this disease.

Localized Form

In comparison to the generalized form, defects in neutrophil and monocyte function in the localized form are less frequent, less severe, and do not occur simultaneously.

Refractory Periodontitis
CLINICAL FINDINGS

For many years it has been obvious that periodontitis could not always be successfully treated. A small number of patients suffer continued periodontal breakdown. This is called refractory periodontitis, as the disease does not respond to current conventional therapy. It is assumed that this breakdown is a response to poorly understood bacterial factors or host factors, or both.

BACTERIAL FINDINGS

Several microorganisms commonly are isolated from refractory periodontitis pockets. In active sites, these include *P. forsythus, P. gingivalis, C. rectus,* and *P. intermedia.* Inactive sites are characterized by increased numbers of aerobic bacteria, including *S. sanguis* and *Actinomyces.* The numbers of *S. sanguis* also increase in treated pockets.

IMMUNOLOGIC FINDINGS

Refractory periodontitis appears to have a reduced neutrophil chemotaxis. This has not been well studied. In addition, patients exhibit elevated serum antibodies to *A. actinomycetemcomitans, P. gingivalis,* and *Eikenella corrodens.*

Acute Necrotizing Ulcerative Gingivitis (ANUG)
CLINICAL FINDINGS

ANUG is a disease with rapid onset characterized by painful, necrotic, ulcerative gingival lesions. In most cases, particularly during the early stages, the lesions are limited to the tips of the gingival papillae. Occasionally in longstanding disease, the necrotic ulcerative lesions may extend into the attached gingiva and alveolar mucosa. Patients with ANUG frequently have associated physiologic stress or psychologic stress, or both. Two stereotypical candidates for ANUG are military personnel under battle conditions (leading to an early name of the disease of "trench mouth") and college students studying for examination. Patients with ANUG often have a history of lack of sleep, poor eating patterns, and failure in plaque control.

The stress in ANUG patients leads to elevated serum cortisol levels.

Treatment is focused on reinstitution of proper plaque control procedures and debridement, usually with ultrasonic instrumentation, to remove the necrotic tissue and reduce the bacterial counts. If there is systemic involvement, such as fever, antibiotics may be prescribed. Several follow-up appointments are necessary for thorough scaling and root planing and to assess whether there are residual soft tissue craters that would necessitate periodontal surgery.

BACTERIAL FINDINGS

There is ample evidence to demonstrate that bacteria play an important role in the pathogenesis of ANUG. While rarely recommended for treatment, antibiotics such as penicillin lead to almost complete healing within a matter of days.

Early observations of smears from ANUG patients suggested that ANUG was caused by an intermediate-sized spirochete called *Borrelia vincentii* and fusiform bacilli. Ultrastructural classification of spirochetes by Listgarten (1965) indicated that this spirochete was found only superficially rather than within the lesion.

The principal bacteria now found to be associated with ANUG are *P. intermedia* and an unnamed intermediate-sized spirochete. *P. intermedia* constitutes a significant part of the microflora in ANUG, making up 8 to 15 percent of the total cell counts.

Ultrastructurally, the disease is characterized by four major zones extending from the surface to the depths of the lesions:

1. *Bacterial Zone*—This is the most superficial zone and contains small, intermediate-sized and large spirochetes, as well as other bacteria.

2. *Neutrophil-Rich Zone*—This zone contains numerous spirochetes and rod-shaped bacteria interspersed between neutrophils.

3. *Necrotic Zone*—In addition to necrotic tissue, there are numerous spirochetes and rod-shaped bacteria in this zone.

4. *Zone of Spirochetal Infiltration*—In this deepest area, intermediate-sized and large spirochetes are located between areas of normal collagen fibrils. The intermediate-sized spirochetes in this zone, however, are not *Borrelia vincentii*.

Although the roles of the microorganisms in the pathogenesis are not fully understood, both direct bacterial effects and indirect host responses may be important. Along with the direct invasion of the gingival tissues, the bacterial counts and associated endotoxin concentrations may be important. The host responses are considered subsequently.

IMMUNOLOGIC FINDINGS

In ANUG, both the cellular and humoral responses are affected. Sera collected from patients within a few days after onset of ANUG (acute phase) have elevated IgG and IgM antibody titers to intermediate-sized oral spirochetes and elevated IgG titers to *P. intermedia*. These elevated titers suggest that these organisms proliferated weeks to months before the development of the lesions and indicate that they are pathogenically significant agents. The significance of the elevated bacterial antibody titers in the pathogenesis of ANUG is unknown. The histopathology, the large numbers of bacteria within the tissues, and the elevated levels of antibodies suggest the possibility of an immune complex type of disease. However, further studies are necessary.

Cellularly, patients with ANUG have reduced PMN chemotaxis and phagocytosis. Although not proven, such dysfunction could play a role in the pathogenesis of ANUG. Whether the leukocyte dysfunction results from the bacterial infection in ANUG or develops first, thus allowing the "explosion" in the bacterial flora to occur, is unknown.

Desquamative Gingivitis

Desquamative gingivitis is a chronic gingival disease characterized by erythematous, erosive, vesiculobullous, and/or desquamative lesions of the free and attached gingivae. Instead of a single etiology, it is a clinical manifestation of several disease processes, as summarized in Table 28–16. Because of the multiple etiologies, desquamative gingivitis may be better called desquamative gingival lesions. The majority of cases or approximately 75 percent are dermatologic diseases. Among the total cases, approximately one half are cicatricial pemphigoid, one quarter are lichen planus, and less than 10 percent are pemphigus, chronic ulcerative stomatitis or psoriasis. The remainder have an unknown or nondermatologic etiology. Among the dermatologic diseases, pemphigus and pemphigoid are autoimmune diseases, psoriasis and chronic ulcerative stomatitis have characteristics of an autoimmune disease, and lichen planus with an unknown etiology has characteristic immunopathology (Table 28–17).

Clinically, most desquamative gingival lesions occur in middle-aged females. Half the time, lesions are localized solely to the gingivae and in the others, lesions concurrently involved other intraoral and extraoral sites including the buccal mucosa, palate, tongue, lips, skin, and the conjunctiva of the eye.

The diagnosis and treatment of desquamative gingivitis is dependent on identifying the under-

TABLE 28–16 ✦ Diseases Associated with Desquamative Gingivitis

I. Dermatoses (75.4%)
   Cicatricial pemphigoid
   Lichen planus
   Pemphigus
   Psoriasis
   Bullous pemphigoid
   Epidermolysis bullosa acquisita
   Contact stomatitis
II. Endocrine imbalance
   Estrogen deficiencies following oophorectomy
   and in postmenopausal women
   Testosterone imbalance
   Hypothyroidism
III. Aging
IV. Abnormal response to bacterial plaque
V. Idiopathic
VI. Chronic infections
   Tuberculosis
   Chronic candidiasis
   Histoplasmosis

lying etiology through (1) clinical observation, (2) histologic examination, and (3) immunologic examination (direct immunofluorescence tests on biopsies and sometimes indirect immunofluorescence tests on sera) (see Chapter 34). The rapid identification of patients with cicatricial pemphigoid and pemphigus is of the utmost importance, since cicatricial pemphigoid can cause blindness and pemphigus is a life-threatening disease.

The examination of sera from patients with desquamative gingivitis by indirect immunofluorescence usually yields negative results, except in pemphigus and in less than one third of the cases of cicatricial pemphigoid. Because of this, serum tests are not usually recommended.

TABLE 28–17 ✦ Immunopathology in Dermatoses Associated with Desquamative Gingivitis

DISEASE	IMMUNOPATHOLOGY
Cicatricial Pemphigoid	Basement membrane deposits of IgG and C3*
Lichen planus	Globular deposits of cytoid bodies and/or fibrin deposits along the basement membrane zone†
Pemphigus, all forms	Intercellular IgG in gingival epithelium*
Chronic ulcerative stomatitis	Stratified-epithelium specific antinuclear antibody*
Psoriasis	Stratum corneum deposits†

*Findings are diagnostic.
†Findings are suggestive but not diagnostic.

DESQUAMATIVE GINGIVITIS ASSOCIATED WITH CICATRICIAL PEMPHIGOID

Histologically, the presence of a subepithelial blister is indicative of the pemphigoid group of diseases.

Immunologically, immunofluorescence yields diagnostic findings in both gingival biopsy specimens and sera. In biopsy specimens, basement membrane zone deposits of IgG and C3 are most common. In approximately 10 percent of the cases, IgG antibodies to the basement membrane occur in the sera.

DESQUAMATIVE GINGIVITIS ASSOCIATED WITH PEMPHIGUS

While most pemphigus vulgaris cases first develop intraorally, the gingiva does not appear to be a major intraoral site.

Histologically, acantholysis of epithelial cells with the resultant intraepithelial blisters occur.

Immunologically, desquamative gingivitis associated with pemphigus is identical to pemphigus involving any part of the body. Biopsies have intercellular deposits of IgG in the gingival epithelium and sera contains IgG antibodies reactive with the intercellular substance of squamous epithelium in most if not all specimens.

DESQUAMATIVE GINGIVITIS ASSOCIATED WITH LICHEN PLANUS

Histologically, there is a band-like infiltrate below the epithelium, degeneration of the basal cells, and a "saw-tooth" interdigitation of the epithelium and lamina propria.

Immunologically, desquamative gingivitis associated with lichen planus reveals characteristic but not diagnostic findings including cytoid bodies in the epidermis and dermis and fibrin (fibrinogen) deposits along the basement membrane.

DESQUAMATIVE GINGIVITIS ASSOCIATED WITH PSORIASIS

A few rare cases of desquamative gingivitis are associated with psoriasis.

Histologically, there is epithelial hyperplasia with a thickened stratum corneum, parakeratosis, hyperplasia of the stratum malpighi, and epidermal microabscesses.

Immunologically, desquamative gingival biopsy specimens reveal antibodies and complement bound in vivo to the stratum corneum antigen.

Diagnostic Tests for Periodontal Disease

Numerous assays have been used in studies of periodontal disease (Table 28–18). Details on test

TABLE 28–18 ✦ Assays for Studying Periodontal Disease

Plaque Assays

Phase and dark field microscopy
Culture and isolation
Identification of bacterial enzymes and products in
  subgingival specimens
Immunofluorescence
Latex agglutination
Immunoperoxidase
ELISA
Immunoblotting

Indirect Assays on Sera

Immunofluorescence
ELISA

methodology are provided in Chapter 34. Several of these assays may also have applications as clinical tests. Based on current knowledge, assays on plaque appear to have more clinical relevance than immunologic tests on sera (with the exception of desquamative gingivitis). Commercial laboratories are already offering cultural and immunofluorescence tests. Second generation tests that can be performed in the clinical office with minimal training, are under consideration. These include a rapid test to identify specific bacteria, groups of bacteria, bacterial enzymes, and tissue enzymes. Adequate studies of their efficacy in determining diagnosis, prognosis, disease activity or treatment selection is incomplete. Their roles in clinical practice are still to be established. These and other tests will emerge to help dental personnel in the future.

BIBLIOGRAPHY

Altman, L. C., Page, R. C., Vandesteen, G. E., Dixon, L. I., and Bradford, C.: Abnormalities of leukocyte chemotaxis in patients with various forms of periodontitis. J. Periodont. Res. 20:553, 1985.

Asikainen, S.: Occurrence of *Actinobacillus actinomycetemcomitans* and spirochetes in relation to age in localized juvenile periodontitis. J. Periodontol. 57:537, 1986.

Bick, P. H., Carpenter, A. B., Holdeman, L. V., Miller, G. A., Ranney, R. R., Palcanis, K. G., and Tew, J. G.: Polyclonal B-cell activation induced by extracts of Gram-negative bacteria isolated from periodontally diseased sites. Infect. Immun. 34:43, 1981.

Bolton, R. W., Kluever, E. A., and Dyer, J. K.: In vitro immunosuppression mediated by an extracellular polysaccharide from *Capnocytophaga ochracea*. J. Periodont. Res. 20:251, 1985.

Chung, C. P., Nisengard, R. J., Slots, J., and Genco, R. J.: Bacterial IgG and IgM antibody titers in acute necrotizing ulcerative gingivitis. J. Periodontol. 54:557, 1983.

Cogen, R. B., Stevens, A. W. Jr., Cohen-Cole, S., Kirks, K., and Freeman, A.: Leukocyte function in the etiology of acute necrotizing ulcerative gingivitis. J. Periodontol. 54:402, 1983.

Christersson, L. A., Slots, J., Zambon, J. J., and Genco, R. J.: Transmission and colonization of *Actinobacillus actinomycetemcomitans* in localized juvenile periodontitis patients. J. Periodontol. 56:127, 1985.

Ebersole, J. L., Taubman, M. A., Smith, D. J., and Haffajee, A. D.: Effect of subgingival scaling on systemic antibody responses to oral microorganisms. Infect. Immunol. 48:534, 1985.

Frank, R. M. and Voegel, J. C.: Bacterial bone resorption in advanced cases of human periodontitis. J. Periodont. Res. 13:251, 1978.

Genco, R. J.: Host responses in periodontal diseases: Current concepts. J. Periodontol. 63:338, 1992.

Greiner, D.: Inactivation of human serum bactericidal activity by a trypsinlike protease isolated from *Porphyromonas gingivalis*. Infect. Immunol. 60:1854, 1992.

Holt, S. C.: Bacterial surface structures and their role in periodontal disease. In Genco, R. J., and Mergenhagen, S. E. (eds.): Host-Parasite Interactions in Periodontal Diseases. Washington, DC, American Society of Microbiology, 1982, p. 139.

Killan, M.: Degradation of immunoglobulins A1, A2, and G by suspected principal periodontal pathogens. Infect. Immunol. 34:757, 1981.

Kornman, K. S. and Loesche, W. J.: The subgingival microbial flora during pregnancy. J. Periodont. Res. 15:111, 1980.

Kornman, K. S.: Age, supragingival plaque, and steroid hormones as ecological determinants of the subgingival flora. In Genco, R. J., and Mergenhagen, S. E. (eds.): Host-Parasite Interactions in Periodontal Diseases. Washington, DC, American Society of Microbiology, 1982, p. 132.

Listgarten, M. A.: Electron microscopic observations on the bacterial flora of acute necrotizing ulcerative gingivitis. J. Periodontol. 36:328, 1965.

Loesche, W. J., Syed, S. A., Laughon, B. E., and Stoll, J.: The bacteriology of acute necrotizing ulcerative gingivitis. J. Periodontol. 53:223, 1982.

Loesche, W. J., Syed, S. A., Schmidt, E., and Morrison, E. C.: Bacterial profiles of subgingival plaques in periodontitis. J. Periodontol. 56:447, 1985.

Magnusson, I., Marks, R. G., Clark, W. B., Walker, C. B., Low, S. B., and McArthur, W. P.: Clinical, microbiological and immunological characteristics of subjects with "refractory" periodontal disease. J. Clin. Periodontol. 18:291, 1991.

Malberg, K., Molle, A., Streuer, D., and Gangler, P.: Determination of lymphocyte populations and subpopulations extracted from chronically inflamed human periodontal tissues. J. Clin. Periodontol. 19:155, 1992.

Mashimo, P. A., Yamamoto, Y., Slots, J., Park, B. H., and Genco, R. J.: The periodontal microflora of juvenile diabetics: Culture, immunofluorescence, and serum antibody studies. J. Periodontol. 54:420, 1983.

Newman, H. N. and Addison, I. E.: Gingival crevice neutrophil function in periodontosis. J. Periodontol. 53:578, 1982.

Newman, M. G., Socransky, S. S., Savitt, E. D., Propas, D. A., and Crawford, A.: Studies of the microbiology of periodontosis. J. Periodontol. 47:373, 1976.

Newman, M. G., Grinenco, V., Weiner, M., Angel, I., Karge, H., and Nisengard, R.: Predominant microbiota associated with periodontal health in the aged. J. Periodontol. 49:553, 1978.

Newman, M. G. and Sims, T. N.: The predominant cultivable microbiota of the periodontal abscess. J. Periodontol. 50:350, 1979.

Nisengard, R. J.: The role of immunology in periodontal disease. J. Periodontol. 48:505, 1977.

Nisengard, R. J. and Neiders, M.: Desquamative lesions of the gingiva. J. Periodontol. 52:500, 1981.

Nisengard, R. J. and Blann, D. B.: Detection of immune complexes in gingiva from periodontitis patients. J. Dent. Res. 64:361, 1985.

Novak, M. J. and Cohen, H. J.: Depolarization of polymorphonuclear leukocytes by *Porphyromonas (Bacteroides) gingivalis* in the absence of respiratory burst activation. Infect. Immunol. 59:3134, 1991.

Oshrain, H. I., Telsey, B., and Mandel, I. D.: A longitudinal study of periodontal disease in patients with reduced immunocapacity. J. Periodontol. 54:151, 1983.

Page, R.: The role of inflammatory mediators in the pathogenesis of periodontal disease. J. Periodont. Res. 26:230, 1991.

Page, R. C., Altman, L. C., Ebersole, J. L., Vandesteen, G. E., Dahlberg, W. H., Williams, B. L., and Osterberg, S. K.: Rapidly progressive periodontitis: A distinct clinical condition. J. Periodontol. 54:197, 1983.

Page, R. C., Bowen, T., Altman, L., Vendesteen, E., Ochs, H., Mackenzie, P., Osterberg, L., Engel, D., and Williams, B. L.: Prepubertal periodontitis. I. Definition of a clinical disease entity. J. Periodontol. 54:257, 1983.

Preus, H. R.: Possible exogenous source of Aa in rapid destructive periodontitis in man (abstr). J. Dent. Res. 66:709, 1987.

Saglie, R., Newman, M. G., Carranza, F. A., Jr., and Pattison, G. L.: Bacterial invasion of gingiva in advanced periodontitis in humans. J. Periodontol. 53:217, 1982.

Seymour, G. J., Cole, K. L., Powell, R. N., Lewins, E., Cripps, A. W., and Clancy, R. L.: Interleukin-2 production and bone-resorption activity *in vitro* by unstimulated lymphocytes extracted from chronically-inflamed human periodontal tissues. Arch. Oral Biol. 30:481, 1985.

Schenkein, H. A.: Complement factor D-like activity of *Porphyromonas gingivalis* W83. Oral Microbiol. Immunol. 6:216, 1991.

Schenkein, H. A.: The complement system in periodontal disease. In Genco, R. J., and Mergenhagen, S. E. (eds.): Host-Parasite Interactions in Periodontal Diseases. Washington, DC, American Society of Microbiology, 1982, p. 299.

Shenker, B. J. and DiRienzo, J. M.: Suppression of human peripheral blood lymphocytes by *Fusobacterium nucleatum*. J. Immunology 132:2357, 1984.

Slots, J.: Importance of black-pigmented *Bacteroides* in human periodontal disease. In Genco, R. J., and Mergenhagen, S. E. (eds.): Host-Parasite Interactions in Periodontal Diseases. Washington, DC, American Society of Microbiology, 1982, p. 27.

Slots, J. and Rosling, B. G.: Suppression of the periodontopathic microflora in localized juvenile periodontitis by systemic tetracycline. J. Clin. Periodontol. 10:465, 1983.

Slots, J. and Genco, R. J.: Black-pigmented *Bacteroides* species, *Capnocytophaga* species, and *Actinobacillus actinomycetemcomitans* in human periodontal disease: Virulence factors in colonization, survival, and tissue destruction. J. Dent. Res. 63:412, 1984.

Slots, J., Bragd, L., Wikstrom, M., and Dahlen, G.: The occurrence of *Actinobacillus actinomycetemcomitans, Bacteroides gingivalis* and *Bacteroides intermedius* in destructive periodontal disease in adults. J. Clin. Periodontol. 13:570, 1986.

Socransky, S. S. and Haffajee, A. D.: Microbial mechanisms in the pathogenesis of destructive periodontal diseases: A critical assessment. J. Periodont. Res. 26:195, 1991.

Socransky, S. S. and Haffajee, A. D.: The bacterial etiology of destructive periodontal disease: Current concepts. J. Periodontol. 63:322, 1992.

Sundqvist, G., Carlsson, J., Herrmann, B., and Tarnvik, A.: Degradation of human immunoglobulins G and M and complement factors C3 and C5 by black-pigmented *Bacteroides*. J. Med. Microbiol. 19:85, 1985.

Suzuki, J. B., Collison, B. C., Falker, W. A., Jr., and Nauman, R. K.: Immunologic profile of juvenile periodontitis. II. Neutrophil chemotaxis, phagocytosis and spore germination. J. Periodontol. 55:461, 1984.

Taubman, M. A., Ebersole, J. L., Smith, D. J.: Association between systemic and local antibody and periodontal disease. In Genco, R. J., and Mergenhagen, S. E. (eds.): Host-Parasite Interactions in Periodontal Diseases. Washington, DC, American Society of Microbiology, 1982, p. 283.

Taubman, M. A., Yoshie, H., Ebersole, J. L., Smith, D. J., and Olson, C. L.: Host response in experimental periodontal disease. J. Dent. Res. 63:455, 1984.

Tew, J. G., Marshall, D. R., Moore, W. E. C., Best, A. M., Palcanis, K. G., and Ranney, R. R.: Serum antibody reactive with predominant organisms in the subgingival flora of young adults with generalized severe periodontitis. Infect. Immunol. 48:303, 1985.

Van Dyke, T. E., Horoszewicz, H. U., Cianciola, L. J., and Genco, R. J.: Neutrophil chemotaxis dysfunction in human periodontitis. Infect. Immun. 27:124, 1980.

Van Dyke, T. E., Schweinebraten, M., Cianciola, L. J., Offenbacher, S., and Genco, R. J.: Neutrophil chemotaxis in families with localized juvenile periodontitis. J. Periodont. Res. 20:503, 1985.

Vandesteen, G. E., Williams, B. L., Ebersole, J. L., Altman, L. C., and Page, R. C.: Clinical, microbiological and immunological studies of a family with a high prevalence of early-onset periodontitis. J. Periodontol. 55:159, 1984.

Whal, S. M.: Mononuclear cell-mediated alterations in connective tissue. In Genco, R. J., and Mergenhagen, S. E. (eds.): Host-Parasite Interaction in Periodontal

Disease. Washington, DC, American Society of Microbiology, 1982, p. 132.

Whitney, C., Ant, J., Moncla, B., Johnson, B., Page, R., and Engel, D.: Serum immunoglobulin G antibody to *Porphyromonas gingivalis* in rapidly progressive periodontitis: Titer, avidity, and subclass distribution. Infect. Immunol. 60:2194, 1992.

Wilson, M. E. and Hamilton, R. G.: Immunoglobulin G subclass response of localized juvenile periodontitis patients to *Actinobacillus actinomycetemcomitans* Y4 lipopolysaccharide. Infect. Immunol. 60:1806, 1992.

Wilson, M. E., Zambon, J. J., Suzuki, J. B., and Genco, R. J.: Generalized juvenile periodontitis, defective neutrophil chemotaxis and *Bacteroides gingivalis* in a 13-year old female. J. Periodontol. 56:457, 1985.

Zambon, J. J., Christersson, L. A., and Slots, J.: *Actinobacillus actinomycetemcomitans* in human periodontal disease—Prevalence in patient groups and distribution of biotypes and serotypes within families. J. Periodontol. 54:707, 1983.

29 Control and Prevention of Periodontal Disease

Sebastian G. Ciancio and Russell J. Nisengard

CHAPTER OUTLINE

Plaque control
Chemotherapeutic agents for treatment of periodontal disease
Agents for control of calculus

With the significant reduction in dental caries during the past decade, attention has turned to new methods of control, prevention, and treatment of periodontal disease. This chapter will focus on chemotherapeutic and immunologic approaches to periodontal therapy. (See Chapter 28 for further details.)

PLAQUE CONTROL

The role of plaque in the etiology of gingivitis and periodontitis has been known for several decades. While the exact organisms causing periodontal diseases and their mechanisms of action have not been conclusively identified, plaque control aids in the prevention and treatment of these diseases. This has been the backbone of preventive dentistry whereby plaque is removed by mechanical means—brushing and flossing by patients, scaling and root planing by dental professionals.

Because of the relatively high incidence of periodontal disease indicating a failure in prevention by traditional (demonstrably successful but difficult to motivate) mechanical means, other methods of plaque control are being explored. The major thrust so far has been toward finding a chemical agent that would control plaque. This could be incorporated in a mouthwash, toothpaste, pill, or other delivery system. The chemotherapeutic agents would be (1) nonspecific, affecting all plaque bacteria uniformly and leading to a quantitative reduction in plaque, or (2) specific, acting as a "silver bullet" to qualitatively reduce only the periodontopathic plaque bacteria. The simpler approach of reducing all plaque is closer to reality. Chemical agents could reduce plaque by (1) affecting initial colonization, (2) inhibiting plaque development and metabolism, or (3) reducing existing plaque.

The Council on Dental Therapeutics of the American Dental Association (ADA) has established guidelines for accepting an agent for control of plaque and gingivitis. To receive the seal of approval of the ADA, an agent must not only reduce plaque, particularly supragingival plaque, it must also reduce gingival inflammation when used in conjunction with routine home care procedures such as brushing and flossing. It is quite possible that some agents that reduce plaque quantitatively would not significantly reduce the periodontopathic bacteria and therefore have little, if any, effect on gingival inflammation. Agents should be evaluated not only in terms of efficacy, but also on the basis of specificity, substantivity (i.e., adherence to teeth or gingival tissue), penetrability (i.e., ability to penetrate into plaque), selectivity (i.e., effectiveness on specific bacteria), safety, and stability. Two brand name mouth rinses are currently approved by the ADA for control of plaque and gingivitis: Peridex and Listerine, chlorhexidine and phenolic solutions, respectively as well as generic copies of Listerine made by two manufacturers, Perigo Labs and Vijohn Labs. The characteristics of an ideal agent are listed in Table 29–1.

Delivery Systems

Topical, local delivery of chemotherapeutic agents for control of periodontal disease is considered most desirable, since the incidence of side effects is far less than by the systemic route. Mouthwashes offer advantages in ease of use; however, they mainly affect supragingival plaque with

TABLE 29–1 ✦ Ideal Chemotherapeutic Agent

Clinically effective in plaque control
Clinically effective in control of inflammation
Maximum effect on pathogens
Highly substantive to minimize dosage
Minimal adverse effects
No bacterial resistance
Stable for prolonged time periods

little subgingival activity. This may limit their efficacy to treatment of gingivitis with minimal value for periodontitis. Delivery directly into the gingival crevice using various types of devices has been evaluated. Additionally, antibiotics have been placed into fibers that are positioned subgingivally, leading to some improvement in periodontal health; antimicrobials also have been placed on acrylic strips inserted subgingivally; and the subgingival area has been irrigated with chemotherapeutic agents. These systems offer promise for future therapy.

Korman divided chemotherapeutic agents into first-generation and second-generation agents, based on their efficiency in plaque control and substantivity. These are nonspecific, affecting all plaque similarly, or have minimal specificity, such as antibiotics. A third-generation agent may be developed with high specificity for periodontal pathogens. Some topical agents currently of interest are listed in Table 29–2.

First-Generation Agents

These agents demonstrate limited substantivity and are therefore not retained intraorally for any significant time after use. This group includes topical antibiotics, quaternary ammonium compounds, phenolic compounds, and sanguinarine.

Second-Generation Agents

These agents demonstrate significant substantivity and are retained and released for a prolonged time. Chlorhexidine and its analogues, and possibly stannous fluoride, are included in this group. Tetracycline, an antibiotic with substantivity, also may be in this group.

Third-Generation Agents

These agents have yet to be developed and will be effective against only one or a few periodontopathogens. Considerable research into the pathogenesis of periodontal diseases and nature of antibacterial agents would be necessary before third-generation agents could be given serious consideration.

Antibiotics

Some systemic and topical antibiotics inhibit plaque and plaque-induced disease for short time periods. In limited situations, their use has been advocated for treatment of some types of periodontal diseases (see Chapter 28). However, the potential for hypersensitivity reactions and microbial antibiotic resistance limits their long-term use for plaque control. Even more important, since antibiotics are essential for treatment of serious infections, their use may best be reserved for treatment of systemic infection rather than plaque control.

A number of systemically administered antibiotics have been evaluated for periodontal therapy, such as tetracyclines, clindamycin, and metronidazole (see Chapter 33). These drugs offer some promise as adjuncts to periodontal therapy but, as with any antibiotic, it is necessary to monitor various body functions for adverse effects. For instance, tetracyclines have reportedly caused kidney and liver disorders; clindamycin can cause serious gastrointestinal disorders including colitis; and metronidazole initiates tumors in rats and causes bacterial mutagenicity. The risk-benefit ratios of these and other antibiotics must be evaluated before use in periodontal therapy.

As more antibiotics are employed, the development of resistance is an increased probability. With the tetracyclines, the development of multidrug–resistant bacteria (termed plasmid factor resistance) has been documented with *Escherichia coli*. In view of this, microbiologic monitoring of bacterial resistance may be part of future therapy.

Local Delivery of Antibiotics

The most researched product is a tetracycline-loaded, 0.5 mm-diameter ethyl vinyl acetate fiber (Actisite), which is well tolerated by oral tissues. When packed subgingivally into a periodontal

TABLE 29–2 ✦ Chemotherapeutic Agents for Control of Plaque*

First-Generation
    Antibiotics
    Cetylpyridinium chloride
    Essential oils
    Fluorides
    Salicylanilides
    Sanguinarine
    Zinc compounds
Second-Generation
    Alexidine
    Chlorhexidine
    Antibiotics (tetracyclines)

*Agents are listed in alphabetical order. (See text for efficacy.)

pocket, antibiotic concentrations in excess of 1300 μg/ml are sustained for at least ten days in gingival crevicular fluid that is well beyond levels required to inhibit the growth of periodontal pathogens and more than five times greater than that obtained following systemic tetracycline administration. Therefore, local delivery can achieve a bacteriostatic affect at approximately 1/1000 of the dose administered systemically.

Tetracycline containing fibers with or without scaling and root planing reduced pocket depth, increased attachment level, reduced bleeding on probing and reduced periodontal pathogens significantly better than scaling and root planing alone or placebo fibers. This product may represent the first locally delivered antibiotic system approved by the FDA.

Chlorhexidine

Chlorhexidine, a bisbiquanide, in a concentration of 0.2 percent has been available in Europe for over 20 years in toothpastes and mouthwashes. Its efficacy has been clearly demonstrated in short- and long-term trials. In a long-term study, plaque and gingivitis scores were reduced by approximately 50 percent for 2 years. It may be of value as an agent for selected populations requiring short-term plaque control. Tooth staining, mucosal irritation (especially in children), and a bitter taste are common side effects. The brownish stain can be removed by a routine dental prophylaxis.

Chlorhexidine is available as a mouthwash (Peridex) at a concentration of 0.12 percent in the United States. This lower concentration minimizes the side effects without altering its effectiveness on plaque and gingivitis. Peridex is marketed by Proctor and Gamble as a prescription drug. It has Food and Drug Administration (FDA) and ADA approval for treatment of gingivitis. Six-month studies have shown clinically significant reductions in plaque and gingivitis with the use of this agent. In addition, chlorhexidine is also effective in treatment of oral candidiasis.

Alexidine, another drug with a similar chemical structure, has shown promise in short-term studies but has not been adequately investigated. As with chlorhexidine, tooth staining and taste alteration can occur.

Dentifrices

Most dentifrices claim to be of value in plaque reduction. These claims are based not on chemotherapeutic agents but on the observation, from clinical studies, that brushing with a dentifrice is more effective in plaque removal than brushing without a dentifrice.

The incorporation of effective chemotherapeutic agents into dentifrices must overcome the problems of bioavailability of the agent and compatibility with other dentifrice ingredients.

Enzymes

At present, enzymes directed against pellicle, plaque, or its components have not been effective.

Fluoride

The efficacy of fluorides in control of caries is without question. While the relative effectiveness for caries prevention of stannous fluoride versus sodium fluoride is not clear, short-term data suggest a distinct advantage of stannous fluoride. Fluorides also have been recently investigated in short-term studies for efficacy as antiplaque and antigingivitis agents. Stannous fluoride, which has some substantivity, may be of value at 0.4 to 1.64 percent for control of plaque. Tooth staining and an unpleasant taste have been reported as frequent side effects of some fluoride preparations. Long-term studies have not shown consistent benefits for reduction of plaque and gingivitis.

Essential Oils

Listerine and Cool Mint Listerine, mouthwashes that contain a mixture of phenolic compounds and methylsalicylate, has moderate antiplaque activity with no reported side effects other than a temporary burning sensation. They are accepted by the ADA as are two generic copies marketed under a variety of proprietary names. Two long-term 6-month trials in conjunction with routine oral hygiene have shown plaque reduction. In another study of 9 months' duration, lower gingivitis scores were seen after 9 months but not after 6 months. The average plaque reduction has been 25 percent and gingivitis reduction has been 30 percent. The effect of phenols on gingival inflammation must be further evaluated. This product has also been shown to control candidiasis in the oral cavity.

Quaternary Ammonium Compounds

Quaternary ammonium compounds such as cetylpyridinium chloride mouthwashes exhibit moderate antiplaque activity, reducing plaque by an average of about 25 percent. They rapidly absorb to the tooth surface in high concentrations but have limited substantivity and are quickly released. Some side effects include burning tongue, mucosal irritations, and minor reversible tooth staining. Cepacol (Merrill-Dow), Scope (Proctor and Gamble), and a number of proprietary products contain these agents.

Oxygenating Agents

Oxygenating agents that raise the oxygen tension of the gingival sulcus were proposed to reduce the anaerobic periodontopathogens. Short-term studies have been contradictory, and long-term studies have not been performed. Serious questions of safety also have been raised with concentration of hydrogen peroxide of 3 percent or greater in view of reports of burns and tissue irritation with chronic use and co-carcinogenic effects in animals.

Sanguinarine

Sanguinarine, a benzophenanthradine alkaloid, has been evaluated in several short-term studies, generally of 6 weeks or less. The agent appears to reduce plaque and gingival inflammation from 20 to 60 percent in short-term studies, but its long-term effectiveness on plaque and disease reduction is unclear. In one study evaluating sanguinarine's effects on the development of experimental gingivitis, no differences from the placebo were observed. More recent studies in which both the dentifrice and mouthrinse have been used as combined therapy suggested beneficial effects on plaque and gingivitis. Viadent mouthwash, commercially available from Vipont Laboratories, contains 0.03 percent of sanguinarine extract (0.01 percent pure sanguinarine). It also is manufactured as a dentifrice.

TRICLOSAN

Triclosan, a 2,4,4'-trichloro-2'-hydroxydiphenyl ether, is approximately 65 percent as effective as chlorhexidine. By itself, triclosan does not have good substantivity, but when in special formulations, it is non-ionic and compatible with dentifrice ingredients. It is marketed in Europe by Colgate, Proctor & Gamble, and Unilever under the respective trade names Colgate Gum Protection Formula, Crest Gum Health, and Mentadent P. Clinical studies of six months or longer have shown reductions in plaque ranging between 0 and 30 percent and reductions in gingivitis ranging between 20 and 75 percent.

SODIUM BENZOATE

This chemical, found in Plax, has surface-active properties and may aid plaque removal by mechanical methods. However, most published studies have suggested minimal benefit over placebo.

COMPARATIVE DATA

Comparisons among antiplaque agents are sometimes difficult to make, as their actions are usually compared with placebos rather than with other antiplaque agents. Some comparisons have been made and more will certainly follow. Table 29–3 compares the effectiveness of several agents on plaque formation and development of gingivitis, in studies of 6 months' duration or longer. Chlorhexidine was significantly more effective than phenolic compounds, quaternary ammonium compounds, and sanguinarine, earning its reputation as a second-generation agent. Another concern with mouthwashes is their alcoholic content. Table 29–4 summarizes the alcoholic concentrations, which range approximately 11 to 27 percent and their pH's.

Since chemotherapeutic agents have resulted in significant plaque reduction, they definitely have a role in periodontal therapy. At this time they can be recommended as adjuncts to oral hygiene in patients experiencing difficulty in mechanical plaque control, those with extensive splinting of teeth, and those with refractory cases or who are considered unsuitable for periodontal surgery.

Immunologic Control of Plaque

Numerous animal studies have demonstrated the effectiveness of immunization as a means of controlling *S. mutans* caries (see Chapter 27). Secretory IgA is stimulated by local sensitization in the salivary glands or intestinal tract with *S. mutans* antigens. Currently, there are several human clinical trials of this novel approach to prevention. Secretory IgA occurs only in saliva and not in crevicular fluid. Thus, if immunization were considered for blocking the colonization of periodontopathogens in plaque, two routes of immunization may be required: salivary stimulation for supragingival plaque and systemic stimulation for subgingival plaque.

CHEMOTHERAPEUTIC AGENTS FOR TREATMENT OF PERIODONTAL DISEASE
Antibiotics

Antibiotics have demonstrable efficacy for the treatment of some forms of periodontal disease. For example, tetracyclines are now part of the routine therapy for patients with localized juvenile periodontitis (see Chapter 33) presumably because of their effects on *A. actinomycetemcomitans*.

Golub and coworkers have demonstrated another potentially important role for tetracycline in addition to its antibacterial activity. Tetracyclines inhibit tissue collagenase and therefore retard the breakdown of collagen that normally occurs in periodontal disease. This decreased collagen breakdown may reduce the chemotactic effect of collagen fragments; this reduces polymorphonuclear leukocytes and inflammation in gingival crevicular

TABLE 29–3 ✦ **Comparison of Chemotherapeutic Agents in Studies 6 Months or Longer**

	FREQUENCY OF USE	NUMBER OF SUBJECTS	PLAQUE REDUCTION	GINGIVITIS REDUCTION
Cetylpyridinium chloride	Twice daily	99	14%	24%
Chlorhexidine 0.2%	Twice daily	150	50%	50%
0.12%	Twice daily	430	61%	45%
0.1%	Once daily	158	60%	67%
Essential oils	Twice daily	145	20%	28%
	Twice daily	109	34%	34%
	Twice daily	85	20%	24%
	Twice daily	104	25%	28%
Sanguinarine	Twice daily	100	0%	0%*
	Twice daily	115	0%	0%
	Twice daily†	204	35%	35%
Stannous fluoride	Twice daily	268	0%	0%
	Twice daily‡	145	40%	50%
Triclosan	Twice daily§	583	30%	35%

*In this dentifrice study, the gingival index scores increased by 71% in the placebo group and 49% in the sanguinarine group.
†Use of dentifrice and mouthrinse in three studies.
‡Data from two studies: one in orthodontic patients and one on abutment teeth.
§Data from five studies.

fluid. Agents such as these may become a part of therapy in the "defense of collagen."

Anti-Inflammatory Agents

Animal and human studies have demonstrated that flurbiprofen, a nonsteroidal anti-inflammatory drug, may arrest bone loss and aid in bone regeneration. Since this substance is a prostaglandin inhibitor, further studies may prove it to be useful in therapy. In contrast, nonsteroidal anti-inflammatory drugs appear to have no significant effect on gingival inflammation. One possible conclusion is that these agents may be effective in diseases of oral hard tissues but not oral soft tissues.

Reattachment Agents

Coronal reattachment of connective tissue and epithelium in patients with periodontitis would be

TABLE 29–4 ✦ **Alcohol and pH of Mouthwashes**

	ALCOHOL	pH
Cepacol	14.0%	6.0
Listerine	26.9%	4.2
Cool Mint Listerine	22%	4.2
Peridex	11.6%	5.6
Scope	18.5%	5.5
Viadent	11.5%	4.5

beneficial. Citric acid, fibronectin, and tetracycline have been evaluated as topical agents to be applied to root surfaces during periodontal surgery as aids in soft tissue reattachment. Tetracyclines have the added benefit of being substantive and maintaining their bacteriocidal activity for some time after topical application.

Results of studies of various root surface modifiers to date have been mixed, with some demonstrating reattachment and others showing no differences from untreated controls. Some studies have even reported irreversible resorption and ankylosis of the root. Longer time periods are needed to answer the question of their therapeutic value.

AGENTS FOR CONTROL OF CALCULUS

The incidence of calculus formation ranges from 45 to 66 percent, depending to some degree on sex and age. Some patients are "calculus formers" and appear to form heavy calculus in spite of reasonable plaque control. Recently, dentifrices and mouth rinses have been introduced that reduce calculus *formation* to a limited extent (approximately 30 to 40 percent). They are not effective against calculus already present nor do they affect gingival inflammation, as do antiplaque agents.

Crest Tartar Control, Colgate Tartar Control, and Prevent toothpastes are advertised as reducing the formation of dental calculus. The active ingredients in Crest are 3.4 percent tetrasodium pyrophosphate and 1.37 percent disodium, dihydrogen pyrophosphate. Colgate's active agent is 5 percent tetrasodium pyrophosphate. Similar ingredients are found in Crest and Colgate Tartar Control mouth rinses. Prevent contains 2 percent zinc chloride as its tartar-reducing ingredient. These chemicals block receptor sites on enamel for calcium phosphate (found in food and saliva), and inhibit crystal growth of calculus. All of these dentifrices contain sodium fluoride and are formulated so that the fluoride is available.

The practitioner must decide if calculus formation is an esthetic problem for the patient, or if it interferes with good oral hygiene, or both. For selected patients, especially those with intracoronal splints or extensive fixed bridgework, a reduction of calculus by 30 to 40 percent might be of value.

BIBLIOGRAPHY

Accepted Dental Therapeutics, ed. 39. American Dental Association, 1982.

Addy, M., Rawle, L., Handley, R., Newman, H. N., and Coventry, J. F.: Development and in vitro evaluation of acrylic strips and dialysis tubing for local drug delivery. J. Periondontol. 53:693, 1985.

Braatz, L., Garrett, S., Claffey, N., and Egelberg, J.: Antimicrobial irrigation of deep pockets to supplement non-surgical periodontal therapy. II. Daily irrigation. J. Clin. Periodontol. 12:630, 1985.

Caffesse, R., Holden, M., Kon, S., and Nasjleti, C.: Citric acid/fibronectin in treating periodonitis in beagle dogs. IADR Progr. Abstr. J. Dent. Res. 63:221, 1984.

Ciancio S. G., Mather, M. L., and Bunnell, H. L.: Clinical evaluation of a quaternary ammonium-containing mouthrinse. J. Periodontol. 46:397, 1975.

Ciancio, S. G., Slots, J., Reynolds, H. S., et al.: The effect of short-term administration of minocycline HCl on gingival inflammation and subgingival microflora. J. Peridontol. 53:557, 1982.

Ciancio, S. C.: Chemotherapeutic agents and periodontol therapy—Their impact on clinical practice. J. Periodontol. 57:108, 1986.

Crigger, M., Renvert, S., and Bogle, G.: The effect of topical citric acid application on surgically exposed periodontal attachment. J. Periodontol Res. 18:303, 1983.

Dunn, R. K., Perkins, B. H., and Goodson, J. M.: Controlled release of tetracycline from biodegradable fibers. IADR Progr. Abstr. J. Dent. Res. 62:289, 1983.

Flota, L., Gjermo, G., Rolla, G., and Waerhaug, J.: Side effects of chlorhexidine mouth washes. Scand. J. Dent. Res. 79:119, 1971.

Golub, L. M., Ramamurthy, N., McNamara, T., et al.: Tetracyclines inhibit tissue collagenase activity: A new mechanism in the treatment of periodontal disease. J. Periodontal Res. 19:651, 1984.

Gordon, J., Walker, C., Lamster, I., et al.: Evaluation of clindamycin in refractory periodontitis. IADR Progr. Abstr. J. Dent. Res. 63:268, 1984.

Gordon, J. M., Lamster, I. B., and Seiger, M. C.: Efficiency of Listerine antiseptic in inhibiting the development of plaque and gingivitis. J. Clin. Periodontol. 12:697, 1985.

Kornman, K. S.: The role of supragingival plaque in the prevention and treatment of periodontal diseases: A review of current concepts. J. Periodontal Res. 21(Suppl):5, 1986.

Lang, N. P. and Brecx, M. C.: Chlorhexidine digluconate—An agent for chemical plaque control and prevention of gingival inflammation. J. Periodontal Res. (Suppl.):74, 1986.

Linde, J., Heijl, L., Goodson, J. M., and Socransky, S. S.: Local tetracycline delivery using hollow fiber devices in periodontal therapy. J. Clin. Periodontol. 6:141, 1979.

Mazza, J. E., Newman, M. G., Perry, D. A., and Carranza, F. A. Jr.: The effect of daily self-applied SnF_2 on clinical parameters of periodontitis. IADR Progr. Abstr. J. Dent. Res. 63:268, 1984.

Menaker, L., Weatherford, T. W., III, Pitts, G., et al.: The effects of Listerine antiseptic on dental plaque. Ala. J. Med. Sci. 16:71, 1979.

Nygaard, P., and Persson, I.: Evaluation of sanguinarine chloride in control of plaque in the dental practice. Comp. Cont. Educ. Dent. (Suppl)5:s90, 1984.

Valtonen, M. Y., Valtonen, Y. Y., Salo, O. P., et al.: The effect of long-term tetracycline treatment for acne vulgaris on the occurrence of R factors in the intestinal flora of man. J. Dermatol. 95:311, 1976.

Vogel, R. I., Cooper, S. A., Schneiders, L. G., and Goteiner, D.: The effects of topical steroidal and systemic nonsteroidal anti-inflammatory drugs on experimental gingivitis in man. J. Periodontol. 55:247, 1984.

Wikesjo, U. M. E., Baker, P. J., Christersson, L. A., et al.: A biochemical approach to periodontal regeneration: Tetracycline treatment conditions dentin surfaces. J. Periodontal Res. 21:322, 1986.

Zacheryl, W. A., Pfeiffer, H. J., and Swancar, J. R.: The effects of soluble pyrophosphates on dental calculus in adults. J.A.D.A. 110:737, 1985.

30

Periapical Infections

Russell J. Nisengard, Anthony D. Goodman,* and
Benjamin Schein

CHAPTER OUTLINE

Diagnosis
Microbiology
Immunology
Treatment
Summary

The dental pulp is a loose connective tissue composed of collagen fibers, amorphous ground substance, intercellular fluid, arterioles, venules, lymphatics, and a nerve supply. Once the tooth is fully developed, the pulpal communication with the periapical tissues maintains normal physiologic health, which is particularly dependent on the pulpal blood supply and a normal tissue osmotic and hydrostatic pressure.

The dental pulp is surrounded by unyielding, calcified dentinal walls of the tooth, which physically restricts the tissue. Even minimal inflammation with edema and cellular infiltrates causes pressure which cannot be easily alleviated. In some cases, pain and pulpal necrosis may ensue.

Periapical infections of endodontic origin are subdivided into acute and chronic disease. A common acute form is acute apical periodontitis also known as acute alveolar abscess. The chronic forms include periapical granulomas and periapical cysts, which are not distinct entities, but a continuum of pathologic processes.

Periapical infections result from pulpal trauma by bacteria, temperature extremes, and physical forces. *The most common cause is bacterial contamination of the pulp from carious lesions that extend through the enamel and dentin.* Bacteria and their products also may penetrate the pulp via accessory foramina, which communicate with periodontal pockets. Restorative dental procedures also

can traumatize the dental pump by temperature generated during tooth preparation, impression-taking, and chemicals in some restorative materials. Physical trauma such as a sudden blow to the face can compromise the pulpal blood supply leading to pulpal death and subsequent bacterial colonization of the root canal. This phenomenon, termed *anachoresis*, is the attraction of bacteria via the bloodstream into inflamed and/or necrotic tissue.

The host response begins when bacteria invade the dentin and becomes more acute and intense after cariogenic bacteria invade the pulp. Because the pulp is enclosed by unyielding dentin, continued presence of bacteria and their antigens rapidly leads to pulpal necrosis.

While the inflammatory response is often protective, it also may cause unwanted, deleterious effects. Accompanying the inflammatory infiltrate is complement and immunoglobulins. These lesions are also surrounded by type II collagen, as the body attempts to wall off the area. The specific means by which bacteria cause pulpal inflammation, degeneration, and destruction is not completely understood but involves host-bacterial interactions. Once degeneration occurs, large numbers of viable and nonviable bacteria accumulate in the root canal system leading to high concentrations of toxins and enzymes. Periapical disease is an infectious process with direct and indirect microbial damage to tissue cells and blood vessels, leading to release of inflammatory substances.

*Deceased.

391

If the bacterial irritant is removed early (e.g., excavation of caries and restoration with a filling), pulpal tissue may return to normal. However, if the caries is untreated, the inflammatory response may reach a critical, irreversible, self-sustaining stage with necrosis extending in an apical direction.

DIAGNOSIS

Periapical infections are diagnosed by clinical symptoms, radiographic findings, and "pulp testing." Radiographs of chronic cases usually show apical or lateral bone loss, while those of acute cases often show little or no abnormality.

Pulp testing performed by applying an electrical stimulus, heat, or cold to the crown of a tooth is a clinical method for determining pulp vitality. Pulp testing elicits a sensation with vital pulp and no response in nonvital pulp. Teeth with acute, painful symptoms commonly respond to lower levels of stimuli or are hyper-responsive to pulp testing.

Restorative procedures on asymptomatic teeth with either chronic periapical lesions or necrotic pulps may cause pain during, or immediately following treatment from acute pulpal inflammation and edema. In some cases, restorative procedures on vital teeth can also evoke pulpal inflammation with acute, painful symptoms. In such situations, the pulp either heals or becomes necrotic within a period of a few months, leading to cessation of symptoms.

Microbiology

Bacteria and their products are the main causative factors in pulp disease. Kakehashi and co-workers (1965), in a classic study with gnotobiotic animals, conclusively demonstrated the role of bacteria in pulpal disease. Exposure of the pulp to the oral environment in germ-free animals elicited minimal inflammation. Pulpal necrosis and abscesses occurred only after exposure to bacteria.

Periapical infections have been examined microbiologically for (1) identification of microorganisms as etiologic agents for root canal infections, and (2) sterility testing of the root canal system as an end point for therapy prior to obturation (filling the root canal space).

Early studies of root canal infections enumerated only the aerobic and facultative anaerobic bacteria. In the 1970s, the advent of strict anaerobic culturing techniques led to the isolation of a significantly greater percentage of the flora in necrotic canals. Prior to this, many dental abscesses were reported as sterile when they probably contained obligate, anaerobic bacteria.

Microorganisms Associated With Root Canal Infections

Root canal infections are mixed bacterial infections with organisms from salivary contamination, carious lesions, and gingival crevices/pockets. These infections are predominantly by anaerobic bacteria, with gram-negative anaerobic bacilli being the most common. Facultative anaerobes and to a lesser extent, aerobic bacteria also are isolated. The selective colonization of pulpal tissues by anaerobic bacteria has been demonstrated experimentally by exposing pulpal tissue to salivary contamination. Although a spectrum of bacteria initially had access, eventually obligate anaerobes dominate. Table 30–1 summarizes six reports on the incidence of anaerobes. Anaerobic bacteria were isolated from approximately 97 percent of the cases and were exclusively isolated in 40 percent of the cases. Among the anaerobic bacteria, *Prevotella* and *Porphyromonas* species occur in 4 to 67 percent of necrotic canals (Table 30–2) and 14 to 90 percent of periapical abscesses (Table 30–3). The development of apical purulent inflammation appears to be induced by a mixed flora that includes *Porphyromonas endodontalis, P. gingivalis,* or *Prevotella intermedia.* The apical portion of root canals from teeth with necrotic pulp and periapical lesions regularly contain bacteria, mainly anaerobes (68 percent). These include species of *Actinomyces, Lactobacillus, Porphyromonas, Prevotella, Peptostreptococcus, Veillonella parvula, Enterococcus faecalis, Fusobacterium nucleatum,* and *S. mutans.*

Black-pigmenting bacterial species, particularly *Porphyromonas endodontalis,* have been singled out as potentially important pathogens in periapical infections. The black-pigmenting bacteria possess potent lipopolysaccharides or endotoxins; a bacterial capsule that can inhibit their phagocytosis; enzymes such as collagenase, hyaluronidase, and fibrinolysin, which can affect the connective tissue stroma; and antigens capable of inducing cellular and humoral immune responses.

In acute endodontic lesions, large numbers of obligate anaerobic bacteria are present. These include *Prevotella, Porphyromonas, Veillonella parvula, Actinomyces,* and *Peptostreptococcus. Porphyromonas endodontalis* and *P. gingivalis* commonly are isolated from teeth with acute symptoms of pain, swelling, open sinus tract, and tenderness to percussion. This association suggests an important role for these bacteria in the pathogenesis of acute infections. In contrast, *P. denticola* is mainly isolated from asymptomatic infections. In some acute periapical abscesses in children, *P. melaninogenicus* and *P. oralis* that produce beta-lactamase were found which could be resistant to pen-

TABLE 30–1 ✦ Aerobic Versus Anaerobic Bacteria in Periapical Infections

ROOT CANAL SPECIMEN	NO. OF CASES	ANAEROBIC AND OTHER BACTERIA (%)	ANAEROBIC BACTERIA EXCLUSIVELY (%)	FACULTATIVE BACTERIA EXCLUSIVELY (%)
Necrotic teeth with peri-apical lesions	94	91 (97%)	38 (40%)	4 (4%)
Residual periapical lesions post–root canal treatment	6	5 (83%)	5 (83%)	1 (17%)

icillin. Periapical lesions that fail to heal following endodontic therapy sometimes harbor *Arachnia propionica* or *Actinomyces isrealii*.

Periapical infections can extend beyond the alveolar bone into the contiguous soft tissue, creating an orofacial infection. The incidence of bacteria in 50 cases of dentoalveolar abscesses is summarized in Table 30–4. *Streptococcus milleri, Peptostreptococcus* species, *Peptococcus* species, and *Prevotella, Porphyromonas* species were most commonly isolated. Anaerobic gram-negative rods, particularly *Prevotella, Porphyromonas* and fusobacteria, are more common in severe orofacial infections, whereas gram-positive cocci and rods are more frequent in mild infections. *F. nucleatum* appeared to be most closely associated with the severe infections.

Bacterial Role in Periapical Lesions

Experimentally, bacteria isolated from periapical infections can directly cause tissue damage. Combinations of isolates from infected root canals can induce purulent "mixed infections" including either transmissible, subcutaneous abscesses or experimental apical periodontitis with periapical bone loss. Pure cultures of single isolates usually were incapable of producing such lesions. *Prevotella asaccharolyticus* (possibly *endodontalis*) in combination with *Peptostreptococcus micros* appeared to be necessary components of this mixed infection.

Microorganisms in necrotic root canal systems can produce inflammatory disease. These microorganisms have the capacity for invasion, production of enzymes that cause adverse tissue reactions, and toxins that can directly and indirectly damage the tissue. The cell wall lipopolysaccharides or endotoxins of gram-negative bacteria are directly toxic for a variety of host cell types including fibroblasts. These substances can also cause osteoclastic bone loss and activate complement via the alternate pathway (Table 30–5). Complement activation leads to the generation of chemotactic peptides, accumulation of leukocytes, and an inflammatory reaction (see Chapter 2). Endotoxin has been measured in infected root canal systems and periapical lesions of teeth with necrotic pulps. Higher concentrations of endotoxin can be detected in symptomatic pulpless teeth than in asymptomatic pulpless teeth.

Microbiologic Cultures in Treatment of Root Canal Infections

With the identification of microorganisms in the etiology of periapical lesions, culture techniques were introduced as part of clinical therapy in the 1960s and 1970s. The root canal system was sampled and cultured prior to and during endodontic therapy as a means of determining the end point of therapy. Until a negative culture was achieved, indicating that no viable microorganisms could be cultured from root canal samples, the root canal

TABLE 30–2 ✦ *Prevotella* and *Porphyromonas* in Necrotic Root Canals

	INCIDENCE
Positive culture	60–80%
Black-pigmenting species	4–67%
P. endodontalis	1–16%
P. gingivalis	5–11%
P. intermedia	5–28%
P. melaninogenicus	4–50%

TABLE 30–3 ✦ *Prevotella* and *Porphyromonas* in Periapical Abscesses

	INCIDENCE
Positive culture	89–100%
Black-pigmenting species	14–100%
P. denticola	38%
P. endodontalis	2–69%
P. gingivalis	5–10%
P. intermedia	8–20%
P. melaninogenicus	30–50%

TABLE 30–4 ✦ Incidence of Bacteria Isolated from Periapical Abscesses

	% ISOLATES*
Facultative Anaerobes	
Streptococcus millereri	15
Streptococcus mitior	2
Streptococcus sanguis	2
Streptococcus mutans	1
Lactobacillus fermentum	1
Lactobacillus salivarius	1
Actinomyces odontolyticus	1
Actinomyces naeslundii	1
Actinomyces meyeri	1
Arachnia proprionica	1
Haemophilus parainfluenzae	1
Capnocytophaga ochracea	1
Eikinella corrodens	1
Strict Anaerobes	
Peptostreptococcus sp.	8
Peptococcus sp.	19
Streptococcus intermedius	2
Streptococcus constellatus	1
Propionibacterium acnes	1
Eubacterium lentum	1
Veillonella parvula	2
Porphyromonas oralis	12
Porphyromonas gingivalis†	8
Bacteroides melaninogenicus	7
Prevotella intermedia	3
Other *Bacteroides* sp.	6
Fusobacterium nucleatum	4
Fusobacterium mortiferum	1

*Percent isolates out of 166 isolates.
†Probably *P. endodontalis*.
Adapted from Lewis et al., J. Med. Microbiol. 21:101, 1986.

system was not filled or obturated. Careful appraisal of the culture procedure suggested numerous false-positive and false-negative cultures. These resulted from inadvertent contamination of the paper points used for collection, residual disinfectants used to medicate the canals being transferred to the paper point, inadequate chairside culture techniques particularly for anaerobes, and inappropriate culture media. As a consequence, the use of bacterial culture in endodontic therapy declined. Today, proper sampling, cultivation, characterization, and antimicrobial susceptibility permit the acquisition of clinically important and useful information.

IMMUNOLOGY

As in other soft tissues, the pulp and periapical tissues develop host responses to bacterial infections. Although such responses may be beneficial by eliminating, preventing, or minimizing the spread of bacteria, they may be harmful by inducing hypersensitivity reactions or excessive responses to the bacteria. A hypersensitivity reaction manifested as an inflammatory response in the confined root canal system may lead to further tissue destruction.

Sensitization Via the Pulp

Bacterial infection of the pulp sensitizes the host to bacterial antigens. Experimental topical application of antigen to pulpal tissue of animals first sensitizes and then induces a local immune response. Once host sensitization occurs, severe pulpal inflammation and bone destruction result from subsequent topical exposure to the sensitizing antigen. The pulpal route of sensitization also induces serum antibodies to the antigen.

Similarly, in an immunocompromised host, minimal inflammation may occur in pulpal infections. In one patient with an immunologic deficiency, extensive microbial invasion of the pulp failed to cause the usual cellular inflammatory infiltrate.

Immunopathology of Pulpal Disease

The pulpal and periapical tissues respond to the bacterial antigens by mounting a cellular and humoral response. Depending on the stage of disease, the tissues may be infiltrated by neutrophils, plasma cells (immunoglobulin containing cells), T-helper lymphocytes, T-suppressor lymphocytes, B lymphocytes, macrophages, and mast cells (Table 30–6). The T cells are more numerous than the B cells with approximately equal numbers of T-helper and T-suppressor cells in chronic lesions.

The neutrophils provide one of the first lines of defense against the bacteria by phagocytosing whole bacteria and their antigens. This phagocytosis is enhanced by antibodies reacting with the bacteria. Sensitized T lymphocytes respond to the bacterial antigens by releasing soluble mediators or cytokines, which can not only potentiate the protective host response, but can also cause tissue destruction. Some cytokines possibly important in periapical infections are chemotactic for macro-

TABLE 30–5 ✦ Factors Leading to Bone Loss

Bacterial Factors
   Lipopolysaccharides
Host Factors
   Interleukin 1β (IL-1β)
   Interleukin 1α (IL-1α)
   Tumor necrosis factor α (TNFα)
   Tumor necrosis factor β (lymphotoxin or TNFβ)
   Prostaglandin E_2 (PGE$_2$)

TABLE 30–6 ✦ Immune Components in Pulpal and Periapical Tissues

	IgG	IgE	IgA	IgM	COMPLEMENT COMPONENTS	LYMPHOCYTES T	B
Normal pulp	−	−	−	−	−	−	−
Inflamed pulp	+ + +	+ +	+ +	+	+ +	+	+ + +
Periapical lesions	+ + +	+ +	−	+	+ + +	+ + +	+

+ + + = large numbers present; + + = moderate numbers; + = few; − = not present.

phages, neutrophils, basophils, and eosinophils; inhibit migration of macrophages and leukocytes; activate macrophages; act as mitogens by inducing blast formation of nonsensitized lymphocytes; are cytotoxic for fibroblasts; and activate osteoclasts (IL-1β, IL-1α, TNFα, and TNFβ, which constitute what was previously called osteoclast activating factor) (Table 30–5). Sensitized B lymphocytes also produce some cytokines on exposure to the sensitizing antigen and evolve into plasma cells. The plasma cells elaborate antibodies. Antibody-antigen interactions, sometimes with activation of serum complement, may be either protective by lysing bacteria and promoting phagocytosis or destructive through immune complex disease and immediate hypersensitivity. Mast cells in the tissue contribute to immediate hypersensitivity reactions by release of histamines and other active substances upon reaction of antigens with mast cell IgE. Macrophages in the tissues play a role in processing of antigens for the lymphocytes and in phagocytosis.

Based on current knowledge, it is difficult to assess the contribution of immunity to the pathogenesis of periapical infections and whether it has a net protective or destructive result. It may be postulated to play more of a destructive than a protective role in most cases. This results from the restricted environment imposed by the surrounding calcified structures, which leads to tissue necrosis when there is extensive inflammation and continuous exposure to large numbers of bacteria from carious lesions.

The elements necessary for immunopathology are present in inflamed pulp tissue, periapical granulomas, and periapical cysts. In the inflamed human dental pulp, plasma cells containing IgG, IgA, IgM, and IgE commonly occur, with 60 percent of the cells containing IgG. The concentrations of IgG and IgA are elevated in inflamed pulps compared with normal pulps. The inflammatory response in periapical granulomas is characterized by lymphocytes, plasma cells, polymorphonuclear leukocytes, mast cells, and macrophages. Plasma cells containing IgG are most common, with IgA, IgM, and IgE less frequently found. Antibodies commonly are found in periapical biopsies and explants, which react with microorganisms associated

with root canal infections. These frequently include antibodies to *P. intermedia, P. gingivalis, P. endodontalis, Peptostreptococcus micros, Actinomyces israelii* and *Fusobacterium nucleatum.* Immunoglobulins are also extracellular along with complement; C3c occurs within and adjacent to blood vessels.

The association of IgE with mast cells in periapical lesions also allows consideration of IgE hypersensitivity reactions within the lesions. Proposed sources of allergens have included not only the bacteria and their products but also denatured host tissues. Ultrastructurally, many of the mast cells demonstrate cell degranulation and discharge from the surface of granules suggesting histamine release as a result of immediate hypersensitivity reactions in periapical infections. This is consistent with elevated serum IgE levels in patients with acute apical abscesses.

Immune complex disease has been considered in the immunopathology of periapical lesions. Experimentally, immune complexes induce rapidly evolving periapical lesions characterized by bone loss, collagen breakdown, and leukocytic infiltration. In periapical infections, complement is frequently closely associated with IgG, IgA, and IgM, suggesting possible immune complexes of bacterial antigens with the immunoglobulins. Such reactivity could be protective and accelerate phagocytosis and bacterial lysis or could be destructive in the form of immune complex disease.

Cell-mediated immune reactions in periapical lesions have been suggested by the fact that macrophages and lymphocytes constitute a majority of the inflammatory infiltrate. Prostaglandin and other arachidonic acid metabolites, as well as OAF, a lymphokine involved in bone resorption, have also been identified in human periapical disease.

TREATMENT

Irreversible pulpitis with subsequent pulpal necrosis does not normally heal. As a result, endodontic therapy is directed toward removal or extirpation of the necrotic pulpal tissue, chemotherapy to reduce or eliminate the bacterial contamination, and filling the root canal system with an inert material such as gutta-percha to allow healing in the periapical area. When biologic principles are adhered to, endodontic therapy is a highly successful and dependable procedure for retaining teeth.

Successful endodontic therapy does not appear to depend on complete absence of all microorganisms but on significant reductions in their numbers and on complete seal of the canals, preventing further bacteria invasion. However, obligate anaerobic bacteria can sometimes be isolated from asymptomatic periapical lesions that previously had root canal therapy. When persistent infections occur following root canal therapy, enterococci are frequently isolated.

Penicillin or amoxicillin is the drug of choice for a serious periapical infection based upon clinical responses and their cost effectiveness. For patients who fail to respond to penicillin, or who are allergic to it, the drug of choice is clindamycin. It is estimated that close to 70,000 patients per year receive clindamycin for serious odontogenic infections. Recent studies have demonstrated that some bacteria, including *Prevotella* and *Porphyromonas*, may be resistant to penicillin.

SUMMARY

It is clear that the predominant bacteria in periapical infections are obligate anaerobic bacteria. Many cases are exclusively made up of obligate anaerobic bacteria, while very few cases are made up exclusively of facultative bacteria. Gram-negative rods such as *Porphyromona, Prevotella,* and *Fusobacterium* seem to be the most common.

Treatment must be directed at the removal of the necrotic substrate, the establishment of drainage as atraumatically as possible, and the use of support of antimicrobial agents. Because bacterial resistance is frequent, therapy in the absence of culture/susceptibility testing is a questionable practice.

BIBLIOGRAPHY

Aderhold, L.: Bacteriology of dentogenous pyogenic infections. Oral Surg. 52:587, 1981.

Baumgartner, J. C. and Falkler, W. A.: Reactivity of IgG from explant cultures of periapical lesions with implicated microorganisms. J. Endodontol. 17:207–212, 1991.

Baumgartner, J. C. and Falkler, W. A.: Bacteria in the apical 5 mm of infected root canals. J. Endodontol. 17:380–383, 1991.

Brook, I., Grimm, S., and Kielich, R. B.: Bacteriology of acute periapical abscesses in children. J. Endodontol. 7:378, 1981.

Fabricius, L., Dehlen, G., Holm, S. E., and Moller, A. J. R.: Influence of combinations of oral bacteria on periapical tissues of monkeys. Scand. J. Dent. Res. 90:200, 1982.

Goodman, A. D.: Isolation of anaerobic bacteria from the root canal systems of necrotic teeth by the use of a transport solution. Oral Surg. 43:766, 1977.

Haapasalo, M.: *Bacteroides* sp. in dental root canal infections. Endod. Dent. Traumatol. 5:1–10, 1989.

Heimdahl, A., von Konow, L., Satoh, T., and Nord, C. E.: Clinical appearance of orofacial infections of odontogenic origin in relation to microbial findings. J. Clin. Microbiol. 22:299, 1985.

Johannessen, A. C., Nilsen, R., and Skaug, N.: Deposits of immunoglobulins and complement factor C3 in human dental periapical inflammatory lesions. Scand. J. Dent. Res. 91:191, 1983.

Kakehashi, S., Stanley, H. R., and Fitzgerald, J. R.: The effects of surgical exposure of dental pulps in germfree and conventional laboratory rats. Oral Surg. 20:340, 1965.

Kantz, W. E. and Henry, C. A.: Isolation and classification of anaerobic bacteria from intact pulp chambers of non-vital teeth in man. Arch. Oral Biol. 19:91, 1974.

Kettering, J. D.: Specificity of antibodies present in human periapical lesions. J. Endodontol. 17:213–216, 1991.

Kuntz, D. D. and Genco, R. J.: Localization of immunoglobulins and complement in persistent periapical lesions. J. Dent. Res. 53:215, 1974.

Lewis, M. A. O., MacFarlane, T. W., and McGowan, D. A.: Quantitative bacteriology of acute dento-alveolar abscesses. J. Med. Microbiol. 21:101, 1986.

Morand, M., Schilder, H., Blondin, J., Stone, P., and Franzblair, C.: Collagenolytic and elastolytic activities from diseased human dental pulps. J. Endodontol. 7:156, 1981.

Morse, D. R.: The endodontic culture technique: An impractical and unnecessary procedure. Dent. Clin. North Am. 15:793, 1971.

O'Grady, J. F.: Periapical Actinomycosis involving *Actinomyces israelii*. J. Endodontol. 14:147–149, 1988.

Oguntebi, B., Slee, A. M., Tanzer, J. M., and Langeland, K.: Predominant microflora associated with human dental periapical abscesses. J. Clin. Microbiol. 15:964, 1982.

Pantera, E. A., Jr., Zambon, J. J., Reynolds, H. S., and Shih-Levine, M.: Identification of black-pigmented *Bacteroides* sp. in human dental pulp by indirect immunofluorescence microscopy. J. Dent. Res. 64 (Sp. Iss.):176, 1985.

Perrini, N. and Fonzi, L.: Mast cells in human periapical lesions: Ultrastructural aspects and their possible physiopathological implications. J. Endodontol. 11:197, 1985.

Pulver, W. H., Taubman, M. A., and Smith, D. J.: Immune components in normal and inflamed human dental pulp. Arch. Oral Biol. 22:103, 1977.

Schonfeld, S. E., Greening, A. B., Glick, D. H., Frank, A. L., Simon, J. H., and Herles, S. M.: Endotoxin activity in periapical lesions. J. Endodontol. 8:10, 1982.

Sjogren, U., Happonen, R. P., Kahnberg, K. E., and Sundqvist, G.: Survival of *Arachnia proprionica* in periapical tissue. Int. Endodont. J. 21:277–282, 1982.

Stabholz, A. and McArthur, W. P.: Cellular immune responses of patients with periapical pathosis to necrotic dental pulp antigens determined by the release of LIF. J. Endodontol. 4:282, 1978.

Stashenko, P.: The role of immune cytokines in the pathogenesis of periapical lesions. Endod. Dent. Traumatol. 6:89–96, 1990.

Sundqvist, G. K., Eckerbom, M. I., Larsson, A. P., and Sjogren, U. T.: Capacity of anaerobic bacteria from necrotic dental pulps to induce purulent infections. Infect. Immun. 25:685, 1979.

Sundqvist, G.: Prevalence of black-pigmented *Bacteroides* species in root canal infections. J. Endodontol. 15:13–19, 1989.

Torabinejad, M., Eby, W. C., and Naidorf, I. J.: Inflammatory and immunological aspects of the pathogenesis of human periapical lesions. J. Endodontol. 11:479, 1985.

Trenstad, L., Barnett, F., Flax, M., and Slots, J.: Anaerobic bacteria in periapical lesions of human teeth. J. Endodontol. 12:131, 1986.

Williams, B. L., McCann, G. F., and Schoenknecht, F. D.: Bacteriology of dental abscesses of endodontic origin. J. Clin. Microbiol. 18:770, 1983.

Zavistocki, J., Dzink, J., Onderdonk, A., and Bartlett, J. G.: Quantitative bacteriology of endodontic infections. Oral Surg. 49:171, 1980.

31

Medical Infections of Interest

Russell J. Nisengard, Joseph J. Zambon, and
Michael G. Newman

CHAPTER OUTLINE

Systemic diseases caused by oral bacteria
Systemic diseases with multiple etiologies

Many systemic infections of medical importance have been described throughout this text. Two facets not adequately discussed elsewhere are systemic diseases caused by oral microorganisms and systemic diseases that can be caused by more than one pathogen.

SYSTEMIC DISEASES CAUSED BY ORAL BACTERIA

Many oral, indigenous bacteria have significant pathogenic capabilities. Infections and tissue destruction can result from (1) direct effects of bacteria on the tissues including bacterial cell surface constituents, enzymes, toxins, and invasive ability; and (2) indirect effects on the host immune system by microbial factors. When oral microorganisms gain access to other locations of the body, they no longer are held in check by the complex oral ecology and may produce disease. Among the more significant systemic diseases caused by the oral flora are subacute bacterial endocarditis, infections in joints, abscesses, and human bite infections.

Subacute Bacterial Endocarditis

Subacute bacterial endocarditis (SBE) is a potentially life-threatening heart disease resulting from bacterial colonization of previously damaged heart tissues, particularly the valves. Conditions predisposing to SBE include rheumatic fever (when there has been cardiac damage), congenital heart disease (including ventricular septum defects), mitral valve prolapse (when there is insufficiency), aortic stenosis and persistent ductus arteriosus, prosthetic heart valves, and previous endocarditis. Patients with vascular grafts are sometimes at risk as well.

The oral cavity is the most common source for the bacteria that colonize the heart in SBE. Bacteremias usually occur following dental procedures that cause bleeding, such as periodontal probing, scaling and root planing, extractions, gingival surgery, endodontic therapy, biopsies, and impressions for crowns and bridges. The relatively high numbers of bacteria that gain access to the alveolar blood and circulate throughout the body are usually eliminated by the host defenses. However, in patients with predisposing factors that have damaged the heart tissue or the heart valve, the bacteria can rapidly colonize, leading to SBE.

Bacteremias can also occur following toothbrushing and chewing hard substances, particularly in patients with periodontal disease. While brushing and chewing have not been reported to cause SBE, the risk should be minimized by preventing and controlling periodontal disease in patients with predisposing factors for SBE.

Several microorganisms have been identified as causing SBE. These include the alpha-hemolytic streptococci or viridens group of streptococci *(S. mitior, S. sanguis* and *S. mutans), Staphylococcus epidermidis*, and *Actinobacillus actinomycetemcomitans. A. actinomycetemcomitans*, a known pathogen in periodontal disease, also has been identified as a causative agent in SBE. There are now numerous reported cases of SBE caused by this organism, including at least two cases in patients taking penicillin for prevention of SBE. SBE caused by *Staphylococcus epidermidis* is more common in intravenous drug users.

Bacterial factors that facilitate adherence to heart tissue result in colonization and rapid growth. At times, bacterial aggregates or emboli break away from the colonized heart tissue and lodge in other organs, leading to further systemic complications. In SBE, death results from heart failure, hemorrhage, and emboli affecting other organs.

As in many other diseases, prevention of SBE is far easier and simpler than its treatment. Patients with predisposing factors for SBE should be prophylactically premedicated with an antibiotic prior to any dental treatment in which the gingival tissue is manipulated resulting in *any* bleeding (see Chapter 33).

Patients who have localized juvenile periodontitis (LJP), and others with *A. actinomycetemcomitans* infections, should be managed differently if they are at risk of developing SBE. These patients have two types of bacteria capable of causing SBE: gram-positive bacteria that are usually sensitive to penicillin class drugs and gram-negative bacteria that are minimally affected by many penicillins. In these cases, it is recommended that patients first be given a therapeutic course of tetracycline to suppress the *A. actinomycetemcomitans*. This is then followed by the usual prophylactic regimen of Amoxicillin (see Chapter 33) starting 1 hour before the dental procedure.

Infections in Joint Implants Following Dental Procedures

Joint replacements, particularly of the hip, are increasingly common and must be considered prior to any dental treatment in which there may be bleeding leading to bacteremias. As with damaged heart tissue, joint replacement sites are prone to bacterial colonization, infection, and subsequent injury. Such infections are often difficult to treat and may lead to crippling.

Patients with hip replacements who will undergo dental procedures in which bacteremias may occur require prophylactic antibiotics to prevent joint infections. The current practice is to use the same antibiotic regimen employed for prevention of SBE.

Lung Abscesses/Infections

Aspirating dental materials contaminated by the septic oral environment (including saliva and plaque) into the lungs can lead to lung abscesses. Pieces of fillings or crowns that are inadvertently aspirated can be responsible for severe, sometimes life-threatening, lung infections. These are often caused by the gram-negative, subgingival, anaerobic bacteria including black-pigmenting species, *Actinobacillus actinomycetemcomitans*, *Actinomyces* species, and *Eikenella corrodens*.

Abscesses of this type are best prevented by exercising caution when performing dental procedures. At times, rubber dams and gauze can aid in blocking the posterior part of the oral pharynx. Usually, swallowing of dental materials is of no consequence. However, if aspiration of a crown or filling is suspected, the patient should immediately be referred to a hospital emergency room, where radiographs of the lungs should be taken to confirm the aspiration. If confirmed, antibiotics usually are given immediately as a prophylactic measure.

A. actinomycetemcomitans can cause other extraoral infections in addition to abscesses of the lungs, including thyroid gland abscesses, urinary tract infections, brain abscesses, and vertebral osteomyelitis. These extraoral infections occur as a result of both direct and hematogenous transmission of bacteria residing in the oral cavity.

Infections as a Result of Human Bites

Infections of hands, fingers, and other tissues can result from exposure of cuts to the oral flora. Bites, particularly human bites, leading to puncture wounds, fights with blows to the mouth causing abrasions and cuts on hands, fingernail biting, and inadvertent oral exposure of previous cuts on the hands of dental practitioners during dental treatment can all cause infections.

The causative agents in these types of traumatic infections are generally considered to be anaerobic microorganisms. As expected with the complex flora in the mouth, many infections are mixed infections involving more than one organism. Anaerobes isolated include *Bacteroides*, *Clostridium*, *Fusobacterium*, *Arachnia*, and *Peptostreptococcus;* aerobes isolated include staphylococci, streptococci, and diphtheroids.

The pathogenicity of oral bacteria has been demonstrated in studies of periodontal disease. Human plaque subcutaneously injected into experimental animals can cause a transmissible, mixed anaerobic infection mainly involving gram-negative bacteria. These infections are sometimes fulminating, causing death.

Because of the pathogenicity of the oral flora, lesions resulting from bites and related trauma should be immediately treated. The area should be thoroughly washed and debrided, and a topical antibiotic or antiseptic applied. Depending on the depth of the wound, a systemic antibiotic also may be considered. Consultation with an infectious disease physician is necessary. Preventive measures, particularly the use of gloves, should be employed by dental personnel with cuts on their hands.

SYSTEMIC DISEASES WITH MULTIPLE ETIOLOGIES

Many systemic diseases can be caused by more than one microorganism. The practitioner must recognize this in the differential diagnosis and ultimate treatment of a disease. This section focuses on five of the diseases with multiple etiologies: venereal disease, meningitis, food poisoning, pneumonia and osteomyelitis. The predominant organisms causing these diseases are listed, but it should be recognized that other bacteria have occasionally been associated with these diseases. Further discussion is provided in chapters dealing with the specific etiologic agent.

Venereal Disease

Venereal diseases are a group of diseases transmitted by direct genital-to-genital, genital-to-oral, or oral-to-oral routes. These include both bacterial and viral agents (Table 31–1). While not considered a venereal disease in the classic sense of transmission by contact with a lesion, the AIDS virus, or HIV-1, should be included.

Meningitis

Meningitis, a sometimes life-threatening disease of the nervous system, can also be caused by several microorganisms (Table 31–2). Commonly, meningitis follows pharyngitis or a sore throat.

Food Poisoning

Food poisoning can occur immediately or several hours after ingestion of contaminated food containing high concentrations of bacterial toxins. Depending on the organism and degree of contamination, the disease may be relatively mild with nausea and vomiting, or it may lead to death. Several bacteria are associated with food poisoning (Table 31–3). The most common form of food poisoning occurs following ingestion of poorly refrigerated foods leading to bacterial growth. An

TABLE 31–1 ✦ Microorganisms Associated with Venereal Disease

Neisseria gonorrhoeae
Treponema pallidum
Chlamydia trachomatis
Haemophilus ducreyi
Herpesvirus type 2

TABLE 31–2 ✦ Microorganisms Associated with Meningitis

Neisseria meningitidis
Haemophilus influenzae
Streptococcus pneumoniae
Group B streptococci
Escherichia coli

TABLE 31–3 ✦ Microorganisms Associated with Food Poisoning

Clostridium perfringens
Staphylococcus aureus
Vibrio cholerae
Escherichia coli
Vibrio parahaemolyticus
Bacillus cereus
Salmonella sp.

TABLE 31–4 ✦ Microorganisms Associated with Pneumonia

Streptococcus pneumoniae
Staphylococcus aureus
Klebsiella pneumoniae
Proteus sp.
Pseudomonas aeruginosa
Escherichia coli
Serratia sp.

example would be food containing dairy products that has been left in the sun for several hours. More recently, raw or incompletely cooked meat and fish or improperly canned foods have been implicated.

Pneumonia

A large number of bacteria, including some oral bacteria, can cause pneumonia (Table 31–4). Because both gram-positive and gram-negative organisms may be involved, cultural identification is necessary prior to effective treatment.

Osteomyelitis

Osteomyelitis or infections of the bone can also be caused by several microorganisms (Table 31–5). This disease is particularly difficult to treat and often amputation is necessary. Many patients continue to harbor bacteria for months or years after clinical healing, which may eventually lead to reactivation of the infection. Patients with compromised resistance to infections, such as those with diabetes, are more prone to develop osteomyelitis.

TABLE 31–5 ✦ Microorganisms Associated with Osteomyelitis

Staphylococcus aureus
β-hemolytic streptococci
Haemophilus influenzae
Escherichia coli
Pseudomonas sp.

BIBLIOGRAPHY

Ciancio, S. G. and Bourgault, P. C.: Clinical pharmacology for dental professionals. PSG Publishing, Littleton, Mass., 1984, p. 361.

Finegold, A. M.: Anaerobic bacteria in human disease. Academic Press, New York, pp. 428–432, 1977.

O'Connell, C. J.: Microbiology in the practice of medicine. In Milgrom, F., and Flanagan, T. D. (eds.): Medical Microbiology. Churchill-Livingstone, New York, 1982, pp. 697–716.

32 *Sterilization and Asepsis*

W. Eugene Rathbun

CHAPTER OUTLINE

Infectious diseases
Prevention and control of autogenous infections
Practical asepsis
Sterilization
Sterilization Assurance
Conclusions

Dental health care workers including dentists, hygienists, assistants, and laboratory personnel are frequently exposed to life-threatening microorganisms. Current methods of sterilization and asepsis in the dental office and laboratory can significantly decrease the risk of infectious disease for the patient, dentist, and staff.

Concern about the transmission of disease has been expressed for thousands of years. Written guidelines for "disease control" are found in the Bible, especially in the books of Leviticus and Numbers. The Israelites were required to follow principles of heat sterilization, hand washing, and isolation. Early records indicated the use of chemicals for wound-cleansing hygiene and methods of food preservation.

More effective chemical disinfectants were introduced in the mid-19th century. Iodine as a wound dressing was recommended by Davies in 1839. Chlorine water was introduced by LeFerne in 1843 and later in 1847, Sammelweis, who began using chlorinated lime to dramatically reduce the incidence of childbirth infections. Heat sterilization by heated water in a pressurized vessel was first utilized in 1832 by William Henry.

The field of asepsis and sterilization has undergone considerable growth and development in the last 100 years with the discovery of numerous chemical and physical agents and barrier techniques to prevent the transmission of infective organisms.

The major impetus for the current interest in asepsis has been the concern about hepatitis B beginning in the early 1970s and the AIDS epidemic beginning in the 1980s. Since 1990 there has been considerable professional and public interest in the transmission of HIV to six patients of an AIDS-infected dentist in Florida. These cases are the only documented instances of transmission of HIV from an infected health care worker to patients in spite of numerous studies of patients treated by infected health care workers.

The "standard of care" now includes universal precautions, exposure control plans, barrier protection, immunization, instrument sterilization, and unprecedented needs for awareness and frequent educational updates in this critical area. The federal government through OSHA adopted stricter laws in 1991 that provided specific regulations about safety for health care employees concerning bloodborne pathogens. During 1992, at least six states mandated specific infection control procedures such as heat sterilization of high speed handpieces and sterilizer monitoring.

The goals of this chapter are to develop an awareness of diseases that may be transmitted in the dental environment and the present methods of sterilization, disinfection, and asepsis that will help students and practitioners develop a safe, efficient, and medicolegally acceptable clinical practice.

INFECTIOUS DISEASES

Many infectious diseases may be transmitted during dental care. A goal of dental and medical practice is to do no harm. By "infection control," serious infections and even death may be prevented. Many sources of potential infection exist in the dental office (Fig. 32–1). Hands, saliva, nasal secretions, blood, clothing, and hair as well as dental instruments and equipment all need to be studied to minimize the risk of disease.

Contamination of the oral cavity and open wounds may be caused by air-, water-, dust-, aerosol-, respiratory secretion-, or spatter-borne organisms. These sources may lead to contamination of hands, instruments, or dental supplies. The patient's microorganisms may be transmitted to the clinician and staff by aerosols, splatters or droplets, respiratory secretions, and plaque, calculus, tooth restorative materials, and debris. The patient's pathogenic oral flora may be transmitted to other tissues or organs (**"autogenous infection"**) such as susceptible heart valves, artificial joints, and adjacent soft tissue or bone.

PREVENTION AND CONTROL OF AUTOGENOUS INFECTIONS
History

Patients with a history of rheumatic heart disease, endocarditis, mitral valve prolapse, heart murmur, heart valve prosthesis, or joint prosthesis are especially susceptible to infection. Prophylactic antibiotics as recommended by the American Dental Association and the American Heart Association should be given in consultation with the patient's physician whenever the treatment will cause bleeding, especially prophylaxis and surgery. Although the risk of infective endocarditis or arthritis is minimized by appropriate antibiotics, a wide range of bacteria and fungi may infect the damaged heart valve or joint. Patients should be instructed to contact their dentist and physician should changes in health occur after dental care. Topical antibacterial therapy is frequently recommended for susceptible patients prior to dental treatment. These may include plaque removal by the patient or staff, and vigorous mouth rinsing with an antimicrobial such as 0.12 percent chlorhexidine gluconate.

Patients with a history of diabetes or immunodeficiency should be treated after consultation with their physician to minimize their risk of infection.

Bacterial or fungal infections after dental therapy require careful diagnosis and therapy. Laboratory studies including aerobic and anaerobic culture and antibiotic sensitivity frequently are necessary. With infective endocarditis or infective arthritis, hospitalization and intense prolonged care are often required. The infected valve or joint may need to be replaced surgically. The diagnosis of endocarditis is often not made for several weeks to months after the infection begins, and the mortality approaches 30 percent.

CROSS INFECTIONS

The dentist, staff, and patients are at significant risk of exposure to pathogenic bacteria, viruses, and fungi during dental treatment. Table 32–1

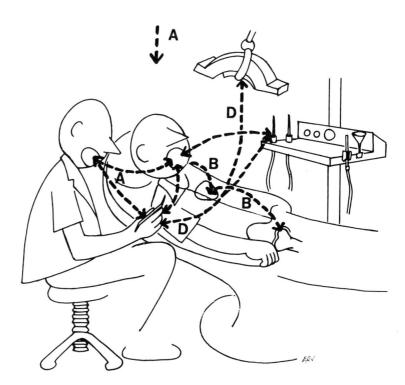

FIGURE 32–1 ✦ Examples of sources of infection in the dental operatory. *A* = Airborne–aerosols, secretions. *B* = Blood-borne–autogenous: to heart valves or joint prosthesis. *D* = Direct contact—blood and saliva or hand pieces, instruments, charts, telephones, and so on.

TABLE 32–1 ✦ Representative Cross-Infections in Dentistry

AGENT/DISEASE	ROUTES	INCUBATION PERIOD	ESTIMATED SURVIVAL AT ROOM TEMPERATURE
Bacterial			
Mycobacterium tuberculosis	Saliva Sputum	To 6 mo	Months
Staphylococcus aureus Staphylococcal infections	Saliva Exudates Skin	4–10 days	Days
Streptococcus pyogenes Streptococcal Wound infections Endocarditis	Open wound Blood-borne	1 day–1 wk	Hours–days
Treponema pallidum Syphilis	Direct contact with lesions	1–10 wk	Seconds
Viral			
Respiratory viruses Flu, colds	Saliva Secretions	1–14 days	Hours
Hepatitis A virus Hepatitis A	Blood Feces Saliva	2–6 wk	Days
Hepatitis B virus Hepatitis B	Blood Saliva Semen	6 wk–6 mo	Months
HIV, formerly HTLV III/LAV AIDS, ARC	Blood, semen Secretions	To 10 yr	Days
Herpes simplex I and II Recurrent herpes Whitlow Conjunctivitis	Saliva Secretions	2 wk	Minutes

Adapted from Crawford, J.: Clinical Asepsis in Dentistry, ed. 3. R. A. Kolstad, Mesquite, Tex, 1986, p. 23.

summarizes some of the principal pathogens and diseases that they cause.

Hepatitis B

One of the most serious pathogens to the dentist is hepatitis B (see Chapter 22). Hepatitis B produces the most significant illness, practice disruption, and death of any of the pathogenic agents transmitted in dentistry. The incidence of hepatitis B after accidental exposure by a cut with a sharp instrument or a needle stick from a hepatitis BsAg–positive patient is approximately 20 percent compared with an estimated 0 to 0.5 percent incidence of AIDS following a similar exposure to HIV. The prevalence of antibodies to hepatitis B among general dentists ranged from 12.9 percent in 1976 to 30 percent in 1984. The prevalence of HBV carrier states for dentists and dental students has been reported from 0.8 to 3.9 percent.

The risk of acquiring hepatitis B in dentists is six times that in the general population and appears related to the frequency of contact with patients' blood. Dental hygienists have a slightly lower prevalence than general dentists, followed by laboratory technicians, dental assistants, and dental clerical workers.

There have been at least nine reported outbreaks of hepatitis B involving 3 to 53 patients who were infected by hepatitis B carrier dentists. In one outbreak, 2 of 27 patients died of fulminating hepatitis and one patient was paralyzed. Most often the dentist was not aware of his or her hepatitis B exposure, illness, or carrier status.

Pre-exposure active immunization against hepatitis B is required to be offered within 10 days of employment at no cost to the health care worker who might be exposed to bloodborne pathogens. (See Chapter 22 for recommendations.) If possible, this should be accomplished at the beginning of professional education. Hepatitis B immunization requires a series of three intramuscular injections in the arm, at 0 time, 30 days, and 180 days. It is recommended that immunized persons be tested after the series to determine that the immunization was effective. The vaccine has been proven to be very safe and approximately 96 percent effective.

Medical histories will usually only reveal approximately 20 percent of individuals who have had hepatitis B. Therefore, all patients should be presumed to be active hepatitis B carriers. The ethical, legal, and financial costs of a dentist developing hepatitis B are very serious, including transmission to spouses, vertical transmission to newborn offspring, as well as transmission to patients and staff. The usual time lost from practice is 2 to 3 months by the infected health care worker. Continuous evaluations of the frequent recommendations from the CDC and the ADA will be very helpful in avoiding disastrous medical and legal complications.

Herpes

Herpes simplex viruses I and II are frequently in the mouth of dental patients and may lead to serious infections for the dentist or staff. (See Chapter 22.) The most serious infection, "ocular herpes," may cause blindness. Another troublesome herpes infection is a viral whitlow of the operator's finger causing severe pain on pressure and inability to practice dentistry.

In one report, 20 patients developed herpes gingivostomatitis from a dental hygienist with herpes simplex virus I infection on her fingers. Most developed serious illnesses and lost several days of work or school.

AIDS

Infection by human immunodeficiency virus (HIV) is extremely serious (see Chapter 22) and for those who develop AIDS it is uniformly fatal. The AIDS "epidemic" has accelerated research, politics, and interest in "dental asepsis." Since 1985, dentists have rethought and updated their asepsis programs to protect their patients, their staff, themselves, and their practices. Even the best informed and conscientious practitioners are challenged by the fact that hepatitis B and AIDS follow very long incubation periods and most infected individuals are not identifiable. Studies underway and reported to date suggest the incidence of infection after exposure via needle stick or cut with HIV-infected blood or serum is 0 to 0.5 percent. The fact is that many AIDS patients have oral symptoms and diseases. Federal, state, and local laws make it mandatory that the whole dental profession be prepared technically and emotionally to serve those individuals. As of December 12, 1992, 249,301 AIDS cases were reported in the U.S. It is estimated that between 1.0 and 1.5 million individuals in the United States are HIV-positive. There were 8,467 health care workers reported with AIDS as of June 30, 1992, including 233 dental workers. Of these dental workers, 173 have died. After five years of ADA screening of 6,451 dentists, only one dentist who denied any high risk behavior was confirmed positive for HIV antibodies. The estimated risk of HIV infection to the dentist is estimated at 0.02 to 0.04 percent. Although the number of HIV viruses per milliliter of infected blood is 10,000 to 1 million times less than in hepatitis B, there will be great distress among those dentists who puncture themselves while treating any AIDS patient or who refuse to wear gloves during treatment and later discover that their patient had AIDS.

Tuberculosis

Tuberculosis is again becoming a problem. Since 1985 the incidence of TB rose 18.3 percent after decades of decline and continues to increase at an alarming rate, especially among the young in minority populations. The resurgence is a major public health concern and considered epidemic in New York and New Jersey. While TB control is very difficult, it also is difficult to become infected with TB. It is estimated that to develop TB usually takes 6 to 8 months of 8-hour-a-day contact with a person who has active TB and is not undergoing treatment. Coughing is the only likely source of infective aerosols. Dental workers are not at significantly increased risk of TB.

During 1992 and 1993 there have been numerous professional publications and television "exposés" bringing dental infection control procedures, regulations, and recommendations before the general public and dental health care workers. Patients are aware of the potential for disease transmission in the dental office and are interested in the specific procedures in each office. OSHA regulations are designed specifically to protect the "employee" health care worker. ADA, CDCP, and several state laws require procedures protecting the patient as well as the health care worker. A major change in recommendations for universal precautions is that all patient's blood and several body fluids, including saliva, are to be considered infectious.

The definitions in Table 32–2 will be useful in understanding the material that follows.

PRACTICAL ASEPSIS

Practical asepsis includes barrier techniques, sterilization, disinfection, and monitoring office

TABLE 32–2 ✦ Definitions

Antiseptics:	Agents that prevent the growth or action of microorganisms on living tissue.
Asepsis:	(1) The opposite of sepsis, i.e., freedom from infection.
	(2) The prevention of contact with pathogens. In dentistry this includes the techniques of barrier protection, sterilization, and disinfection.
Cold sterilization:	Sterilization at room temperature usually with an aqueous solution of a chemical. This type of sterilization is subject to serious drawbacks including dilution, cutting short the required exposure time, organic contamination, or inactivation.
Cross infections:	The transmission of pathogenic microorganisms from one patient to another.
Disinfectants:	Chemicals capable of killing pathogenic organisms when applied to inanimate objects. Frequently, the range of activity, directions for use, and conditions are cited by the manufacturer on the label.
Disinfection:	The destruction of pathogenic agents by directly applied chemical or physical means.
Nosocomial:	Office or hospital-acquired infections.
Sepsis:	The presence of pathogens in the blood or other tissues.
Sterilization:	The destruction of all life. Practically, sterilization denotes the use of physical or chemical agents to eliminate all viable microorganisms, including bacteria, fungi, viruses, and spores.

procedures. To be effective, the dentist must assume that all patients and dental staff are carriers of hepatitis B, AIDS, or TB and follow universal precautions.

More than 100 years ago, Joseph Lister remarked that "you must be able to see (the contamination) with your mental eye as distinctly as with the corporeal eye." No asepsis program will achieve maximal effectiveness without the exercise of this ability.

Many have found it helpful to demonstrate the areas in a dental operatory needing disinfection procedures by substituting red poster paint for saliva. By seeing the red paint on all instruments, charts, chairs, equipment, cabinets, telephones, pens, and other objects that would normally be handled when working on a patient, one can gain an appreciation of the extent of the need for disinfection. Many dental schools have slides or videotapes of this type of procedure that are available for loan.

Essential Infection Control Guidelines

The following procedures should be routinely used to minimize the risk of transmitting infectious disease in the dental office setting. (See Table 32–3.)

Personal Asepsis

HANDS

The major route of transmission of respiratory and oral microorganisms is by the hands. Nails should be kept short and all rings and bracelets be removed prior to patient contact. Before the first patient contact, clean hands thoroughly with a brush and hand cleaning "soap." Lather and rinse a total of three times using cool water, and dry with disposable paper towels. Each hand scrubbing should take at least 10 seconds.

Sinks are now available with either foot-operated or "electronic eye"–operated faucets to break the cycle of contaminating the faucet when turning the water on and off by hand (Fig. 32–2). As an alternative, a paper towel may be used over the faucets to adjust or to turn off the water.

Hand cleansers are available containing antimicrobial agents that contain iodophors (about 1 percent iodine), chlorhexidine gluconate (2 to 4 percent), parachlorometa-xylenol (PCMX) (0.5 to 3 percent), or alcohols (i.e., 70 percent isopropyl alcohol foam) and other ingredients. Several commercial products should be evaluated for practicality and acceptability in each office situation. A broad-spectrum antiseptic may be chosen such as one containing chlorhexidine for the first scrub of the day, before and after lunch, and before leaving for the day. A less effective hand soap may be used between regular patient visits.

The ADA and CDC recommend and OSHA *requires* that "for protection of personnel and patients, gloves must always be worn when touching blood, saliva, or mucous membranes, blood-soiled items, body fluids, or secretions, as well as surfaces contaminated by them. Gloves also must be worn when examining all oral lesions. The hands must be washed and regloved before performing pro-

TABLE 32–3 ✦ Essential Infection Control Guidelines

Especially for the Patient

Health history
Plaque removal
Pretreatment antiseptic mouth rinse
Protective eyewear
Rubber dam when appropriate
Sterile handpieces, instruments
Disinfected equipment
Disposable covers
Flush waterlines

General

Use high volume evacuation when appropriate
Ultrasonic cleaning of instruments when possible
Appropriate packaging
Heat sterilization
Sterilizer monitoring
Surface covers
Surface cleaners and disinfectants (kill TB)
Sharps and waste disposal system

Especially for the Dental Staff

Immunization
Handwash
Wear single use gloves
Wear disposable mask and glasses or chin length
  face shield
Wear protective clinic gown
After treatment remove contaminated protective
  attire and wash hands
OSHA posters and regulations posted

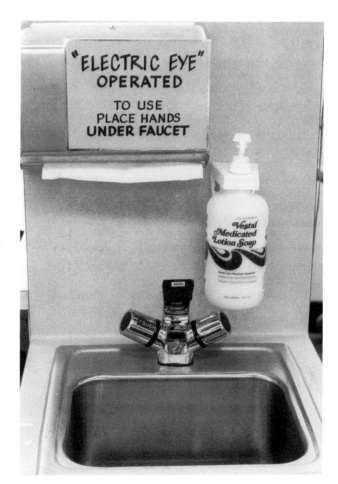

FIGURE 32–2 ✦ "Electronic eye"–operated faucet.

cedures on another patient. Repeated use of a single pair of gloves is *not* recommended, since such use is likely to produce defects in the glove material, which will diminish its value as an effective barrier."

Most individuals are able to use latex gloves. Hypoallergenic gloves and various vinyl gloves are available for those with allergies to the typical latex gloves.

It is further recommended that heavier utility gloves be used when disinfecting the operatory or when handling infected instruments or debris. Hands should be washed after removing gloves to cleanse the hands of skin bacteria and reduce possible contamination if the gloves were cut or punctured during treatment. The bacteria that entered such defects may multiply rapidly and should be removed before regloving for the next patient.

Dental health care workers who have exudative lesions or weeping dermatitis on their hands should refrain from direct patient care and from handling dental patient-care equipment until their condition resolves.

FACIAL PROTECTION

The face should be protected by surgical masks and protective eyewear or chin-length plastic shields when exposed to splashing or splattering blood or other body fluids. This includes rinsing, polishing, scaling, ultrasonic or sonic scaling, and the use of rotary burs or stones with either high- or low-speed handpieces. Masks should also be worn whenever the operator or patient has a respiratory infection. Masks should be discarded when wet or after approximately 20 minutes of use.

Either tied or formed masks are effective at reducing the risks of aerosol or splatter. There are significant differences between brands and types as to fit, comfort, and effectiveness. Choose a style and brand that feels good to your face. High filtration masks provide the best defense against penetration. A close peripheral fit is needed to provide the best aerosol blockage. It is a good idea to wash your glasses or protective eyewear frequently and at least before leaving the office to decrease the likelihood of taking pathogens home to friends or family.

High-velocity evacuation greatly decreases aerosols and splatter. These may be further reduced by using a rubber dam whenever possible. Thorough removal of plaque with a brush and floss followed by a rinse with a broad-spectrum mouthwash such as chlorhexidine gluconate (0.12 percent) provides further reduction.

CLOTHING AND HAIR

Reusable and disposable gowns, laboratory coats, or uniforms must be worn when clothing may be soiled with blood of other body fluids such as saliva. If reusable gowns are worn, they should be washed in hot water with a detergent and chlorine bleach either on site or by a commercial laundry. They are not to be taken home. Gowns should be changed at least daily or when visibly soiled with blood. Contaminated office clothing must not be taken home because of their hazard to children and other family members. Hair should be kept away from the treatment field and may be protected by a hair covering from splatter and aerosols. It is a good idea to wash your face before lunch and face and hair before bed. Pathogenic bacteria and some viruses, particularly hepatitis B virus, can survive for days to weeks on clothing.

Operatory Asepsis

What is not contaminated does not need to be disinfected or sterilized.

During the course of treatment, many objects, surfaces, instruments, and equipment become contaminated either directly by hands or via splatter and aerosols. Decide as a staff the minimal objects necessary in the operatory or treatment room and then determine which can be (1) covered or (2) sterilized, and what must be (3) disinfected (the poorest choice). Develop a plan for daily or weekly cleaning and disinfection as needed for floors and other horizontal flat surfaces.

COVERINGS

Covers eliminate the need for disinfection by allowing the removal of contaminated surfaces. The most useful and simple coverings for surfaces are paper, plastic, or foil cut into the desired shape before use and stored where they will remain clean. A new cover is used for each patient. Some areas to consider include:

1. *Instrument trays:* cover with a plastic backed patient bib, or plastic film to reduce contamination of the tray and cart or table. Place a paper tray cover, if desired, on top of the bib onto which instruments and supplies are placed. After the procedure, instruments can be removed to the "clean-up" area wrapped in the bib or plastic cover.
2. *Radiograph cone and head:* cover with plastic wrap or paper secured with tape.
3. *Switches and controls:* cover when possible, with plastic secured by double-faced tape or small pieces of aluminum foil.
4. *Headrest:* cover with plastic or paper covers or bags.
5. *Triplex (air/water) syringes:* cover with small plastic sleeves to save a great deal of cleaning time. This is especially helpful when using cements and impression mate-

rials. Replaceable, disposable, or sterilizable triplex syringe tips are available for most syringes (Fig. 32–3).

6. *High-velocity vacuum valves and hose:* cover with a 2-inch by 6-inch (or larger) plastic bag slit in the end for insertion of the vacuum tip (Fig. 32–4).

7. *Lamp handles:* cover with foil, paper, or 4-inch by 4-inch gauze sponges. Sterilizable lamp handles are available for some units (Fig. 32–5).

8. *Light "guns" for curing composite restorations:* cover the tip, handle and control trigger with plastic wrap secured with masking tape (See Fig. 32–6).

What you do not cover or remove will have to be disinfected or sterilized. Make it easier on your staff! With proper planning and covers, an operatory can be cleaned and disinfected in approximately 10 minutes.

Surface Disinfection

Disinfectants are capable of destroying pathogens on inanimate objects. They are frequently separated according to their efficacy in killing certain groups of organisms: "high-level" disinfectants being synonymous with sterilization; "intermediate-level" capable of destroying all forms of life except bacterial spores; and "low level" destroying such viruses as influenza and herpes but not polio,

hepatitis B, or *Mycobacterium tuberculosis* (Table 32–4).

For surface disinfection of operatory surfaces, one of three disinfectants are commonly used. Each is an effective intermediate level disinfectant when surfaces are kept wet for 10 minutes.

1. Iodophors may be diluted according to manufacturers' directions. They should be diluted fresh daily in soft or distilled water. Only an iodophor registered as a surface disinfectant by the EPA should be used. These are not to be confused with surgical hand-scrubs regulated by the FDA and used undiluted. Iodophors are loose complexes of iodine bound to synthetic carriers, such as povidone. In their "tamed" and diluted form, they are still effective disinfectants but are much less liable to stain cloth or plastic.

2. Phenolic derivatives (O-phenyl phenol 9 percent, and O-benzyl-P-chlorophenol 1 percent) are diluted 1:32, and at least one product is stable after dilution for 60 days. Other claimed advantages are residual phenolic effect and lack of discoloration of instrumentation or hard surfaces.

3. Sodium hypochlorite (laundry bleach) diluted 1:10 to 1:100 is inexpensive and very effective. Caution should be exercised during use because sodium hypochlorite is corrosive for some metals, particularly aluminum. Sodium hypochlorite has the additional

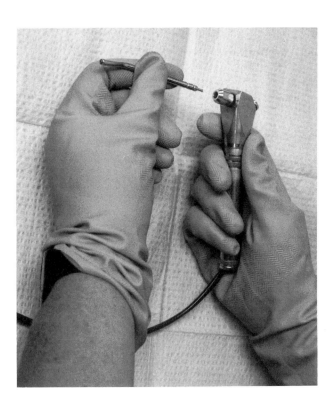

FIGURE 32–3 ✦ Replaceable triplex syringe tips.

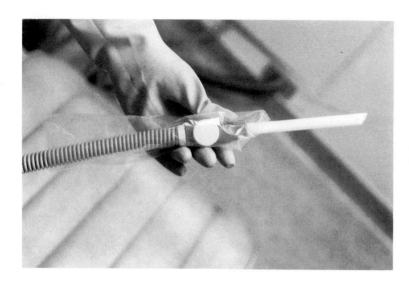

FIGURE 32–4 ✦ Cover difficult to clean high-velocity vacuum valve.

FIGURE 32–5 ✦ Cover light handles with foil.

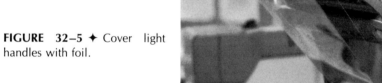

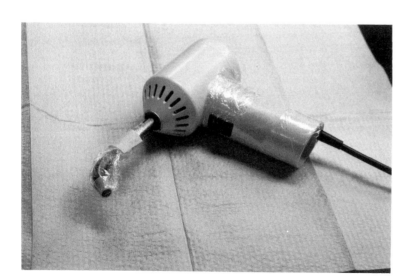

FIGURE 32–6 ✦ Cover composite light-curing "gun" with plastic wrap.

TABLE 32–4 ✦ **A Comparison of Three Levels of Disinfection and Test Groups of Organisms**

| | BACTERIA | | | | | VIRUSES | |
	GRAM-POSITIVE	GRAM-NEGATIVE	*MYCOBACTERIUM TUBERCULOSIS*	SPORES	FUNGI	LIPID	NONLIPID
High	+	+	+	+	+	+	+
Intermediate	+	+	+	−	+	+	+
Low	+	+	−	−	±	+	−

From Crawford, J.: Clinical Asepsis in Dentistry, ed. 3. R. A. Kolstad, Mesquite, Tex, 1986, p. 28.

disadvantage of bleaching fabrics and making the office smell like a swimming pool.

SUGGESTED STEPS FOR SURFACE DISINFECTION

Scrub exposed items such as the triplex syringe head or vacuum valve thoroughly and rinse them clean. At best, utilize a sink, scrub brush, and running water. Otherwise, use 4-inch by 4-inch sponges or paper towels.

Wet items or surfaces to be disinfected with the disinfectant for the time specified by the manufacturer, usually about 10 minutes.

Specific Techniques

There are two methods to disinfect and prepare the dental unit. *Technique I* (Dr. James Crawford, UNC 1986) utilizes paper towels and a fine-mist spray bottle. Paper towels are cheaper, larger, and faster to use than gauze sponges.

First, put on utility gloves. Remove instruments, tip of air-water syringe, and so forth. Discard any used covers. Wash the gloves.

Second, disinfect smooth surfaces and controls. (Control switches should not be sprayed directly because excess fluid may cause short circuits.) To do this, moisten a paper towel with disinfectant spray and scrub smooth surfaces and controls. Wipe each item clean. Spray another paper towel and wipe them again, leaving them moist so the disinfectant will continue to act.

Third, hoses and attached instrumentation must be disinfected.

1. Hold a paper towel behind items in the forked holders to catch excess spray. Spray both sides of the items with disinfectant; for example, suction hose ends, air-water syringe handle (Fig. 32–7).
2. Use a clean brush to scrub each item with irregular surfaces and lay the item across the support or empty instrument tray.
3. Spray supports and wipe them clean with a paper towel.
4. Spray another towel and wipe each hose end and attached instrumentation. Wipe each hose along its most accessible length; place it back in its support.
5. When all items are replaced, hold a paper towel behind them to catch excess spray. Spray and leave them wet until they are ready

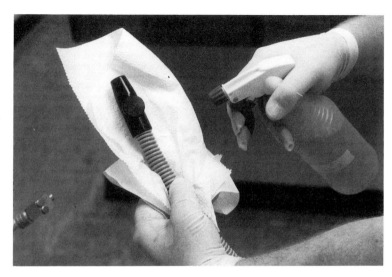

FIGURE 32–7 ✦ Example of surface disinfection of suction hose end using spray mist technique.

to use. Ten minutes is specified on most labels. Any items still wet can be dried with a paper towel before use.

6. Moisten a paper towel with disinfectant and wipe the areas of the chair that have become contaminated, controls, and arms. Leave the chair to dry.

Fourth, disinfect trays and lamp handles. To do this, wipe trays clean and dry and cover with film backed covers. Place foil or film covers on the lamp handles. (There is no need to disinfect anything that has been covered.) Spray and clean outside, then inside of cuspidor. Wash gloves, disinfect faucet handles, remove gloves, and wash hands.

The final step after each appointment is to put on utility gloves; remove instruments, tip of air-water syringe, and so on; discard any used covers; wash gloves; and clean the unit as described. Do *not* replace covers when vacating the unit.

In *Technique II,* three-by-three-inch or four-by-four-inch gauze sponges wet with disinfectant solution are used. Gauze sponges can be soaked ahead in solution of synthetic phenols but not iodophor. Put on "heavy-duty" utility gloves and remove instruments, tips of air-water syringes, and other such items. Discard any used covers; wash gloves. Next, moisten each item and surface to be disinfected, and scrub or brush to remove all debris. Remove each air-water syringe, handpiece, and the vacuum hose form its holder to clean forks (Fig. 32–8). Then, with a second soaked sponge, thoroughly wet the items and leave wet for the required time. Some clinicians like to wrap gauze around the item to be disinfected until needed for the next patient. After each appointment, put on utility gloves, remove instruments, tip of air-water syringe, handpieces and so on. Discard any used covers, wash gloves, and clean the unit as described earlier. Do not replace the covers when vacating the unit.

Handpieces and air-water syringe tips are subject to heavy contamination. The required method for decontaminating the hand-piece and the air-water syringe tip is sterilization. Follow the manufacturer's instructions for cleaning, lubricating and sterilizing *very carefully.* Proper technique is essential to maximize the useful working life of dental handpieces. When purchasing equipment, especially handpieces, choose heat sterilizable units. All handpiece manufacturers in the United States market handpieces that can be sterilized by either an autoclave at 121°C or a chemiclave at 132°C.

Units, controls, and hoses of smooth material are much easier to disinfect than those with knurled knobs, recesses, and corrugations. Operatory floors of seamless vinyl or similar products are relatively easy to clean and disinfect, whereas carpeting is impossible to adequately clean and disinfect.

Dental Water Systems

Dental unit water systems typically contain significant lengths of small diameter plastic tubing. This tubing is conducive to the formation of biofilms such as plaque on the inside of our arteries. These biofilms multiply during periods of non-use such as overnight or weekends, possibly causing the water delivered from the high-speed handpiece or ultrasonic scaler to be highly contaminated with numerous bacteria, especially *Pseudomonas* and *Legionella* species. Only rarely has infection of patients been reported from waterline contamination. However, many dental workers, especially dentists and hygienists, have developed much higher levels of antibodies to *Pseudomonas* and to

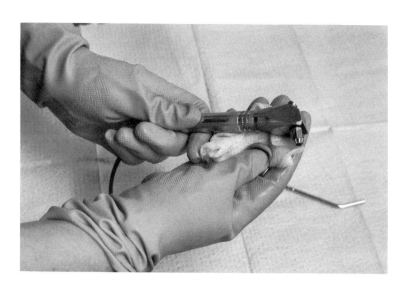

FIGURE 32–8 ✦ Surface disinfection using 4 × 4 sponge to clean and disinfect triplex syringe. *Note* heavy gloves.

Legionella than dental technicians or the general public, suggesting a higher exposure.

To reduce contamination in dental waterlines, the ADA recommends a minimum 2-minute flush of each waterline prior to the first patient of the day and then a 20- to 30-second flush between each patient. Newer systems are being studied to reduce the biofilm problems such as constant water recirculation, filtration, and chemical disinfection between patients.

Impressions

Laboratory technicians and other patients are frequently exposed to pathogens from dental impressions, stone casts, and appliances. The ADA recommends that all impressions be rinsed to remove saliva, blood, and debris followed by disinfection before being cast in die stone or sent to a dental laboratory. Disinfection of irreversible hydrocolloid may be more difficult than other materials since virus is apparently absorbed by alginate. Note that no single disinfectant is compatible with all impression materials. Alginate impression materials and dental stone with disinfectant properties are now being marketed. (See Table 32–5.) An alternative to impression disinfection is to sterilize or disinfect the stone cast. Stone casts may be sterilized in an ethylene oxide sterilizer or disinfected by immersion for 10 minutes in diluted iodophor or diluted hypochlorite. At the minimum, impressions should be rinsed carefully of saliva and debris and then immersed for 10 minutes in an approved disinfectant, such as diluted iodophor.

Appliances

Prosthodontic and orthodontic appliances should be disinfected or sterilized before delivery and before and after any laboratory adjustments. The simplest techniques utilize a disposable plastic drinking cup or zip-lock baggie. Ultrasonic clean-

TABLE 32–5 ✦ Guide for Selection of Disinfectant Solutions

	GLUTAR-ALDEHYDES*	IODOPHORS†	CHLORINE COMPOUNDS‡	COMPLEX PHENOLICS*	PHENOLIC GLUTAR-ALDEHYDES§
Impressions					
Alginate	−	+	+	−	−
Polysulfide rubber base	+	+	+	+	+
Silicone rubber	+	+	+	+	+
Polyether	−	−	+	−	−
ZOE Impression paste	+	+	−	?	+
Reversible hydro-colloid	−	+	+	?	+
Compound	−	+	+	−	+
Prostheses‖					
Fixed (metal/porcelain)	+	+/−	−	?	+
Removable (acrylic/porcelain)	−	+	+	−	−
Removable (metal/acrylic)	−	+/−	+/−	−	−

Impressions/prostheses should be rinsed under running tap water and then immersed for the time recommended for TB disinfection with the selected product. Thorough rinsing of impressions and prostheses under running tap water following disinfection is necessary to remove any residual disinfectant.

+ = recommended method; − = not recommended; +/− = use with caution to avoid damage to metal; ? = data not available or inconclusive.

*Prepared according to the manufacturer's instructions.
†1:213 dilution.
‡1:10 dilution of commercial bleach or prepared according to the manufacturer's instructions.
§Diluted as per the manufacturer's instructions for disinfection.
‖May also be ethylene oxide sterilized.

From Merchant, V.: Update on disinfection of impressions, prosthesis, and costs. J.C.D.A. 10:33, 1992.

ing for 3 to 5 minutes will greatly aid the removal of debris of heavily contaminated appliances. The appliance is scrubbed free of debris and then immersed in the chosen disinfectant for 10 minutes.

Freshly diluted iodophor or chlorine compounds are the disinfectants most widely recommended. The clinician must be careful to rinse the appliance thoroughly with water prior to delivery to remove corrosive and toxic agents.

Rag wheels, felt wheels, points, and bristle brushes can be easily sterilized with the steam autoclave or chemiclave. One should use fresh pumice delivered in a disposable paper or plastic tray and moistened with a disinfectant. After adjustment and polishing, the appliances are disinfected, rinsed carefully, and delivered to the patient.

Recommendations for the commercial laboratory are similar to those for the dental office and are addressed in guidelines published by the ADA in August 1992.

STERILIZATION

All instruments that contact saliva or blood should be sterilized, using ADA-accepted methods of sterilization, before storage or subsequent patient use (Table 32–6). Since 1974, and certainly since the 1985 AIDS "epidemic," the standard of care in the United States is for sterilization according to the ACA/CDC guidelines rather than disinfection. At least six states enacted laws in 1992 requiring heat sterilization of dental instruments and handpieces. It is considered unethical to ignore the recommendations of the ADA and the CDC; in addition, ignoring those guidelines leaves the practitioner defenseless in court regarding post-treatment infections.

Cleaning

The first step before instrument sterilization is removal of most organic debris, blood, and saliva.

TABLE 32–6 ✦ A Comparison of Sterilization Methods

METHOD	ACTIVITY	CONDITIONS	LIMITATIONS	ADVANTAGES	SPORE TESTING
Steam auto-clave	Protein denatur-ation	20 min. at 121°C (250°F) 132°C 3–7 min. (270°F)	Rust and corro-sion (Protect with 2% so-dium nitrite), some plastic and rubber items may be damaged	Time efficient, good pene-tration, can sterilize wa-ter based liquids	*Bacillus stear-othermophi-lus* strips
Unsaturated chemical vapor	Protein denatur-ation and al-kylation	20 min. 132°C (270°F)	May damage some plastic and rubber items	Time efficient, no rusting	*Bacillus stear-othermophi-lus* strips
Dry heat	Oxydation	60–120 min., 160°C (320°F)	May damage some plastic and rubber items	No rusting, large capac-ity, low cost	*Bacillus sub-tilis* strips
Rapid heat transfer		6–12 min., 190°C (375°F)	Small capacity	Time efficient	
Ethylene oxide	Alkylation	3 hrs, 49°C (120°F)	Slow—may re-quire up to 24 hours areation	No damage to heat sensi-tive items	*Bacillus sub-tilis* strips
		12 hrs am-bient	Toxic and car-cinogenic		
Glutaral-dehyde	Alkylation	6–10 hrs, 20°C (68°F)	Requires rinsing and han-dling, no proof of ster-ilization, NOT for handpieces	No damage to heat sensi-tive items, low cost	None possible

Instruments and other reusable items from the operatory are removed to a central cleaning and sterilizing area, where the assistant wears heavy-duty rubber gloves to discard disposable items and either clean instruments immediately or submerge in a holding disinfecting solution to prevent drying of organic debris before cleaning. Holding for a short period of time (30 to 60 minutes) can be accomplished using soap solutions or immersion in disinfectants such as iodophor or phenolics. For periods more than 60 minutes, synthetic phenols would be the agents of choice owing to their antirust and disinfectant properties.

Regardless of the choice of holding solution, thorough cleaning requires the operator to wear heavy rubber gloves and brush visible debris from individual instruments under running water. Attempting to scrub several instruments at a time may lead to punctures or cuts. Continue cleaning with an ultrasonic cleaner with detergent specifically designed for these cleaners. Ultrasonic cleaning is generally thought to be much safer, efficient, and more effective than handscrubbing (Fig. 32–9). Operate the ultrasonic cleaner with closed cover for at least 10 minutes. Following cleaning, the instruments are rinsed under running water and carefully dried before sterilizing.

The cleansing action of ultrasonic cleaners frequently decreases with time, so it is useful to test its action periodically. Recommended user testing requires filling the ultrasonic cleaner with detergent solution and running the cleaner until it is warmed up. A piece of regular-strength aluminum foil is one-half immersed by holding it vertically into the solution for exactly 20 seconds. It is then inspected for the evidence of minute bubbles and holes in the immersed half of the foil by holding it up to a light. If there are holes or bubbles, the ultrasonic cleaner is still operating efficiently; if not, it needs to be repaired or replaced.

Drying instruments before sterilization is important for proper sterilization function and for rust inhibition.

Packaging

Proper packaging of instruments prior to sterilization depends on the method chosen for sterilization. Generally, packaging instruments prior to sterilization is preferred because handling and storage after sterilization is simplified and chances of contamination are minimized. There are numerous systems for instrument packaging including trays and cassettes that fit specific sterilizers and simplify packaging and reuse. Several manufacturers make sterilizing bags and wraps from a variety of paper and plastic materials. Packaging guidelines from the ADA and the sterilizer manufacturers should be followed. The following is a summary of ADA-approved sterilization methods (Table 32–6).

Storage

Storing sterilized instruments in packages in cassettes or packed on trays has several advantages over "loose" storage (Fig. 32–10). The safest, most efficient handling of storage is to use separate cassettes of instruments for each anticipated procedure. These are stored after sterilization in closed cabinets and opened just prior to the procedure. Obtaining and handling of "loose," or cabinet-stored, instruments requires sterile pick-up forceps, overgloves, or paper towel, being careful not to contaminate doors or drawers.

Disposable items are best stored in covered containers and dispensed in appropriate numbers anticipated for the immediate procedure.

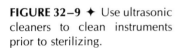

FIGURE 32–9 ✦ Use ultrasonic cleaners to clean instruments prior to sterilizing.

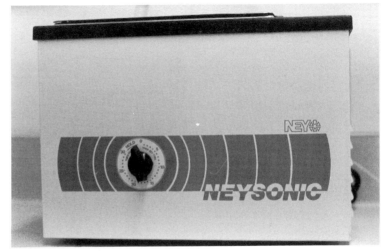

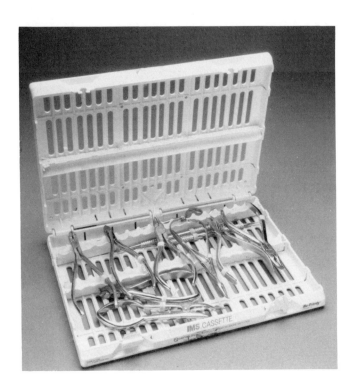

FIGURE 32–10 ✦ Instrument cassette.

Autoclave Sterilization

The word "autoclave" means self-locking and is used to denote an apparatus that sterilizes by the use of steam under pressure. Autoclaves operate on the same principle as pressure cookers (Fig. 32–11). Saturated steam is much more efficient for destroying microorganisms than either boiling water or dry heat. At 100°C, there is at least seven times as much available heat from saturated steam as from boiling water. Thus, the presence of air in packages hinders the penetration of steam and delays or prevents sterilization. The following section summarizes the different holding times required for sterilization.

PARAMETERS

The parameters are 121°C (250°F), for 15 minutes, at 15 psi; or 132°C (270°F), for 3 to 7 minutes, at 30 psi for unwrapped instruments. Add 5 minutes for moderately wrapped packs.

RECOMMENDED PACKAGING

The instruments should be packaged either "loose" or wrapped in muslin cloth, paper, nylon, aluminum foil, steam permeable plastic; there should be no impermeable closed containers.

ADVANTAGES

Autoclaving provides the most efficient and reliable sterilization available. Autoclaves are usually quite simple to operate and are relatively inexpensive. Most dental instruments and devices can be safely autoclaved (Table 32–7). Flexibility of packaging, loading and cycles for liquids, and cloth goods are advantageous.

DISADVANTAGES

Nonstainless metal instruments may oxidize (rust) unless protected by a reducing agent or "emulsion" dip prior to packaging and autoclaving. Two percent sodium nitrite is an effective rust inhibitor. Low-melting plastics and rubber cups may melt or distort. Items that retain moisture take time to dry, thus extending the cycle time.

MONITORING AUTOCLAVE STERILIZATION

Biologic indicators available as spore strips and glass ampules should be used at least weekly as recommended by the ADA and CDC to assure the efficacy of the sterilization procedure. Process and dosage indicators also are available to indicate processing or gross errors in technique.

Dry Heat Sterilization

When used properly, dry heat is an effective and accepted method of instrument sterilization. This method requires more time to sterilize (10 to 90 minutes per cycle), owing to warm-up time.

Ovens are manufactured specifically for medical and dental use (Fig. 32–12). However, a number of commercial, home, laboratory, and industrial ovens will be suitable. Mechanical convection

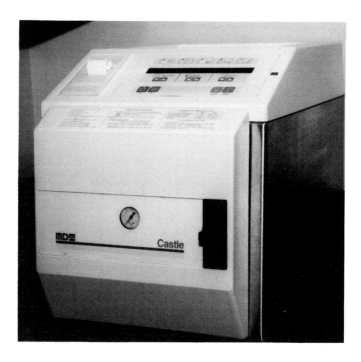

FIGURE 32–11 ✦ Steam autoclave.

ovens, usually available, provide more even and rapid heating.

The efficiency of dry heat ovens depends mainly on the power available per cubic foot of the chamber. The minimum for a 30-minute warm-up time is 550 watts per cubic foot.

An accurate pyrometer, thermocouple, or thermometer is needed to verify the actual temperatures for determining cycle time.

A newer dry heat "rapid head transfer" device has gained wide acceptance in dentistry due to short cycle and convenience.

PARAMETERS

The parameters are as follows: 170°C (340°F) for 60 minutes cycle time. For the rapid heat transfer device, the temperature is 375°F (190°C). The time is 12 minutes for packaged instruments or 6 minutes for unwrapped instruments. Even shorter cycles are being studied for hand piece sterilization.

RECOMMENDED PACKAGING AND LOADING

Instruments should be packaged "loose" (or bare) and loaded a finger's space apart for minimum warm-up time. Lightly wrapping with paper or aluminum foil increases time required from 45 to 60 minutes.

ADVANTAGES

The advantages include large volume capacity, low-cost equipment and operation, and no rusting or dulling of dry instruments.

DISADVANTAGES

The disadvantages are:
1. Careful loading, packaging, and temperature monitoring are essential.
2. Temperatures above 175°C (350°F) may melt solders in instruments and impression trays.
3. Dry heat is not suitable for rubber plastics, and most high-speed handpieces.
4. Longer, long-cycle times compared with autoclave.

STERILIZATION MONITORING

Spore strips should be used weekly as a biologic indicator. Color change strip labels and bags are available as process indicators. Stick-on labels are available as dosage indicators.

Unsaturated Chemical Vapor

A mixture of formaldehyde, alcohol, ketone, water, and acetone heated under pressure forms a gas that can sterilize instruments. The Chemiclave requires the use of a solution, "Vapo-steril." The Chemiclave is in widespread effective use in offices and clinics at present (Fig. 32–13).

PARAMETERS

For this method, heat at 270°F (132°C), at 20 to 40 psi for 20 minutes. The unit must be preheated before use.

RECOMMENDED PACKAGING

Pack instruments bare or in muslin, paper, steam-permeable plastic, or nylon. Avoid paper or

TABLE 32–7 ✦ Sterilization and Disinfection of Dental Instruments, Materials, and Some Commonly Used Items*

	STEAM AUTOCLAVE	DRY HEAT OVEN	CHEMICAL VAPOR	ETHYLENE OXIDE	CHEMICAL AGENTS	OTHER METHODS & COMMENTS
Angle attachments*	+	+	+	+ +	+	
Burs						
Carbon steel	−	+ +	+ +	+ +	−	Discard
Steel	+	+ +	+ +	+ +	−	Discard
Tungsten-carbide	+	+ +	+	+ +	−	Discard
Condensers	+ +	+ +	+ +	+ +	+	
Dappen dishes	+ +	+	+	+ +	+	
Endodontic instruments (broaches, files, reamers)	+ +	+ +	+ +	+ +	−	
Stainless steel handles	+	+ +	+ +	+ +	+	
Stainless w/plastic handles	+ +	+ +	−	+ +	−	
Fluoride gel trays						
Heat-resistant plastic	+ +	=	−	+ +	−	
Nonheat resistant plastic	=	=	−	+ +	−	Discard (+ +)
Glass slabs	+ +	+ +	+ +	+ +	+	
Hand instruments						
Carbon steel	−	+ +	+ +	+ +	−	
	(Steam autoclave with chemical protection [2% sodium nitrite])					
Stainless steel	+ +	+ +	+ +	+ +		
Handpieces*	(+ +)*	−	(+)*	+ +		
Contra-angles	+ +	−	+ +	+ +		
Prophylaxis angles* (disposable preferred)	+	+	+	+		Discard (+ +)
Impression trays						
Aluminum metal	+ +	+	+ +	+ +	−	
Chrome-plated	+ +	+ +	+ +	+ +	+	
Custom acrylic resin	=	=	=	+ +		Discard (+ +)
Plastic	=	=	=	+ +	+	Discard (+ +) preferred
Instruments in packs	+ +	+ Small packs	+ +	+ + Small packs	=	
Instrument tray setups						
Restorative or surgical	+ Size limit	+	+ Size limit	+ + Size limit	=	
Mirrors	−	+ +	+ +	+ +	+	
Needles						
Disposable	=	=	=	=	=	Discard (+ +) Do not reuse

+ + Effective and preferred method.
+ Effective and acceptable method.
− Effective method, but risk of damage to materials.
= Ineffective method with risk of damage to materials.
* Since manufacturers use a variety of alloys and materials in these products, confirmation with the equipment manufacturers is recommended, especially for handpieces and their attachments.
From Infection control recommendations for the dental office and laboratory. J.A.D.A. 123:4–5, 1992.

TABLE 32–7 ✦ Sterilization and Disinfection of Dental Instruments, Materials, and Some Commonly Used Items *Continued*

	STEAM AUTOCLAVE	DRY HEAT OVEN	CHEMICAL VAPOR	ETHYLENE OXIDE	CHEMICAL AGENTS	OTHER METHODS & COMMENTS
Nitrous oxide						
Nose piece	(+ +)*	=	(+ +)*	+ +	(+)*	
Hoses	(+ +)*	=	(+ +)*	+ +	(+)*	
Orthodontic pliers						
High-quality stainless	+ +	+ +	+ +	+ +	−	
Low-quality stainless	−	+ +	+ +	+ +	−	
W/plastic parts	=	=	=	+ +	+	
Pluggers & Condensers	+ +	+ +	+ +	+ +	+	
Polishing wheels & disks						
Garnet and cuttle	=	−	−	+ +	=	
Rag	+ +	−	+	+ +	=	
Rubber	+	−	−	+ +	−	
Protheses, removable	−	−	−	+	+	
Rubber dam equipment						
Carbon steel clamps	−	+ +	+ +	+ +	−	
Metal frames	+ +	+ +	+ +	+ +	+	
Plastic frames	−	−	−	+ +	+	
Punches	−	+ +	+ +	+ +	+	
Stainless steel clamps	+ +	+ +	+ +	+ +	+	
Rubber items						
Prophylaxis cups	−	−	−	+ +	−	Discard (+ +)
Saliva evacuators, ejectors (plastic)	−	−	−	−		Discard (+ +) (single use/disposable)
Stones						
Diamond	+	+ +	+ +	+ +	−	
Polishing	+ +	+	+ +	+ +	−	
Sharpening	+ +	+ +	+ +	−	−	
Surgical instruments						
Stainless steel	+ +	+ +	+ +	+ +	−	
Ultrasonic scaling tips	+	=	=	+ +	+	
Water-air syringe tips	+ +	+ +	+ +	+ +	−	(Discard (+ +)
Radiographic equipment						
Plastic film holders	(+ +)*	=	(+)*	+ +	+	
Collimating devices	−	=	=	+ +	+	

tape with a high sulfur content due to blackening of the interior of the chamber and possible damage to the valve.

ADVANTAGES

The advantages of this method are rapid efficient cycle time, lack of rust and corrosion, and availability of good instructions and services.

DISADVANTAGES

Unsaturated chemical vapor does not penetrate heavily wrapped packages as well as steam. The high temperature necessary may melt some plastics and rubber goods. Chemiclaves may not be safe to sterilize some autoclavable handpieces. Consult the handpiece manufacturer.

MONITORING STERILIZATION

Biologic indicators—spore strips—must be used weekly to determine sterilization. Instrument bags are available that include a process indicator. The process indicator's color change does not ensure sterilization has occurred.

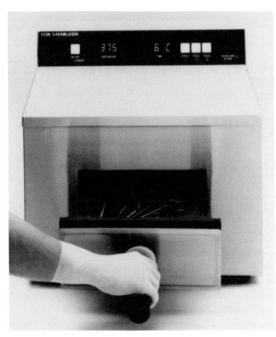

FIGURE 32–12 ✦ Rapid heat transfer device.

Ethylene Oxide Sterilizers

Gas sterilization with ethylene oxide at ambient temperatures is useful for sterilizing virtually any material including plastics, rubber, handpieces, casts, and appliances. Ethylene oxide gas is toxic to all bacteria, fungi, viruses, and spores at room temperature.

PARAMETERS

Heat at 120°F for 2 to 3 hours for sterilization. At room temperature, sterilization time is 12 hours. Aeration of permeable materials, plastics, rubber, or cloth requires 12 to 24 hours. Adequate humidity is required for sterilization. Ventilation to the outdoors is required.

ADVANTAGE

This method sterilizes virtually anything, except liquids, at room temperature.

DISADVANTAGES

The EPA and OSHA monitor carefully the use or misuse of ethylene oxide sterilizers, since the gas is potentially mutagenic and carcinogenic and is directly toxic to skin. The manufacturer's instructions must be followed exactly including venting to the outside by a hood and blower device (Fig. 32–14). Total cycle times vary from 2½ to 36 hours.

MONITORING STERILIZATION

Spore strips and ampules are available for biologic monitoring. Tape and labels are available for process indicators. Glass ampules and paper strips are available for dosage indicators.

Glutaraldehyde Sterilization

Several glutaraldehyde solutions are available that are registered with the EPA for sterilization. Depending on their use, glutaraldehydes are effec-

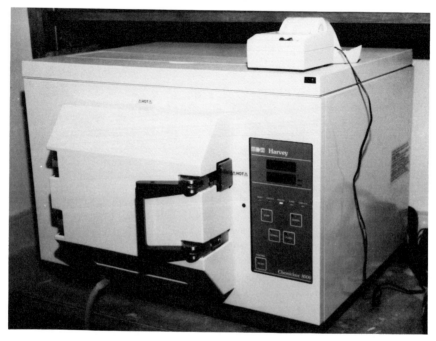

FIGURE 32–13 ✦ Chemiclave sterilizer.

tive up to 28 days after activation. Products are available in alkaline, neutral, and acidic pH ranges (see Table 32–8). Glutaraldehydes are useful as immersion solutions for instrument and product sterilization.

PARAMETERS

For this method, 6 to 10 hours are required for sterilization at room temperature. Dilution by water limits the useful life to 28 days or less in most examples.

ADVANTAGES

Heat sensitive plastics, rubbers, and fiber optics can be safely sterilized. No expensive equipment is required. The cost for use is relatively low.

DISADVANTAGES

Postexposure rinsing and handling are required. Skin and mucous membrane toxicity requires gloves while handling. Dilution is difficult to detect except by test kits or indicator strips that monitor the concentration of glutaraldehyde. Chemical disinfection is not recommended for high-speed handpieces, prophy angles, or most dental instruments and devices.

MONITORING STERILIZATION

Monitoring sterilization is very difficult because there are no biologic monitors available. Concentration test strips and indicator solutions are now available to monitor glutaraldehyde concentration.

Solution should be discarded below 1 percent glutaraldehyde.

Other sterilization methods are being studied and evaluated for possible dental use. They include microwave irradiation and chlorine gas generators. (See Table 32–8 for a summary of sterilization and disinfection methods and materials.)

STERILIZATION ASSURANCE

It is very important to know and record that sterilization has occurred. Surveys using biologic indicators (spore strips) have shown that from 15 to 51 percent of sterilizers in unmonitored private practices fail to sterilize when tested with standard spore strips.

Theoretically, sterilizers function properly when used according to the manufacturer's directions. In clinical use, there are many ways to reduce the effectiveness of sterilization procedures, including improper packaging and loading and lack of water in autoclaves (or solution in chemiclaves) resulting in normal temperature readings but no sterilization. Carefully read and follow all the manufacturer's instructions for your sterilizer including varying time required for various materials, packaging, and loading.

Sterility assurance requires the use of bacterial spores. These are required when setting up new or repaired equipment and at regular intervals. The ADA and CDC recommend and several states require weekly spore tests. Process or dosage indi-

TABLE 32–8 ✦ A Comparison of Chemical Disinfecting/Sterilizing Agents

CHEMICAL CLASSIFICATION	TB DIRECTIONS	STERILANT	REUSE (DAYS)
Surface Only			
Chlorine compounds	1:10 10 min 20°C	No	None
Phenylphenol + ethanol	10 min.	No	None
Surface/Immersion			
Iodophor (1.75% titratable iodine)	1:213 10 min.	No	None
Complex phenols	1:32 10 min.	No	None
Phenylphenol + benzylchlorphenol			
Immersion Only			
Glutaraldehyde + phenolics	1:20 10 min.	FS 6 hrs	30 days
Glutaraldehyde, 2% neutral	FS 10 min.	FS 10 hrs	30 days
Glutaraldehyde, 2% acidic	FS 30 min.	FS 10 hrs	30 days
Glutaraldehyde, 2% alkaline	FS 10–90 min.	FS 6–10 hrs	30 days

The American Dental Association *does not* endorse any disinfectant or sterilization product.
Always look for EPA registration and directions for killing TB on the bottle.
Always make sure the solutions are compatible with your instruments or equipment.
None of the solutions is acceptable for disinfection of high-speed handpieces. ADA, 5/92.
Sources of information as to which products are available in the above categories can be obtained from OSAP, 1 (800) 243-1233.

cators are used for each load to verify sterilizing conditions or to detect gross errors.

Biologic Indicators

Biologic monitors or spore tests use paper strips containing a measured number of heat-resistant, harmless, bacterial spores. These strips are packaged in envelopes, capsules, or ampules (Figs. 32–14 and 32–15). Usually, two test strips and one control are needed for each testing procedure. The procedure should be performed in the following manner.

The test strips are placed in the sterilizing load in the center of the load or in a large pack. The control strip is left outside the sterilizer. The sterilizer is operated according to the manufacturer's instructions including times, temperatures, and solution required.

After the sterilizing cycle is completed, the test monitor strips are removed and, with the control strip, are cultured and incubated for growth. This may be done in the office, by the manufacturer, or at a commercial or university laboratory. The results of each test are recorded and maintained for future reference.

If the results indicate that sterilization has not occurred, the unit should be retested immediately and instruments should be sterilized by alternate methods until the results of further testing indicate that sterilization has occurred. If the second test fails, the sterilizer needs to be repaired by qualified service personnel.

Advantage. The results are proof of sterilizing conditions at time of test.

Disadvantage. The results are not available for several days to a week after culturing.

PROCESS INDICATORS

Process indicators are used to indicate sterilizer processing for each load cycled. They do not prove sterilization, but are useful for indicating processing and gross handling problems or sterilizer failure to heat.

Process indicators are found on bags, tags, and strips, as well as the familiar "autoclave tape," and indicate processing by color change. The results of process indicator tests should be recorded and saved for future reference.

Advantages. The advantages to process indicators include that they afford "instant" results and can be used for each load.

Disadvantage. The disadvantage is that process indicators do not verify sterilization, only processing.

DOSAGE INDICATORS

Dosage indicators indicate heat or gas penetration into packs or instrument loads but do not indicate precise conditions of sterilization. Stick-on labels, paper strips, or glass ampules are supplied for various techniques. The results of dosage indicators should be retained for reference.

Advantages. Dosage indicators can be read immediately and provide more useful information than process indicators.

Disadvantages. These indicators are not a biologic monitor of sterilization and are not considered an acceptable substitute for spore strips.

CONCLUSIONS

Dental care providers must seek the best for our patients and not be the source of serious illness among patients, coworkers, or family. However, it

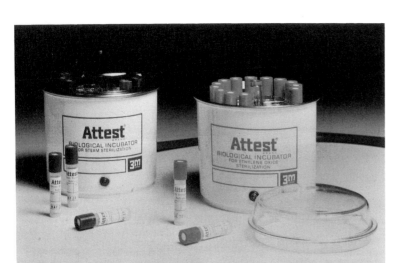

FIGURE 32–14 ✦ Biologic indicator ampules and incubators.

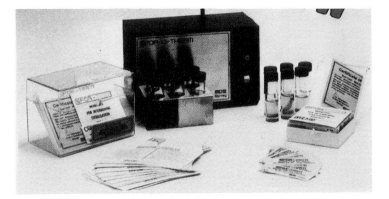

FIGURE 32–15 ✦ Biologic monitors and incubator using spore strips.

is difficult to significantly change the approach to everyday asepsis in the office. The technology now is available to decrease, to a large degree, the risk of infection for the patient and the dental staff.

First, and perhaps most importantly, steps should be taken to wash hands carefully and to wear gloves whenever there is any contact between the hands and saliva. Second, sterilization methods known to kill all life forms should be used on dental instruments. Third, surfaces, units and controls should be cleaned and disinfected. Patients and the general public should be assured that dental care is extremely safe.

BIBLIOGRAPHY

Block, S. S.: Disinfection, Sterilization and Preservation, ed. 3. Lea and Febiger, Philadelphia, 1983.
American Dental Association: OSHA: What You Must Know. American Dental Association Regulatory Compliance Manual. American Dental Association, Chicago, 1990.
American Dental Association: OSHA: What You Must Know. American Dental Association, Chicago, 1992.
C.D.A. J.-1992(10): Major Issue on Infection Control.
CDC: Recommendation for prevention of HIV transmission in health-care settings. MMWR (Suppl.) 36:25, 1987.
CDC: Current trends—Recommended infection-control practices for dentistry. MMWR 35:237, 1986.
Centers for Disease Control: Protection against viral hepatitis. MMWR 39:1-26, 1990.
Centers for Disease Control: Recommendations for preventing transmission of human immunodeficiency virus and hepatitis B virus to patients during exposure-prone invasive procedures. MMWR 40:1–9, 1991.
Clinical Research Associates Newsletter, 307 North Canyon Road, Suite 6, Provo, Utah, 84604.
Control: The Infectious Newsletter. Infection Control Publications, 850 N. Highway 91, Suite 7-K, P.O. Box 541, North Salt Lake, Utah 84054.
Cottone, J. A., Tevezhalmy, G. T., and Molinari, J. A.: Practical Infection Control in Dentistry. Lea & Febiger, Philadelphia, 1991.

Cottone, J.: Hepatitis B. Transmission and Epidemiology in the Dental Profession. Proceedings of National Conference on Infection Control in Dentistry, U.S. Dept. of Health Care and Human Services. Atlanta, Ga, 1986, pp. 12, 13, 16.
Council on Dental Materials, Instruments and Equipment, Council on Dental Therapeutics, Council on Dental Research, and Council on Dental Practice: Infection control recommendations for the dental office and the dental laboratory. J.A.D.A., 123:8 (suppl), 1992.
Crawford, J.: Clinical Asepsis in Dentistry, ed. 3. R. A. Kolstad, Mesquite, Tex, 1986.
Division of Scientific Affairs of the ADA Facts About AIDS for the Dental Team, ed. 3, Chicago, J.A.D.A., 122: supplement, 1991.
J.A.D.A.-1992: 123(1) Infection Control Update.
J.A.D.A.-1993: 124(1) Infection Control Update.
Manuella, J. P., et al.: An outbreak of herpes simplex virus type I gingivostomatitis in a dental hygiene practice. J.A.M.A. 252:2019, 1984.
McCray, E.: Special report, occupation risk of the acquired immunodeficiency syndrome among health care workers. N. Engl. J. Med. 314:1131, 1986.
Merchant, V.: Update on disinfection of impressions, prosthesis, and costs. J.C.D.A. 10:31–35, 1992.
Miller, C. H.: Cleaning, Sterilization and Disinfection: Basis of microbial killing for infection control. J.A.D.A. 124:48–56, 1993.
O.S.A.P. (office sterilization and asepsis procedures research foundation). 2150 West 29th Avenue, Suite 500, Denver Col., 80211.
OSHA Department of Labor, Occupational Safety and Health Administrator, 29, CFR Part 1910, 1030 occupational exposure to bloodborne pathogens: Final rule. Fed. Reg. 56:235, 64004–64182, 1991.
Runnels, R.: Infection control in the wet finger environment. Publishers Press, Salt Lake, Utah, 1984.
Russell, A. D., Hugo, W. B., and Ayliffe, G. A. J.: Principles and Practice of Sterilization. Blackwell Scientific Publications, Oxford, 1982, pp. 3–6.
Schafer, M. E.: Practical Infection Control in the Dental Office. Henry Scheiss, Port Washington, N.Y., 1985.
Whitaker, R. J., Robins, S. K., Williams, B. L., and Crawford, J. J.: Dental Asepsis. Stoma Press, Seattle, 1979.

33 *Antimicrobials and Antibiotics*

Sebastian G. Ciancio

CHAPTER OUTLINE

Basic principles
Use in dentistry
Management of the patient with various cardiac problems

Antimicrobial agents either suppress the growth of microorganisms or destroy them. They are divided into three categories: antibiotics, sulfonamides, and antiseptics. In dentistry, antibiotics are currently the most frequently used.

Antimicrobial drugs were first used by Paul Ehrlich, who treated syphilis with salvarsan, an organic chemical. Much later, in 1936, sulfonamides were introduced. Antibiotics became available in 1941 with the clinical introduction of penicillin. Since then, numerous antibiotics have been introduced and new ones are constantly being evaluated. Topical "antiseptics" were considered as early as the 1800s, but with the introduction of chlorhexidine in the 1960s in Europe and in 1986 in the United States, considerable dental interest has been stimulated in antiseptic agents.

This chapter focuses on antimicrobial agents of clinical importance in dentistry. Other antimicrobials are discussed elsewhere in this book.

BASIC PRINCIPLES

Antibiotics originally were isolated from microorganisms and either retarded the growth or killed other microorganisms. Today many antibiotics are chemically synthesized.

Depending on the antibiotic, there are several mechanisms of action, including inhibition of bacterial cell wall synthesis, alteration of bacterial cell membrane permeability, alteration in the bacterial synthesis of cellular components, and inhibition of bacterial cell metabolism.

General Concepts

Certain terms and concepts are necessary for understanding the pharmacology of antibiotics.

RESISTANCE

Microorganisms are sometimes resistant or unaffected by an antibiotic. Resistance can be (1) natural (present before contact with the antibiotic) or (2) acquired, developing during exposure to the drug. Acquired resistance via a plasmid is a result of a change in the microorganism's DNA, which is genetically inherited by subsequent generations. Therefore, once resistance develops, a new antibiotic must be found to control the resistant bacteria.

Microorganisms resistant to one antimicrobial agent frequently are resistant to other chemically-related drugs. This is referred to as *cross-resistance*. Occasionally, cross-resistance to two chemically dissimilar drugs occurs. Resistance usually results from antibiotic inactivation by bacterial enzymes, development of alternate bacterial metabolic pathways unaffected by antibiotics, or biochemical alterations in the bacteria preventing uptake or binding of the antibiotic.

Antibiotic ineffectiveness results not only from resistance but also from inadequate therapy that does not control the large numbers of microorganisms. At other times, low antibiotic doses only destroy the more susceptible microorganisms and allow the more resistant to survive. This phenomenon is called *selective pressure*. The process of selecting increasingly less susceptible or resistant microorganisms occurs in a stepwise manner over a period of time. Therefore, it is imperative that the initial antibiotic dose is sufficient and given long enough for successful therapy. Finally, antibiotics can also be ineffective if they are antagonized by interacting with other drugs.

SPECTRUM OF ACTIVITY

No antibiotic is effective against all microorganisms encountered in oral infections. Instead, they have a certain spectrum of activity. Some antibiotics affect only a few microorganisms and have a very limited spectrum of activity and others affect a wide variety and have a broad spectrum of activity. Broad-spectrum antibiotics are only necessary for infections caused by a mixed flora. Because of the limited range of activity of antibiotics, it is important to select one effective against the infecting microorganism. The ideal method is to isolate the microorganism from the lesion or infected site and culture it to determine its susceptibility to different antibiotics (culture and sensitivity) (Chapter 34). At times, selection of an antibiotic is based on clinical experience, which sometimes leads to mistakes.

SUPERINFECTIONS

Suppression of one group of microorganisms by an antibiotic may permit the growth or "superinfection" by another group that is normally present but usually does not cause disease.

TYPE OF ACTION

Antibiotics are either bacteriostatic or bactericidal. Bacteriostatic antibiotics inhibit the growth and multiplication of microorganisms, permitting the host defenses to deal with their removal. Bactericidal antibiotics directly kill or destroy microorganisms. In general, bacteriostatic antibiotics alter metabolic pathways or synthesis of cellular components that do not destroy the cell. In contrast, bactericidal drugs cause cell death by interfering with the synthesis or function of the cell wall, the cell membrane, or both.

When two bactericidal antibiotics are given together, they may exert a greater effect than when given separately. This is called antibiotic synergism. Sometimes, however, when a bacteriostatic

and a bactericidal antibiotic are given together, their effectiveness is negated or reduced. This is called antibiotic antagonism.

ANTIBIOTICS AND PREGNANCY

During pregnancy, antibiotics should be used with caution. For example, tetracycline given during the last of pregnancy may slow down bone growth, alter enamel formation, and result in permanent tooth discoloration. In addition, many antibiotics appear in the milk of lactating females. However, no adverse effects have been reported with the most commonly used antibiotics.

USE IN DENTISTRY

The antibiotics currently used in dentistry are summarized in Table 33–1.

Penicillin

Penicillin, derived from a mold, *Penicillium notatum,* was the first antibiotic used in humans in 1941. Research has resulted in quantity production not only by biosynthetic *Penicillium* but also by semisynthetic methods.

TYPES OF PENICILLIN

The first penicillin, penicillin G, is still the most effective penicillin against susceptible microorganisms that do not produce penicillinase. Penicillinase, an enzyme produced mainly by staphylococci, breaks down penicillin and renders it inactive. Newer semisynthetic penicillins are not inactivated by penicillinase and are therefore effective against penicillinase-producing bacteria. Augmentin, a combination of amoxicillin and clavulanate potas-

TABLE 33–1 ✦ Antibiotics of Use in Dentistry

	ACTION	
ANTIBIOTIC	**BACTERIOSTATIC**	**BACTERICIDAL**
Penicillin V		✔
Penicillin G		✔
Ampicillin		✔
Erythromycins	✔	
Tetracyclines	✔	
Oxacillin, nafcillin		✔
Cephalosporins		✔
Metronidazole		
Nystatin	✔	
Bacitracin		✔
Lincomycin	✔	
Vancomycin		✔
Streptomycin		✔

From Ciancio and Bourgault, Clinical Pharmacology for Dental Professionals, 1989.

sium, is an example and has been found to be of value in some cases of refractory periodontitis.

MECHANISM OF ACTION

Penicillin is a bactericidal drug that inhibits the synthesis of cell walls of some bacteria leading to high osmotic pressure with swelling, membrane disruption, and subsequent cell death. Because penicillin acts during the synthesis of cell walls, it is most effective against multiplying bacteria.

Once absorbed, penicillin is widely distributed throughout the body including, in small amounts, saliva and gingival crevicular fluid. It crosses the placenta but does not pass the blood–brain barrier in healthy individuals, although it does so in those with meningitis. Penicillin is rapidly eliminated from plasma by the kidneys.

Penicillins are excreted in breast milk in low concentrations. Although significant problems have not been documented, the risk-benefit ratio must be considered before their use by nursing mothers, which in the infant could lead to sensitization, diarrhea, and candidiasis.

ADVERSE EFFECTS

Penicillin toxicity is extremely low and, except for allergic reactions, is one of the safest drugs known.

The incidence of allergic reactions to penicillin has been estimated at 1 to 5 percent. Topical and aerosol preparations of penicillin are more likely to lead to allergic reactions. The oral route is the least likely to cause penicillin allergy.

Patients allergic to one penicillin are likely to be allergic to all other penicillins. Also, those with a history of hypersensitivity to cephalosporins, griseofulvin, or penicillamine may also be allergic to penicillin.

Various procedures have been attempted to determine if a person is allergic to penicillin. The most promising is a skin test with a small amount of penicillin combined with various penicillin derivatives. However, 5 percent of patients with a negative reaction to this skin test still have allergic reactions to penicillin (Chapter 34).

Cephalosporins

These antibiotics are semisynthetically derived from a mold, *Cephalosporium acremonium,* and are structurally related to penicillin.

TYPES OF CEPHALOSPORINS

The cephalosporins are of interest to dentists. Usually, the one advantage of using these antibiotics rather than other antibiotics for treating dental infections is that they may be safe for patients with penicillin allergies. However, there have been reports of cross-hypersensitivity between cephalosporins and penicillin.

MODE OF ACTION

Cephalosporins are bactericidal and inhibit bacterial cell wall synthesis in a manner similar to penicillin. They also inhibit cell division and growth so that lysis of some bacteria occurs. Cephalosporins are broad-spectrum antibiotics and are effective against most gram-positive microorganisms, including staphylococci. They also are effective against strains of gram-negative *Proteus mirabilis, Escherichia coli, Klebsiella,* and *Enterobacter.*

The cephalosporins are recognized as the first drug of choice for non-hospital acquired *Klebsiella* infections and secondly as a substitute for penicillin.

Some bacteria produce cephalosporinases, which inactivate cephalosporins, rendering the bacteria resistant to them.

METABOLISM

Most cephalosporins are widely distributed throughout the body. However, they do not easily cross into the cerebrospinal fluid and are therefore not indicated in meningitis. Most of the administered dose is excreted unchanged in the urine within 4 to 6 hours after administration.

These antibiotics occur in low concentrations in breast milk and do cross the placenta.

ADVERSE EFFECTS

The incidence of allergic reactions is almost as high as with penicillin. Although patients allergic to penicillin may not be allergic to the cephalosporins, the possibility of an allergic reaction to cephalosporins is higher in these patients than in others. Also, cephalosporins can cause erythrocyte hemolysis. Because of this, in long-term therapy, tests for hemolysis should be performed. On occasion, renal damage has occurred as well as local pain and tissue sloughing at the site of injection. Oral moniliasis has been reported in patients on long-term therapy. Other side effects include rash, urticaria, fever, gastrointestinal disorders, glossitis, neutropenia, and superinfections (especially with *Pseudomonas* and *Enterobacter*).

Erythromycin

These drugs are classified as macrolide antibiotics. They are one of the safer antibiotics in use today and often are a satisfactory alternate for penicillin, particularly in patients who are allergic to penicillin. They are derived from *Streptomyces.*

Azithromycin, a new type of macrolide, recently has been introduced and shows great promise in treating upper respiratory infections. This drug concentrates in white blood cells that migrate to the infection.

MECHANISM OF ACTION

Erythromycins are bacteriostatic or bactericidal, depending on the dose and microorganism. They produce their antibacterial effect by inhibiting the synthesis of bacterial protein. Usually with dental infections, low doses are bacteriostatic and high doses are bactericidal.

SPECTRUM OF ACTIVITY

Erythromycin is effective against most gram-positive microorganisms sensitive to penicillin G. It is also effective against *Staphylococcus aureus* but not as effective as the "antistaphylococcal penicillins." In general, its antibacterial spectrum lies between those of penicillin and the tetracyclines.

Bacterial resistance appears relatively early in patients taking erythromycin for prolonged periods of time.

METABOLISM

Erythromycin rapidly diffuses throughout the body, and the brain contains higher concentrations than are found in plasma. As with penicillin, it passes into cerebrospinal fluid in patients with meningitis.

This antibiotic is concentrated in the liver and is excreted in bile, urine, and feces. Although the kidneys remove erythromycin from the body, non-renal mechanisms are more important. A large amount can be found in bile and only about 15 percent in urine. During pregnancy erythromycin passes the placental barrier but does not appear to harm the fetus.

ADVERSE EFFECTS

Following oral administration, gastrointestinal irritation often occurs including nausea, vomiting, and abdominal pain. This can be minimized if erythromycin is taken with food. Tablets with acid-resistant coatings (enteric coated) are available and should be prescribed if taken with food to prevent inactivation by stomach acids. Cholestatic hepatitis has also been associated with the use of the estolate form. Symptoms of this disorder include nausea, vomiting, and abdominal pain followed by jaundice, fever, and a disturbance in white blood cells. Because of this, the estolate form should be avoided in patients with a history of liver disease.

The incidence of allergic reactions to erythromycin is low and is manifested as fever, eosinophilia, and skin eruptions.

Tetracycline

The tetracyclines are a group of broad-spectrum antibiotics initially obtained from soil microorganisms. They are useful in a number of dental infections and are often used in place of penicillin or erythromycin. However, they are not acceptable substitutes for the prophylaxis of patients with a history of rheumatic fever.

TYPES OF TETRACYCLINES

Seven basic types of tetracyclines are currently in use. They are all similar chemically, possess similar antibacterial spectra, and have cross-hypersensitivity. When resistance or hypersensitivity to one tetracycline occurs, it also occurs to all. The types of tetracyclines are summarized in Table 33–2. Although topical sensitization is possible, this is infrequent.

While all tetracyclines have a similar spectrum of activity, minocycline is the most effective in treatment of meningococcal infections. Most of the tetracyclines—but doxycycline and minocycline to a lesser extent—are bound to metal ions. Dairy products and antacids that contain calcium limit the gastrointestinal absorption of tetracycline so that minimal therapeutic benefits can be expected. A similar interaction has been reported with products containing iron, magnesium, and aluminum. Therefore, patients should be told to refrain from these products for at least 1.5 hours prior to or following administration of oral tetracycline.

MECHANISM OF ACTION

The tetracyclines are bacteriostatic and inhibit protein synthesis in susceptible bacteria. Since they all have the same mechanism of action, resistance to one implies resistance to all tetracyclines.

Tetracyclines can block or inhibit the antibacterial effect of penicillin. Penicillin is most effective on multiplying, growing bacteria, while tetracyclines slow down the rate of bacterial growth and multiplication. Therefore, concomitant administration of these drugs is contraindicated.

SPECTRUM OF ACTIVITY

The tetracyclines are broad-spectrum antibiotics that are effective against a number of gram-negative and gram-positive bacteria. They are also effective against a few viruses, treponemata, mycoplasma, chlamydia, and rickettsia. Minocycline also may be effective against staphylococci not affected by other tetracyclines.

METABOLISM

These antibiotics pass into most body fluids and tissues. They also pass through the placenta and occur in low doses in milk of lactating mothers.

TABLE 33–2 ✦ Various Tetracyclines

GENERIC NAME	TRADE NAME	ROUTE OF ADMINISTRATION	AFFECTED BY METAL IONS
Chlortetracycline HCl	Aureomycin	po, IV	+
Demeclocycline HCl	Declomycin	po	+
Doxycycline and salts	Vibramycin	po, IV	−
Methacycline HCl	Rondomycin	po	+
Minocycline HCl	Minocin	po, IV	−
Oxytetracycline and salts	Tetramycin	po, IM, IV	+
Tetracycline and salts	Achromycin V, Cyclopar, Panmycin, Robitet, SK-Tetracycline, Tetra-cyn, Sumycin, Tetrex	po, IM, IV	+

po = orally, IV = intravenous, IM = intramuscular.
From Ciancio and Bourgault, Clinical Pharmacology for Dental Professionals, 1989.

However, no adverse effects on the newborn have been reported when the child receives low doses in the mother's milk. This antibiotic also concentrates in gingival crevicular fluid and is therefore in intimate contact with plaque in the gingival crevice.

They have an affinity for and occur in higher concentrations in rapidly growing and metabolizing tissue such as liver, tumors, bone, and developing teeth.

Tetracyclines are excreted mainly by the kidneys and can be recovered from the urine in the unchanged form.

ADVERSE EFFECTS

Treatment with tetracyclines can adversely alter the normal oral and intestinal flora, resulting in gastrointestinal problems including diarrhea. Some patients also have developed monilial infections of the gastrointestinal tract, oral cavity, and vagina due to alterations in the flora. Tetracyclines also have been reported to adversely affect the efficacy of birth control pills.

The side effects associated with tetracycline therapy are varied. A number of side effects have resulted from the use of outdated tetracyclines. Side effects are also more common in pregnant patients (in addition to the tooth-staining problem). Therefore, these drugs are contraindicated during pregnancy.

Although the incidence of allergy is low, allergy to one tetracycline usually means allergy to all other forms. A reliable allergy test is not available.

Another side effect is the discoloration of dentin of teeth during their formation. The stain is permanent and is only correctable by covering the tooth with a restorative material. This is another reason that tetracycline should be avoided during pregnancy.

PRIMARY INDICATIONS FOR NONDENTAL CONDITIONS

Since their introduction in 1948, tetracyclines have been widely used, particularly for the treatment of acne. This widespread use has led to frequent antibiotic resistance, decreasing the effectiveness of the tetracyclines.

Several species of *E. coli*, beta-hemolytic streptococci, *S. pneumoniae, Neisseria gonorrhoeae, Bacteroides, Shigella,* and *S. aureus* are resistant to the tetracyclines. However, tetracyclines remain the drug of choice for a variety of rarely occurring infections.

INDICATIONS FOR DENTAL CONDITIONS

Tetracyclines have been suggested as an adjunct for periodontal therapy, in prevention of some forms of subacute bacterial endocarditis, for treatment of acute necrotizing ulcerative gingivitis (ANUG), and for treatment of periodontal abscesses. Their use for treating ANUG and periodontal abscesses, however, has not been substantiated. Tetracycline commonly is administered systemically but is currently under active investigation for topical application in fibers or gels placed in periodontal pockets where it is released slowly.

Adjunct to Periodontal Therapy

Tetracyclines improve the healing after periodontal surgery and minimize postsurgical discomfort and infection. Clinical studies on humans indicate that tetracycline enhances bone formation and possibly reattachment. In addition, animal studies demonstrate early crestal bone repair and reversal of a form of periodontal disease in the rice rat. Part of the effectiveness of tetracyclines following oral administration results from their occurrence in gingival crevicular fluid in higher concentrations than in serum. A novel role of tetracycline in the treatment of periodontal disease has been suggested because of its demonstrated effects on collagen stabilization. Unrelated to its antibacterial activity, tetracycline inhibits the dissolution of collagen in connective tissue.

Prevention of Subacute Bacterial Endocarditis

Tetracyclines are not drugs of choice for prevention of subacute bacterial endocarditis (SBE) since group A streptococci frequently are resistant to tetracyclines. The American Heart Association and the American Dental Association recommend that the drug of choice for the prevention of subacute bacterial endocarditis is penicillin, and the second drug of choice is erythromycin.

Recent reports have indicated that nonstreptococcal subacute bacterial endocarditis is often caused by *Actinobacillus actinomycetemcomitans,* an organism strongly associated with localized juvenile periodontitis (LJP). This bacterium is only weakly susceptible to penicillin or erythromycin. For this reason, therapy of patients with LJP who are predisposed to subacute bacterial endocarditis may consist of 2 to 3 weeks' therapy with 1 g daily of a tetracycline (to eliminate *A. actinomycetemcomitans* prior to dental treatment) followed by the penicillin or erythromycin therapy to control the streptococci (Table 33–3). Therapy with either penicillin or erythromycin cannot be simultaneous with tetracyclines, as these drugs are antagonistic to each other because of their differing modes of action.

Metronidazole

Metronidazole, a systemic trichomonacide, is highly effective in the treatment of *Trichomonas vaginalis* infections. The drug is biologically active in semen and urine and, therefore, is active against trichomonads in extravaginal as well as vaginal foci. However, it is *ineffective* against *Candida albicans* and other yeasts or bacteria that cause vaginitis. It is also recommended by some investigators as an adjunct to periodontal therapy, because it is active against plaque bacteria, primarily because of its effect on anaerobes and spirochetes.

ADVERSE EFFECTS

This drug should be used with a degree of caution, as it is carcinogenic in mice and possibly also in rats. It is also mutagenic to some bacteria in concentrations found in individuals receiving therapeutic doses of the drug. Because the drug has not also been shown to be carcinogenic in other animal species so far studied, or in humans, other authorities believe that the risk of using the drug is justified.

The incidence of adverse effects with metronidazole is low and no serious reactions have been reported clinically. The most frequent reaction is nausea. Diarrhea occurs less commonly.

Temporary leukopenia can occur following metronidazole therapy; therefore, total and differential white cell counts should be performed once a week if the drug is given for longer than 7 days, especially in very young, very old, and debilitated patients or if a second course of therapy is necessary because of relapse or reinfection. Metronidazole should be used with caution in individuals who have or are prone to blood dyscrasias, since it has a potential for depressing bone marrow activity. Similarly, it should be used cautiously in individuals with any pronounced central nervous system disorder. No adverse reactions affecting the fetus have been reported. There is evidence, however, that the drug readily crosses the placenta, and has mutagenic activity against certain bacteria at con-

TABLE 33–3 ✦ Recommended Standard Prophylactic Regimen

DRUG	DOSING REGIMEN*	COMMENT
Amoxicillin	3 g 1 hour before procedure; 1.5 g 6 hours after initial dose	Especially for high-risk patients
Penicillin V	2 g 1 hour before procedure; 1 g 6 hours after initial dose	For other than high-risk patients—amoxicillin regimen (above) preferred
Erythromycin stearate	1 g 2 hours before procedure; 500 mg 6 hours after initial dose	Only for patients allergic to penicillin
Erythromycin ethylsuccinate	800 mg 2 hours before procedure; 400 mg 6 hours after initial dose	Same as for erythromycin stearate
Clindamycin	300 mg 1 hour before procedure; 150 mg 6 hours after first dose	For patients who cannot take penicillin or erythromycin—protection as good as with erythromycin

*For children amoxicillin or penicillin V 50 mg/kg, erythromycin 30 mg/kg, and clindamycin 10 mg/kg. Follow-up doses are half of these doses.
Adapted from Ciancio, S. G.: Biological Therapies in Dentistry, vol. 6. Littleton, MA, PSG Publishing, 1991.

centrations obtainable following therapeutic doses. Therefore, metronidazole should definitely *not* be used during the first trimester of pregnancy and should be avoided throughout pregnancy. Metronidazole is excreted in breast milk, but no adverse effects have been observed in nursing infants. It is also found in crevicular fluid in levels slightly below those found in serum.

Metronidazole has been administered concomitantly with either amoxicillin or augmentin. This combination has been found to be of value in localized juvenile periodontitis and refractory periodontitis. The rationale for this combination is that amoxicillin is more active against *Actinobacillus actinomycetemcomitans* than metronidazole and metronidazole is more effective than amoxicillin against anaerobes. Also, this combination is synergistic, enhancing the bactericidal effect of each antibiotic. The major adverse effect of this combination is gastrointestinal distress.

Lincomycin and Clindamycin

These antibiotics were discovered in 1962 in soil samples from Lincoln, Nebraska. Their use should be reserved for patients who cannot take penicillin or erythromycin. Since their adverse effects can be severe, they are seldom used in dental patients.

TYPES OF ANTIBIOTICS

Lincomycin (Lincocin) and its semisynthetic derivatives, clindamycin hydrochloride (Cleocin) and other salts, have similar spectra of activity. Clindamycin is better absorbed and more potent than lincomycin but has more frequent adverse effects. These antibiotics inhibit bacterial protein synthesis and are usually bacteriostatic, but in high doses they are bactericidal.

SPECTRUM OF ACTIVITY

Their antibacterial spectra are similar to those of the erythromycins. Because of their ability to penetrate bone, however, they are particularly useful in treating osteomyelitis involving alveolar bone. They also are the drugs of choice for serious infections caused by anaerobic microorganisms. Their use is primarily for microorganisms resistant to penicillin and erythromycin or for patients who cannot tolerate other antibacterial agents.

METABOLISM

Lincomycin is only partially absorbed from the gastrointestinal tract, while clindamycin is almost completely absorbed. These drugs are excreted in feces, urine, and bile, with the biliary route being the most important.

Both drugs are widely distributed in body tissues, including bone. They also cross the placental barrier. Although lincomycin will pass through inflamed meninges as in meningitis, clindamycin does not.

ADVERSE EFFECTS

The incidence of diarrhea with these drugs is high. However, a more serious problem is the development of a severe, sometimes fatal, hemorrhagic colitis. This has been termed antibiotic-associated colitis (AAC). This severe diarrhea has sometimes been successfully treated by the restoration of fluid and electrolyte balance and vancomycin (500 mg every 6 hours). In view of this side effect, serious consideration should be given before using this drug. Other side effects include glossitis, stomatitis, nausea, vomiting, skin rashes, vaginitis, and changes in blood cells. The incidence of hypersensitivity reactions to these drugs is low.

Quinolones

Quinolones such as ciprofloxin have been reported to be of value in refractory periodontitis, particularly if infections with enterococci is expected or confirmed by microbiologic testing.

MECHANISM OF ACTION

These antibiotics interfere with synthesis of bacterial DNA. They are bacteriostatic in low concentrations and bactericidal in high concentrations.

SPECTRUM OF ACTIVITY

They are effective against gram negative bacteria, particularly those associated with urinary tract infections, and some gram positive bacteria (enterococci, some staphylococci, gonococci), and chlamydia.

METABOLISM

Absorption following oral administration ranges between 50-98% and is decreased by the concomitant adminsitration of food, antacids, and products containing iron and zinc. They pass into most body fluids, appear in breast milk, and cross the placenta.

ADVERSE EFFECTS

The main adverse effect of dental interest is xerostomia, increased gag reflex, and increased nausea and vomiting. Additionally, some patients have complained of insomnia, anorexia, headache, dizziness, drowsiness, photophobia, and white blood cell and blood glucose disorders. Hypersensitivity reports are rare.

Vancomycin

Vancomycin, discovered in 1956, is a glycopeptide with an unknown chemical structure. It is useful in both preventing and treating bacterial endocarditis and antibiotic-associated colitis. The only commercially available derivative is Vancocin.

MECHANISM OF ACTION

Vancomycin is bactericidal and exerts its effect by inhibiting cell wall synthesis.

SPECTRUM OF ACTIVITY

This drug is bactericidal for gram-positive bacteria. Cross-resistance with other antibiotics has not been reported.

METABOLISM

It is poorly absorbed following oral administration. Therefore, the intravenous route is preferred. It penetrates most body fluids, including cerebrospinal fluid, when the meninges are inflamed. Its main route of excretion is via the kidney. The drug is poorly absorbed through oral mucosa, and some studies have reported improvement in gingivitis following topical application.

ADVERSE EFFECTS

Side effects are severe. Therefore, it should be restricted to bacterial endocarditis prophylaxis and gram-positive infections in which no other antibiotic is effective.

The untoward effects include phlebitis and pain at the injection site, deafness, toxic changes in the kidney, anaphylaxis, skin rashes, and fever. No adverse effects have been reported from the topical route of administration.

Nystatin

Nystatin (Candex, Mycostatin, Nilstat, O-V Statin), a polyene antibiotic is excellent for treatment of fungal infections.

It is most useful for the treatment of both oral and vaginal candidiasis (thrush).

METABOLISM

This drug can be given orally but is poorly absorbed from the gastrointestinal tract. Also, it is not absorbed from skin and mucous membranes. When taken orally, large amounts are found in feces. It exerts its main effect via the topical route in most cases.

ADVERSE EFFECTS

Adverse effects are rare and include nausea, vomiting, and diarrhea following ingestion. However, no adverse effects have been reported via the topical route. Neither hypersensitivity reactions nor resistance have occurred.

Ketoconazole

Ketoconazole (Nizoral) is one of the newest drugs approved for oral treatment of systemic fun-

gal infections. It is also useful for the treatment of oral candidiasis (thrush).

Ketoconazole interferes with the synthesis of chemicals needed to form the plasma membrane of fungi, resulting in disorganization of the membrane.

METABOLISM

Its absorption from the gastrointestinal tract is better than that of nystatin. It is metabolized in the liver, and only small amounts are found in urine and feces. Since data are lacking for use in pregnancy, it is not recommended at that time. It does appear in maternal milk.

ADVERSE EFFECTS

The most common adverse effects are nausea and pruritus. Headache, dizziness, gastrointestinal problems, nervousness, and liver dysfunction have occurred less frequently.

Streptomycin

Streptomycin is useful to dentistry only in the prophylaxis of certain patients with a history of complications from rheumatic fever and will be discussed only in this respect. It is also used in the treatment of tuberculosis and bacterial endocarditis. Because of its severe toxicity, the drug has limited usefulness.

Streptomycin is bactericidal, inhibiting bacterial protein synthesis.

SPECTRUM OF ACTIVITY

It is effective against gram-positive, gram-negative, and acid-fast microorganisms. Unfortunately, bacterial resistance develops rapidly, thus limiting its usefulness.

METABOLISM

Since it is not absorbed from the intestinal tract, the injectable form must be used. It distributes throughout plasma and all extracellular fluids before being excreted mainly unchanged by the kidneys.

ADVERSE EFFECTS

Severe eighth nerve damage is common, causing loss of both balance and hearing. Its use can also cause blood disorders and severe kidney damage. Allergic reactions may occur, ranging from rashes to shock.

Bacitracin

Bacitracin is sometimes used topically for dental infections. It is effective against gram-positive cocci and bacilli, *Actinomyces,* and *Fusobacterium.* Rarely, hypersensitivity reactions have been reported after topical application. It is available as an ointment containing 500 units per gram for topical use and often is combined with other topical antibiotics such as neomycin and polymyxin, which have some broad-spectrum properties. It has been placed in some periodontal dressings, but its value is questionable. It is not used parenterally, since kidney damage is common following such usage.

Sulfonamides

The first sulfonamide was synthesized in 1908 as para-aminobenzoicsulphonamide but was not used as an antibacterial agent until 1936. Since that time many sulfonamides have been synthesized. Although they are effective in some infections of dental origin, antibiotics are more effective and safe. The sulfonamides are contraindicated for topical application on oral mucosa because they are highly allergic. However, they are sometimes used topically for minor eye infections and over burn areas.

The sulfonamides are bacteriostatic. Since the sulfonamides are structurally similar to para-aminobenzoic acid, they interfere with its uptake by bacteria. Para-aminobenzoic acid is important to bacterial metabolism because bacteria use it to make folic acid, which is essential to the vitality of most microorganisms.

SPECTRUM OF ACTIVITY

The sulfonamides are effective against many gram-positive and some gram-negative bacteria. They are also effective against some large viruses of trachoma and lymphogranuloma venereum. They are mainly used to treat lower urinary tract infections.

METABOLISM

Once sulfonamides enter plasma, they are rapidly concentrated in urine. Some are excreted unchanged, while others are metabolized in the liver. The sulfonamides can be classified as short-, intermediate-, and long-acting on the basis of duration of effect in the body.

Many bacteria develop a high degree of resistance to sulfonamides. Resistance to one sulfonamide leads to resistance to all others. Because the sulfonamides concentrate in urine, crystals may form in the urinary tract as a complication of therapy. Therefore, sulfonamides are usually administered with large amounts of fluid and in combination with other sulfonamides to decrease the concentration of any one agent.

ADVERSE EFFECTS

A number of adverse effects are associated with sulfonamide therapy, the most common being allergic reactions. The most frequent allergic reactions include urticaria, rash, fever, pruritus, dermatitis, and photosensitivity. Less frequent allergic reactions include Stevens-Johnson syndrome, erythema nodosum, and exfoliative dermatitis. Sensitivity to one sulfonamide usually indicates sensitivity to all sulfonamides.

Other adverse effects include nausea, vomiting, diarrhea, headache, dizziness, vertigo, tinnitus, and mental depression.

Sulfonamide therapy may result in toxic effects in the urinary tract owing to the formation of sulfonamide crystals in urine. Adequate urinary volume is important to minimize this effect. Also, since some sulfonamides are not soluble in alkaline media, agents such as sodium bicarbonate are given concurrently to make urine more alkaline.

Blood dyscrasias also have occurred with sulfonamide therapy. Clinical signs associated with these are sore throat, fever, pallor, or jaundice. These drugs cross the placenta and are excreted in milk. Therefore, since sulfonamides can cause problems in infants, they should not be given to pregnant or lactating females.

MANAGEMENT OF THE PATIENT WITH VARIOUS CARDIAC PROBLEMS

Patients may have histories of cardiovascular problems such as those associated with rheumatic fever which require antibiotic prophylaxis prior to dental therapy that produces bleeding from oral tissues.

The occurrence and extent of bacteremias following dental procedures vary with the extent of the procedure and the amount of trauma and health of the gingival tissues. Prophylactic antibiotic therapy is recommended for dental procedures that are likely to cause gingival bleeding to minimize the risk of bacteremias leading to subacute bacterial endocarditis. *Streptococcus viridans,* a microorganism found in the gingival crevice, has an affinity for diseased heart valves or weakened cardiac tissues. This microorganism can lodge in heart tissues and produce bacterial endocarditis, a life-threatening disease. Therefore, these patients must be premedicated with antibiotics, as outlined in Tables 33–3 to 33–5. The question of prophylactic antibiotics in a patient who has a history of rheumatic fever but no signs of cardiac damage should be based on the judgment of the physician. If the dentist is certain that a physician has examined the patient with such a history and has found no sign of cardiac damage, prophylactic therapy should not be necessary. It is noteworthy that, since December 1990, the American Heart Association recommends oral administration with the exception of

TABLE 33–4 ✦ Parenteral Regimen for Low to Moderate Risk Patients Unable to Take Oral Medication

DRUG	DOSING REGIMEN*
Ampicillin	2.0 g intravenously or intramuscularly administered 30 minutes before procedure; 1.0 g intravenously or intramuscularly or 1.5 g orally administered 6 hours after initial dose.
Clindamycin (if penicillin allergic)	300 mg intravenously administered 30 minutes before procedure; 150 g intravenously or orally administered 6 hours after initial dose.

*For children, ampicillin 50 mg/kg and clindamycin 10 mg/kg. Follow-up doses are half of these doses.
Adapted from Ciancio, S. G.: Biological Therapies in Dentistry, vol. 6. Littleton, MA, PSG Publishing, 1991.

TABLE 33–5 ✦ High-Risk Patients and Those Not Candidates for Other Regimens

DRUG	DOSING REGIMEN*
Ampicillin, gentamicin, and amoxicillin	2.0 g ampicillin intravenously or intramuscularly administered and 1.5 mg/kg of gentamicin intravenously or intramuscularly administered (not to exceed 80 mg) 30 minutes before procedure; 1.5 g amoxicillin taken orally 6 hours after initial dose. Alternatively, the parenteral regimen may be repeated 8 hours after initial dose.
Vancomycin (if penicillin allergic)	1.0 g intravenously administered over 1 hour, starting 1 hour before procedure. A repeat dose is not necessary.

*For children, ampicillin or amoxicillin 50 mg/kg, gentamicin 2.0 mg/kg, and vancomycin 20 mg/kg. Follow-up doses are half of these doses.
Adapted from Ciancio, S. G.: Biological Therapies in Dentistry, vol. 6. Littleton, MA, PSG Publishing, 1991.

those who cannot take oral medications or those considered by their physician to be at high risk such as patients who have had a recent episode of bacterial endocarditis. *Actinobacillus actinomycetemcomitans*, a microorganism often found in pa-tients with localized juvenile periodontitis, also has an affinity for diseased heart valves or weakened cardiac tissue. No definite therapeutic regimen has been developed, but a number of clinicians pre-medicate these patients with tetracyclines followed by the prophylactic regimen shown in Tables 33–3 to 33–5. However, the use of amoxicillin, which is effective against *A. actinomycetemcomitans* may eliminate the concept of premedication with tetracyclines.

ACKNOWLEDGMENT

This chapter has been partially adapted from *Clinical Pharmacology for Dental Professionals*, Third Edition, by Sebastian G. Ciancio and Priscilla C. Bourgault, copyright 1989 by C.V. Mosby Company, St. Louis, Missouri, used with permission.

BIBLIOGRAPHY

Archard, H. O., and Roberts, W. C.: Bacterial endocarditis after dental procedures in patients with aortic valve prosthesis. J.A.D.A. 72:648, 1966.

Ariaudo, A. A.: The efficacy of antibiotics in periodontal surgery: A controlled study with Lincomycin and placebo in sixty-eight patients. J. Periodontol. 40:150, 1969.

Baer, P. N., Sumner, C. F., and Miller, G.: Periodontal dressings. Dent. Clin. North Am. 13:181, 1969.

Breloff, J. P., and Caffesse, R.: Effect of achromycin ointment on healing following periodontal surgery. J. Periodontol. 54:368, 1983.

Ciancio, S. G., Mather, M. L., and McMullen, J. A.: An evaluation of minocycline in patients with periodontal disease. J. Periodontol. 54:530, 1980.

Ciancio, S. G.: Tetracyclines and periodontal therapy. J. Periodontol. 43:155, 1976.

Ciancio, S. G., Slots, J., Reynolds, H. S., Zambon, J., and McKenna, J.: The effect of short term administration of minocycline HCl on gingival inflammation and subgingival microflora. J. Periodontol. 53:557, 1982.

Cunha, R. A., and Stucca, A. M.: Third generation cephalosporins. Med. Clin. North Am. 66:283, 1982.

Kannangara, D. W., Thadepalli, H., and McQuirter, J. L.: Bacteriology and treatment of dental infections. J. Clin. Pharmacol. 50:103, 1980.

Sabbath, L. D.: Drug resistance in bacteria. N. Engl. J. Med. 280:291, 1969.

Slots, J., Rosling, B., and Genco, R.: Suppression of penicillin-resistant oral *Actinobacillus actinomycetemcomitans* with tetracycline: Considerations in endocarditis prophylaxis. J. Periodontol. 54:193, 1983.

Stahl, S. S.: The healing of a gingival wound in protein-deprived, antibiotic-supplement adult rats. Oral Surg. 17:443, 1964.

Tedesco, F. J., Barton, R. W., and Alpers, D. H.: Clindamycin associated colitis. Ann. Intern. Med. 81:429, 1974.

Walker, C. B., Gordon, J. M., McQuikin, S. J., Niebloom, T. A., and Socransky, S. S.: Tetracycline: Levels achievable in gingival crevice fluid and in vitro effect on subgingival organisms. J. Periodontol. 52:613, 1981.

Weinstein, L.: Antimicrobial agents, penicillins, and cephalosporins. In Goodman, L. S., and Gilman, A. (eds.): The Pharmacological Basis of Therapeutics. New York, MacMillan, 1975.

34 Diagnostic Microbiology and Immunology

Michael G. Newman and Russell J. Nisengard

CHAPTER OUTLINE

Identification of bacteria
Identification of antibodies
Other diagnostic tests

Numerous microbiologic and immunologic tests are currently available with new assays continually being introduced. This chapter focuses on diagnostic tests of value in dentistry that are currently offered by clinical laboratories as well as tests used in dental research and practice.

The fields of microbiology and immunology have been rapidly expanding with a virtual explosion of two diverse types of diagnostic tests: (1) those dependent on increasingly sophisticated techniques and instrumentation requiring highly trained personnel, which are available in clinical laboratories; and (2) those employing relatively simple procedures and requiring less skill to perform, which lend themselves to a clinician's office. The greatest growth in the next decade will be in diagnostic tests designed for office use.

IDENTIFICATION OF BACTERIA

In dentistry, many oral infections are successfully treated empirically without identification of the specific etiologic agent. For example, most abscesses respond to penicillin and many types of periodontal diseases are alleviated to some degree by tetracycline therapy. This empirical approach is not always successful, as antibiotic resistance can occur or the wrong antibiotic may be selected. In clinical microbiology, the best approach is first to identify the etiologic microorganism and then to select the appropriate therapy. Several methods of identifying bacteria have been used in dental research (Table 34–1).

Direct Examination

Many clinical specimens are directly examined under light, phase contrast, or darkfield micros-

copy, preferably as soon as they are collected from the patient. This provides a rapid assessment of the relative morphotypes and numbers of bacteria. Most culture techniques require a minimum 24-hour incubation.

If the oral sample is very concentrated, as occurs with plaque, it must be diluted in sterile culture media or physiologic saline before microscopic examination.

Bacterial samples can be examined microscopically as either stained or unstained preparations. A variety of stains have been developed to aid in the differentiation of bacteria.

PHASE CONTRAST AND DARKFIELD MICROSCOPY

Fresh, unstained, wet oral samples are frequently examined by either phase contrast or darkfield microscopy. These "wet mount" techniques allow evaluation of the relative numbers of bacterial morphotypes and bacterial motility. Spiro-

TABLE 34–1 ✦ Identification of Bacteria

Direct examination—microscopy
Culture and sensitivity assays
    Culture techniques—aerobic and anaerobic
    Speciation techniques—GLC, DNA homology, and so on
    Antimicrobial susceptibility—requirements and interpretation
Immunologic assays
    Immunofluorescence
    Latex agglutination
    Immunodot/blot
    Flow cytometry
Other assays
    DNA probes

chetes, other motile bacteria, and trophozoites or parasites can be identified by these techniques.

Both phase and darkfield microscopy require special microscope condensers, which alter the way the light is reflected or refracted off the bacterial cell surface. The outline of the bacterium is black against a light background in phase contrast microscopy and light against a black background in darkfield microscopy.

GRAM STAIN

The Gram stain, first developed by Hans Christian Gram in the late 19th century, is one of the most important procedures in the diagnostic laboratory. While normally it does not allow species identification, it is usually the first step in identification of unknown bacteria. The Gram stain is a differential stain that divides all bacteria into two groups: gram-positive bacteria, which stain blue-violet, and gram-negative bacteria, which stain pink-red.

Method. The Gram stain consists of sequential application of four reagents: (1) crystal violet as the primary stain; (2) iodine to chemically bind the alkaline crystal violet to the cell wall; (3) alcohol as a decolorizer that increases the permeability of the cell wall, allowing the crystal violet stain to be washed out of gram-negative bacteria and those gram-positive bacteria that have lost cell wall integrity from antibiotics or autolysis; and (4) safranin as a counterstain to allow visualization of gram-negative bacteria as red to pink in color.

ACID-FAST STAIN

This stain primarily identifies tubercle bacilli. Cells of some bacteria and parasites contain long-chain fatty acids, which resist destaining of basic dyes by acid alcohol. These microorganisms are thus called "acid-fast." Mycobacteria such as *M. tuberculosis* and *M. marinum* are characterized by their acid-fast stain.

Method. The bacteria are stained with hot carbol-fuchsin, decolorized with acid alcohol, and counterstained with methylene blue. Acid-fast bacteria maintain the initial red color or carbol-fuchsin, while non-acid fast bacteria stain blue from the methylene blue counterstain.

Culture and Susceptibility

A specimen is usually sent to the microbiology laboratory to culture and identify the organism(s), as well as to determine its susceptibility and resistance to various antimicrobial agents.

Although future trends in clinical microbiology point to the rapid, non-growth dependent methods for detecting infectious agents, the isolation and identification of viable pathogens is still the current

"gold standard." The major advantages of culturing are the elucidation of most major microorganisms and determination of the antimicrobial susceptibility of pathogens.

GUIDELINES

Microbial sampling from orofacial infections is often necessary for effective patient management. **The dental clinician should be aware that each infection has specific sampling and processing requirements and laboratory procedures are constantly updated.**

Methods of specimen collection and transport are important because many diagnostic tests for infectious diseases depend on the selection, timing, and method of specimen collection. These factors are often more critical for microbiologic specimens than for chemical or hematologic laboratory tests.

The following general rules apply to all specimens:

1. A sufficient quantity of specimen must be provided to permit thorough study.
2. The sample should be representative of the infectious process.
3. Only sterile equipment and aseptic techniques should be used to prevent specimen contamination.
4. The specimen must be transported to the laboratory and examined promptly. Special transport media may be helpful or required (i.e., anaerobes).
5. The specimen should be accompanied by a request form indicating the genera suspected. Separate samples must be submitted for aerobic and anaerobic cultures. Depending on the laboratory, duplicate request forms may be required for the aerobic and anaerobic laboratory if they are processed in separate locations.

Types of Specimens
MUCOSAL SURFACES

Since bacterial infections of mucosal surfaces are often mixed infections involving anaerobes, aerobes, or facultative bacteria, both aerobic and anaerobic culturing may be necessary.

BLOOD SAMPLES

Blood specimens are rarely collected by the dentist. Such samples are taken to determine the causative agent(s) of a septicemia.

PERIODONTAL POCKETS

With increased understanding about specific bacteria associated with different types and stages of periodontal disease, culture of periodontal pathogens is becoming more common.

Sampling Methods. The most common sampling devices for periodontal pockets are periodontal curettes (that normally are used for scaling and root planing) and paper points (that are normally used for endodontic therapy) (Table 34–2). Paper points are being increasingly used but may selectively remove the loosely adherent tissue-associated, gram-negative microorganisms and leave the tooth-adherent, gram-positive microorganisms in the pocket. A wash of a pocket obtained with an irrigating device has also been used for darkfield microscopic analysis. By this technique, a predetermined volume of liquid is introduced into the sulcus, and then part of it is removed for analysis.

PROCESSING PLAQUE SPECIMENS

To identify plaque microorganisms, it is imperative that proper transport and processing of the specimens takes place. Important parameters are

1. *Anaerobiosis.* Since plaque—especially subgingival plaque—contains many anaerobic bacteria, it is important to provide an anaerobic transport medium.
2. *Viability during transport.* The transport medium must preserve the microbial viability until the specimen is processed at the laboratory. At the same time, it should not allow selective growth of some species, leading to distorted results.
3. *Dispersion.* Because clumping of bacteria in plaque is common, the plaque must be dispersed prior to culturing in order to obtain representative results. This is usually accomplished by sonification, stirring with glass beads, or vigorous agitation.
4. *Dilution.* Since the numbers of microorganisms in plaque samples are usually quite high (ranging from 10^4 to 10^8), the specimen must be diluted before culturing on solid media to allow accurate colony counts.
5. *Incubation.* Most oral isolates are anaerobic and must be incubated in an anaerobic environment. If aerobic or microaerophilic microorganisms are suspected, however, the specimen must be cultured in one of these environments.

Cultural Microbiology
ATMOSPHERE OF CULTURE

Organisms are (1) *aerobic,* utilizing oxygen as a terminal electron acceptor, and growing very well at normal room atmosphere; (2) *anaerobic,* growing in the absence of oxygen; (3) *microaerophilic,* growing best in an atmosphere of reduced oxygen; or (4) **facultative** *anaerobic,* growing in an aerobic **or** anaerobic environment. Most clinically significant "aerobic" organisms are actually facultative anaerobes. Strict aerobes include *Pseudomonas*

TABLE 34–2 ✦ Subgingival Plaque Sampling Methods

Nickle-plated curette-scaler
Paper points
Irrigation
Surgical

species, members of the Neisseriaceae family, *Brucella* species, *Bordatella* species, *Francisella* species, *Mycobacterium,* and filamentous fungi. Organisms that require greater concentrations of carbon dioxide are **"capnophilic."** An example is *Actinobacillus actinomycetemcomitans.*

ARTIFICIAL MEDIA

Many ingredients necessary for the growth of pathogens can be supplied by (1) human or animal hosts, (2) cell or tissue culture, and (3) synthetic or semisynthetic media in the form of dehydrated media powder and prepared media, which are commercially available. A combination of enriched, supportive, nonselective, selective, and differential media is used for the isolation and presumptive identification of bacteria from clinical material.

1. *Enriched* media encourage the growth of organisms found in large numbers in normal flora.
2. *Supportive* media allow growth of most nonfastidious organisms at their natural rates without permitting a growth advantage for any organism.
3. *Nonselective* media permit the growth of most oral microorganisms without specific inhibitory agents (Table 34–3).
4. *Selective* media contain dyes and antibiotics that are inhibitory to all organisms except those being sought. Many selective media are available (Table 34–4).
5. *Differential* media allow selective morphologic identification of certain microbial colonies.

The most supportive, differential media is blood agar, which allows growth of many microorgan-

TABLE 34–3 ✦ Typical Nonselective Media

Trypticase soy agar
5% sheep blood
Brain heart infusion agar
Trypticase soy agar
5% sheep blood supplemented with hemin and menadione
Columbia base agar
Trypticase soy agar
5% rabbit blood supplemented with hemin and menadione

TABLE 34–4 ✦ Selective Media for Periodontal Bacteria

Bacteria	Media (main ingredients)	References
Black-pigmenting bacteria *Bacteroides gingivalis*	Tryptic soy agar, 5% rabbit blood BGA media (Columbia agar base + 5% sheep blood)	Zambon et al., 1981 Hunt et al., 1986
Fusobacterium	CVE (trypticase agar + 5% sheep blood)	Walker et al., 1979
	FEA (brucella agar + 2.5% egg yolk)	Morgenstein et al., 1981
Actinobacillus actinomycetemcomitans	TSBV (tryptic soy agar, 10% serum)	Slots et al., 1982
	Modified MGB (tryptic soy agar, 5% sheep blood)	Mandell et al., 1986
Capnocytophaga	TBBP (tryptic soy agar, 5% sheep blood)	Mashimo et al., 1977
	CAP (G-C agar, 10% hemoglobin)	Rummeus et al., 1985
Eikenella corrodens	Todd-Hewitt agar	Slee and Tanzer, 1978
Actinomyces	GMC	Kornman and Loesche, 1978
	CFAT (trypticase soy agar, 5% sheep blood)	Zylber and Jordan, 1985
Streptococcus	Mitis salivarius agar	Difco Laboratories, Detroit, MI
Spirochetes	Brain-heart infusion broth and ingredients	Fiehn and Frandsen, 1984

isms and separation on the basis of red cell hemolysis, colony morphology, and production of pigment. Because of this, most specimens sent to a clinical laboratory are plated onto media containing blood and a source of protein such as tryptones or soybean-protein digest. Bacteria produce extracellular enzymes that cause complete red blood cell lysis *(beta hemolysis)*, a greenish discoloration around the colony *(alpha hemolysis)*, or no hemolysis (sometimes called *gamma hemolysis*). Hemolysis is controlled by many environmental factors, including pH and atmosphere of incubation.

The colony morphology and type of hemolysis are initial screening tests to determine further steps in identification of an isolate. In some cases, rabbit blood rather than sheep blood is selected for enhancement of organisms of black-pigmenting bacteria.

ANAEROBIC CULTURE TECHNIQUES

Several techniques are available for the anaerobic growth of microorganisms.

Jar Techniques. Anaerobic jars are used to control the atmosphere with two methods that yield comparable numbers of anaerobes.

One common method utilizes commercially available H_2- and CO_2-generator envelopes. An envelope is placed in the jar with the inoculated agar plates, water is added, and the jar is sealed. Along with the gas mixture generated, residual oxygen is removed to establish anaerobiosis by catalytic re-

action with hydrogen to form water. A catalyst composed of palladium-coated aluminum pellets within a wire mesh container is preferred, as it is convenient and there is no explosion hazard. Reduced anaerobic conditions as demonstrated by an indicator of methylene blue or resazurin are achieved in 1 to 2 hours.

The second technique is an evacuation-replacement system whereby air within the jar is removed by vacuum followed by replacement with an oxygen-free gas containing 80 to 90 percent N_2, 5 to 10 percent H_2, and 5 to 10 percent CO_2. Flushing with this anaerobic gas is repeated twice.

Bio-bag Technique. This technique utilizes a clear, gas-impermeable bag into which is placed an ampule containing resazurin as an anaerobic indicator, and a gas generator ampule. One or two plates are placed inside the bag (Bio-bag type A), which is then sealed with a heat sealer. Reduced conditions are achieved in one-half hour. The viability of organisms can be maintained within the bag for up to 1 week. These bags are particularly convenient for incubation of primary plates and whenever only a few plates are used.

Prereduced Anaerobically Sterilized (PRAS) Roll Tubes. PRAS tubes are prepared by dissolving the medium constituents, boiling the medium to remove dissolved air, and then flushing with oxygen-free gas. The tubes can be inoculated by either closed or open methods. The closed or Hungate method utilizes a syringe and needle to inoculate the medium through a seal. By the open method, the tube is opened, a cannula or blunt needle is inserted into the tube, and the medium is constantly flushed through the cannula with oxygen-free gas until the medium is inoculated and the tube is capped. Platinum wires and loops should be used for inoculation, since tungsten wire may oxidize the PRAS medium.

Anaerobic Chamber Techniques. Rigid gastight cabinets or flexible, gas-impermeable plastic bags are used as anaerobic chambers. All materials used in the chamber are introduced through a series of air locks and access to perform culture procedures in the box is through sealed gloves. Anaerobiosis is initially achieved by flushing with 5 to 10 pecent H_2, 5 to 10 percent CO_2, and 80 to 90 percent N_2 in the presence of an active palladium catalyst and maintained by use of a palladium catalyst and 3 to 10 percent H_2.

Enzyme Reduction Techniques. Newly developed primary isolation plates containing enzymes that scavenge oxygen show promise as an enhanced method for culturing anaerobic bacteria.

GAS-LIQUID CHROMATOGRAPHY

Anaerobic bacteria produce a variety of metabolic end products that are often unique enough to serve as markers for identification (Table 34–5). Because the nutritional composition of the medium, particularly the carbohydrate-to-peptide ratio, affects the metabolic products, the medium for determining end points must be standardized. Although different species produce a variety of end products, the majority form acetic and succinic acids. The gram-positive bacilli produce large amounts of propionic acid. *Actinomyces* produces succinic acid, and *Fusobacterium* produces butyric acid.

The fatty acid end products are measured by different detectors in the gas chromatograph. Thermal conductivity (TC) and flame ionization detectors (FID) require helium as a carrier gas and can measure both volatile and nonvolatile end products. The separation of fatty acids is achieved by injecting the prepared samples through a siphon into a column in a heated oven. The high temperature volatizes the sample, and the flow of the carrier gas moves the sample down the length of the column, separating the fatty acids according to molecular weight and polarity. When a fatty acid reaches a detector, it causes an electrical response, which creates a peak on a chart. The more fatty acid present, the larger the height and width of the peak. The retention line (the length of the line from the injection of the sample to the detection of the peak) determines the identity of the peak as compared with a standard of known fatty acid composition.

TABLE 34–5 ✦ Metabolic End Products of Commonly Encountered Anaerobes

Gram-Positive Cocci	
Peptostreptococcus anaerobius	Acetic acid, isobutyric acid, isovaleric acid, isocaproic acid
Peptostreptococcus micros	Acetic acid
Gram-Negative Cocci	
Veillonella	Acetic acid, propionic acid
Gram-Positive Bacilli	
Actinomyces	Acetic acid, succinic acid, lactic acid
Lactobacillus	Lactic acid
Eubacterium	Acetic acid, isobutyric acid, butyric acid, isovaleric acid, valeric acid, caproic acid
Gram-Negative Bacilli	
Fusobacterium	Acetic acid, butyric acid, lactic acid
Porphyromonas Prevotella	Acetic acid, propionic acid, isobutyric acid, butyric acid, isovaleric acid, lactic acid, succinic acid

DNA-DNA HYBRIDIZATION

This method, which determines the similarity between two different bacterial clones, is based on the ability of single-stranded DNA to bind complementary sequences. Clones from a single colony of a known bacterium are grown in a medium containing radiolabeled substrates that are incorporated into the bacterial DNA during growth. The bacteria are then lysed and the released DNA cleaved into small fragments with endonucleases. The fragments dissociate into single-stranded DNA after heating or chemical treatment.

The unknown or test bacteria are cultured in unlabeled media, attached to a filter matrix, and treated to dissociate their double-stranded DNA into single strands. The labeled single-stranded DNA of the known bacteria are reacted with the DNA of the unknown strain on the filter matrix. The filter is then washed to remove unbound DNA. Labeled DNA pieces will only bind (hybridize) to complementary DNA so the amount of label remaining on the filter after washing indicates the relatedness of the known and unknown bacteria. Bacteria with similar morphologic and biochemical characteristics exhibit approximately 70 percent genetic relatedness.

Antimicrobial Susceptibility

Cultivation and isolation of clinically important anaerobic bacteria are relatively slow requiring at least 2 to 4 days. Susceptibility tests are necessary for isolates from patients with serious infections and infections that persist or recur despite appropriate empiric antimicrobial therapy. The susceptibility to antimicrobial agents cannot always be predicted, since strain differences occur, and testing of the isolated pathogen is required. The effects of antibiotics or chemotherapeutic agents against pathogenic or potentially pathogenic microorganisms can be measured qualitatively, semiquantitatively, or quantitatively.

There are three degrees of susceptibility:

1. A microorganism is *susceptible* if it is inhibited by the concentration of an antimicrobial agent that can be achieved in the blood or tissues of patients taking the recommended doses.

2. A microorganism is *resistant* if the concentration of antimicrobial agent required for inhibition is greater than that obtained in the blood or tissues during therapy.

3. A microorganism is *intermediate* in susceptibility if the inhibitory concentration is equal to or slightly higher than normally obtained in the blood. Only a small group of organisms are intermediate.

Antimicrobial susceptibility is determined as either the **minimum *inhibitory* concentration (MIC)** or the **minimum *bactericidal* concentration (MBC)**. The MIC is the lowest chemotherapeutic concentration that inhibits microbial growth in broth as defined by lack of visual turbidity. The MBC is the lowest concentration of the antimicrobial agent that allows less than 0.1 percent microbial survival.

BROTH DILUTION TESTS

Broth dilution tests allow determination of the bactericidal and bacteriostatic activity of a drug. Bactericidal end points are determined by streaking 0.1 ml sample from each diluted broth culture onto agar plates. Microdilution tests are a miniaturized version of the broth dilution procedure. Various manual, semiautomated, and automated devices that improve the economy and speed of the tests are available. Until recently, automated systems did not lend themselves to testing of oral bacteria because of these organisms' fastidious nature.

BROTH DISK TEST

Disks with various concentrations of antimicrobial agents are placed in broth, which is then inoculated with 0.1 ml of an actively growing culture and incubated for 18 to 24 hours. A tube without the chemotherapeutic agents serves as a positive control, and a tube without bacterial inoculation serves as a contamination control.

BACTERIAL DISK DIFFUSION TEST

Several methods have been developed for evaluating susceptibility to multiple antimicrobial agents. The most important is the bacterial disk method of Bauer and colleagues (1966), which has been standardized and correlated with MICs. First, the test organism is inoculated onto the surface of agar, and then disks impregnated with different agents are placed on the surface. The antimicrobial agents diffuse into the agar, creating concentration gradients with the highest concentrations closest to the disks. The zone of growth inhibition around the disk indicates the relative susceptibility to the chemotherapeutic agent. The degree of susceptibility (susceptible, intermediate, or resistant) is determined according to the criteria of the National Committee for Clinical Laboratory Standards (NCCLS). Proper interpretation of this test is influenced by factors such as (1) agar depth, pH, cation content, and media supplements; (2) age and turbidity of the bacterial inoculum; (3) method of inoculating onto the agar; (4) atmosphere of growth; (5) time of incubation; and (6) antimicrobial content of the disks, as well as their age and method of storage.

RAPID TEST FOR ANTIMICROBIAL SUSCEPTIBILITY

Certain bacteria such as gonococci, *Staphylococcus aureus,* and black-pigmenting bacteria may be resistant to the beta-lactam antibiotics such as penicillin and cephalosporin due to production of the enzyme beta-lactamase. This enzyme binds antibiotics possessing a beta-lactam ring and usually opens the ring leading to inactivation of the antibiotic.

The most sensitive method for detection of this enzyme is to test the microorganism on a chromogenic cephalosporin, which turns red when its beta-lactam ring is broken. This cephalosporin called nitrocefin is commercially available in impregnated filter paper disks and strips. The disks or strips are moistened with sterile water, smeared with isolated colonies, and incubated for 5 to 10 minutes. A positive reaction is indicated by a color change from yellow to red.

Immunologic Assays

Several immunologic assays have been used clinically as "stains" to identify microorganisms in clinical specimens. These include immunofluorescence and enzyme immunoassays.

IMMUNOFLUORESCENCE

Immunofluorescence combines the sensitivity and specificity of an immunologic assay with that of microscopic localization. This permits the identification of specific bacteria in bacterial smears such as subgingival plaque samples. Two types of immunofluorescence assays have been employed for the identification of specific bacteria in clinical samples: direct and indirect immunofluorescence (Fig. 34–1A and B).

By **direct** immunofluorescence, antisera to a microorganism is conjugated to a fluorescent dye such as fluorescein. When this conjugate is incubated on a clinical smear containing the organism and then washed off, the antibodies attach to their corresponding bacterial antigen and the organism is

DIRECT IMMUNOFLUORESCENCE

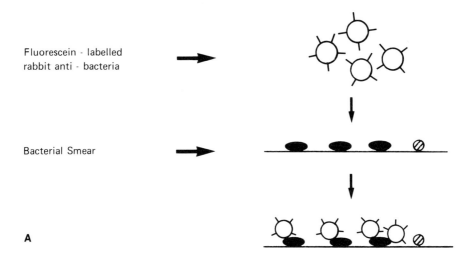

Fluorescein - labelled
rabbit anti - bacteria

Bacterial Smear

A

INDIRECT IMMUNOFLUORESCENCE

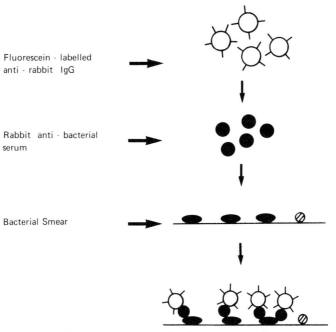

Fluorescein - labelled
anti - rabbit IgG

Rabbit anti - bacterial
serum

Bacterial Smear

B

FIGURE 34–1 ✦ Direct immunofluorescence **(A)** and indirect immunofluorescence **(B)** for identification of bacteria in clinical samples.

visualized by its fluorescent outline when viewed with a microscope equipped with special filters and light source (Fig. 34–2). If that organism is not present, the conjugated antibodies will not attach to any bacteria and will be removed by washing so that the smear will appear dark with no fluorescence.

Indirect immunofluorescence is similar to direct immunofluorescence but is a two-step test. In an indirect immunofluorescence test, antiserum to a microorganism is incubated on the clinical smear and washed off. Then a conjugate of a fluorescent dye and an antiserum to the first antiserum are incubated on the smear and then washed off. For example, rabbit antisera to *Propyromonas gingivalis* would be first incubated on a clinical smear followed by fluorescein-labeled, goat antirabbit IgG.

Direct and indirect immunofluorescence assays have proven to be useful laboratory tests for the diagnosis of specific bacterial pathogens. Studies of periodontopathogens have demonstrated the advantages of identifying the percentage of the pathogen in the plaque smears. These have been determined by dividing the total specific fluorescent bacteria by the total number of bacteria counted with phase contrast microscopy or counter-stain.

ENZYME IMMUNOASSAYS

Horseradish peroxidase, a small enzyme, is conjugated to specific bacterial antibodies in this assay and incubated on bacterial smears. An orange-brown color is developed by incubation with a substrate for the peroxidase. This can be visualized by examination with a regular light microscope. Such tests are commonly available for detection of *cytomegalovirus* and other viruses and bacteria.

LATEX AGGLUTINATION

Latex agglutination is an immunologic assay with moderate sensitivity that is based on the binding of protein to latex and its agglutination or clumping on exposure to its specific antigen or antibody.

Latex agglutination tests are commercially available for identifying antigens or antibodies in clinical specimens including Group A, B, C, D, F, and G streptococci, *H. influenzae, S. pneumoniae, N. influenzae.* They have been particularly useful in detection of bacteria but have also been used in tests for viruses and antibodies to bacteria or tissue. The sensitivity level of these tests is similar to those of traditional culture techniques for microorganisms, but the results are available in minutes rather than hours or days. The latex tests are considered to be qualitative or semiquantitative.

The two major types of latex agglutination tests are the indirect (passive) assay and the inhibition assay. The indirect assay is illustrated in Figure 34–3. The **indirect assay** is the most common latex agglutination test for bacteria. Either bacterial antigens or antibodies to bacterial antigens can be determined.

In the indirect test, antibody is either passively or covalently bound to latex for detection of bacterial antigens. In performing the tests, a suspension of the sample is mixed with the sensitized latex and gently agitated for 3 to 5 minutes. The test is then examined for clumping or agglutination indicative of a positive test for the bacteria being tested for in Figure 34–4.

The latex **inhibition assay** is based on the principle of inhibiting the expected agglutination reaction between known antigen and known antibody as a result of competition. For example, known

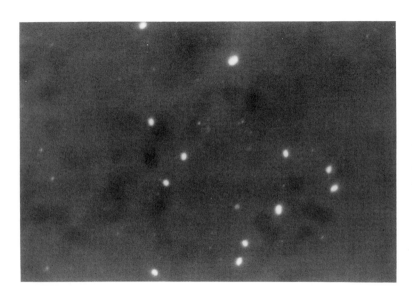

FIGURE 34–2 ✦ Indirect immunofluorescence for *Actinobacillus actinomycetemcomitans* in a subgingival sample from a first molar site in a patient with localized juvenile periodontitis.

Latex   Antibody   Sensitized Latex

+

Agglutination   Bacterial Sample

FIGURE 34–3 ✦ Principle of the latex agglutination test.

antibody is mixed with a sample thought to contain bacteria (antigen). The mixture is then reacted with latex coated with antibody to bacteria. If the clinical sample contains the organism, then the antibody will be bound, preventing the expected agglutination. If it is absent from the clinical sample, the antibody would bind with the antigen on the latex, leading to agglutination. Thus, the occurrence of agglutination indicates that the clinical sample does not contain the bacteria tested for, and lack of agglutination indicates that the organism is present.

FLOW CYTOMETRY

Flow cytometry, or fluorescence-activated flow cytometry permits identification and quantification of cell populations. It has been applied to lympho-

cyte subsets and to bacteria. Cells in suspension are reacted with monoclonal antibodies to a cell-surface constituent(s) that is labeled with one or more fluorescent dyes such as fluorescein. After incubation, the cells are passed through a focused beam of laser or lamp arc light. The cells scatter the light at low and wide angles, which is then measured. Each type of cell generally has a characteristic volume and scatter pattern. "Gating" allows the selection of a single scatter parameter permitting identification of a limited population of cells.

Flow cytometry techniques have recently been applied to identification of oral bacteria. However, many technical questions must be solved to demonstrate the efficacy of this technique for identification of specific bacteria in plaque.

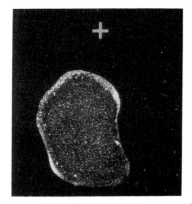
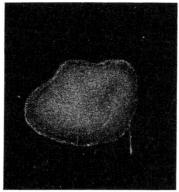
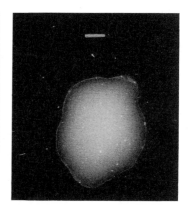

FIGURE 34–4 ✦ Latex agglutination test for *Actinobacillus actinomycetemcomitans*. The square on the *right* is the positive control and the square on the *left* is the negative control. The *middle* well with the clinical sample is positive indicating the presence of the organism.

ENZYME-LINKED IMMUNOSORBENT ASSAY (ELISA)

ELISA is similar in principle to radioimmunoassays but an enzymatically derived color reaction is substituted as the label in place of a radioisotope. The assay is very sensitive and relatively economical to run. ELISA assays detect either antigens or antibodies. Similar to immunofluorescence, both direct and indirect techniques can be employed for detection of bacteria. Tests for serum antibodies usually employ an indirect assay, as illustrated in Figure 34–5. Bacterial antigens are assayed in a similar fashion. Antigen is incubated in wells in a plastic plate (or occasionally in test tubes) to allow absorption or coating by the material. After washing to remove free antigen, the plates are ready for tests. Samples containing suspected antibodies and controls are then incubated in separate wells to allow antibodies to bind to the antigen on the surface of the wells. After washing to remove unbound serum components, antisera to the immunoglobulin (for example, goat antihuman IgG) conjugated to either alkaline phosphatase or horseradish peroxidase is then incubated in the wells. A positive reaction is visualized by the addition of a chromogen, which changes from a colorless to a colored solution. The intensity depends on the concentration of reactants. Tests are usually read photometrically for optimal quantitation. Sensitivity of the assays has frequently been improved by the use of the avidin-biotin system.

ELISA assays have been used primarily as research tools in dentistry but are commercially available in other countries for detection of periodontopathogens.

Other Assays for Bacterial Identification

DNA PROBES

In recent years, DNA probe technology has progressed from a research technique to a practical clinical laboratory assay. It is particularly important for identification of pathogens that are difficult to grow, those present in a mixed flora and those present in relatively low numbers. It is expected that the use of this methodology will greatly expand because of its exquisite specificity and sensitivity. Potential uses for these probes include identification of (1) bacteria and antibiotic resistance of bacteria, (2) viruses, (3) specific cancer, (4) genetic diseases, (5) tissue typing, and (6) susceptibility to disease. Clinical assays for periodontopathogens are now available in dentistry.

DNA probe technology developed as an offshoot of genetic engineering. Assays with DNA probes are based on the ability of DNA to hybridize or bind to complementary strands of DNA or RNA having exactly the same base sequence. A portion of DNA from a bacterium, virus, cancer, and so on, is isolated with the aid of restriction endonucleases, enzymes that cut the DNA molecule at

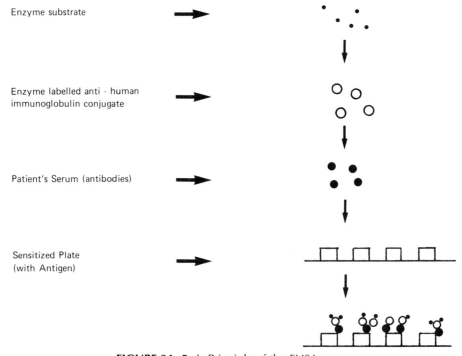

Enzyme substrate

Enzyme labelled anti · human immunoglobulin conjugate

Patient's Serum (antibodies)

Sensitized Plate (with Antigen)

FIGURE 34–5 ✦ Principle of the ELISA assay.

specific locations. The DNA plasmid is then spliced into a bacterial plasmid and propagated in large volumes in bacteria such as *E. coli*. The desired cloned DNA fragment is isolated from the bacterial genome with the aid of restriction endonucleases and then dissociated into single strands. The single-strand DNA fragments serve as the probe for complementary sequences in an unknown specimen. To identify a complementary fragment, the DNA probe is labeled with a radioactive isotope or an avidin-biotin enzyme system. Depending on the assay, DNA or RNA in the clinical sample is denatured to form single strands and then incubated on a membrane such as nitrocellulose to allow binding. The labeled DNA probe is incubated on the membrane to allow hybridization and then washed. If the specimen contains complementary DNA or RNA, hybridization or binding of the two single strands occurs, which is visualized via the label on the probe.

IDENTIFICATION OF ANTIBODIES

Antibodies to bacteria and other antigens can be measured in serum, saliva, and crevicular fluid. Antibody determinations for oral bacteria are primarily a research tool although a commercially available test recently has been introduced. Serum tests for viruses are of practical clinical significance but rarely are ordered by dentists. Tests for autoantibodies (discussed separately further on) are also clinically relevant and are requested by dentists whenever autoimmune disease is suspected (desquamative gingivitis).

The main antibody assays in dentistry are the ELISA, immunofluorescence, and precipitation assays. The ELISA and immunofluorescence assays have been described earlier in this chapter for detection of bacterial antigen. Substitution of antigen for antibody in the assays allows determination of antibody titers or units of antibody.

OTHER DIAGNOSTIC TESTS
Allergy Testing

Various allergy tests are used for the diagnosis of dental patients with suspected allergies (Table 34–6).

IMMEDIATE HYPERSENSITIVITY (ANAPHYLACTIC REACTIONS, REAGENIC ALLERGY, AND IgE-MEDIATED REACTIONS)

A major concern in dentistry is an allergic reaction to a drug or dental medicament. An anaphylactic reaction occurs very rapidly within minutes and could be life-threatening.

TABLE 34–6 ✦ Allergy Tests in Dentistry

Patch tests
Skin tests
Serum tests
RAST test
Histamine release

The immediate hypersensitivity reactions occur within minutes after exposure in a sensitized individual and frequently occur in response to chemicals, drugs, dust, pollens, and so on. In a person with an allergy, IgE antibodies specific for the allergen or antigen are formed. (See Chapter 2.) These homocytophilic antibodies fix to or sensitize mast cells and basophils. Subsequent antigenic exposure to the allergen forms complexes of the antigen with two antibody molecules and results in the degranulation of the mast cell or basophil with release of biochemically active mediators including histamine, slow-reacting substance of anaphylaxis, prostaglandins, and eosinophil chemotactic factor. These mediators cause smooth muscle contraction, edema resulting from increased capillary permeability, constriction of small venules, platelet aggregation, and mobilization of phagocytes.

The assays for immediate hypersensitivity reactions include skin tests, assays for histamine release from basophils, and assays for the concentration of IgE specific for an allergen. Skin tests are office procedures usually performed by an allergist. The histamine-release assay is performed on freshly drawn blood and the assay for specific IgE antibodies on serum; both assays must be performed by a laboratory.

Skin Tests. The two types of skin tests are the intradermal skin test, in which small volumes of the test material are injected into the skin, and the prick test, in which a drop of the test material is applied to the surface of the skin and then a needle is used to prick the area. Both are performed with dilute solutions of antigen, usually on the skin of the arm or back. After 15 to 20 minutes, the site is examined for a wheal (localized, circumscribed area of edema) and flare (irregular, often poorly defined erythema) indicative of a positive reaction. Often positive reaction sites itch because of the localized histamine release. Multiple tests can be performed simultaneously. Frequently, several dilutions of the test material are also tested. Usually, positive immediate skin test reactions are indicative of an allergy to the test substance. However, false-positive and false-negative reactions can occur. Because of the possibility of an anaphylactic reaction which can be life-threatening and the complexity of interpretation, skin testing should be performed by an allergist. A practical consideration in dentistry is a patient with a suspected allergy to penicillin. This will be discussed in greater detail further on.

Histamine Release From Peripheral Blood Basophils. The measurement of histamine released by basophils in peripheral blood upon challenge or exposure to an antigen is an in vitro assay for immediate hypersensitivity. Basophils sensitized with IgE antibodies on their surfaces are stimulated to secrete histamine upon challenge with complementary antigen. The amount of histamine released is directly proportional to the extent of antigen-IgE antibody concentration and can be quantitated as to the percentage of histamine release relative to the total cellular histamine content. The concentration of blocking antibody or antigen-neutralizing antibody developed by desensitization also can be measured by this method. Blocking antibodies are a measure of protection against a specific allergen.

RADIOALLERGOSORBENT TEST (RAST)

The RAST test is a solid phase immunoassay that provides quantitative data on the concentration of IgE in serum specific for an allergen or antigen (Fig. 34–6). The antigen is first coupled with an insoluble particle. The serum to be tested is then incubated, with the particle allowing the specific antibody to bind to the antigen. After washing to remove the unbound serum components, the particles are reacted with radiolabeled or enzyme-labeled anti-IgE. The amount of radioactivity or enzyme-generated color is directly proportional to the concentration of specific IgE antibodies. The RAST test takes 24 to 48 hours to obtain results.

The common occurrence of penicillin allergies and the frequent use of penicillin in the treatment of oral diseases necessitates a consideration of allergy testing for penicillin. An allergy to penicillin is primarily an IgE-mediated response and is detected by means of a skin test. Early studies using penicillin alone as a skin test reagent frequently yielded false-negative results. It now appears that the reason many patients with penicillin allergies had negative reactions when tested with penicillin was that the pencillin acted as a hapten. Allergic reaction to this low molecular weight substance only resulted when the molecule covalently bound in vivo to larger carrier proteins to form penicilloyl-protein complexes or was partially metabolized. Two types of skin test reagents are now available to detect the major and minor antigenic determinants. A commercially available reagent composed of penicillin linked to a polylysine chain to form penicilloyl polylysine (PPL) detects the major antigenic determinant, and a reagent composed of penicillin and one or more of its highly reactive metabolites detects the minor antigenic metabolites in a mixture called minor determinent mixture (MDM). Skin testing may be used in patients with a suspected penicillin and cephalosporin allergy, particularly in a life-threatening situation in which penicillin is the drug of choice, and in patients with a suspected but uncertain reaction during penicillin therapy.

DELAYED HYPERSENSITIVITY

Delayed or cell-mediated hypersensitivity is also important in dentistry. This type of hypersensitivity reaction occurs when sensitized small lym-

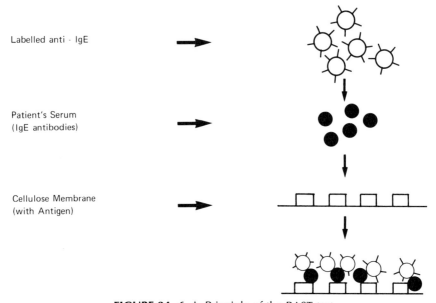

Labelled anti - IgE

Patient's Serum
(IgE antibodies)

Cellulose Membrane
(with Antigen)

FIGURE 34–6 ✦ Principle of the RAST test.

phocytes are exposed to the sensitizing antigen with the release of lymphokines. The major assays for this are the skin test (intradermal and patch tests), lymphocyte proliferation, and lymphokine production assay. The skin test is an in vivo assay, whereas the latter two are in vitro assays. The two in vivo assays are primarily used for research purposes.

Skin Tests. The skin tests are performed either as an intradermal injection (e.g., tuberculin test) or as a topical application of the suspected allergen (patch test) held in contact by a bandage. The sites are examined in 24 to 48 hours. Positive intradermal injections exhibit induration (hardness) and edema. Positive patch test results exhibit eczematous reddened areas and are compared with areas to which just a bandage was applied. In dentistry, a patch test would be indicated for suspected allergies to metals, medicaments, and so on, and could be performed by the dentist. The skin tests are usually used for the diagnosis of a systemic disease such as mycobacterial infections and are usually performed by a physician.

Tests for Oral Autoimmune Diseases

Several autoimmune diseases have oral manifestations. These include pemphigus, pemphigoid, systemic lupus erythematosus (SLE), discoid lupus erythematosus (DLE), and some forms of desquamative gingivitis. The most common clinical immunologic tests for these include direct immunofluorescence for in vivo deposits of immune reacts in biopsy specimens, indirect immunofluorescence for tissue reactive antibodies in serum, and gel precipitation tests for serum antibodies to tissue components.

DIRECT IMMUNOFLUORESCENCE
(Fig. 34–7)

Immunoglobulins, complement, and fibrin are localized in biopsy specimens by direct immunofluorescence. Biopsy specimens are either placed in a special holding solution for transport to the laboratory or quick frozen in liquid nitrogen and transported on dry ice. Frozen sections 2 to 4 microns thick are cut with a cryostat and stored frozen until tested. Sequential sections are incubated with fluorescein-labeled IgG, IgA, IgM, C3, or fibrin. After washing off the specimens to remove the unreacted antisera, the slides are examined with a microscope equipped with a special light source and fluorescent filters. A green fluorescence indicative of the antigen in the tissue is interpreted as to tissue location and pattern of staining.

INDIRECT IMMUNOFLUORESCENCE
(see Fig. 34–1A)

Antibodies in serum to tissue components are determined by indirect immunofluorescence. Frozen sections of tissue, depending on the antibody to be detected, are prepared (e.g., monkey esophagus for pemphigus and pemphigoid antibodies and mouse kidney for antinuclear antibodies associated with connective tissue disease). Dilutions of the sample serum are incubated on sections and then washed off. Fluorescein-labeled antihuman IgG is then incubated on the sections and washed off. Antibodies in the sample serum to a specific tissue

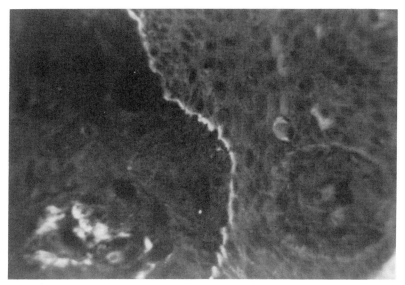

FIGURE 34–7 ✦ Example of a direct immunofluorescence test for the third component of complement (C3) on oral mucosa. Identification of the C3 along the basement membrane is diagnostic for cicatricial pemphigoid.

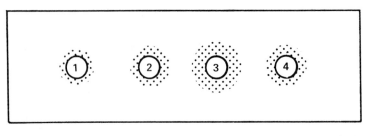

FIGURE 34–8 ✦ Principle of the RID assay. The diameter of precipitation is proportional to the antigen concentration. The concentration of the unknown sample is extrapolated from the line formed by graphing the three diameters of the three known concentrations.

Gel Containing Antibody

Wells No. 1 - 3: known concentrations of antigen
Wells No. 4: unknown sample

constituent are then microscopically visualized as a green fluorescence.

GEL PRECIPITATION

Double diffusion gel precipitation tests are employed to identify serum antibodies to nuclear constituents, which are of significance in systemic lupus erythematosus. Partially purified nuclear antigens are placed in wells and allowed to diffuse toward wells containing serum. Precipitation lines are indicative of an antigen-antibody reaction.

Tests for Immunoglobulins and Complement

Several methods are currently employed for quantitation of serum proteins. These are divided into two major groups: (1) assays that measure the physical properties of the immune complexes formed when antisera specific for the serum protein react with the protein (precipitation in gel, turbidimitry, and light scattering); and (2) assays that measure the amount of labeled antibody bound to the antigen. The two most common clinical methods are radial immunodiffusion (RID) and rate nephelometry.

In the **RID assay,** antibodies specific for the protein to be quantitated are incorporated into a gel. Serum or other fluid samples to be assayed are added to wells in the gel and allowed to incubate. A ring of precipitation forms as the antigen diffuses into the gel and reacts with the antibodies. The ring is directly proportional in size to the concentration of antigen. The protein concentration of the sample is determined from a line formed by graphing the ring diameters against protein concentrations of three controls with different protein concentrations (Fig. 34–8).

Rate nephelometry is based on the principle that soluble immune complexes formed by the reaction of antibody with antigen scatters incident light. Since the antibody is constant, the amount of scatter is proportional to the antigen concentra-

tion. The concentration in samples are calculated from a dose response curve generated with reference control sera.

The quantitation of immunoglobulins and complement in serum, saliva, and crevicular fluid has been a research tool in dentistry for some time, particularly for studies of periodontal disease and caries. It is also of clinical relevance in such diseases as systemic lupus erythematosus, in which decreased C3 levels correlate with disease activity.

ACKNOWLEDGMENT

The authors wish to thank Sushma Nachnani for her contributions to this chapter.

BIBLIOGRAPHY

Adkinson N. F., Jr.: Tests for immunological drug reactions. In Rose, N. R., DeMacario, E. C., Fahey, J. L., Friedman, H., and Penn, G. M.: Manual of Clinical Laboratory Immunology, ed. 4. American Society of Microbiology, Washington, D.C., 1992, p. 717.

Anonymous: Products of microbiology: technical manual. Madison, Wisconsin: GIBCO Laboratories, 1983.

Appelbaum, P.C., Kaufman, C. S., Keifer, J. C., and Venbrux, M. J.: Comparison of three methods for anaerobic identification. J. Clin. Microbiol. 18:614, 1984.

Aranki, A., Syed, S. A., Kenney, E. B., and Freter, R.: Isolation of anaerobic bacteria from human gingiva and mouse cecum by means of a simplified glove box procedure. Appl. Microbiol. 17:568, 1969.

Bauer, A. W., Kirby, W. N. M., Sherris J. C., and Torck, M.: Antibiotic susceptibility testing by a single disc method. Am. J. Clin. Pathol. 45:493, 1966.

Bonta, Y., Zambon, J. J., Genco, R. J., and Neiders, M. E.: Rapid identification of periodontal pathogens in subgingival plaque: comparison of indirect immunofluorescence microscopy with bacterial culture for detection of *Actinobacillus actinomycetemcomitans*. J. Dent. Res. 64:793, 1985.

Campbell, S. M., Fiedler, P. N., and Pershing, D. H.: Nucleic acid amplification in clinical diagnostics. In Rose, N. R., DeMacario, E. C., Fahey, J. L., Friedman, H., and Penn, G. M.: Manual of Clinical Laboratory Immunology, ed. 4. American Society of Microbiology, Washington, D.C., 1992, p. 27.

Carlone, C. M., Valadez, M. J., and Pickett, M. J.: Methods for distinguishing gram-positive from gram-negative anaerobic bacteria. J. Clin. Microbiol. 13:444, 1983.

Check, I. J., Piper, M., Papadea, C.: Immunoglobulin quantitation. In Rose, N. R., DeMacario, E. C., Fahey, J. L., Friedman, H., and Penn, G. M.: Manual of Clinical Laboratory Immunology, ed. 4. American Society of Microbiology, Washington, D.C., 1992, p. 71.

D'Amato, R. F., Bottone, E. J., and Amsterdam, D.: Substrate profile systems for the identification of bacteria and yeasts by rapid and automated approaches. In Ballows, A., Hauser, W. J. Jr., Herrmann, K. L., Isenberg, H. D., and Shadomy, H. J.: Manual of Clinical Microbiology, ed. 5. American Society of Microbiology, Washington, D.C., 1991, p. 128.

Dowell, V. R., Jr. and Lombard, G. L.: Reactions of anaerobic bacteria in differential agar media. U.S. Dept. of Health and Human Services, Public Health Service, Centers for Disease Control, Atlanta, GA, 1981.

Dzink, J. L., Socransky, S. S., Ebersole, J. L., and Frey, D. E.: ELISA and conventional techniques for identification of black-pigmented *Bacteroides* isolated from periodontal pockets. J. Periodontal Res. 18:369, 1983.

Hamilton, R. G., and Adkinson N. F., Jr.: Measurement of total serum immunoglobulin E and allergen-specific immunoglobulin E antibody. In Rose, N. R., DeMacario, E. C., Fahey, J. L., Friedman, H., and Penn, G. M.: Manual of Clinical Laboratory Immunology, ed. 4. American Society of Microbiology, Washington, D.C., 1992, p. 689.

Holdeman, L. V., Cato, E. P., and Moore, W. E. C.: Anaerobe Laboratory Manual, ed. 4. Anaerobe Laboratory, Virginia Polytechnic Institute and State University, Blackburg, VA, 1977.

Kornman, K. S., Patters, M., Kiehl, R., and Marucha, P.: Detection and quantitation of *Bacteroides gingivalis* in bacterial mixtures by means of flow cytometry. J. Periodontal Res. 19:570, 1984.

Lanier, L. L., and Jackson, A. L.: Monoclonal antibodies: Differentiation antigens expressed on leukocytes. In Rose, N. R., DeMacario, E. C., Fahey, J. L., Friedman, H., and Penn, G. M.: Manual of Clinical Laboratory Immunology, ed. 4. American Society of Microbiology, Washington, D.C., 1992, p. 157.

MacFaddin, J. F.: Media for isolation—cultivation identification. In Maintenance of Medical Bacteria, Vol. 1. Williams and Wilkins, Baltimore, 1985.

Mulcahy, L.: DNA probes: an overview. Am. Clin. Prod. Rev. 5:14, 1986.

Norman, P. S.: Skin testing. In Rose, N. R., DeMacario, E. C., Fahey, J. L., Friedman, H., Penn, G. M.: Manual of Clinical Laboratory Immunology, ed. 4. American Society of Microbiology, Washington, D.C., 1992, p. 685.

Nichols, W. S., and Nakamura, R. M.: Agglutination and agglutination inhibition assays. In Rose, N. R., Friedman, H., and Fahey, J. L.: Manual of Clinical Immunology, ed. 3. American Society of Microbiology, Washington, D.C., 1986, p. 49.

Nisengard, R. J., and Neiders, M.: Desquamative lesions of the gingiva. J. Periodontal. 52:500, 1981.

Roit, I., Brostoff, J., and Male, D.: Immunology. St. Louis, C.V. Mosby, 1985, p. 191.

Smith, R. F.: Microscopy and Photomicrography: A Practical Guide. Appleton-Century-Crofts, New York, 1982.

Sutter, V. L., Citron, D. M., Edelstein, M. A. C., and Finegold, S. M.: Wadsworth Anaerobic Bacteriology Manual, ed. 4. Star Publishing, Belmont, Calif, 1985.

Tinghitella, T. J., and Edberg, S. C.: Agglutination tests and *Limulus* assay for the diagnosis of infectious diseases. In Ballows, A., Hauser, W. J. Jr., Herrmann, K. L., Isenberg, H. D., Shadomy, H. J.: Manual of Clinical Microbiology, ed. 5. American Society of Microbiology, Washington, D.C., 1991, p. 61.

Index

Note: Page numbers in *italics* refer to illustrations; page numbers followed by t refer to tables.

Cell envelope, of gram-negative bacteria, 58, 59, 60-61, *63*, *65*
Cell wall, 57-61, *57*, 59t
  lipopolysaccharide of, 60-61, *63*
  peptidoglycan of, 59, 59t, *60*, *61*
  synthesis of, 84-85, *86*
  teichoic acids of, 59-60, 59t, *62*, *63*
Cellobiose, in clostridial species, 207t
Cementum, calculus attachment to, 336, *336*, *337*
  caries of, 343
Cepacol, in plaque control, 387
Cephalosporins, 425t, 426
Cerebrospinal fluid, normal flora of, 121t
Cetylpyridinium chloride, in plaque control, 387, 389t
Chancroid, 163
Chemical, mutagenic, 102, 102t
Chemical vapor sterilization, 414t, 417, 418t–419t, 419, *420*
Chemiosmotic hypothesis, of ATP production, 73, *74*
Chemoattractants, 31, 33t
Chemokinesis, phagocytic, 31, *33*
Chemotaxis, 31, *33*, 33t
  defects of, in periodontal disease, 367, 368, 368t
  in pulpal disease, 394-395
Chemotaxonomy, in bacterial classification, 118
Chemotroph, 72
Chicken pox, 265
Chlamydia pneumoniae, 239t
Chlamydia psittaci, 239t, 240
Chlamydia trachomatis, 239-240, 239t
Chlamydiae, 239-240, 239t
  diagnosis of, 240
Chlorhexidine (Peridex), anticaries activity of, 356, *356*
  in plaque control, 387, 389t
Chlorosome, prokaryotic, 66t
Cholecystitis, gangrenous, clostridial, 208-209
Cholera, 113t, 189t, 190
Choleragen, 113t
Cicatricial pemphigoid, desquamative gingivitis in, 381, 381t
Citrate reaction, of *Enterobacter aerogenes*, 186t
  of *Enterobacter cloacae*, 186t
  of Enterobacteriaceae, 180t
  of *Escherichia coli*, 186t
Citric acid, in periodontal disease, 389
Citric acid cycle, 73, 75, *76*
Citrobacter diversus, 189
  biochemical reactions of, 180t
Citrobacter freundii, 189
  biochemical reactions of, 180t
Clark, J. K., 4
Cleanser, hand, 406
Clindamycin, 430
  in subacute bacterial endocarditis, 429t
  prophylactic, 433t
Clostridium, 205-206, 205-210
  classification of, 210
  clinical features of, 208-209
  colonial morphology of, 210
  fermentation in, 78-79, 79t
  identification of, 206t–207t, 210
  immunity to, 208
  in AIDS, 225t
  of gastrointestinal tract, 127, 127t
  pathogenesis of, 208

Clostridium (Continued)
  treatment of, 208t–209t, 210-211, 211
Clostridium baratii, 206t–207t, 210
Clostridium bifermentans, 206t–207t, 210
Clostridium botulinum, 208, 210
  toxins of, 113t, 208
Clostridium butyricum, 206t–207t, 210
Clostridium cadaveris, 206t–207t
Clostridium carnis, 205
Clostridium clostridiiforme, 206t–207t
  in AIDS, 225t
Clostridium difficile, 206t–207t, 210
Clostridium hastiforme, 206t–207t
Clostridium histolyticum, 205, 206t–207t, 210
Clostridium innocuum, 206t–207t
Clostridium limosum, 206t–207t
Clostridium novyi, 206t–207t, 208, 210
  exotoxin of, 113t
Clostridium perfringens, 206t–207t, 210
  clinical features of, 208-209
  exotoxin of, 113t
  invasive factors of, 111t
  toxins of, 208
  treatment of, 208t–209t, 210-211
Clostridium putrificum, 206t–207t
Clostridium ramosum, 206t–207t, 210
Clostridium septicum, 206t–207t, 208, 210
  exotoxin of, 113t
Clostridium sordellii, 206t–207t, 210
Clostridium sphenoides, 210
Clostridium sporogenes, 210
  exotoxin of, 113t
Clostridium subterminale, 206t–207t
Clostridium tertium, 205, 206t–207t
Clostridium tetani, 206t–207t, 210
  exotoxin of, 113t
  toxins of, 208
Clothing, asepsis for, 408
Clumping factor, of staphylococci, 149
CMV. See *Cytomegalovirus (CMV)*.
CNM group, 173
Coaggregation reaction, in plaque formation, 326, 326t
Coagulase, of staphylococci, 149
Cocci, shape of, 48, *51*
Coccidioides immitis, 293-294, *294*
Coccidioidomycosis, 293-294, *294*
Coenzyme Q, of electron transport system, 76
Colitis, hemorrhagic, *Escherichia coli* in, 185
  pseudomembranous, *Clostridium difficile* in, 210
Colon, normal flora of, 121t
Colony-stimulating factors, 36-39, 37t–38t
Combinatorial diversity, in antibody generation, 11
Competency, bacterial, 98-99
Complement, 26-29
  activation of, biologic effects of, 28-29, *29*
    IgG in, 25, 25t, *26*, *27*
  alternative pathway of, *26*, 27-28
  classical pathway of, 26-27, *26*
  in periodontal disease, 373
  regulation of, 29
  tests for, 448
Complement fixation test, in viral antibody identification, 256
Condylomata acuminata, 271

Haemophilus influenzae (Continued)
  invasive factors of, 111t
  lipooligosaccharides of, 161
  of nose, 125, 125t
  of oropharynx, 126, 126t
  outer membrane proteins of, 161-162, 162
  type b, 162
  vaccine against, 162
Haemophilus parainfluenzae, 160, 161t, 162, 163t
  normal distribution of, 121t
  of eye, 125t
  of nose, 125, 125t
  of oropharynx, 126, 126t
Haemophilus paraphrophilus, 160, 161t, 162, 163t
Haemophilus segnis, 160, 161t, 162, 163t
Hafnia alvei, 189
  biochemical reactions of, 180t
Hair, asepsis for, 408
Hands, asepsis for, 406-408, *407*
Hansen's bacillus, 173t, 176-177
Haustoria, 288
Hay fever, 42
Head, Joseph, 6
Healing, in periodontal disease, 367-368
Heart disease, management of, 432-433, 433t
Heat sterilization, 414t, 416-417, 418t-419t, *420*
Heavy chain gene, 11-13, *11*
Helicobacter, 227
Helicobacter cinaedi, 227
Helicobacter fennelliae, 227
Helicobacter mustelae, 227
Helicobacter pylori, 227
Hemagglutination inhibition test, in viral antibody identification, 256
Hematopoiesis, cytokine regulation of, 38, 38t
Hemocuprine, 312
Hemolysin, of *Clostridium*, 208
  of *Pseudomonas aeruginosa*, 194
  of staphylococci, 149
Hemolysis, streptococci and, 129-130
Hemolytic anemia, drug-induced, 44
Hemorrhagic colitis, *Escherichia coli* in, 185
Henle, Jacob, 3
Hepatitis, delta-associated, clinical illness of, *267*
Hepatitis A, 250t, 266, 266t
  clinical illness of, *267*
  dental treatment in, 270
  in cross infection, 404t
  in health care professionals, 269-270
Hepatitis A virus, 251t
Hepatitis B, 250t, 252t, 266, 266t, 268-269, *269*
  antigens of, 268-269
  clinical illness of, *267*, 268
  Dane particles of, *267*, *268*
  dental treatment in, 270
  in health care professionals, 269-270, 404-405, 404t
  vaccine for, 269, 270t
Hepatitis C (non-A non-B hepatitis), 266t, *267*, 269
Hereditary fructose intolerance, caries in, 352-353
Herpes encephalitis, 261
Herpes genitalis, 261
Herpes keratitis, 261, *264*
Herpes labialis, 261, *263*, *264*

Herpes simplex virus (HSV), 252t, 261-262
  clinical disease with, 261, *263*, *264*
  diagnosis of, 262
  electron micrograph of, *249*
  in cross infection, 404t, 405
  latent, 258, 261-262
  pathogenesis of, 261
  plaque of, *257*
  recurrence of, 261-262, *264*
  replication of, *262*
Herpesviruses, 250t, 252, 252t, 261-265
Heterolactic fermenters, 343
Heteropolysaccharide, 83
Heterotroph, 72
Hfr cells, 97-98
Hip replacement, infection with, 399
Hippocrates, 1
Hippurate test, of *Campylobacter*, 226
Histamine, in allergy, 446
  in immediate hypersensitivity reaction, 43t
Histoplasma capsulatum, 292-293, *293*
Histoplasmosis, 292-293, *292*
HIV. See *Human immunodeficiency virus (HIV)*.
Holdfast, bacterial, 55
Homolactic fermenters, 343
Homopolysaccharide, 83
Hormones, *Bacteroides* infection and, 213
  in subgingival plaque, 317
Host-bacteria inter-relationships, 309-310
Hot-cold hemolysin, of staphylococci, 149
H_2S, of *Campylobacter*, 226
  of Enterobacteriaceae, 180t
HSV. See *Herpes simplex virus (HSV)*.
Human bite, infection from, 399
Human immunodeficiency virus (HIV), 251t, 275, *276*. See also *Acquired immunodeficiency syndrome (AIDS)*.
  CD4-bearing T cell binding to, 15
  in cross infection, 404t, 405
  periodontitis with, 363
  replication of, 275
  transmission of, 275
Human leukocyte antigen (HLA) complex, 16-18, *17*
Human papillomavirus, 252t, 270-271
Human polyoma virus, 252t
Hunter, John, 5
Hutchinson's triad, 234
Hyaluronidase, of periodontal pockets, 366-367
  of staphylococci, 149
  of streptococci, 133
Hydrogen peroxide/povidone-iodine, anticaries activity of, 356
Hydrophobic interactions, in plaque formation, 324, *324*
Hydroxyapatite, demineralization of, 345, *345*
  structure of, 344, *344*
Hydroxylamine, in mutation, 102, 102t
Hypersensitivity reaction, 41-45, 42t
  type I (immediate), 41-43, 42t, 43t
    in periodontal disease, 373
  type II (cytolytic), 43-44
  type III (immune complex), 44-45
    in periapical infections, 395
    in periodontal disease, 374
  type IV (delayed), 45